NURSING IN THE COMMUNITY

NURSING
IN THE COMMUNITY

Edited by

Victoria Schoolcraft, R.N., M.S.N.

Assistant Director, Baccalaureate Program
Associate Professor
College of Nursing
University of Oklahoma
Oklahoma City, Oklahoma

A WILEY MEDICAL PUBLICATION
JOHN WILEY & SONS
New York • Chichester • Brisbane • Toronto • Singapore

Cover Design: Wanda Lubelska

Production Supervisor: Audrey Pavey

Library of Congress Cataloging in Publication Data:

Main entry under title

Nursing in the community.

    (A Wiley medical publication)
    Includes bibliographies and index.
    1. Community health nursing. I. Schoolcraft, Victoria.
II. Series. [DNLM: 1. Community health nursing.
2. Community health services. WY 106 N9755]
RT98.N88 1984   610.73'43   83-21592
ISBN 0-471-86409-9

Printed in the United States of America

10 9 8 7 6 5 4 3 2 1

If you can imagine it,
You can achieve it;
If you can dream it,
You can become it.

William Arthur Ward

To the Universal Father, who gave me my imagination

To Helen McInish, R.N., who gave me my dream

Contributors

Thomas S. Allen, B.S.N., R.N.
Instructor
Department of Nursing
Oklahoma State University Technical
  Institute
Oklahoma City, Oklahoma

Marilyn M. Bagwell, R.N., M.A.
Assistant Professor
College of Nursing
Arizona State University
Tempe, Arizona

Dorothy Jacobson Baker, M.N., R.N.
Assistant Professor
Community Health Nursing
School of Nursing
Yale University
New Haven, Connecticut

Mary Ellen Banks, R.N., M.S.N.
Assistant Professor
School of Nursing
The University of Wisconsin-Milwaukee
Milwaukee, Wisconsin

Thomas H. Cook, M.S.N., R.N.-C.
Assistant Professor
Community Health Nursing
School of Nursing
Yale University
New Haven, Connecticut

Jo Frazer, R.N., M.S.
Assistant Professor
College of Nursing
University of Oklahoma
Oklahoma City, Oklahoma

Elsie Maxwell Hamm, R.N., Ph.D.
Consultant
Programs in Aging
Lawton, Oklahoma

Judith Belliveau Krauss, R.N., M.S.N.
Associate Dean
Assistant Professor
School of Nursing
Yale University
New Haven, Connecticut

Carolyn J. Leman, R.N., M.S.
Assistant Professor
Briar Cliff College
Sioux City, Iowa

Diane J. Mancino, M.A., R.N.-C.
Director of Program
National Student Nurses' Association
New York, New York

Myrtle P. Matejski, R.N., Ph.D.
Assistant Dean
Associate Professor
College of Nursing
University of Rhode Island
Kingston, Rhode Island

Mary Ann McClellan, R.N., M.N.
Assistant Professor
College of Nursing
University of Oklahoma
Oklahoma City, Oklahoma

Martha Primeaux, R.N., M.S.N., F.A.A.N.
Assistant Dean and Director
Baccalaureate Program
Associate Professor
College of Nursing
University of Oklahoma
Oklahoma City, Oklahoma

Evelyn E. Ramming, M.S.N., R.N.-C.
Associate Professor
College of Nursing
University of Oklahoma
Oklahoma City, Oklahoma

Estelle H. Rosenblum, R.N., Ph.D.
Professor
College of Nursing
The University of New Mexico
Albuquerque, New Mexico

Victoria Schoolcraft, R.N., M.S.N.
Assistant Director
Baccalaureate Program
Associate Professor
College of Nursing
University of Oklahoma
Oklahoma City, Oklahoma

**Sherry L. Shamansky, Dr. P.H., R.N.,
F.A.A.N.**
Chairperson, Community Health Nursing
Associate Professor
Nursing and Public Health
School of Nursing
Yale University
New Haven, Connecticut

Yoshiko Shimamoto, R.N., M.P.H.
Assistant Professor
School of Nursing
University of Hawaii at Manoa
Honolulu, Hawaii

Gloria R. Smith, R.N., Ph.D., F.A.A.N.
Director
Michigan Department of Public Health
Lansing, Michigan

Janet Sullivan Wilson, R.N., M.A.
Assistant Professor
College of Nursing
University of Oklahoma
Oklahoma City, Oklahoma

Ruth Kramer Young, R.N., M.S.
Associate Professor
College of Nursing
University of Oklahoma
Oklahoma City, Oklahoma

Preface

Current health problems increasingly illustrate the fact that human progress has been purchased at a great cost. Indeed, the accounting mechanisms of history may never accurately document the price that has been paid for urbanization, technological advances, and human comforts, since not all societal changes have served to promote health. People are not effectively responding to the rapidly changing times. The onslaught of societal stimulation and change has affected both physical and emotional coping mechanisms.

Thus, the community health nurse must be prepared to meet the demands of a constantly changing environment. Nursing must become increasingly future-sighted in developing roles and practice areas. Such a view encompasses the importance of several key variables, including a knowledge of public health tradition and principles and the current and evolving characteristics of the health care system with a keen awareness of the role and responsibilities of nurses.

This text provides nursing students and practitioners with a comprehensive source-book that can serve as a foundation for designing community health nursing strategies for individuals, families, and communities. The unifying theme of the book is health promotion, encompassing the three target areas delineated by The Surgeon General's Report on Health Promotion and Disease Prevention (1979): life-style, environment, and services. This book offers traditional, contemporary, and futuristic points of view and includes perspectives on the knowledge and skills that can be used to enrich the practice of professional nursing in the community.

What does this mean for the nurse? In an era emphasizing health promotion and disease prevention, nursing's challenge is to evolve fully as the central unifying force in the health care system. By definition, community health nursing is "a synthesis of nursing practice and public health practice applied to promoting and preserving the health of populations" (ANA, 1980, p. 2). The practice is continuing, comprehensive, directed toward all age groups, takes place in a wide variety of settings, and includes health education, maintenance, and the coordination and evaluation of individuals, families, groups, and communities.

It is hoped that this textbook will help the reader understand the development and operation of the present system and the implications of future trends.

Victoria Schoolcraft

Acknowledgments

Even though it is difficult to thank adequately all the people who have supported me during the development of this book, I would like to acknowledge the assistance of some of those who did facilitate this project. First of all, without the willingness of the contributors to share their expertise, the book would never have become such a rich compilation of knowledge. I am indebted to these people for their time and effort in developing such worthwhile additions to this book.

I consider myself fortunate to be a part of the faculty of the University of Oklahoma College of Nursing. I would like to thank former Dean Gloria Smith, Assistant Dean Martha Primeaux, and Interim Dean Lorraine Singer for their support, both professionally and personally. Many other faculty members helped by giving advice, reading drafts, and encouraging me throughout the process.

I am grateful to Bonnie Morris Garcia for typing the bulk of the manuscript. She not only typed flawlessly but also provided extra help with her encouragement and good humor. The talented people of the Wiley editorial staff, Jim Simpson and Andrea Stingelin, encouraged and guided me in undertaking and completing this project.

I want to thank my wonderful family for their timely words and gestures, which kept me going. This includes my parents, Barbara and R A, as well as all the other Schoolcrafts—Bob, Mike, Mary Chloe, Frances Anne, and Suzie. I am especially grateful to some of my friends for their loving encouragement—Evelyn McKennon, Caryn Hess, Ruth Young, Clare Delaney, Rose Marie Smith, and Tom Allen; and to two special little friends, C. C. and V. C., who were there when no one else was and provided much comfort.

It has been a privilege to be a teacher. Through that role, I have had the opportunity to watch many fine people develop into excellent nurses. My association with students and faculty members has continually inspired me to develop an interesting and forward-looking reference to facilitate learning for nursing in the future.

Victoria Schoolcraft

Contents

PART I
PROFESSIONAL NURSING

xiii

PART II
NURSING WITH INDIVIDUALS AND SMALL GROUPS

PART III
NURSING WITH AGGREGATE POPULATIONS

PART I
PROFESSIONAL NURSING

Part I, "Professional Nursing," introduces some general theoretical and practical areas of knowledge useful for the successful practice of nursing in the community.

Chapter 1 introduces concepts of futurism and presents ways of integrating futuristic thinking into nursing practice. The chapter provides a basis for understanding and developing future-oriented applications in other parts of the book.

Chapter 2, "Historical Foundations and Trends in Community Health Nursing," describes where nursing in the community began and how it has evolved. The chapter identifies problems that will continue to challenge the current and future practitioners of nursing.

It would be impossible to consider nursing and the future without understanding something about change theory. Chapter 3, "Change: A Continuum of Events," provides fundamental concepts of change and gives examples of how these can be used in nursing.

"Role Theory," Chapter 4, helps explain the importance of roles in understanding why people function as they do. This chapter describes how people take on and fulfill roles and how this affects nursing and health.

Chapters 5 through 10 deal with specific skills, activities, and principles that enrich professional nursing practice. Two of the chapters describe concepts of ethics and standards of practice and relate them to nursing. The other four chapters discuss particular kinds of behavior that are useful to nursing practice: assertiveness and leadership, political action, consultation, and effective and creative thinking. These chapters describe the processes involved in these kinds of behavior and discuss particular ways that the relevant activities can be used by nurses.

Chapter 11, "Nursing in the Community," discusses the nurse's role and the focus of nursing outside of acute care settings. The chapter provides a basis for using the remainder of the content in the book.

1

Futurism and Nursing

Victoria Schoolcraft

We should all be concerned about the future because we will
have to spend the rest of our lives there.
CHARLES FRANKLIN KETTERING

OBJECTIVES

After reading this chapter, you should be able to:

- ☐ Define futurism and other related concepts.
- ☐ Describe how futurism is related to learning about and practicing nursing.
- ☐ Identify ways in which to become more future sighted.
- ☐ Identify some of the major trends affecting the future of nursing.

INTRODUCTION

Nursing students of today will be faced with many changes that will affect their practice. These will include increasingly complex technology; breakthroughs in short- and long-term treatment of illness and disease; changes in role expectations for nurses and their colleagues in health and illness care; and the advent of new physical, psychological, and spiritual needs and problems that will result from other changes in the social environment. These are but some of the issues that will affect the nursing practice of those who are to be part of the nursing force of the future.

Our world is changing so rapidly that people may become overwhelmed with "future shock." This term has become a permanent part of our language thanks to Alvin Toffler and his book *Future Shock*. He describes the concept of *future shock* as the "shattering stress and disorientation that we induce in individuals by subjecting them to too much change in too short a time" (Toffler, 1971). This notion has implications not only for nurses themselves but also for their work with clients and patients.

Although we can find predictions describing the future in terms of overpopulation and diminished resources, economic col-

3

lapse, and various natural disasters, we can also find many positive thinkers who see us as architects of our own lives. The work of these futurists provides the underpinnings and frameworks for this chapter and by and large for the entire book.

There are many possible futures and the future in which we live will be determined by a combination of change and human choice (Van Avery, 1980). R. Buckminster Fuller (1981) has described the function of human life as being "co-creative" with the universe. He has an optimistic view of the future and of the ability of people to improve the condition of the world. Toffler (1981) used a metaphor of waves to describe the ways in which society changes. He projected a "third wave" that will help us preserve the parts of the past that should be retained and yet provide for necessary change. The "Aquarian Conspiracy" described by Marilyn Ferguson (1980) is another approach to looking at the autonomy and power of each individual to make a future that will be an adventure rather than an accident.

FUTURISM

Once past a certain age, we all know that the word *future* means a time yet to come. However, the introduction into our language of such words as "futurism," "futuristics," and "futurology" may create some confusion. The word *futurism* usually refers to the philosophical systems used to study the future. *Futuristics* refers to the subject matter of futurism, and *futurology* is the science or branch of knowledge concerned with futurism. For the scope of this chapter and of this book, more concise differentiations among these terms are unimportant.

Futures research is concerned with the identification of new developments, the probability of certain events occurring in a given period of time, consequences of alternatives, and the impact of one alternative on another (Pulliam & Bowman, 1974). Such research is concerned with the relationships among many fields and events. The approaches used assume the ability of human beings to "invent" the future by increasing or decreasing the probability of alternative futures. The principal function of futures research is to project and examine alternative futures and their consequences in order to evaluate them before they become reality (Pulliam & Bowman, 1974).

One way of conceiving of the future is as a direct projection of the past or present. This is called the *extrapolist* approach. For example, we might look at the population of the United States and project that if the population has grown at a certain rate in the past it will continue to grow at the same rate. *Alternative forecasting* is another conception of projecting possible futures. Using the population example, we could project several different outcomes, such as an increase in the rate of population growth, a continuation of the same rate of growth, and a drop in the rate of growth. A third way of looking at the future is *cross-impact projection*. This involves examining the ways in which various alternative futures in one area might affect another area. Instead of studying population growth as if it were a distinct entity, we might project the interaction between population changes and advances in technology. For example, medical research has not only increased population levels by means of improved treatment of illness, it has also controlled population levels by means of improved conception-control devices and drugs.

Another way of using futures research is to describe a desirable future and then plan how to bring it about. This kind of pursuit requires imagination and an interdisciplinary approach. For example, we might design a future in which professional nurses are principally found outside of acute care settings and are typically the health care professionals who manage health promotion activities and minor disruptions in health. To arrive at such a future, many changes are needed, not all of which have to do directly with nursing practice. The public would have to come to value such services, physicians would have to be willing to discontinue these pursuits, and economic systems would have to evolve to support health care. Changes within the nursing profession might include clear differentiation between technical and professional practice; in addition, nurses who were considered professionals would have to value giving such care and wish to function outside of acute care settings, and educational systems would have to be devised to prepare such professionals.

As this example indicates, even though we may have the intellectual and technical ability to plan for such a future, the crucial consideration is determining what is "desirable." The future that is desirable to one group of professionals might be quite unsatisfactory to another, even within the same profession. Dissatisfaction within a group is often related to differences in concepts of desirable futures. The greater the number of people to be affected by the implementation of plans to bring about a certain future, the more likely it is that disruption will result from disagreements about outcomes. In nursing, for example, there is the continuing stress that results from the commitment of some professionals to the eventual differentiation of technical and professional nursing. Unless most nurses agree on the same future, we will continue to suffer upheaval within our profession.

FUTURE SHOCK

When Toffler (1971) coined the phrase "future shock," he gave the world a name to put to a long-observed phenomenon. *Future shock* is what happens when people are subjected to change without adequate time to adjust to it. Kenneth Boulding accounts for this phenomenon by describing the way in which time has become "telescoped" as our culture has progressed (Boulding, 1962). He points out that human beings had centuries to adjust to the changes brought about by the use of agriculture and the domestication of animals. The next major change was the Industrial Revolution; society had nearly a century to adjust to this change and related societal responses. The new revolution is what Boulding calls the "Computer-Cybernation Revolution" and Naisbitt (1982) refers to as the "Information Society." The effects of this revolution are occurring so quickly that many people feel overwhelmed by them. People are developing new physical and psychological responses to the advances contained within the information revolution. Some perceive that human beings are becoming outmoded or that privacy is becoming a thing of the past. Boulding projects that from now on, we are likely to undergo a new revolution with each generation.

As this chapter is being written, the popular media are featuring stories about the space shuttle and about Pac Man "fever." Many people find it difficult to cope with the excitement and anticipation surrounding such exploits as extraterrestrial travel and the fears and misgivings about our own priorities here on earth. Most of us are not prepared by our educations or experiences to know how to respond to these events or to perceive how they can affect our own lives.

In the past, our forebears learned ways of

coping with daily life and assumed attitudes about the world around them that saw them through a lifetime. It is no longer possible to find that kind of security. The things we learn today to help us cope with today and tomorrow may not see us through enough tomorrows. When we are confronted with new situations, we tend to try to fit them into familiar molds. When this does not work, we respond in a variety of ways. When we are unprepared for change, we may react with psychological withdrawal or denial or we may experience physical reactions in the form of real or feigned illness. Unfortunately, however, the more we use inappropriate adaptive responses to deal with changes, the less able we become to deal with future changes.

By understanding and anticipating the future, one can become better able to cope with the changes that will inevitably occur. There will of course always be unpredictable occurrences, but certain skills will go far to forestall the more disastrous effects of future shock.

Attenuating and Preventing Future Shock

Many of the other chapters in this book are designed to give the student knowledge and skills to mitigate future shock. For example, one way of lessening maladaptive response to a change is to become more flexible and creative. This enables us to reframe experiences that may seem to be problems and to consider them as opportunities and challenges. The chapters on creativity, change theory, political activity, and assertiveness provide information and specific recommendations that will help a nurse meet a new experience with an open mind and a ready repertoire of skills.

Our greatest challenge is to prepare ourselves to cope with change. We can best be prepared by the acquisition of knowledge and the transformation of that knowledge into wisdom. According to Cleveland (1982, p. 34), "*Wisdom* is integrated knowledge—information made super-useful by creating theory rooted in disciplinary knowledge but crossing disciplinary barriers to weave into an integrated whole something more than the sum of the parts." We must keep well informed, but we must also know what to do with what we know. One student said, "I guess it will take a long time for me to reach a true understanding of 'understanding.'" What she was summing up is that process we must all go through—that leap beyond mere "knowing" to knowing what we know. Although people may share the wisdom they have developed, each of us must earn his or her own wisdom.

A teacher can give students lectures, reading assignments, and papers to write, and thereby facilitate the students' knowledge and promote their achievement of wisdom. An individual can strive to attain knowledge in many ways, but all of us must make that knowledge useful to ourselves. That commitment to learn and understand is the best thing an individual can do to prepare for the future.

ELEMENTS AFFECTING FUTURE HEALTH CARE

The elements that will affect health care in the future can be placed in the following categories: socioeconomic and sociopolitical forces, population forces and available resources, automation and cybernation, human determinants, and communications. An understanding of the relevance of each of these elements will help the student project and prepare for the future.

Socioeconomic and Sociopolitical Forces

One forecaster sees the decline of individualism as one of the main effects of American society as it has progressed (Lesse, 1981). In order to survive today and in the future, the individual must be willing and able to cooperate with groups of people. Frequently, the individual must subjugate his or her own wishes to the will of a larger group. In the earlier part of this century, individualism was extolled as a value; this ideal helped bring about reform in labor practices and social welfare. Ironically, such advances were accomplished precisely because the previous inequities did not affect individuals only. These enlightened changes occurred because *groups* were affected. Changes were brought about not by the isolated efforts of single individuals but by groups of people working for common goals. Individualism in the past was concerned with "one's expression of uniqueness on an *interpersonal* basis" (Lesse, 1981, p. 33). In the future, this will be counterproductive to the person involved in most enterprises. At this time, people who tend to become successful, although they seem to have done it "on their own," are standing on the shoulders of many others who preceded them or assisted them.

Describing or advocating a move away from individualism may sound as if the basic worth of an individual is being denied. A distinction between "individualism" and "individuality" may be useful. *Individualism* is a doctrine that individual interests are or ought to be ethically paramount. This clearly elevates any one person above the state, the community, the family, and even above the Supreme Being, however that force is conceived. By simply examining this definition, one can see how unproductive such a philosophy is in a group-oriented society. How can a group, whether it is a family, a community, a business, or a government, function effectively if everyone's interests are paramount to everyone else's? Obviously it is an untenable situation. What individualism means is that the strongest individuals get their interests taken care of above and before others and that many people's interests, let alone needs, are never met or even addressed.

Individuality refers to the total character peculiar to and distinguishing of one person from others. Within this philosophical definition, each person is valued because of his or her individual traits and abilities. Beyond their uniqueness, all people are valued because they are human and because they are individuals. This is consistent with philosophical systems that elevate the interests of the group or of a Supreme Being. Many religious forms advocate the service to others as a way to serve God. Therefore, within a theistic system, it is consistent to serve the interests of the group and to become fulfilled through such service and through the advantages that accrue to the individual because of the resulting welfare of the group.

The passage of the era of individualism is a predictable event given the growth of the three "bigs"—"big business, big labor, and big government" (Lesse, 1981, p. 31). Survival has necessitated the identification of individuals with groups and a willingness to accomplish personal goals through group involvement. Lesse gives the example of the women's movement to illustrate the difficulty of social revolution when the model being used is outdated. Many women have used the model of individualism to characterize their struggle at a time when men have learned to succeed by using group or team models (Harragan, 1977; Lesse, 1981).

The 1980s will see the last efforts to seek

self-fulfillment at any expense and the beginning of the movement toward achieving fulfillment of personal goals by advancing society's well-being (Yankelovich, 1982). However, this era will be marked by confusion and a feeling that things are out of control. Although it is uncomfortable to those who must live and work through it, this upheaval is necessary to the advancement of our culture.

After the consideration of individuals, we must consider the institutions on which our society has come to rely. Lesse (1981) has cited the move from nationalism, which was an extension of the individual need for security, to a federated society, structured to satisfy individual needs by promoting the general welfare of the country and its citizens. The move from the emphasis on individuals and their dealings is reflected by the trends in legislation relevant to the rights and needs of citizens in groups.

Our educational institutions are in great need of an overhaul. When this finally comes about, it will affect every aspect of our society. In the past, our educational system has encouraged students to accumulate an enormous fund of facts. As available information has increased, more and more time has been spent in trying to make students learn data. This is no longer functional. Schools at all levels must prepare students to understand what they know and to be able to use it. The educational system must prepare people to learn more effectively, to know how to think, and to be able to adapt to change (Lesse, 1981; Pulliam, 1981; Seif, 1981; Yankelovich, 1982).

Many of the systems that have held our society together were appropriate for the ages in which they developed. Such groups as labor unions helped to raise the laborer out of a state of exploitation. With enlightened management and commitment to quality, new approaches to working with employees make the unions outmoded in many settings. However, such groups and the people who earn their own livings by running them foster the schism between labor and management with a seeming regard for the individual. Many of the gains made to benefit the individual in these situations have resulted in decreases in productivity and no apparent change in job satisfaction. Yankelovich is only one of the critics who point out the unwieldiness of this archaic system. Phillip Crosby is another who has made great strides in looking at how quality can be defined in a way that results in satisfaction of individual goals as well as the goals of the organization (Anderson, 1983). Crosby's definition of *quality* is "conformance to requirements" (Anderson, 1983, p. 21). By accepting an error rate of 5 percent (in a sometimes misguided effort to protect individuals), industry and service organizations have incurred heavy costs that affect everyone involved, including the individual who was being protected in the first place. If we continue to condone less than the best in our education, political, and business institutions, our society will not be able to survive.

The institutions of religion and family are also undergoing change. With a desire to meet their needs by involvement in a group commitment, people are recognizing the importance of higher spiritual needs. Religious institutions are responding at present by providing shelter for those who are adrift or overwhelmed by the events of the world. The upheaval seems to encourage the pessimists who accept a fast-approaching end to our world. Our society as we have known it is coming to an end, but not with a blast and the destruction of human beings. The end is that of the outmoded, cumbersome, anachronistic devices that are finally being recognized for the burdens they are. The future will see a resurgence of the need for spiritual fulfillment, but this will be expressed in a variety of ways and will come to be an integral part of daily life and of the society as a whole.

The family is always responsive to societal changes. Revolutions tend to include as a first phase the swing to the opposite of the previous order. Therefore, it is no surprise that there has been a vast change in family configurations. Families today are frequently comprised of single parents with one or more children as well as of two parents with some or all of their children from previous marriages. More households than ever before are occupied by one adult. The old family configuration with the male breadwinner, housewife, and two children comprises only 7% of the population (Naisbitt, 1982). Families are small, because children are valued as a continuation of the family and not so much as a resource for inexpensive labor, as they were in the near past. A great deal of thought and money goes into the rearing of most children, even among the disadvantaged. In the future, with less opportunity for self-expression through individualism on a societal scale, there will be an increased need for the expression of individuality within oneself or within the family group. Many people have expressed concern about the small number of close friends they have (Yankelovich, 1983). This has come about because of the diffuseness of commitment and the emphasis on meeting personal needs. With an evolution of society toward restoring and promoting the quality of life, people will return to the valuing of the work involved in establishing and maintaining meaningful relationships among friends and family.

Many science fiction stories concern a society that has become so group oriented that the rights and needs of the individuals are submerged. In such stories, the protagonists are the rebels who see that this must be reversed. Quite often, the heroes and heroines of these stories are ultimately defeated. Now is the time to ensure that such scenarios do not occur. The new "groupism" described here is a way of saving the group and the individual by bringing their needs and values into concert.

Population Pressures and Available Resources

If the size of the population exceeds the earth's ability to sustain it, there will be no long-term future for this planet. More than ever before, Americans are facing the realities of being citizens of the world. Our economy and other manifestations of our nation's strength reflect the impact that events and decisions in other parts of the world have on our daily lives. The need for grain in Russia determines agricultural practices in Kansas. The need for water in India has nearly led to war with Pakistan and Bangladesh. The efficiency of Japanese management affects domestic automobile sales in Europe and America. Decisions in the Middle East change the speed limits on U.S. highways. There are many examples of the interrelationships among the governments and the economy in all populated areas.

Lesse (1981) has suggested that diminishing rural land area and the reliance of most people on housing within urban areas may require even larger and taller structures than in our modern cities today. Buildings providing housing may tower to 30 or more stories. Then people within such swelling centers may constitute a community of their own, relatively independent of the world outside except for work. The buildings will include shopping malls and food stores, enabling residents to conserve time and energy by such ready access to products. Some cities are already increasing the available space in downtown centers by developing underground areas for shopping malls and other businesses.

There has been a significant exodus from the cities to the rural communities (Naisbitt, 1982). Although this has eased some of the swelling metropolises of their numbers, it is having an impact on the rural areas which is not altogether pleasant. Even though the shift has afforded some relief from overcrowding, if population figures continue to soar, the new communities will become as large as the communities that were left behind. There is a limit to the amount of habitable land on each continent. A certain amount of land is necessary for greenery—forests and the like—not only for its resource value but also for its contribution to the ecology of the planet.

One solution to the decrease in amounts of habitable land is for people to build and inhabit floating cities. Such a proposal has been designed by Fuller (1981). Many major cities are near large bodies of water that could accommodate the type of structure Fuller proposed. These self-sufficient communities would offer all the usual advantages of urban dwelling. They would be located near other major population areas with easy access via water to other parts of the country. Major private and governmental groups have been giving these possibilities serious consideration. For such land-poor countries as Japan, this solution could provide great relief.

Another resource that is not always sufficient is water. The viability of any community is affected by the availability of usable water. Decreasing supplies in the Sun Belt and the South may forestall continued growth in those areas. Much research will be devoted to desalinating and rerouting sea water to make it usable and available to those who need it (Lesse, 1981).

The continual quest for inexpensive, accessible energy sources has dominated scientific and governmental agendas for much of the last 15 years. Suddenly we have had to come to grips with the fact that our energy resources are dwindling and that those we have used so freely in the past are not renewable. The debate goes on about the use of nuclear energy for domestic purposes and the practicality of solar energy for general use. In the meantime, most people, particularly in the United States, continue to behave as if energy supplies are never-ending. Because most of us have witnessed great technological developments within our lifetimes, we tend to believe that science and technology can solve any problem. Therefore, people continue to squander and misuse resources. The greater the number of people who have this approach, the faster our world will be depleted.

Automation and Cybernation

Automation is the technique of making an apparatus, a process, or a system function automatically; that is, operating without human intervention. *Cybernation* is the employment of computers in bringing about automation. Many people fear automation and the intrusion of computers into our human world because of the sense that automated or computer systems are mysterious and potentially malevolent. Another factor in the fear and distrust of such systems is the belief that human workers will be replaced by machines. There is also the fear that computers threaten our rights to privacy. To some extent, these concerns are justified. Automated systems and computers have made it possible for factories to function with fewer unskilled laborers. Many who have no skills or low-level skills have already been supplanted by automated systems. Furthermore, the complex systems do have the potential for being invaded and misused by people who wish to take unfair advantage of their fellows.

With the decade of the 1980s, we are beginning to value the computer for what it can do for us, not fearing so much what it can do to us. The computer has liberated people from many burdensome tasks (Naisbitt, 1982). Naisbitt cites several examples in which the computer has permitted more individualization rather than depersonalization in industry. For example, some companies can tailor contracts to each of their thousands of workers because a computer can retain the necessary information and produce individualized agreements suiting the mutual needs of the employee and the company. Naisbitt mentions a trend in health care: the technology used in sustaining life has brought about an intense interest in the quality of life and the investigation of many philosophical issues long ignored by health care professionals.

Naisbitt characterizes the trends in this area as "high tech/high touch" (1982). By this he is describing the need that people seem to have for increased interpersonal contact as their lives are influenced by technology. People are more satisfied with technological changes in their lives when there is a concomitant increase in their contact with others. Although various futurists have prophesied about the so-called electronic cottage from which people will be able to conduct their every activity (O'Toole, 1982; Sutherland, 1982; Toffler, 1971; Tydeman, 1982), Naisbitt emphasizes that people are unlikely to rely on computers for all these activities unless they have replacement opportunities to be with people. People may opt to work or learn in their homes in order to conserve time that they can spend in other pursuits with other people.

As more and more people become conver-sant with computers, much of the fear and distrust of technology will fall away. As people are released from boring, ungratifying jobs, they will be able to pursue more people-oriented occupations and professions. Service workers already comprise about 50 percent of the workforce, and this general category is sure to increase as technology advances (Edelhart et al., 1982). Technology affords opportunities for such specialization in medicine and nursing, and this will have implications for professionals in these fields. Nurses who are clinically competent and who have technological skills may be able to design their own positions.

Human Determinants

Human determinants are the primary forces which result in human needs. Lesse (1981, p. 72) defines *human needs* as

those factors which, when satisfied, permit and aid an individual to function either alone or in a group, in a given milieu, with optimum ability to adapt to or modify the human–environmental equilibrium, in order to guarantee survival with pride and pleasure.

These determinants fall into the categories of individual, societal, and environmental. The *individual determinants* include the genetic makeup of each person and the ontogenetic determinants, such as developmental stages. In addition are the human rhythms, both biological and emotional.

Societal determinants include the influences of demographic patterns and institutional structures, such as the family, the community, the nation, and the world. The customs and demands of each of these groups play a part in determining what the individual will perceive to be his or her needs.

Environmental determinants include climate, ecology, and technological factors. These factors determine such things as the resources available to the individual and the quality of the environment.

The basic needs for nutrition, water, air, and sunlight will persist. However, the ways in which these needs are met will change. The degree to which people can cope with those changes will be influenced by a wide variety of determinants.

Communication and Information

Information has become the most valuable commodity in the modern world (Cleveland, 1982; Ferguson, M., 1980; Naisbitt, 1982; Weil, 1982). Gathering it, storing it, and retrieving it are the essential processes involved in handling this resource. When we share this resource, we engage in communication. Human beings seem to have an innate need to communicate with one another, and technology is enhancing this process. Already our personal and professional lives are marked by the efforts we expend to communicate with one another.

Our increasingly sophisticated means of communication will make the process much more efficient. As technology makes new information almost instantaneously available, events in distant places can become available to us in as little time as it takes to record them. Computer systems and relationships among their owners already make it possible for people to communicate quickly and inexpensively. At present, there is a lag time of a several months to a year between the time a professional article is written and when it published. The lag time for textbooks is one to two years. In the near future, this time will be cut down considerably, making contributions to professional literature much more timely. Electronic submission of material from authors to editors and from editors to typesetters is already in use on a limited basis (Skarnulis, 1982). Some forms of "electronic publishing" have virtually eliminated lag time by bypassing typesetters and printers entirely; consumers receive the latest publications directly through word-processing terminals at home or at work.

FUTURISM AND NURSING

Nursing is now at a pivotal point, just as the rest of society is. We are in a position to determine the real future of our profession. If we are unimaginative and individualistic, we not only may hold the profession back, but we may participate in its demise. If we continue to expend energy warring among ourselves, we will not have the energy to participate in the health care planning that is vital for the future. In 1971, Esther Lucille Brown made the following statement:

No one needs to be a social scientist or a follower of the women's liberation movement to realize that one of the basic causes for the inadequacy of present health services is the fact that the nursing role was cast from too small a mold to encourage, or even permit, a profession twice the size of medicine to maximize its potential contribution. (p. 493)

If we are starting at too low a level, we have far to go to attain a place in determining the needs for a healthy public. Nurses have succumbed to individualism. They have taken jobs rather than positions. They have allowed one group after another to determine nursing practice. Nurses have been guilty of putting patient or client needs after ego needs. We, as nurses, are certainly not the only ones who have had difficulty in defining and implementing our profes sional goals, but we seem to have been struggling with the problem for too long.

The only thing that will change the public's view of the nurse's role is for the amorphous body of people who constitute the profession to think and act in unity. Unity is not the same as uniformity. *Uniformity* means having the same form and being undiversified. *Unity* is a totality of related parts; an entity that is a complex or systematic whole. Unity allows for differences as long as the final result is continuity. The most significant aspect of the lack of unity within nursing is the current educational "system," which is really a nonsystem. Virginia Cleland made a succinct declaration of the situation in 1976:

Nursing should not continue to tolerate a system of education which cannot be defended logically, which is incomprehensible to the general public, which is restrictive to individuals, and which is on the threshold of producing too many nurses for first-hand positions. Through an evolutionary process nursing is moving toward a two, four, six, eight pattern of education. The fact that it is evolving without direct professional pronouncements may mean that the pattern makes a lot of sense educationally and professionally in our culture. (p. 5)

Dr. Cleland advocates a clear definition of the conceptual base of each type of educational program and an agreement within the profession about what should be taught at what time and how the various programs should be articulated. Too much energy has been spent arguing about whether the graduates of one program are as "good" as the others. If quality means meeting requirements, then nursing should delineate the requirements for each kind of nurse and hold practitioners to those requirements. Nurses should not be asked to do things for which they have not been educated; they also should not accept responsibility for doing things that are inappropriate given

their levels of education. For example, a nurse with no experience and only a baccalaureate degree should not be asked to become a director of nursing. Furthermore, it should be so clear that this is an inappropriate role that no new graduate would consider filling such a position.

Earlier in this chapter, the societal factors that will have a bearing on the future of the health sciences were discussed. However, some more specific factors will affect nursing and the other health professions. The broad areas under which these issues can be classified deal first with client population and second with the nature of nursing practice.

Client Population

Our population is gradually changing to one that is heavily represented by older people. People are living longer and healthier lives. It has been projected that by 1990 the life expectancy for men in the United States will be 71.9 years and for women 80 years ("Six Population Surprises," 1982). The same source projects that the proportion of nonwhites surviving into old age will continue to increase. This will place a great demand on health and illness care services. A variety of approaches will be necessary to meet the needs of these people in order to preserve the quality of their later years. By the time that the average reader of this book reaches the age of 65, around the year 2030, 18 to 20 percent of the world's population will be that age or older, and the proportion of people in that age group will be even higher in developed countries (Bezold, 1982). This has implications not only for the care systems that nurses will help to develop and implement but also for consumers of the health care system. Those who set the patterns of care for and the attitudes toward the older population will eventually reap the benefits of deficiencies of the climate they have created.

The nature of health problems has changed over the years, requiring changes in the manner in which people learn about and give care to clients and patients. For example, cancer is a more common problem than in the past for a variety of reasons. For one thing, our ability to diagnose cancer has increased dramatically. Perhaps the most significant factor, however, is that people live longer and therefore are more likely to develop cancer and other diseases. People who would have succumbed to pneumonia, tuberculosis, small pox, diphtheria, and so on are either cured of such diseases or never contract them. Therefore, because they live longer, they may later develop cancer, renal problems, or cardiovascular disabilities.

Treatment of many illnesses is easily managed outside the hospital setting, so those who require episodic care within a hospital are critically ill and require intensive support to ensure their survival and recovery. More people in the community require some type of supportive care while recovering from illnesses as well as for promoting their health status. In the past, it was taken for granted that people would age at a prescribed rate and would gradually deteriorate and eventually die from "old age." Now people are finding that quality as well as length of life can be increased by many preventive efforts that forestall the physical and mental deterioration formerly considered to be unavoidable concomitants of getting older.

Nurses are well prepared to help clients plan and manage a healthy life-style and to determine when their concerns or problems warrant other kinds of intervention, such as attention from a physician (Henry, 1979; Schlotfeldt, 1981). The movement toward self-help and self-care will persist (Bezold, 1982; Naisbitt, 1982). If clients are to be successful at their individual efforts in this area, they can use the input and guidance of nurses.

Nurses can not only provide education and information for clients but also can help monitor the unscrupulous practitioners within the community. In such a wide-open atmosphere, many people are easy targets for those who attempt to profit from consumers' concerns for their health. This does not mean that all those who do not have formal credentials should be disregarded. There is a need to investigate the many different approaches that crop up and are used by people from all kinds of backgrounds. Nurses must be informed about available alternative health care activities in order to be effective resources to their clients.

With people relying less on episodic care, nursing practice will take place more frequently in distributive settings (Henry, 1979; Leininger, 1973; Thurston, 1972). Leininger advocated an open system that would permit clients to get quick and effective care without a great deal of bureaucratic interference. Such a system would be facilitated if consumers had access to nurses or other caregivers who could help potential clients define their needs and identify appropriate resources. Access could be enhanced by the use of computer information services and cable television health networks.

As we increase the depth and breadth of our understanding of the interrelationships of mind, body, and spirit, we will be able to design and implement ever more holistic approaches to working with clients. We are already seeing a resurgence and acceptance of cultural diversity. No longer is everyone expected to ascribe to the norms of the homogenized society. The move from individualism toward collectivism has encouraged the spread and acceptance of the unique aspects of various cultural groups that make up American society. With the move toward a world orientation rather than a national orientation, many of us are being brought into frequent contact with people of different nationalities. For the United States to remain in a global leadership role, the majority of its citizens must be willing and able to interact with temporary and permanent residents from other countries. Immigration of legal and illegal aliens accounted for nearly one and a quarter million new United States residents in 1981, and this source of population growth is predicted to continue ("Six Population Surprises," 1982).

In the future, nursing practice will be much more complex, because of holistic approaches and the need to be knowledgeable about so many variables within the population. Nurses working in the community may come into contact with one or more clients every day who have different customs, health care expectations, and languages than the nurse. It will be useful for nurses to understand and speak more than one language. There are already small computer translators that assist people in communicating when they travel, and some health care settings already maintain these devices for use with clients. Although this provides some assistance, personal interaction based on true understanding of the other person's tongue and customs is the best way to foster a meaningful relationship.

Some nurses have expressed concern about the move away from the concept of "public health nursing" to the notion of "community health nursing" (Barkauskas, 1982; Dreher, 1982). *Public health nursing* is the practice of nursing in relation to aggregates or groups of people; *community health nursing* concerns care given individuals within the community. In the future the skills nurses use to work with entire communities and with health issues that have implications for groups of citizens will need to be revitalized. For example, the use of nuclear power for energy poses some threats to the health of people who live near nuclear power plants. The continued disorganization in the management of the quality of our air and water is another ongoing challenge to any health care professional who wishes to promote well-being within the heavily populated areas where most people choose to live.

Nurses must take responsibility for knowing communities, not just the individuals who reside there. Since people try to meet their own individual needs, it is most efficient for nurses to provide and promote access to health care resources for entire groups rather than to focus on one individual or one family at a time. There will always be a need for nurses who wish to work with individuals and families, but there is an even greater need for people who will obtain advanced educational and experiential training that will enable them to look at large contexts, in order to assess these contexts and design future-oriented interventions to prevent or minimize emerging health care problems.

Naisbitt (1982) identified as one megatrend the desire for multiple options rather than either/or choices. In other words, clients wish to have a selection of resources when they wish to meet some need. If clients have more choices, they will be interested in conserving limited resources such as money and energy when they select a health care professional; thus they will be willing to work with different kinds of professionals and lay people to promote and maintain health. If nurses are geographically closer and have more reasonable fees than other professionals, a client will be likely to select a nurse for assistance. Smith (1980) raised the issue of direct access to patients and clients. She challenged nurses to admit that they are in a position to compete with physicians for clients. Although this role is not yet fully legitimized by the public, if nurses have the courage to persist in providing their skills to clients, the public will eventually be willing to accept and even demand a reorganization of the health care system based on what health care professionals have to offer, rather than continuing to rely on the practice of medicine as the organizing rubric under which all illness and health concerns fall. The future will see a great increase in the areas in which nurses function autonomously, but only if nurses are willing to demonstrate their ability to function autonomously (Smith, 1980).

Nursing Practice

Nursing practice is affected by forces from outside the profession as well as by internal forces. The economic climate of society has an impact on every aspect of our lives. For example, when finances are short there is always a movement to try to fill slots formerly occupied by professional nurses with less skilled and lower-paid workers. With the growing complexity of nursing practice, this is not as frequently done. However, it is up to professional nurses to demonstrate that they make contributions to the health care system that cannot be made by anyone else. Nursing is unique, and nurses are not interchangeable with other people in the health care system.

In times when financial resources are limited, consumers may favor seeking nursing care for some of their needs rather than more expensive physician care. When consumers find that they can meet health care needs less expensively by seeking out nurses, their health care patterns will change, even though their resources may improve. In 1980, health care costs constituted 10 percent of the gross national product. The public seems to have reached its level of tolerance for these ever-increasing costs and to have begun to demand cost-containment measures. People want to know what they are paying for when they visit a physician or are hospitalized. There will be a trend toward programs which will discourage hospitalization and promote health (Edelhart et al., 1982).

The future will favor the development of insurance systems and organizations that will promote healthy practices. Innovative developments, such as direct reimbursements or tax credits for staying healthy, may be seen before the end of this century. People will be able to apply for assistance or credits in undertaking self-initiated health-promotion activities. For example, present tax law permits a deduction for the costs of a weight-reduction program only if a physician has ordered it for a medical condition such as hypertension. In the future, people will demand the right to deduct such costs even if they are self-prescribed. This may lead to the regulation and accreditation of such programs, and this will be a fertile field for the involvement of nurses, both in helping to evaluate such endeavors and also in serving as consultants and participants in health-maintenance programs.

Governmental influence on our daily lives has been increasing for most of this century. The future model for this influence must be oriented in a new direction in order to provide the structure needed for health promotion as a national objective. Hancock (1982, p. 7) contrasts public health policy and a healthy public policy as follows:

Public Health Policy	Healthy Public Policy
Chiefly concerned with health care system	Chiefly concerned with creating a healthy society
Dominated by the hard health path (e.g., medical model, hospital-based, quantity of life, encourages dependence)	Dominated by the soft health path (e.g., focus on prevention, community-oriented, quality of life, promotes self-care)
Sectoral/analytical	Holistic
Present-oriented	Future-oriented
Accepts the givens	Questions the givens

As experts in health and illness care, nurses can facilitate the move from the current model to a new model. The principal factor is for nurses to become more politically knowledgeable and active (Baumgart, 1981; Dreher, 1982; Henry, 1979; Northrop, 1982; Smith, 1980). Nurses have made great strides in becoming politically aware and politically influential over the last two decades. The next two decades will provide the forum for continued growth. This is another area in which collectivism has an impact. One nurse voting for a candidate has little influence, but when nurses become organized to support a given candidate, they become powerful. At present, one in every 44 women voters is a registered nurse. Numbers such as that impress legislators and candidates for office. The relatively new Nurses' Coalition for Action in Politics (N-CAP) has been influential in raising money to support candidates for national offices. Coalitions in various states have followed the lead in races for state and local offices. Legislative committees and lobbyists are commonly sponsored by state nurses' associations. The American Nurses'

Association Government Relations Department in Washington, D.C., has been active in representing nursing interests at the federal level. Such organized efforts are only the beginning if nurses choose to work as a group in acquiring and wielding the power that is within our reach to influence the government in concerns related to the health of our nation.

Both Cleland (1976) and Smith (1980) have articulated the importance of nurses developing more effective models for the relationships between themselves and the organizations within which they function. If nurses are to be accountable for nursing, they must be in control of their own practice (Northrop, 1982; Schlotfeldt, 1981). This issue relates directly to the way in which individual nurses define and practice their profession. As long as nurses function as employees and see themselves as holding jobs, they will continue to be controlled and activated by those who employ them. Professional nurses determine the limits and the scope of their own practice.

A suit was brought against a large hospital by a physician because a nurse had recommended to a patient under the physician's care that the patient seek another opinion about a surgical procedure the physician had recommended. The patient did seek another opinion and subsequently decided not to have the surgery and to discontinue the relationship with the physician who had recommended it. While the suit was pending, the hospital issued a memorandum to the registered nurses that they were not to discuss any patient's condition or options with him or her. The majority of the nurses complained among themselves about this policy, but they did not openly challenge it. One nurse, however, informed the administration in writing that she intended to do whatever she thought was in the best interests of her patients based on her professional judgment. When she told other nurses that she was going to do this, they told her that she would get into trouble and probably lose her job. The administration acknowledged that they had received her memorandum and that they were putting it in her file, but they did not tell her that she was in danger of losing her job. No pressure was exerted to make her do differently than she intended.

Until nursing is willing to take such stands as a collective, not much change will be accomplished. Smith (1980, pp. 541–542) cites a similar situation, in which a client finally died because agency policy superseded the nurse's judgment. Nurses must confront this issue in the near future and mobilize public sentiment to legitimize their responsibility for being accountable for their knowledge when it affects the safety, well-being, and health of clients. This harks back to the issue raised earlier of ownership of the client. In the future, the eventual outcome of a client situation will be determined not by who the client chose first as his or her primary health giver, but by what seems to be in his or her best interests.

Another megatrend Naisbitt (1982) described is the move from hierarchies to networks. This trend promises to provide some way in which clients' needs and rights can be protected. The establishment of a health care network enables clients to seek information from a variety of sources on any given problem or concern. Since the client has established his or her own network, the health care professionals within it are not necessarily part of hierarchy. Clients are becoming more informed consumers of health care, and they are less likely to take any one person's opinion as the final word. As this trend continues, it will support collaboration among health care professionals rather than vertical relationships that put some people in lower positions than others, sometimes with the client actually being the one on the bottom.

A key influence on the future of nursing practice is the willingness of nurses to make a commitment to the advance of nursing as a profession and to the maintenance of the health of the public. Commitment implies risk. Yankelovich (1982) points out that people have withdrawn from the demands inherent in commitment to ideals and to people. However, things are changing, and people are seeking the life enrichment that comes from caring about someone or something beyond one's self. In nursing, this means being willing to take the risk that by asserting one's professional responsibility one may suffer personal consequences, such as losing his or her position. Northrop (1982) stated that nurses may be put in the position of testing employer actions in law suits. For example, in the situation described above, when the nurse informed her employer that she intended to practice nursing unrestricted by nonnursing intervention, she took a considerable risk. If she had been dismissed, she could have contested the employer's right to control her nursing practice. This nurse had a commitment to the care of clients that transcended her concerns about herself, and, her actions were necessary to maintain her comfort and self-respect. She could not have continued to function if she was not willing to take a stand on the practice of nursing.

A related issue has to do with quality. If quality is conformance to standards, in the future, nurses must determine what those standards are. They will delineate the expectations of nursing practice for nurses of all levels of experience and education. Part of the definition of a profession is that it sets its own standards and enforces them. Once nursing frees itself from the nonnursing hierarchy in which it has functioned in the past, nurses will oversee each others' practice. Systems of peer review and quality assurance will be commonplace. This will occur as a result of the efforts toward consensus about standards of nursing practice (Northrop, 1982).

A crucial step in the advancement of professional nursing is the revitalization of professional organizations (Baumgart, 1981; Schlotfeldt, 1981). This brings us back to the importance of collective action. When nurses have functioned collectively within their own organizations, they have been effective on many issues. The main problem has been in promoting and maintaining membership within such organizations. Since many nurses have been individualistic and oriented to nursing as a vocation rather than as a profession, they have looked upon professional association membership as if it were a club. The most frequently raised question is "What are the benefits to me of membership?" When people discontinue their affiliation, it is often because "the organization doesn't do anything for me." One goal of professional associations is to protect the interests of their members. However, in the case of nursing organizations, another equally important charge is to protect and promote the welfare of the public in regard to health and illness care. In order to accomplish such goals, the organization must include and represent a substantial proportion of the members of the profession.

Perhaps new forms of organization are indicated in order to facilitate the function of professional associations within nursing. In 1982, the American Nurses' Association adopted a federation model. It is too early to tell exactly how this will facilitate the accomplishment of the goals of the association. However, it is clear that for the association to be effective and meaningful in the health care arena, professional nurses must be willing to unite as members of the organization. The near future will determine whether or not the present organizations will persist or some new form will arise. Whatever the form, however, it is crucial that some type of association persist. Without an ongoing organization to monitor and channel efforts of nurses, nursing will never realize its potential.

Getting Ready for the Future

If you were going to a party soon, you would make preparations and give some thought to what you needed. For example, you would make plans about how to get there, what to wear, whom to go with, what to take, and so on. Many of us put more time into planning what we are going to do tomorrow than what we are going to do for the rest of our lives. We have to make similar decisions today about the future we want for nursing. Where are we going? How are we going to get there? Whom will we be with? What do we want to do once we get there? The choices each of us makes about such issues determine the course of all our futures. For instance, if too many of us feel that we cannot make a difference even by belonging to the American Nurses' Association, and therefore we do not join, then we will find that that feeling becomes reality. If you think you are helpless, you are helpless. If you believe that you can control the outcome of many events in your life, you will be able to do so.

By investing time, money, and effort in a nursing education, a person is making choices about the future. However, that basic education is only the beginning. One's basic education is just what the word indicates—a base upon which to build everything else. To function even at a safe level, one has to continue to grow and learn. As Will Rogers said, "You may be on the right track, but if you just sit there, you'll be run over." With the world and everything in it changing at an increasingly rapid pace, all of us have to learn things that may be useful to us for only a limited time. It will take skill and courage to give up some of the ideas we are learning today. For example, some of the chapters in this book describe nursing practice as it is to-day. For a nursing student or a nurse to function, such information is necessary. It would be foolhardy to provide young prac-titioners only with skills for a future that has not yet arrived. Therefore, a consider-able amount of time and space must be used to teach how to function today and tomorrow.

At the same time one is learning how to be a nurse in the present, one must also be learning the skills and tools that will make it possible to conform to as well as to set new patterns of nursing practice. This book presents material about the practice of nursing in the community today, but with an eye to possible changes and trends that will affect nursing practice. There are some attempts to predict what may come about in various areas, but generally, the authors have offered possibilities and alternatives in order to indicate the vastness of the pos-sible influences that may affect nursing and health care.

We are at the early stages of a trend to move from short-term to long-term goals and concerns. This is a trend within society and nursing has responded. We must face the future with hope and optimism and a sense that we are in control of our own lives:

The future is what we think it will be. We can make our own future. If we want a future in which nurses are united and able to make a sig-nificant impact on the health care system, we must *make* it happen. We cannot make a differ-ence unless we believe in our own goals and in our personal power to accomplish them. (Schoolcraft, 1983, p. 5)

The greatest challenge to each of us, whether student or nurse, is to take charge of his or her own future.

DISCUSSION TOPICS

1. Give an example from your own life that demonstrates future shock.

2. Imagine where you will be in 10 years. What will you be doing professionally? What will you have accomplished in your personal life?

3. Working backward from the fantasy of your future, what do you have to do to ar-rive at that point?

4. What are your personal goals for your-self as a professional nurse? How will you go about accomplishing those goals?

5. What are your goals or hopes for the nursing profession of the future? How are you going to contribute to realizing those goals and hopes?

6. Identify four ways in which you can be-come more future oriented. What do these things have in common? What makes these things different from each other?

7. Identify a nurse you know or have read about who provides a role model of a fu-ture-oriented person. What makes him or her fit that description? How can you use that role model to enhance your own future orientation?

BIBLIOGRAPHY

Amara, R.: The futures field, which direction now? *The Futurist* 15(3), 42–46, 1981.

Anderson, R.C.: Quest for quality. *Success* 30(1), 21–23, 62, 1983.

Barkauskas, V.H.: Public health nursing prac-tice—An educator's view. *Nursing Outlook* 30(7), 384–389, 1982.

Baumgart, A.J.: Nursing for a new century: a

future framework. Address to the International Council of Nurses Quadrennial Congress, Los Angeles, July 1, 1981.

Bezold, C.: Health care in the U.S.: Four alternative futures. *The Futurist* 16(4), 14–18, 1982.

Boulding, K.: *The meaning of the twentieth century.* New York: Harper & Row, 1962.

Bowman, J., Kierstead, F., Dede, C., & Pulliam, J.D.: *The far side of the future.* Washington, D.C.: World Future Society, 1978.

Brown, E.L.: *Nursing reconsidered: A study of change. Part 2: The professional role in community nursing.* Philadelphia: Lippincott, 1971.

Butz, W.P., McCarthy, K.F., Morrison, P.A., & Vaiana, M.E.: *Demographic challenges in America's future.* Santa Monica, Ca.: The Rand Corporation, 1982.

Clarke, A.C.: *Profiles of the future.* New York: Bantam, 1967.

Cleland, V.S.: *A model for nursing.* In American Nurses' Association, *A look to the future.* Kansas City: ANA, 1976.

Cleland, V.S.: Nurses' economics and the control of nursing practice. In L.H. Aiken, ed., *Nursing in the 1980's.* Philadelphia: Lippincott, 1982.

Cleveland, H.: Information as a resource. *The Futurist* 16(6), 34–39, 1982.

Cornish, E.: An agenda for the 1980's. *The Futurist* 14(1), 5–13, 1980.

Dreher, M.C.: The conflict of conservatism in public health nursing education. *Nursing Outlook* 30(9), 504–509, 1982.

Edelhart, M., Hilts, P., Malone, R., & Schrage, M.: The business sector. In R. Weil, ed., *The Omni future almanac.* New York: Omni Publications, 1982.

Fasano, N.F., & White, M.J.: Futurism scenario: Commencement address to the class of 2010. *Journal of Nursing Education* 21(3), 20–24, 1982.

Ferguson, M.: *The aquarian conspiracy.* Los Angeles: J.P. Tarcher, 1980.

Ferguson, M.: Aquarian conspiracy update. Public address, University of Oklahoma, Norman, Oklahoma, October 20, 1982.

Fuller, R.B.: *Critical path.* New York: St. Martin's, 1981.

Giuliano, V.E.: The mechanization of office work. *Scientific American* 247(3), 149–164, 1982.

Hancock, T.: Beyond health care: Creating a healthy future. *The Futurist* 16(4), 4–13, 1982.

Harragan, B.L.: *Games mother never taught you.* New York: Warner, 1977.

Henry, M.: Futurism: Implications for nursing. *Oklahoma League for Nursing Newsletter*, May 1979.

Hubbard, B.M.: Critical path to an all-win world. *The Futurist* 15(3), 31–37, 1981.

Kelly, L.Y.: Nurses of the third wave. *Nursing Outlook* 28(5), 330, 1980.

Leininger, M.: Health care delivery systems for tomorrow: Possibilities and guidelines. Proceedings, *Health of the Nation—5*, University of Minnesota Hospitals Summer Lecture Series, 1973.

Lesse, S.: *The future of the health sciences.* New York: Irvington, 1982.

Loeb, M.: Changes in the 80's affecting health care. Address to the National League for Nursing Convention, Las Vegas, May 5, 1981.

Naisbitt, J.: *Megatrends.* New York: Warner, 1982.

Northrop, C.: Taking charge of our future. Address to the Oklahoma Nurses' Association Convention, Oklahoma City, October 27, 1982.

O'Toole, J.: How to forecast your own working future. *The Futurist* 16(1), 5–11, 1982.

Pulliam, J.D.: Education priorities for the not-so-gay 90's. *Journal of Thought* 16(3), 33–45, 1981.

Pulliam, J.D., & Bowman, J.R.: *Educational futurism.* Norman, Oklahoma: University of Oklahoma Press, 1974.

Schlotfeldt, R.M.: Nursing in the future. *Nursing Outlook* 29(5), 295–301, 1981.

Schoolcraft, V.L.: A conspiracy within the nursing profession. *Oklahoma Nurse* 27(5), 5, 31, 1982.

Seif, E.: Thinking and education: A futures approach. *Journal of Thought* 16(3), 73–87, 1981.

Six population surprises and the future. *The Futurist* 16(6), 72, 74, 1982.

Skarnulis, L.: Is there an electronic byline in your future? *The Futurist* 16(6), 40–46, 1982.

Smith, G.R.: Nursing beyond the crossroads. *Nursing Outlook* 28(9), 540–545, 1980.

Sutherland, R.A.: Home banking: Electronic money invades the living room. *The Futurist* 16(2), 13–17, 1982.

Thurston, H.I.: Education for episodic and distributive care. *Nursing Outlook* 20(8), 519–523, 1972.

Toffler, A.: *Future Shock.* New York: Bantam, 1971.

Toffler, A.: *The third wave.* New York: Bantam, 1981.

Tydeman, J.: Videotex: Ushering in the electronic household. *The Futurist* 16(1), 54–61, 1982.

Van Avery, D.: Futuristics and education. *Educational Leadership* 37(5), 441–442, 1980.

Weil, R., ed., *The Omni future almanac.* New York: Omni Publications, 1982.

Yankelovich, D.: Toward an ethic of commitment. *AIDE Magazine* 13(2), 17–20, 1982.

2

Historical Foundations and Trends

Gloria R. Smith

If . . . history . . . teaches us anything, it is that man, in his quest for knowledge and progress, is determined and cannot be deterred.

JOHN F. KENNEDY

OBJECTIVES

After reading this chapter, you should be able to:

- [ ] Describe the public health nursing role in the past and the community health nursing role in the present and delineate constraints and opportunities for the role in the future.
- [ ] Discuss characteristic models of nursing practice in the community.
- [ ] Discuss public policy issues affecting the capability of community health nurses to deal with aggregate community health problems.

INTRODUCTION

The Rise of Public Health Nursing

Social trends and health problems have historically shaped public health nursing, the precursor to community health nursing. The field developed with urbanization. With an influx of immigrants inhabiting tenements, dramatic new health problems faced the general public. Public health nursing, including the visiting nurse role, developed in the nineteenth century. Overcoming superstition and adjusting to sanitary conditions often required the public health nurse to actively teach newcomers how to sanitize their environments and how to care for sick family members. With the rise of schools of nursing in the early twentieth century, public health nursing expanded.

Government institutions such as boards of health, further legitimated the public health nursing role. Industrial insurance policyholders were provided with visiting nurses by their insurers in some areas of the country. The physician/nurse distribution of authority was actively debated, primarily in relation to the scope of nurses' roles. Maternal and child care became a focus of attention in the early 1900s, when infant mortality rates were high. The fight against tuberculosis required treatment, education, and environmental modification. Red Cross nursing, which developed in the mid-nineteenth century, was carried to the United States in the late nineteenth century. Exemplary individuals and organizations dramatized the mission of public health nursing. Individuals such as Lillian Wald and Clara Barton and organizations such as the Henry Street Settlement and the Metropolitan Life Insurance Company spread enthusiasm and support for public health nursing. Both rural and industrial nursing thrived in the early twentieth century. The National Organization for Public Health Nursing forged an alliance between nurses and lay people. The visiting nurse was a familiar public health nursing role. Death rates lowered because of public health nurses' application of knowledge of sanitation and new medical discoveries. Significant reduction in the incidence of contagious and infectious illness paralleled an increased incidence of other health problems, such as cancer and heart disease (Kalisch and Kalisch, 1978).

The Phases of Development

The first phase of public health nursing (1877–1911) was marked by the efforts of a few charismatic individuals whose ideals were implemented through new organizational forms, with widespread societal acceptance of the nurse's role in public health. During this period, public health nursing faced enormous unmet demands requiring a greatly increased work force.

Statistics demonstrated the effect of the visiting nurse on the health care status of individuals, especially in an era in which the neediest were not inclined to or could not afford to go to physicians or hospitals. Health assessment and health education were supported by the United States government and private foundations.

The second phase (1912–1930), one of expansion, featured model programs to deal with general health status, specific problems such as trachoma, and newly defined problems such as birth control. Since so few of the sick had previously received much care, improvements were easy to detect and describe statistically (Kalisch and Kalisch, 1978). This second era, one of consolidation of gains, gave way to the Great Depression, when nurses joined the ranks of the unemployed.

Nurses became hospital based with the growth in numbers and influence of hospitals and as a consequence of the control exercised by hospitals upon their education. Nurses had such credibility that people were more inclined to fly on commercial aircraft if nurses were stewardesses. During the 1930s health care payment became an issue, and the debate over third-party payment increased, at a time when there were empty hospital beds and sick patients in the community. Public and private foundation studies provided persuasive documentation of the benefits of third-party payment, and one consequence was that hospital insurance plans with prepayment were backed by insurance companies, civic leaders, hospitals, and some physicians. Blue Cross was developed by the American Hospital Association. The Federal Emergency Relief Administration covered the health care needs of the poor, purchasing services from private agencies. An additional program, the Civil Works Administration, employed a large number of nurses in diversified settings. The Social Security Act funded the training of health care personnel and aided those with unmet health care needs (Kalisch and Kalisch, 1978).

With World War II, once again nurses were in great demand—this time, behind the front lines and as flight nurses. Industrial nursing boomed with the growth of defense industries. The federal government supported civilian hospitals that provided nursing care. Nurses were movie heroines, posters encouraged women to become military nurses, and the drafting of nurses was even suggested. The Cadet Nurse Corps was widely praised and publicized (Kalisch and Kalisch, 1978).

The postwar period was characterized by a nursing shortage, an increased birth rate, and poor wages and work conditions for nurses. The American Nurses' Association (ANA) developed policies designed to enhance the situation of nurses, and the ANA became politically active. Nursing was less popular with young women than in the past, however, and practical nurses took over much of the hospital work. They became a majority of nursing personnel. The Brown Report (1948) from the Russell Sage Foundation called for changes in the conditions of nursing education and nursing practice. Accreditation was instituted, and national health care assistance for facilities, services, and research was debated. Federal aid to nursing was blocked, as was comprehensive national health insurance (Kalisch and Kalisch, 1978).

Until the end of World War II, most nursing was public health nursing. The growing importance of hospitals changed the emphasis of nursing education and of care patterns. In the periods described above, public health nursing care was an instrument of control of the poor by the rich. The poor were taught how to care for themselves to avoid risk to others. Public health nursing was also idealistically tied to the American dream of equality and the perfection of democracy. By 1950, public health nursing was supported by almost everyone (except physician groups at times). It was easy to demonstrate the effects of nursing on health care. Dramatic programs were established by socially powerful organizations, and charismatic leaders abounded. There were no substantial differences among nursing organizations before the establishment of accreditation, and the debate over political activism was simply one of whether to enter the arena at all.

The Rise of Community Health Nursing

The situation has changed markedly as public health nursing has become community health nursing. Social pressures generated in the 1950s restructured health care through legislation by the mid-1960s. The profession of nursing is now characterized by a variety of educational degrees, programs, and specializations. A large number of sometimes conflicting nursing organizations seek to control nursing education and nursing practice. To further understand the context for public and community health nursing from the 1950s to the present, definition of terms in historical context is necessary.

PUBLIC AND COMMUNITY HEALTH NURSING

The difference between public health and community health nursing is more than semantic. Even the formal definitions suggest subtle but real changes in emphasis and mandate. For example, Ruth B. Freeman (1958, p. 30) defined *public health nursing* as:

a special field of nursing in which technical nursing, interpersonal and organizational skills are applied in appropriate relationship to the skills of other members of health and social professions for the conservation of community health. It includes comprehensive nursing care to individuals, families and groups and in addition, public health measures addressed to the community as a whole, such as epidemiologic investigations, law enforcement or organization of the community for health action.

In 1970, Freeman (1970, pp. 31–32) stated that:

the purpose of *community health nursing* is to further community health through the selective application of nursing and public health measures within the framework of the total community health effort. . . . The focus of community health nursing is the community: the direction and nature of the nursing program is shaped by the needs of the community as a whole and by the nature of the total community health effort. (Italics added)

Her definition expands with this statement:

The health of the community is as much the product of its physical and social environment, its institutions, and its interfaces, as it is of the additive health conditions of its population. The interplay between the individual and his environment—whether the micro-environment of family and immediate neighbors or the macro-environment of the city, county, or country—is an essential determinant of family and community health. The betterment of that relationship is one of the major channels for health improvement.

These definitions suggest that public health nursing emphasizes the community as an aggregate, while community health nursing is so broad that it encompasses all nursing activities performed outside of hospitals. Public health nursing seems more specific and community health nursing more general. The transition from public to community health nursing is mainly a re-

sponse to changes in health care financing. Program-based home health care, nurse-practitioner services, and specialized care to individuals and their families are now under the community health nursing umbrella. One consequence is that less time is spent mobilizing communities to deal with community problems. For example, drug abuse, teenage pregnancy, and venereal disease programs employ experts but do not mobilize whole communities to attack these problems as an aggregate. In effect, control for a community's health destiny has shifted from community members to health care specialists who are active in relations with specific individuals and families, while communities are passive as a whole.

PUBLIC AND COMMUNITY HEALTH NURSING: WORLD WAR II TO THE PRESENT

Mobilizing Communities

Public health nursing changed dramatically by the mid-1950s, reflecting societal changes that led to the transition to community health nursing by the mid-1960s. These changes are described in Table 2.1. Public health care's emphasis on mobilizing communities to deal with community problems continued after World War II. Women were readily available in the home in an identifiable community and other group settings that were fixed and predictably stable, making location of a clientele simple. Public health programs emphasized eradicating epidemics and spreading health knowledge and applications. Public health was clearly defined, and practitioners were well educated in public health principles and practice. The clientele was almost entirely the poor. Bureaucracies in-

TABLE 2.1
Public and Community Health Nursing: Post–World War II to Present

Post-World War II Public Health Nursing	Mid-1950s to Present: Social Changes	Mid-1960s to Present: Rise of Community Health Nursing
Emphasis on mobilizing communities to solve community problems	Mobility Suburbanization Family fragmentation	Emphasis on individual and family units solving their own problems
Women readily available in the home in an identifiable community and some group settings (clinics, schools)	Larger proportion of women in the workforce	Loosely structured and varied health care settings
Efforts to eradicate epidemics and spread health care knowledge	Advances in immunology and disease control Dispersion of health knowledge Public money for public health programs through taxes and donations	Emphasis on a broader range of health and illness problems
Single definition, education, and practice of public health nursing	Rise of new health specialties and nursing specializations	Inclusion of all social classes
Public health nursing treats the poor almost entirely		Diversity of specialists in the community
Centralized direction of community health care: aggregates affected by functioning bureaucracies	Societal resistance to centralized direction and existing hierarchies in public health	Public health care dispersed among new and old health specialties with individual clients
	Rise of substantial third-party payment system	
Environmental conditions controlled to eradicate disease	Shifting emphasis in environmental health: individual and group action	No legitimized nurse role in environmental health

fluenced aggregates of people through centralization of administration and by using statistical and epidemiological techniques to reinforce information collected in the field by community health nurses who interacted extensively with each other, constantly comparing their impressions about health care trends. Environmental conditions could be attacked by the individual,

family, or community supported by public health nurses without conflict or confusion about goals, and without social or political censure.

Social Changes

From the mid-1950s to the present, the extent and pace of social change has been enormous. Mobility, suburbanization, and family fragmentation have affected the ability of nurses to define a "community": people with a common identity and welfare. Further, there can be many overlapping communities in an urban environment, where city and county lines do not correspond to air pollution, water control, or industrial waste hazard zones. Large proportions of women are now in the workforce and thus are not available during regular work hours. Advances in disease control and immunology have eliminated many of the diseases that public health nurses fought successfully. Health care knowledge has been dispersed so that even the poor are much more knowledgeable. The public's tax money and donations have financed a variety of specialized programs in which new health specialists who have replaced nurses occupy narrower niches in the system. The number of nursing specialties has increased, dwarfing the generalist role and implying the inferiority of the generalist. Resistance against centralized direction and existing public health hierarchies led to the creation of new, experimental, and potentially short-lived structures. The rise of third-party payments has allowed nonnurses to define nursing activities. The emphasis in environmental health has shifted to individuals and groups who act on their own, not as part of a geographic community.

Community Health Nursing

From the mid-1960s to the present, community health nursing has emphasized individual and family units that deal with their own problems. Loosely structured and articulated health care settings with varied purposes and practitioners have treated a broad range of health and illness problems. People of all social classes have been treated under the community health system, with its diverse specialists. Practitioners of new and old specialties have dealt with clients as individuals. Today's greatest hazard, however, is environmental damage—industrial waste and environmental pollution—problems that cannot be controlled by individual clients. Nurses have barely begun to address this threat. Rather nurses, like other health practitioners, have stressed the limited self-care practices that promote good health, principally among the well-to-do.

Since the mid-1960s, the nurse role has been redefined to fit third-party payment requirements and related federal legislation. Nurse-providers have paid a heavy price for third-party reimbursement. According to Smith (1980):

they had to redefine practice to secure Federal monies. Something called "skilled nursing care" became the quid pro quo. Nursing services are reimbursed in relation to the client's requirement for specific tasks such as injection, catheterization, dressing changes, exercise regimes, and so on. Health assessment, health teaching, family counseling, and other appropriate professional nursing responsibilities were not reimbursable because they did not fall within the definition of skilled nursing care. (pp. 540–541)

Paradoxically, this expansion of the nurse role to include all nonhospital care has not worked to the advantage of nursing: nurses still lack client control and autonomy. They are still faced with an authority gap between what they are qualified and expected to take responsibility for and the power to put their knowledge into practice—to make nursing care decisions unimpeded.

Smith further described these trends in this way:

In no arena do conflicts presented by client ownership appear more clearly or present more problems than with regard to cancer patients.

Today, as in the Fifties, agencies require that all clients be under physician's care, and that the attending physician write the plan for medical care and orders for those portions of the plan which are being delegated to nurses. In the 1950's, there was less awareness of the theoretical basis of thanatology and the implications it provides for therapeutic interventions with the terminally ill. There was great concern about the potential for addicting such clients to drugs; few alternatives were available for minimizing pain. On too many occasions, well-meaning physicians tossed terminally ill cancer clients out of the health–sickness care system because expensive medical care such as surgery or chemotherapy was no longer indicated. Once medical care was withdrawn, however, the client was no longer eligible for the services provided by the agency. A showdown would always lead to the same conclusion—agency policy superseded the nurse's judgment, client needs, and the nurse's accountability to clients. To my knowledge, these conditions still exist. (1980, p. 542)

COMMUNITY HEALTH NURSING AND HEALTH CARE SYSTEM STRUCTURE

Community health nursing today presents the illusion of autonomy and client control without its reality. Changes in structure have occurred because of political and economic decisions that nurses have not recognized and responded to as a professional group. Subtle changes have eroded public health nurses' autonomy and client control vis-à-vis whole communities they serve. The danger is that nurses believe that a battle has been won that is merely in abeyance. Worse yet, aggregate community needs may remain unrecognized and unfulfilled. In fact, economic forces will shape community health as well as other areas of nursing, greatly affecting autonomy and client control. We entered the 1980s with the United States as a government, as a business, and as individuals $5 trillion in debt. During the last decade, individual, government, and corporate debt increased at twice the rate of inflation and four times the rate of the increase in the production of capital goods (Hawken, Ogilvy, & Schwartz, 1982). A decade of mounting inflation, interest rates, and unemployment and declining income, productivity, and economic influence has led to a growing sense of uncertainty about the future (Hawken et al., 1982). In response, the American people have sought, through the office of the president, leadership to restore the economy to the unparalleled growth of the 1950s and 1960s.

In a discussion of cultural economics, Hawken et al. state that although the "supply-side economics" of the 1980s involves a strategy of closing the gap between high demand and low supply by increasing productivity rather than by reducing demand, the primary tools of supply-side economic policy management are the tools inherited from the theories set forth by John Maynard Keynes in the 1920s and 1930s: federal manipulation of interest rates and tax structure in accordance with the diagnoses derived from the traditional economic indicators (Hawken et al., 1982). These authors argue eloquently for an approach that is more consistent with the cultural pluralism and ideological tradition of freedom in America: decentralization. They point out that some of our political, educational, medical, and economic institutions have reached a size at which diseconomics of scale follow from lack of flexibility, failures of communication, and lack of access to relevant information, thus increasing costs of distribution and human alienation.

Although 10 percent of the gross national product in this country is consumed by expenditures for health and sickness care, many segments of the population have not had appropriate access to safe, adequate, humanistic, economical, and culturally relevant care. The United States, as the flagship of the free world, incorporated into its ideology two decades ago the concept that health was a right of all citizens and not a privilege. Underlying this concept was the belief that good health was a key advantage in helping individuals utilize opportunities to share in American prosperity. Good health seemed urgent for quality of survival in a society that emphasized individual production and accomplishment. Although billions of federal dollars have been pumped into the health and sickness care system with the goal of reducing inequalities in access to care, the poor, the aged and children from low income families have not received care in proportion to their health needs (U.S. Department of Health, Education and Welfare, 1976). Rising inflation also has made it difficult for middle-income families to afford escalating medical care costs. Many middle-income families have opted not to purchase essential medical care services. The ushering in of the era of Reagonomics has been viewed by many as a signal of change in government philosophy and policy away from the value of health care as a right and toward the concept that health care is a privilege.

Elazar (1981), suggests that we should seek to understand rather than fear the movement toward decentralization. Elazar argues that the system of government envisioned by the nation's founders was not pyramidal (with channels for giving orders from top to bottom) but rather was a matrix of authoritative government units within a framework provided by the Constitution. Elazar further elaborates that:

this matrix combined a National or general government that could make authoritative decisions, especially on "boundary" questions, with state governments equally authoritative within their areas of constitutional competence. The whole system was based on the Federal principle of redundancy—of more than one authoritative body responsible for the conduct of the government and capable of exercising its responsibility. (p. 17)

Between 1964 and 1966, the Great Society years, numerous programs and social reforms swept through a Democratic-controlled Congress. These new programs asserted the national purpose in such areas as racial equality, educational opportunity, employment, health care, the environment, improving cities, and eliminating poverty (Haider, 1981). The rise of hospital insurance and the introduction of Medicare and Medicaid in 1965 were prime factors in the growth of demand for health and sickness care services. The shift of a greater share of the personal health cost burden to third-party payers resulted in increased utilization of physicians, hospitals, nursing homes, and other health-related services. The 1965 Medicare and Medicaid amendments provided financing, but they also brought with them the burden of complicated federal regulations.

According to Haider (1981), the Nixon and Ford administrations attempted to overhaul, restructure, and redirect intergovernmental policies from 1969 to 1976. President Nixon's New Federalism sought to shift funds, authority, and responsibility from Washington to state and local governments. Haider's analysis shows that state income taxes became the fastest rising revenue component during the 1970s. He predicts that with the decline of the school-age population, states can look forward to shifting future funds into other areas and for other purposes.

The 1970s brought the rise of multihospital systems. According to Ludlam and Christensen (1981), the movement was motivated by regulatory and economic pressures. In the National Health Planning and Resources Development Act of 1974 (PL 93-641), for example, Congress identified three national priorities: the development of "multi-institutional systems for the coordination or consolidation of institutional health services"; the creation of "multi-institutional arrangements for the sharing of [hospital] support services"; and the capacity to provide health care "on a geographically integrated basis." By identifying these priorities, Congress sought to "facilitate the rational allocation of services and facilities and to help contain costs by eliminating duplication and excess capacity" (Ludlam & Christensen, 1981, p. 25). The number of hospital beds represented by multihospital systems has grown to at least one-third of the total. Some projections estimate that by 1985, half of the nation's hospitals will belong to systems (Ludlam & Christensen, 1981).

In recent years, growing attention has been focused on health maintenance, in part indicated by labeling some clinic/hospital institutions "health-maintenance organizations" (HMOs). Health maintenance in this country has been based on the idea that with correct technical information, individuals can control both their behavior and their environment to prevent illness. This approach suggests that one should stress that individuals abstain from smoking cigarettes but ignore industrial pollution in the workplace and in the community. Among the middle class, there is a resurgence of interest in remaining healthy, as health care financing for personal health care becomes increasingly difficult. As yet there are no incentives that would have appeal and utility for the poor. Without identification and formalization of such health care financing mechanisms, the poor will not be affected by the personal health maintenance movement.

The federal government has taken a decreasing role in planning, quality assessment, and access to health care services. Free market competition will become a dominant issue in health care delivery. Since 1965, there has been a major shift in who pays for health care. In 1965, the federal government paid 10 percent, while state and local governments paid 11.4%. In 1979, the federal government paid 30% and state and local governments 12.0%. Increased unemployment carries the corollary of less private health insurance. Employers are reassessing benefit packages with an eye toward saving money. Data are available to prove that there are services that nurses can provide effectively and inexpensively, such as primary health care and maternity care. Whether or not the present era of competition and free enterprise will provide opportunities for the public to have access to more economical and appropriate care remains to be seen.

MODELS FOR HEALTH CARE DELIVERY

Unfortunately, there has never been a conceptual model or policy for health care other than the deficit model, which shows demand for more and newer services without structural change in the system. It is clear that government action has achieved some targeted gains, with residual effects, such as an increased life expectancy, decline in infant mortality, decline in number of cardiovascular deaths, and eradication of smallpox and probably of measles. There has been a striking shift in access, with the poor utilizing the health care system more than the wealthy. There are many more hospitals, physicians, and nurses per capita in the United States now than in the past, so the capacity to meet the health needs of the entire public has expanded immensely.

The future may bring tighter budgeting for health care, limitations on bed supply, rate setting, and greater emphasis on quality assurance and utilization review. At this point, there is the political will to modify the health care system, but not to revolutionize it—power is not being transferred to nurses from physicians, for example. Reimbursement sources and methods may change. How will this affect nursing? Lacking autonomy and legitimacy as primary health care practitioners, nurses are particularly vulnerable to economic tides that encourage or discourage delegation of tasks. The role bargaining that has been so popular in the past decade has never established a long-term mandate for an expanded nurse role in community health or in other areas of nursing.

A variety of models exists for community health nursing, all with different effects upon the nursing role vis-à-vis the aggregate community and segmented groups or families. The future of public/community health nursing depends in part upon the models most in force. These include the domestic service model, the medical outreach model, the independent private corporate model, the health care maintenance organization model, and the purely private enterprise model.

Domestic Service Model

The *domestic service model* in the community is embodied in the school nurse or the industrial nurse who works for a corporation. Nurses are not assigned to specific clients, but rather serve as agents of the employing institution. Domestic service nurses rarely interact intensively or extensively with individual clients because these clients are "owned" by physicians.

Nurses' relations with physicians are characterized by obedience and tend to be relatively peaceful. Since nurses are rarely accountable for the care of individual clients, there is little accountability for nursing care. Physicians are likely to operate separately from nurses and communication occurs primarily through the client's chart.

Consumer groups, health care organizations, the government and other third-party payment sources are likely to overlook nurses or to view them as physician's helpers. Clearly, leadership in the health care system is unlikely for nurses under the domestic service model, since under this model they lack autonomy and legitimacy as professionals. They are perceived as well-trained servants unlikely to take responsibility for an aggregate community with which they have no direct contact.

Predictably, the domestic service model does not fit into third-party payment systems in schools and in industry; thus the number of such positions has dwindled since the mid-1960s.

Medical Outreach Model

Under the *medical outreach model*, an organization collects a fee for nursing service, while the nurse is paid a salary. Services such as hospital home health care may be viewed as medical outreach, as are clinics where physicians bill for nurse-practitioner services (while the nurse-practitioner is an employee).

Nurse/client relationships tend to be warmer and more complete (or holistic) within the Medical Outreach Model. "Sickness care" is emphasized more than "health care." The nurse, or nurse practitioner, is guided by the physician's definition of nursing care, being that of a high-powered physician's assistant.

Consumer groups, health care organizations, the government, and other third-party payment sources are likely to approve of the medical outreach model, because it is cost effective and provides care in situations where physicians are least likely to practice: rural areas and urban ghettos.

Nurses are unlikely to exercise leadership in community health care from a medical outreach base, because in it they are defined as subordinates who are unable to function independently of medical supervision. Further, the outreach into the community is very selective—only those individual clients signed up with the agency or medical practitioner are defined as "the community." There is no recognition of an aggregate community with needs that clients and families reflect in their health care problems.

Nurses functioning under the medical outreach model have the illusion of autonomy while remaining under the control of the medical profession. Their legitimation, as in the domestic service model, depends upon status conferred by members of a more powerful profession, medicine.

Under current economic conditions, we can expect a considerable shrinkage in the number of outreach settings, since many were given short-term funding by the federal government. Few communities have been willing or able to fund outreach clinics on their own. Physicians are likely to oppose the maintenance or expansion of medical outreach settings by nurses, because of the oversupply of physicians and the need to reduce competition in client care provision. Third-party payment sources are likely to experience conflict because nurses' charges are lower than physicians', yet most third-party organizations are controlled by physician reviewers.

Independent Private Practice Model

The *independent private practice model* includes nurses who practice alone or with each other in small clinics, providing and billing for nursing services only. The independent private practice model assumes that treatment is rendered on a fee-for-service basis.

Nurse–client relations are very close under this model, because the nurse retains "custody" of the client during the time of treatment. The client has chosen to visit a nurse, indicating recognition of nurses as autonomous and legitimate health care practitioners. Nurse–physician relations are apt to be cordial, but not intensive, because the nurse is probably engaged primarily in health care rather than sickness care, which remains the province of the physician. The nurse and physician do make referrals to each other, maintaining separate financial and client records.

While individual consumers on a small scale are satisfied with this model, it is difficult and therefore rare for a nurse to establish such a practice. Thus, the independent private practice model has had little impact on highly organized consumer groups, the government, and other third-party payment sources.

Leadership in health care by nurses in independent private practice is highly unlikely, because such nurses suffer from the "left field syndrome." They are so few in number, so lacking in an organizational base or in influence on other nurses, and so likely to spend their energies in generating a nursing practice to survive professionally, that it is unlikely that these nurses will have much impact upon health care delivery systems.

When the economy is retrenching and consumers are spending more cautiously, independent practices may have fewer clients. Further, nurses are likely to be less drawn to the risks of independent private practice during recession, when the insecurity of entrepreneurship is even more apparent than under conditions of expansion.

The so-called community may actually be a defined geographic area, so that aggregate needs are dealt with solely in one-to-one contact with clients and their families. As a lone and vulnerable health care provider, the nurse in private practice is unlikely to call attention to potentially controversial aggregate health problems such as industrial pollution.

Health Care Maintenance Organization Model

The *health care maintenance organization model* assumes that nurses and other health care professionals establish large group practices in which the fees of each individual are billed for separately. The health care practitioners are contractually employed by the health care maintenance organizations and direct the management of such organizations. It is presumed that sickness care organizations, led by physicians, are engaged in cross-referral with health maintenance organizations.

Nurse–client relations are close, but the client must be willing to be treated by other nurses in the absence of a particular nurse. Nurse–physician relations would be egalitarian, since nurses have their own separate power base. Under this model, autonomy, organizational influence, and legitimacy are greatest for members of the nursing profession.

Consumer groups, the government, and third-party payment sources may support HMOs as a long-term means of preventing serious illness and teaching clients self-care. Billing categories and means of evaluating care are worth developing for broad

third-party payment for independent nursing when a sufficient number of practitioners and settings exist (perhaps as a consequence of legislation).

With their large institutional bases, collaboration with other health professionals, and independent clientele, nurses in HMOs would be able to affect legislation and thereby the structure of the health care system. The potential for an alliance of nurses and knowledgeable consumers might provide initial financing for HMOs of the sort described here, but not during a severe recession.

The health care maintenance organization model may encounter difficulties in the 1980s on other than a purely economic level. Government, which has traditionally underwritten innovative structuring of health care settings, is reducing its role in the free marketplace. Most members of the public do not associate nurses with health care; they are viewed as part of the sickness care system. The public seems most concerned about costs, which lent impetus in the past to formation of HMOs, yet several HMOs have recently gone under as a consequence of client overutilization during a period of rising health care costs.

On a purely economic basis, there is no power constituency to advocate and support nursing HMOs during periods of retrenchment. There is no reason to believe that nursing HMOs would reduce health care costs—new organizations are notorious for cost overruns. The idealism of the 1960s and 1970s appears to have run its course and the 1980s are not expected to be a decade of innovation.

While the community is at least more broadly defined under the HMO system, it is still not the general public whose needs are addressed. It is the needs of members, and presently health care is provided in the form of programs for specific purposes for member individuals—weight control, smoking withdrawal, dietary adequacy, and so forth. Such programs are not usually well funded relative to sickness care, and environmental health has been too inflammatory an issue for HMOs to tackle.

Purely Private Enterprise Model

The *purely private enterprise model* is embodied by corporate ownership or contractual management of a large number of health care settings. Another form of this model is when an organization contracts to provide a single service to hospitals, such as nursing, dietary, or physical therapy. These health care settings must operate at a profit to provide a return to investors. The corporation may or may not be owned by nurses or other health care practitioners. The attraction of private corporate ownership is the enhanced focus on efficiency as the prime necessity for survival. Organizational complacency is potentially reduced. Furthermore, the entire history of business indicates that private enterprise, when taking over a formerly public enterprise, restructures the ground rules for organizational performance, including financial relationships with the external environment.

If nurses were employed by large corporations, their traditional mobility would be enhanced by promotional opportunities and by sequential, meaningful, regular, and focused inservice educational experiences. This provides corporate protection because the danger of malpractice suits is potentially reduced. Presumably, physicians would be attracted to hospitals with high professional nursing standards. Consistent with the corporate inclination toward narrowness of organizational roles, greater specialization of nurses would occur under private enterprise. Greater emphasis on de-

grees and credentials would result in differential placement on pay scales, and this would reflect classification of care provided. Nurses in purely administrative positions would acquire degrees in business administration, serving in some instances as bridges to business-oriented corporations.

Nurse–client relations are likely to become standardized and based on corporate policy. Patients would be perceived as clients, and nurses would be part of a closely integrated health care team. Nurse–physician relationships would probably improve. As valuable corporate employees, nurses' satisfaction becomes important. Nursing turnover statistics would be carefully monitored. Nurses might become more credible to physicians as they became more specialized.

Consumer groups, customarily the opponents of corporate expansion, are losing influence. Health care organizations, facing presumably uncontrollable deficits, might be glad to allow private enterprise to manage or buy most hospitals. The present national government would be delighted to see a previously public enterprise go private. Third-party payment sources might fear this potential realignment, which might increase charges, yet the drive toward managerial efficiency could be persuasive.

Leadership roles for nurses in the corporate structure would be entirely dependent upon their willingness to integrate into a multiprofessional environment in which career routes involved either clinical specialization or managerial skills such as finance, accounting, management information systems, and strategic planning. Graduate degrees and credentials in nursing would be assessed in terms of these two career tracks.

Under current economic conditions, the

purely private enterprise model has many advantages. It is consistent with retrenchment and the government's retreat from responsibility for health care systems. Further, it allows restructuring based on competitive dominance. If 90 percent of the hospital beds in the country were controlled by such corporations, changes in the basis for charges could be forced upon third-party payment sources. Nursing costs might then be billed separately, based on complexity-of-care criteria that would increase the incentive to hire professional nurses and also contribute to organizational profit.

The purely private enterprise model might be ideologically favorable to government, the business world, hospitals, and much of the public. In a bureaucratic society the transfer of a public to a private function might appear to occur naturally; thus its visibility as a phenomenon would not be great until an unbeatable power base was consolidated.

Community health nursing, under the purely private enterprise model, would be likely to provide services that could be rendered at a profit to individuals who had third-party payment available. Corporations are notably conservative in the area of environmental health. The emphasis on self-care would provide a smokescreen to prevent serious health problems from becoming publicized.

COMPARISONS OF NURSING SERVICE MODELS

The domestic service model is the most common one today. Medical outreach is familiar to most consumers, as described in the popular press even if it is not part of their experience. The independent private practice form is rare and does not appear to have massive popular support. The health care maintenance organization approach to nursing care delivery exists in concept only and would require substantial effort to become a reality. The purely private enterprise model is rapidly growing in its share of hospital beds controlled. Each model has its advantages. The domestic service model features familiarity and social acceptability outside of nursing. The medical outreach model allows nurses expanded roles without alteration of the structure of health care delivery systems. The independent private practice model provides maximum autonomy. The health care maintenance organization model provides moderate autonomy and maximal legitimation. The purely private enterprise model allocates a professional role for nurses with relatively high legitimation and autonomy, as well as the protection afforded members of large corporations.

The disadvantages of each model are apparent. The domestic service model casts nurses as nonprofessional organizational servants subordinate to physicians and lacking an activist role. The medical outreach model casts nurses as physicians' assistants dealing with a very limited, narrowly defined community. The independent private practice model places nurses outside the mainstream of the profession and too vulnerable to take on industry and government in the industrial health area. The health care maintenance organization model is pure fantasy at the moment and furthermore threatens to divide nurses between "health" and "sickness" care systems, a potential fragmentation of the profession that would render public/community health nursing subject to conflicting definitions and parallel implementation. The purely private enterprise model raises the potential for nursing service provision within and influenced by mercenary goals, with community health care conservatively defined and implemented.

Unless community health nursing is shaped by some vision of the health hazards of the 1980s, then all of the models described above will represent dilutions of the earlier role of the public health nurse. The public health nurse defined health problems and was instrumental in publicizing their existence and in organizing the public to solve them. Concerns for autonomy and client control are relevant to the original role of the public health nurse with clients, not merely the advancement of the profession.

The nursing profession would do well to study the implications of each model in depth in order to decide which to support for optimal public/community health. Alliances may be developed with other health care or non-health care personnel to facilitate nursing autonomy and control of nursing care in emergent and expanding structures where public health problems can be dealt with in the aggregate. Further enhancement of the professional nurse's role in the community involves strategic planning and evaluation of alternative future scenarios for public/community health care nationwide. Nurses' level of awareness and future orientation vis-à-vis the direction of health care organization, and not merely nurses' roles, is crucial. Without this, nurses will be "talking to themselves" while health care systems change at a rapid rate—and perhaps in directions unaffected by nurses and not in the best interests of nurses or of client care. A full understanding of other potential participants in the health care system—business and the general public—is essential. The premises and resources of non-health care providers

should be examined carefully—their future impact may be significant for the ways in which the nursing role is structured in the 1980s and 1990s.

SUMMARY

The Philosophy and Mandate of Public Versus Community Health Nursing

There has been a change in philosophy and mandate with the change in public health nursing's definition. Community health nursing is a catchall for all non-hospital provided nursing services. With such a diffuse mandate, it is impossible to evaluate success or to measure progress toward a higher health status for the general public. Nurses are diverted from this issue by the many types and levels of practice available in a new array of settings. Community health nursing is an unmeasurable abstraction, while public health nursing was quantifiable, centralized, activist, and relatively autonomous within public health departments in state and federal agencies.

If nurses today were involved in public health as it was defined before the social changes of the 1950s, there would be greater professional and personal risks. Everyone supports cleaning up a garbage dump, but industrial health hazards—the major health hazards of this decade—are viewed by powerful organizations and their employees as the cost of progress. Cleanup may be opposed. For public/community health nurses to be effective public health nurses, they need tools that have perhaps fallen into disuse—in-depth knowledge of health care financing, epidemiology, statistics, law, government, corporate policies and practices. Such needs are not met comprehensively in undergraduate nursing education.

Context for the Programmatic Bias

Unfortunately, community health nursing is likely to continue in its current pattern, with a programmatic bias supported by new institutions serving partial publics. It would probably take new diseases that required nursing care, or environmentally induced physical mutations among large numbers of people, as well as an alliance between nurses and environmentalists, to stem the current tide and change the course of community health nursing. Political alliances are usually social-class based, and many nurses have customarily been passive but upwardly mobile female members of the lower middle class. Environmentalists are usually upper-middle-class and upper-class men and women with little tolerance for subservient or dependent individuals in any profession or field of work.

To examine aggregate health care, community health nurses in the future should look at potential changes in health care policy and financing. Differences between the rich and poor are nowhere more obvious than in health care and life-style. Quality programs for diet, exercise, smoking/alcohol/drug withdrawal, and venereal disease prevention and treatment are now widely available for a fee and are affecting the lives of the upper middle class only. Who will develop and teach such programs to the poor?

In the past, public health nurses helped people form community organizations within a defined area. Without specialization based on age of client or type of condition, the public health nurse was able to identify problems before heavy statistical verification, due to interaction with

people of all ages with many different health problems in a geographically and often ethnically or culturally defined community. Early action was possible. If nurses do not plan with communities, who will? How can extensive problems be identified otherwise for early treatment? Can outside experts, each treating a small, well-defined group, coordinate such knowledge with other busy health care providers? Much will fall between the cracks.

An erosion of the preparation of public health nurses lessens the probability of future change. In the 1950s, public health nurses were generalists, not specialists, and they had or were actively pursuing baccalaureate degrees. Now they are often RNs with inadequate education, supporting the watered-down role of the community health nurse.

Dilemmas in Public/Community Health Nursing

In the future, the prospects for public/community health nursing are most directly linked to financing. Ideally there should be: (1) better public financing of aggregate health needs, (2) better education for public/community health nurses, (3) more work through existing public health structures within state and local government, (4) reexamination of the concept of the district, (5) reassessment of the nursing-generalist role in the community, (6) evaluation of the risks and benefits of organizing the poor for the benefit of their health, and (7) projections of the future of the community health nursing role with technological advances, particularly in video- and computer-related areas.

To address the dilemmas of public/community health nursing practice in the early 1980s, we must explore the current role of nurses, delineate modifications in old structures, and propose new structures to enhance the impact of nurses on the health care system. A central assumption is that nursing has the potential for effective leadership in health care—a potential that has been latent recently but that can be reactivated. Another crucial assumption is that public/community health nursing provides the traditional kernel from which the profession can develop methods and strategies for autonomous practice and an independent relationship to clients.

If nurses are to shape the health care system in the near future, they must first be able to provide health care services upon the request of clients or other health care practitioners or representatives of institutions (hospitals, work organizations, social service agencies, governmental units). At present, nursing services are usually invoked by physicians under the auspices of bureaucracies, and these services may be revoked at any point. In hospitals, nursing services are billed as "room and board." Thus nurses are not independent providers but are physician- and organization-dependent (Smith, 1980).

Alternatives to Medicaid, coverage of long-term care through national health insurance, and comprehensive and systematic attention to financing the total needs of the poor require attention. In this context, the nurse ought to be more than the specialist, manager, or liaison person in relation to the clients who make up a private caseload. Thus issues such as hospital and practitioner reimbursement, health planning, and utilization review should be addressed in terms of an agreed-upon role for the public/community health nurse in a definable community. The bewildering array of state, federal, local government, and private programs must be sorted within the context of the nursing role in public policy. Some redefinition of nursing knowledge and the requirements of public/community health practice must occur.

DISCUSSION TOPICS

1. What should be the future role of the community health nurse?

2. How can the role of the community health nurse be implemented for an entire community?

3. What sort of relationship should community health nurses form with environmentalists?

4. What characteristics will nurses need in order to become activist leaders in a future where correction of community health hazards requires involvement in politics and controversy?

BIBLIOGRAPHY

Elazar, D.J.: The evolving federal system. In R.M. Pious, ed., *The power to govern.* New York: Academy of Political Science, 1981.

Freeman, R.B.: *Community health nursing practice.* Philadelphia: Saunders, 1970.

Freeman, R.B.: *Public health nursing.* Philadelphia: Saunders, 1958.

Haider, D.H.: The intergovernmental system. In R.M. Pious, ed., *The power to govern.* New York: Academy of Political Science, 1981.

Hawken, P., Ogilvy, J., & Schwartz, P.: *Seven tomorrows.* New York: Bantam, 1982.

Kalisch, P.A., & Kalisch, B.J.: *The advance of American nursing.* Boston: Little, Brown, 1978.

Ludlam, J.E., & Christensen, J.D.: Multihospital arrangements and the federal antitrust laws. In G.E. Bisbee, Jr., ed., *Multihospital systems: Policy issues for the future.* Chicago: The Hospital Research and Educational Trust, 1981.

Smith, G.R.: Nursing beyond the crossroads. *Nursing Outlook* 28(9), 540–542, 545, 1980.

U.S. Department of Health, Education and Welfare. *Trends Affecting U.S. Health Care System.* DHEW Publication #HRA 76-14503, Washington, D.C., U.S. Government Printing Office, 1976.

3

Change: A Continuum of Events

Mary Ellen Banks

The actual future will be what circumstance, the human will, and the human intelligence make it, and we can only hope that all will conspire to produce something good. My role, as a futurist, is to reconnoiter the territory up ahead so that humanity, in its travels through time, may have a better notion of what to aim for and what to avoid.

ISAAC ASIMOV / *Change*, 1981

OBJECTIVES

After reading this chapter, you should be able to:

☐ Define change.
☐ Describe the process of change.
☐ Apply change theory to planned change.
☐ Identify strategies for planned change.
☐ Describe the impact of change on individuals and systems.

INTRODUCTION

Services provided by community health agencies mirror societal response to human needs within its cities and rural areas. Community-based health care programs vary from one region of the country to another, and services available reflect such characteristics as the economic, geographic, racial, and age factors of the people who live within the boundaries, as well as on their endemic level of health. Changes in the manner in which health care is offered are barometers of the planning and direction at leadership levels and the implementation or execution of those plans at the service level of the organization. Leaders who know that change within an organization is manageable are able to construct change strategies with the vital input of the people within the organization. In the case of service organizations, appraisal of needs must extend to consumer viewpoint and demand. Additionally, individuals at entry-level and lower-management positions not only should be cultivated to contribute to reorganizations of structure and function but also must be active supporters of final decisions that affect the overall order and cooperation of agency personnel in meeting new goals.

This chapter presents basic information about the change process and illustrates those concepts with examples found in actual organizational operation. Planned change is a process that implies control over situations such that predictable results can be derived from the efforts exerted to ameliorate unfavorable conditions. Change can occur in an incidental or serendipitous fashion, and the effects of that kind of change may be useful and productive, but such occurrences may at best be only coincidental. In a climate that values cost containment and cost effectiveness, planned change with predictable outcomes and more than a reasonable chance of success have a greater probability of obtaining organizational support and financing. Planned change is also the route for change deemed most suitable in working with people, whether the client is an individual, a family, group, or the community at large. The nature of change as a catalytic phenomenon imbues a quality of dynamic synergy into all situations, and thus examples used here to describe certain concepts may well be obsolete shortly. Kurt Lewin's theory of change will be presented, and the nursing process will be linked to that theory as a tool for effecting change with individuals, families, and groups in the community health nursing environment.

CHANGE

Change is thought of as difficult to design and control, because it requires leadership by those who do not fear the future, who are not too attached to the present, and who are willing to investigate the past. The classic theorist of the change agent is Kurt Lewin. His model for change, constructed in the 1940s, considers behavior as a function of personality and environment in situations that involve three phases: unfreezing, changing, and refreezing. Lewin worked to devise constructs general enough to demonstrate relationships between information and data about people and their environments and the solutions to social problems.

Lewin's model is depicted by the formula

$$B = f(P + E)$$

Behavior = function of personality
and environment

A change in behavior on a human scale is the ultimate goal of a change strategy. Lewin recognized that the function or interreaction between the human aspects of personality and the environment or circumstances of the overall situation would be the dynamic component of any observed change in behavior. It is recognized that the personality element may be the most difficult to control.

Other theorists in the area of change, notably Bennis (1966), look at change models in terms of the relationship between the change and the changer. Collaborative and noncollaborative types of relationships exist; the difference can significantly affect the kind of cooperation that exists among the people involved in a change paradigm. Collaborative means of stimulating change are most appropriate to nursing environments, since collaboration implies mutual goal setting, which is one of the cornerstones of community health nursing. Most nursing theorists project the nurse–client relationship from the viewpoint of the nurse who works to assist the client in attaining an optimal level of functioning. This view is based on the idea that clients are ultimately responsible for their health and personal care.

Lewin's model has been investigated a great deal, since organizational change is an extremely common occurrence and planners and administrators ideally seek the means to make change optimally effective and as painless as possible for all those concerned. Much work has been done on describing the sequence and division of his three stages, and subsequent research stands as testimony to the validity of his original thesis. Outcomes of research in this area suggest the existence of presumed ideal means of dealing with change. Pragmatically, no theory can predict the difficulties that arise in real-life situations, but theory can give useful direction to a project based on an analysis of the most suitable means with which to approach a problem. Lewin's (1958) personal observation about his premise regarding change warns that:

any planned social change will have to consider a multiple of factors characteristic for the particular case. The change may require a more or less unique combination of educational and organizational measures; it may depend upon quite different treatments of ideology, expectation, and organization. Still, certain general formal principles always have to be considered.

The Phases of Change

Unfreezing

In Lewin's scheme, *unfreezing* is a phase representing the recognition of a need for change in a present situation. This phase may be the most difficult in the change process, since most people are creatures of habit. Even if an individual or group is somewhat displeased with a particular circumstance, it is often less stressful to maintain the status quo rather than to face the real or imagined inconveniences that change may bring. Because resistance to change is often regarded as natural in human behavior, it may pose the greatest obstacle to progress and reorganization in many agencies. Lewin spoke of driving and restraining forces within an organization. Very often these forces are dependent upon the personalities in an environment. New and Couillard (1981) discuss five basic reasons why individuals resist change. The number one cause of resistance is that personal costs may outweigh personal benefits. When self-interest is threatened, a person may resist unfreezing. Actions are not necessarily overt; they may be secretive or subtle and difficult to overcome. New and Couillard see other barriers to individuals accepting change: inaccurate perception of the intended change; objective disagreement with the change because of the belief that change will not benefit the organization; psychological reactance to change that is emotionally perceived as a threat or impingement on personal liberties; and a relatively low tolerance for change or even for the ambiguity that often stimulates change because of a wish to retain the security of the present rather than contend with what the future may be.

Creative energy must be generated to face these potential problems so that the work of change may be productive. Therefore, providing change agents with an environment that facilitates free expression enables them to explore options and develop many alternatives that can work to decrease restraining forces caused by the barriers individuals use against change. People may avoid change because of indifference, insecurity, stubbornness, fear, and cognitive dissonance. Any of these factors can be a problem alone, and they often interact in various combinations to affect an individual's response to change. Nothing is more frustrating to someone trying to identify the need for change than to hear phrases like this: "Well, we've always done it this way"; "Traditionally . . ."; "Historically . . ."; "That may work in Niagara County, but I'm afraid it just won't work here"; "I'm all for change (or progress, or the future, or the good of the health department), *but* . . ."; "I believe the state's department of public health policy manual does have the definitive answer to your suggestion."

The term "unfreezing" makes the task of recognition of a need for change sound easy—if the substance in question were water. Human beings, however, are difficult to thaw. Planning to work extensively with the person or group who will be most affected by change is one of the first steps in unfreezing. Resistance to change can be disastrous when changes are actually made, if the people involved move from passive to more active forms of resistance. Employees may imply agreement at the onset of a new project. They may say: "I'm not sure this proposal for getting a health history is practical, but I'll give it a try." Analysis of the employees' use of the new method may ultimately show that they never used the new fact-gathering tool for any number of reasons: lack of time, reputed trouble with form directions, or the awkwardness of form questions interfering with the nurse's established routine. Such stumbling blocks, when unrecognized until after the implementation process, can make results disappointing. Change agents have to pick their cues from such situations so they learn not to repeat disappointing tactics.

Changing

Changing, in the Lewin format, is the implementation of a new idea or plan designed to fit the need for change. This is the moving stage in the process and one that depends on careful organization during the unfreezing and planning stage. During the changing phase, individuals involved in the transition from an established routine must be ready to support changes developed to meet newly perceived priorities. This stage must be conceived in a way to provide for a smooth transition by the investment of time and effort into planning, training, and implementation. It must also include extensive evaluative considerations so that the effects of change can be weighed against desired outcome.

The success of any proposed change is linked to the implementation plan. Change is most expeditious when scientific problem-solving skills are employed to plan a course of action. As unfreezing necessitates careful assessment of driving and restraining forces, planning involves looking at those same forces and using techniques that have proved successful in situations requiring change. New and Couillard (1981) formulated a compendium of strategies that can stimulate personnel involvement in the change process. These include participation, coercion, manipulation, education, use of an external agent, incentives, supportive behavior, and gradual introduction. These techniques range all the way from getting people actively involved in all the processes related to change to providing a reward, such as a cash bonus or compensation time, to employees who participate in a change. For example, financial incentive has been used by hospitals to encourage employees to car pool or use mass transit. A coercive or a manipulative front is often viewed negatively by employees, but it can be effective. For instance, many career military nurses have returned to school to earn BSN degrees because they could not receive promotions unless they continued their formal education. Any of these techniques may have a place in the planning of change, and choosing the correct people-stimulating gambits can be as essential as the goals and objectives of the change project. Personality is a crucial element in Lewin's change formula, and to increase the success quotient of a particular change, energy must be devoted to fighting resistance to change.

The changing phase nears dissolution when evaluative data are collected and analyzed. Generally, evaluation is considered as an integral third step to planning and implementation during the change process. Evaluation can yield valuable data on the effectiveness of the change and provide input for making additional changes or alterations in new procedures before a change is viewed as permanent. The crystallization of a new plan would signal the refreezing stage of Lewin's scheme.

Refreezing

Refreezing is the end state, the settling in and functioning of an organization or group after it has come to a new desired level. This sense of closure is not qualitative, since it does not mean that a change is good or bad, but merely that it is complete. The evaluative process during the change phase might have established that the prior state was better than the changed state, and the group may even have reverted back to its previous manner of functioning. Refreezing simply is a phase in which the group is functioning at a level of operation undisturbed by the mechanisms of change. The organization is either so accustomed to the change that it is no longer perceived as disruptive or inconvenient, or it has elected to return to past procedures in order to accomplish its organizational goals.

In a fast-paced world filled with technological devices, there hardly seems to be a time that an organization is not undergoing some sort of change. This is particularly true in health care facilities, where computer technology is taking over more and more functions. At the same time, nurses are acting more creatively and independently as the body of nursing science knowledge becomes more sophisticated. Nurses are introducing change in health care practices and beliefs as they experiment in constructing and validating nursing theories. In turn this stimulates the development of nursing actions predicated on research grounded in client responses conducive to health promotion, health maintenance, or health restoration. Also, the procurement of machines and devices that scan, control, and measure bodily functions puts great demand on health care providers to keep up with medical technology. Each addition to the armament of the health care professional infuses the system with a new set of rules or guidelines needed to manage the use of the equipment or procedure. Thus even the introduction of new technology can change an established way of dealing with a certain situation. Technological and theoretical changes force the humans who grapple with innovations to ponder their ethical and humanistic ramifications. Nurses, like other professionals, must see change as a tool to be used creatively in managing the people and events in their environments.

THE NURSING PROCESS AS A CHANGE TOOL

The nursing process can be linked with Lewin's change theory as a tool for nurses to use to implement new strategies in their work and client environments (Table 3.1). The nursing process utilizes the scientific method to make a nursing diagnosis predicated on identification of needs. Most needs identified in this process have a final goal of change or modification of behavior aimed at either maintenance or restoration of an optimal level of wellness. The nursing actions initiated with clients should be derived from mutually agreed upon, realistically attainable goals. The nurse ideally should help the client reach a particular goal rather than control the client's circumstances. The community health nurse can serve as a consultant to clients and aid them in choosing the most suitable means to achieve a state of optimal functioning. Establishment of goals and working to

achieve them should be mutual (Hultman 1979), because people are most likely to change if their present values, beliefs, and behavior do not allow them to meet their needs satisfactorily, and if they believe a change will help them meet their needs. Finally, Hultman observes that people are more likely to change if they are actively involved in the change process.

Assessment, Diagnosis, and Planning

In community health settings the assessment phase allows the nurse to look at individual or family circumstances and to explore aggregates in the community to identify situations requiring change. Assessment includes appraising details of the immediate environment and requires investigation of other agency, philanthropic, community, social, and educational resources available that may have bearing upon the client group. For instance, a nurse may be assisting a family grappling with the fact their newborn baby has Down's syndrome. The nurse can work with the family to identify their internal and external strengths and resources as they meet the challenge of providing for the needs of a child with developmental disabilities. The parents may also need direction in determining what resources are available in their area to aid them in this family crisis. The nurse can plan with the family and put them in contact with such agencies or people as the Association for Retarded Citizens, a service organization that operates an infant-stimulation program, or the home-training specialist in the regional office of the state division on mental retardation services. The nurse can work with individuals or families who recognize that their current life situations require change and

TABLE 3.1
Nursing Process and Change Theory

Nursing Process	Lewin's Theory
Realization of a need for change	
Assessment	Unfreezing
Diagnosis	
Plan	
Action related to change	
Implementation	Changing
Evaluation	
Desired behavioral outcome	
Altered level of health	Refreezing

adjustment. Such families may need assistance to accommodate the special needs of family members as they establish objectives using proven strategies for successful attainment of behavior change or modification.

At another level, beyond the individual or family group, a nurse can work with an aggregate of persons identified because of circumstances that link them, such as age or habitat. For example, a group of prisoners may come to the attention of a community health nurse because they form an aggregate due to their confinement within a particular environment. Other examples of aggregates whose health concerns can be viewed in common are schoolchildren, the elderly, migrant workers, refugees, and people from a special occupational group, such as miners or textile workers. A nurse may have to do rather extensive investigation to realize the need for change. This is especially true when the group members share a characteristic such as age or the individuals in question live scattered throughout a large, sparsely populated area. In situations such as this, the nurse will need to make use of other health care professionals. It may be necessary to call upon the assistance of an epidemiologist, biostatistician, sanitarian, nutritionist, physical therapist, and other community health specialists to assess the needs of members of the population who may have needs that are unmet, yet open to change. A group approach to the needs of an aggregate in the community can launch creative efforts. As with individuals or families, such an assessment and planning operation should include key members of the group being studied so that their insight about their needs, strengths and desires are plugged into any plans which may be implemented.

The following problem arose because of the failure to adequately assess, diagnose, and plan for the individuals involved:

It was brought to the attention of the community health department that an inordinate number of elderly persons had been making visits to the emergency department of their neighborhood hospital. Hospital planning reports indicated an expected rise in the number of elderly citizens to be treated or hospitalized after a new high-rise facility for the elderly was built four blocks from the hospital. But six months after the high-rise reached full occupancy, the percentage of self-referrals from the apartment complex far out-distanced the number of visits made by other elderly residents in the neighborhood who lived near the hospital but in other types of residential units. A quick review of resident records at the apartment complex revealed that many of the residents were women in their late sixties and early seventies, who were widowed and had given up the care and maintenance of their own homes or larger apartments. Eighty percent of the women in this group had at least one chronic health problem, and nearly 50% of the group had two or more health problems that interfered in some way with activities of daily living. Residents were interviewed when they made applications to live in these apartments and many verbalized loneliness as their greatest problem. Most of the women had moved at least 15 miles from their former place of residence.

Inclusion of this new group of community residents was not planned for at the inception of the project. Thus six months later the hospital and community health agency had to deal with a problematic situation. Ideally, the apartment complex owners should have assumed responsibility for averting such a problem. In fact, some complexes for the elderly have contractural agreements with official or proprietary health care agencies to provide on-site health promotion services. Other services, such as social and recreational programs, are also beneficial to residents.

To untangle this situation, the nurse used assessment, diagnosis, and planning. To meet the needs of this elderly population and not overburden the emergency department of the hospital, the nurse began this investigation by analyzing the emergency department records of the high-rise complex residents. In addition, the nurse investigated the group's developmental needs and demographic statistics, such as former occupation, sex, marital status, mortality and morbidity data, and educational levels. The nurse determined where the apartment residents had lived before coming to the high-rise facility. This revealed valuable information on problems related to fairly drastic relocation or change of life-style, as well as how close other significant family members and friends lived to the now apartment-dwelling elderly people. After collecting such information, the next steps for the nurse were to work with aggregate leaders, to identify needs, and to plan interventions to make appropriate changes for these apartment residents.

The residents and the nurse identified a desire to increase the residents' level of information on self-care. Planning included proposals that local service clubs organize a regular friendly visitor program to provide parties and gatherings on special holidays, such as Mother's Day, and monthly birthday celebrations. The community mental health association was enlisted to provide on-site clinic services and establish support mechanisms, such as bereavement groups. In addition, two voluntary health organizations, the American Red Cross and the American Diabetes Association, scheduled regular screening clinics at the apartment building. Once needs were identified and possible solutions and ideas for approaches were generated, planning moved at a rapid pace. The community health nurse working in this environment was flexible and creative in order to cope with the situation and thus experienced a sense of usefulness and accomplishment.

Assessment and diagnosis are complicated processes essential to the planning process. In both cases presented here, needs were identified and possible solutions posed to the problems at hand. In the planning phase, details were worked out to determine the feasibility and practicality of the ideas presented. Funding, availability of support personnel, space requirements, and training were all considered as implementation plans got underway.

The more planning that goes into a project, the more likely measurable change will be demonstrated. Getting personnel and clients involved in the change process before implementation allows everyone to become accustomed to the idea of change, to assist in the change, and to understand how the change will affect productivity and service.

Implementation

With the assessment, diagnosis, and planning sequence completed, changes are initiated in the implementation phase. The time for change is now at hand. With adequate planning, the people involved should be sufficiently prepared for change. During implementation a feeling that order is maintained and that upheaval is kept to a minimum will greatly aid in the success of the change. There are various means by which added support can be given to those experiencing change. The transition can at first be experimental, allowing evaluation of steps and effects before proceeding full speed. For example, a health program to be started at a high-rise complex for the elderly may be implemented initially on only one floor so that the receptivity of the residents and the proficiency of the workers providing service can be appraised. In the case of a resident safety program, a general meeting open to everyone and held in the community room may include a film on mugging and home break-ins. The planners, believing that the film will have the greatest impact when residents discuss it in small groups, may at first plan only two or three apartment meetings. They may then wish to see if another approach works better than small-group follow-up before continuing similar gatherings in the rest of the building. The alternatives considered in the planning phase can provide back-up ideas in trial programs if problems are encountered with the initial plans.

In making any change it is best not to interfere with established customs and personalities. Key individuals should be built into the change, especially if they are seen by others as a stabilizing force and as informal leaders. In a high-rise complex for the elderly, even when the agency operating the facility has social service personnel, another person, such as the building manager, may very well be the key leader in working with the residents. A caring, empathetic person who functions in that role very often knows the residents well and has an excellent grasp of the problems of that microcommunity. Including such a person in planning may make the whole planning process proceed more easily than when such a significant person is left out. When implementation time comes, residents who already trust the site manager may feel more trust in the ideas and plans of the agent of change.

When working with the people in the environment, it is important not to disturb peripheral practices. For instance, the health department may recognize that their geriatric clinics would be better utilized if the clinics operated at a site separate from the health department. The realization that the elderly have many transportation problems could lead health department administrators to set up clinics on rotating schedules at senior citizen centers, nutrition sites, and apartment complexes for the elderly. Health department administrators may also identify at the same time a need for some other organizational changes involving daily and monthly time keeping, Medicare and Medicaid billing procedures, mileage reimbursement policies, and the personnel arrangement of the nursing staff. All of these changes may well be necessary, but it is not advisable to introduce them all concurrently. Decide what has the highest priority and begin at that point. Nurses involved in a major reorganization of clinic services should not be unnecessarily burdened with additional details unless such activities are part of the strategy to facilitate the desired outcome.

During the changing phase every effort should be made to provide extra support services to help ease the transition phase. Such supportive behavior from administrative planners is an incentive in itself for persons expected to implement a new plan. Additional secretarial services may be needed for a few weeks while new clinics are being established, to organize a record-keeping system as well as to keep up with the day-to-day admission and client visits, which may be more demanding of clerical time as a new clinic is begun. Using temporary office personnel can make the transition period more tolerable and prevent a backlog of paperwork. Temporary or agency nurses and other health care technicians might also be employed for a short time, particularly if an innovative program includes a large-scale screening clinic at the onset.

Assistance can often be solicited from members of a community service organization or high school students from distributive education classes. These volunteers can be used to register clinic clients or provide and serve refreshments during the first few days of a new clinic. Well-organized and appropriately utilized volunteers can be especially useful in getting a large-scale job done quickly. Another special need may be for computer services and consultation. At the time a new clinic is begun, much information is being gathered and collected, and the evaluation process may well be more efficient if computer analysis is part of the change plan.

Excellent planning not only includes the mechanics of the change itself but also considers the ancillary, auxiliary, and aesthetic particulars that will make the change simpler and more efficient for everyone concerned. A person accustomed to working out the intricacies of change knows how to anticipate the troublesome details as well as how to trouble shoot as problems arise. Attention to detail and the ability to anticipate the vagaries of a situation are talents one wants to consider in choosing a person to lead a change. Working out the best possible plan is essential, but it should be remembered that no perfect plan exists. That realization helps a leader make decisions with expediency and efficiency rather than to procrastinate because of fear, doubt, or lack of confidence.

Evaluation

Evaluation measures are determined during the planning phase and serve to provide feedback to planners and initiators of change on the efficacy of their labors. Evaluation should be linked to measurable goals that are based on objective criteria related to the need or situation being changed. Precision of goals and use of standardized tools wherever indicated make it easier to determine if changes were successful. In choosing evaluation techniques during the planning phase, adequacy and clarity of goals can be judged on the basis of the precision of the evaluation criteria developed. Goals must be specific, not global. For example, a nurse may set a

goal that clinic attendance will improve. But is an increase of three clients a significant success rate? A more explicit goal might state that clinic attendance will increase by 30% in six months. Attendance records can be analyzed to determine success or failure. The following three examples demonstrate the value and appropriateness of goal setting as it is linked to evaluative procedures:

EXAMPLE I

1. Problem: Many black people in this community have undetected and untreated hypertension. Mortality and morbidity data show a higher rate of heart disease and stroke in the black community in comparison to matched groups of white and black people aged 49 to 60 in the area.

2. Plan: Set up screening clinics to reach the at-risk population.

3. Goal: Screen at least 90 percent of 35-to-49-year-old black men and women in the county.

4. Outcome: Special clinics screened 2,000 (10 percent of a known population of 20,000 blacks in the 35-to-49-year-old age range).

5. Evaluation: Success is rated as very poor.

6. Recommendations: Clinic planners should review the practicality of meeting a goal of reaching 90 percent of the known population. Data should be gathered regarding the adequacy of publicity, convenience of clinic hours for working adults, and perceived safety or accessibility of the clinic sites. There is a need to reassess the overall plan and collect data so that any aspect of the project that escaped the scrutiny of the planning committee can be rectified and the clinics tried again.

EXAMPLE II

1. Problem: Clinic attendance in a seaport Florida city is markedly decreased on certain days.

2. Plan: It was found that clinic attendance decreased during rainy weather when people had to wait for their appointments outdoors with no shelter during a cloudburst. As a result staff arranged that a church located next door to the clinic would provide cover on days when the weather was threatening.

3. Goal: Have clinic visits return to usual census on all days of operation.

4. Outcome: Attendance reached a constant level at this free clinic with only slight decreases on days with poor weather.

5. Evaluation: Goal was met successfully.

EXAMPLE III

1. Problem: Senior citizen turnout for a new and well-publicized geriatric clinic in a Wisconsin city is averaging fewer than 15 clients per day.

2. Plan: Gather assessment data from key members of the senior citizen community, clinic and agency staff members, and clinic clients to see why clinic visits were only 25 percent of projections. Interviews reveal that inadequate building access kept potential clients from coming to clinic. Data revealed that even though the building was conveniently located for the population it sought to serve, older people were reluctant to go to the clinic because it was in the basement with primary access down a flight of outside stairs. People were fearful of the steps, particularly in icy and snowy weather.

3. Goal: Have clinic attendance achieve the projected level of 45–60 visits per day by routing clinic users through an existing ground-level entrance equipped with a ramp and direct them to the elevator to the basement level for clinic appointments.

4. Outcome: Attendance reached anticipated levels within two weeks after modifying building and clinic access and providing media coverage of the change. Even though the new route to the clinic was somewhat circuitous, clients responded positively to a change made in the interest of their safety.

5. Evaluation: Goal was met successfully.

Objectively utilized evaluation can prove that changes that are carefully planned and executed are beneficial to those for whom change was necessary. Change in behavior, especially when it relates to health care actions, positively reflects the importance of assisting people to be as independent as possible about meeting their self-care needs.

Desired Behavioral Outcome

After the evaluation process demonstrates that a change is acceptable to clients and staff members, it is necessary to stabilize the situation so that everyone perceives the permanency of the reorganization. By this time any extra support personnel can be withdrawn, and the staff becomes solely responsible for providing services. Permanency, involving reorganization, the provision of new services, or the abolition of one mode of practice in favor of a method deemed to be more efficient, implies that administrative personnel, budgetary support, space allocation, and staff assignment are solidly aligned to ensure the continual operation and provision of services. The need identified and then rectified by the assessment, planning, implementation, and evaluation procedures has been met by the efforts of the organization and becomes an independent, stable function or unit of the organization.

ANTICIPATING OBSTACLES TO CHANGE

Change can be thwarted at any point of the process. Resistance to change can arise from personnel sources at any level of the organizational hierarchy, from budgetary problems, from the nature of the problem or environment, or from the actions of people who are recipients or consumers within the environment. Knowing that a change is not isolated in its application and effects provides the change agent with information needed to anticipate and avoid barriers to change.

One guideline for dealing with the future is to actively plan for change. This should be the highest priority in dealing with the uncertainties ahead. In the early 1980s health and social service programs were plagued by budgetary constraints. Withdrawal of funds, the need to operate programs at zero-budget levels or with decrements and across-the-board budget cuts, and stern retrenchment measures became some of the greatest reasons forcing organizations to implement drastic change. The way an organization deals with financial deficits is a general reflection of how it will handle other difficult matters.

Financial Aspects

Budgetary conditions unfavorable to institutional support constitute serious barriers to change. A need for change may be glaring, but if no money is available, the change may not occur. Fiscal problems force planners to look at change in a manner which may conflict with futurism. Often change is seen as an occurrence that reflects only forward, progressive evolutionary direction. In time of financial exigency, however, change may be necessary to maintain the status quo. Or change may be necessary in order to abandon an aspect of organizational functioning to provide support for the delivery of adequate services in basic areas. For example, some official health agencies are relinquishing home health services and concentrating money and effort on clinics and other health department programs. This has resulted in the development of proprietary home health care agencies to provide home care to clients who need it. The official agencies can then focus on other projects in the community that may be better served by a concentration of staff and resources.

Sometimes the appropriate change is a decision to stand still. This may be particularly true for an agency that has undergone spiraling growth and has frequently added new programs and projects. When the staff of a growth-oriented agency consciously decides not to expand or diversify, this is a significant change from their growth-production orientation.

A more critical regressive change would be to severely curtail programs and staff and provide only essential services for the public welfare, such as sanitarian and environmental service, immunizations, and a prenatal clinic. Other drastic cuts would include trimming back services by a given percentage and having clinics, offices, and other services available only three or four days per week. This saves money on salaries. The staff needs support when such measures are taken, since a cut in their numbers or hours means a concomitant cut in persons available to work or a decrease in pay. If the cut is temporary, most employees, especially if they are happy in their work situations, are able to cope with the inconvenience, because their jobs are otherwise secure. When such cutbacks are permanent, administrative personnel must be honest in informing employees. In the case of one large outpatient clinic, a variety of efforts were undertaken to allow most personnel to work for a full-time salary. Some people were helped to find full-time positions elsewhere, and some combined two part-time positions into one full-time job. Others were able to work in associated inpatient units. With managerial creativity and flexibility on the part of both management and staff, solutions can be found to situations controlled by financial problems.

The Grant Process as a Change Tool

Budgetary problems might indeed cause catastrophe in an agency, particularly in organizations dependent on grants. An administrator must be exceptionally skillful in seeking and securing funding if this source of revenue is the primary means of fiscal solvency, since organizations are facing increased difficulty in acquiring such money. The staff of social service or health care agencies dependent on such funds must work hard to be competitive with other organizations that are endeavoring to secure grant money and philanthropic sources of revenue. Using a proven change strategy involving a cohesive group with a high degree of loyalty to the goals of the organization helps stimulate an environment in which people are creative, cooperative, and achievement directed. Such a staff can be competitive in an effort to obtain scarce or limited funding.

The evaluation process can be vital in obtaining a grant, since it can demonstrate past efficiency and agency success with change in renewal and innovation. As more agencies deal with change imposed by decreasing budgets, there will be greater competition for fewer dollars. A group that employs change strategies creatively can use information collected in that process, as well as outcome data generated by the change process, to remain competitive in grant seeking. Such change tactics were demonstrated in a large urban midwestern school of nursing where many grant proposals are now developed and requested annually. At a time when schools of nursing were experiencing severe cutbacks in federal capitation dollars, this university school of nursing anticipated its need and began to seek out new revenue sources to strengthen its research and community service missions. Faculty members were given strong administrative support to broaden this aspect of their professional expertise. With an increase in grant requests came a concomitant increase in grant awards made to the school of nursing.

Attitudinal Barriers to Change

Change can be hampered by negative thinking as well as by financial exigencies. In the following situation, change was needed to deal with impending crisis. Change is fueled by creativity, and creative expression can be impeded by frustration, prejudice, or a lack of care and concern. The following situation illustrates how such obstacles can make optimal functioning difficult:

In a large Gulf coast city, the county health department used large amounts of federal relief money to assist in the relocation problems of Cuban and Haitian refugees. The directors of the department's medical and nursing services were concerned when a moratorium was placed on monies to be released, because a great need still existed among the Haitian refugees. The Cuban displaced persons had been easily assimilated into the community. Many Cubans had already lived in the area, and they had strong cultural ties and a feeling of responsibility for their compatriots. The newly arrived Cubans were in overall good health, had current immunizations, had values consistent with the prevailing mores of the community, and were basically well educated. In contrast, the Haitians who arrived had a high illiteracy rate, no job skills, and an overall poor level of health, including conditions such as tuberculosis, parasites, poor dental hygiene, mental health problems, and few or no immunizations. In addition, there were no established groups of Haitian residents to cushion the gap between the Haitian homeland and the cultural differences of life in the United States.

The health department was the only resource available to both groups of refugees, but the continued need of the Haitians for assistance had not been foreseen in the emergency planning. Health department administrators were distraught, and their frustration at not having the staff and money required to solve the problem led them to believe that they had neither the time nor the energy for planning any effective change. They reported that their agency was so crisis oriented that change just happened, and they had enough to do just to recognize the phenomenon and try to keep pace with the rules and regulations that were generated. Need identification and goal setting were viewed as nearly impossible.

The agency staff also found themselves in a period of financial exigency, and they felt powerless to mount efforts to increase the flow of funds necessary to meet the health care needs of the Haitians. The agency had had previous success in securing stable local government funds, but that effort had been arduous and time-consuming. The nursing division of the department had identified a need to establish a school health nurse program and had petitioned the city and county governments for the money needed. But in their immediate need for money for the Haitians they did not relish another four-year campaign to secure the funds. Also, the political nature of the plight of the Haitian people made it difficult to approach the local legislators, since the refugee issue was volatile and unpopular in the community. The agency administrators knew that emergency money might be allocated by the state government, and although that money might appear to be a panacea, realistically it would only prolong their organizational crisis.

Often the resistance of a person or the people within the situation to be changed is simplistically viewed as the barrier to change. As this example shows, the political and affective domains must also be assessed in planning for unmet needs. This becomes an exceptional challenge when a condition is interpreted as particularly unfavorable or upsetting. In the case of the Haitian people in this city, fear and prejudice were operating. Such feelings are difficult to combat. The health department in this county understood the magnitude of need and the unpopular climate which prevailed. At the same time, the next level of administrative authority did not allow enough time for the assimilation of the Haitians into their new environment. Their planning was based on unrealistic goals and included no objective criteria to evaluate how well the Haitians were managing. The health department officials at the local level knew that many problems still existed, but they did not have the political clout to effect change at the state and regional decision-making level. The plight of the Haitians in this setting may have been more easily managed if the local health department officials were better versed in penetrating the ascending tiers of bureaucratic administration.

SUMMARY

Although there are many problems associated with change, an understanding of the dynamics of change brings us closer to workable interventions. Application of change concepts in relatively simple situations provides experience and direction for coping humanistically with complex changes and needs. A real challenge is to employ change tactics in difficult situations in which not only cunning, creativity, and cleverness but also compassion and ethical choices are valued. Along with the needs of the poor, the elderly, the disabled, the homeless, the abused, and the disenfranchised, there also exist the unmet needs of the individual who falls into any one or more of those categories. In meeting the needs of any person, the actual steps in the change process are easier to isolate than the limits of the magnanimity of society. Future applications must consider not only these problems but also those that the future will present.

Although future events can be predicted, the future can not be known with accuracy. Change and the management of responses to future situations are important parts of the investment of human and monetary resources in planning and development for people, the environment, business, and any other endeavor of society. Managing and guiding future changes requires built-in contingency plans. Planning for the future requires a comprehensive total view that takes into account all possibilities to provide for the optimal development of our present and future populations.

One thing that seems clear about the future is that all people will become more aware of the process of change. People are learning to cope with more changes in their lives and in their environments within a single generation than our ancestors coped with in a whole century. Educators are introducing change theory into curricula at many levels. This will enable people to appreciate the complexities involved in dealing with changes they did not plan as well as to facilitate changes they wish to bring about. This new way of regarding the advance of one's life will help to contribute to the optimal functioning of each person.

Nurses will be working with many better educated clients who understand change and want to plan for it. Clients will realize that certain events are inevitable, but that these can be met with preparedness. For example, they will have a better understanding of the aging process and an awareness of what aspects of it can be altered. They will seek assistance from health care providers to have a healthier life throughout their lifespans. In turn, nurses can become more sophisticated in planning their own futures and the future of nursing and health care. By understanding change theory, nurses can better anticipate problems and prevent them or arrange for appropriate responses if problems are inevitable. The nurse who is aware of the promises of the future can make suggestions and proposals to take advantage of change rather than be overwhelmed by it.

DISCUSSION TOPICS

1. How can community health nurses facilitate the advent of legislatively mandated health promotion activities, such as annual screening for cancer or periodic mental health assessments? Identify the steps which might take place in the phases of unfreezing, changing, and refreezing.

2. What are the implications for the changes in nursing practice needed to accommodate the increasing acceptance of life-styles formerly labeled as "deviant" (for example, unmarried couples living together; homosexual relationships)?

3. The Australian concept of "granny flats" is being introduced into the United States to provide alternatives to nursing home and high-rise apartment living for the elderly. Small, relocatable modular housing units are placed in the yards of children of elderly people who require support systems. Cottages are moved to new sites when they are no longer needed by a particular family. How would you plan to meet the needs of families if 200 "granny flats" were to be provided in your city (population 20,000) within the next two years?

BIBLIOGRAPHY

Asimov, I.: *Change!* Boston: Houghton Mifflin, 1981.

Bennis, W.G.: *Changing organizations.* New York: McGraw-Hill, 1966.

Bennis, W.G., Benne, K.D., & Chin, R.: *The planning of change.* New York: Holt, Rinehart, & Winston, 1969.

Brown, L.R.: A sustainable society. *The Futurist* 16(1), 12–19, 1982.

Granny flats: Easing the housing crunch for the elderly. *The Futurist* 16(1), 51, 1982.

Hultman, K.: *The path of least resistance.* Austin, Texas: Learning Concepts, 1979.

Kron, T.: *The management of patient care.* Philadelphia: Saunders, 1981.

Lesse, S.: *The future of the health sciences: Anticipating tomorrow.* New York: Irvington, 1981.

Lewin, K.: Group decision and social change. In T.M. Newcomb & E.L. Hartley, eds., *Readings in social psychology* (3rd ed.). New York: Holt, Rinehart, & Winston, 1958.

Longest, B.: *Management practices of the health professional.* Reston, Vir.: Reston Publishing, 1980.

Margulies, N., & Raia, A.O.: *Conceptual foundations of organizational development.* New York: McGraw-Hill, 1978.

Mauksch, I.G., & Miller, M.H.: *Implementing change in nursing.* St. Louis: Mosby, 1981.

New, J.R., & Couillard, N.A.: Guidelines for introducing change. *Journal of Nursing Administration* 11(3), 17–21, 27, 1981.

Schlotfeldt, R.M.: Nursing in the future. *Nursing Outlook* 29(5): 295–301, 1981.

Steele, S.M., & Maraviglio, F.L.: *Creativity in nursing.* Thorofare, N.J., Charles B. Slack, 1981.

4

Role Theory

Ruth Kramer Young

A man who looks a part has the soul of that part.
GUY DE MAUPASSANT

OBJECTIVES

After reading this chapter, you should be able to:

- ☐ Describe the historical development of role theory.
- ☐ Define terms and concepts related to role theory.
- ☐ Discuss role theory as it is related to nursing education.
- ☐ Describe the application of role theory in the practice of community health nursing.
- ☐ Describe the reciprocal role interaction between nurses and physicians.
- ☐ Identify and discuss characteristics of the sick role in our society.
- ☐ Explore ways in which role theory can be used with clients in different developmental stages.

INTRODUCTION

The concept of *role* was part of the common language long before theorists began a systematic study of roles and role theory. People have talked about someone "fitting a role," meaning that their behavior and attitudes were consistent with what others thought they should be. Parents and teachers have taught children about roles. Children have learned about their role as children, about what they can and should do as well as what they should not do. They have learned what to expect from people they interact with. This has been part of the process of *socialization*. The socialization of children has always been considered a basic responsibility of society; the purpose of socialization is to prepare children to live in a given social structure. Social scientists talked and wrote about the phenomena of roles long before they discussed the concept of role and role theory.

The practice of nursing in any setting involves the use of role theory. Role theory helps the nurse understand and organize information related to the socialization process involved in the nurse's professional practice. When a community health nurse changes positions within the same health care facility or moves to another facility, the process of socialization into new roles continues. Role theory provides a framework for looking at what community health nurses do and how they relate to co-workers on the health care team, to clients and their families, as well as to individuals in the nurse's personal life. In nursing practice, role theory helps the nurse understand the roles of clients and how these roles relate to the clients' health and illness. The client has a social network that involves various significant roles. The nurse can use the client's social network system of roles to facilitate the nursing process.

CONCEPTS RELATED TO ROLE THEORY

Derivation of the term "role" is from the Latin *rotula*, which means "little wheel" or "round log." From this, the term came to be used to refer to sheets of parchment assembled into a scroll. In France, the word *role* was used for any volume of papers pertaining to law courts. In the sixteenth and seventeenth centuries, with the emergence of stage plays, the theatrical parts were read from *rôles*, or paper bundles. Later each part came to be called a *rôle* (Moreno, 1960a).

Although the word "role" had commonly been used in English, the psychosocial concept was developed in the early part of the twentieth century when theorists

such as Mead, Moreno, and Linton began writing about role problems. Mead (1934) used the concept of *role taking* to describe the process of learning and demonstrating a role. Moreno (1960b, p. 81) identified three kinds of roles: (1) psychomatic roles, such as sleeper or eater; (2) psychodramatic roles, such as a mother or a teacher; and (3) social roles, such as *the* mother, *the* son, or *the* Christian. A person takes on a role in two stages: first by perceiving the role, then by reacting to the role. Moreno also introduced the concept of *role playing*, which he saw as an experimental procedure or way of learning to perform roles. Role playing occurs before role taking. Linton's (1936), best-known contribution is his classic distinction between *status* and *role*. A *status* is a collection of rights and duties, or a position; a *role* is the dynamic aspect of a status, or actual behavior: what one really does in a role. For example, a status is the position of nursing supervisor, which has specific rights and duties accompanying the title. What the nursing supervisor actually does, the behavior, describes a role. Mead, Moreno, and Linton established a new concept of "role" that laid the foundation for other theorists who built on what had been done to formulate *role theory* (Biddle & Thomas, 1966).

The term and concept of "role" evolved through the work of Cooley (1902), who wrote about the self; Dewey (1899), who analyzed habit and conduct; Sumner (1906), who developed conceptions of mores and folkways; Simmel (1920), who discussed interaction; and Durkheim (1933) and Ross (1908), who wrote about social forces. All of these concepts remain within the domain of role theory.

With the development of role theory, the phenomenon of socialization has been studied. Socialization is the learning of social roles that prepare one for adult and other specific kinds of role performance (Hardy & Conway, 1978). Hardy (Hardy & Conway, 1978, p. 9) states that "in the strictest sense, it would be more accurate to talk about a *role framework* rather than a *role theory*." He differentiates these two phrases in order to indicate the complexity of the phenomenon. Hardy explains that "role theory" refers to a specific orientation toward social structure and social behavior that is used in studying and understanding human interaction patterns.

Role theory includes the terms and concepts for understanding and studying the different aspects of social roles. Theory, in general, is made up of concepts that have a relationship to observable phenomena. Theory uses words, which are symbols of the way we view the world. Words have meaning because people agree about what they mean and have learned their meanings. Concepts are expressed in word symbols. A description of role theory, therefore, includes word symbols, or concepts, that help explain the phenomena of roles as they relate to the structure and function of human interaction.

The *domain* of role theory involves real-life behavior as it is displayed in genuine ongoing social situations. The *perspective* of role theory is a particular way of viewing the factors influencing real-life behavior. The *language* of role theory includes the concepts necessary to describe and study real-life behavior (Biddle & Thomas, 1966).

A role is a pattern of behavior structured around specific rights and duties that are associated with a particular status within a group. There are a number of different kinds of roles. An *achieved role* is one that an individual chooses or earns through his or her own efforts and actions, such as the role of nurse. An *ascribed role* is acquired by an individual automatically at birth or on the attainment of a certain age.

Sex roles are examples, as are those of king, American, adult, or senior citizen. When an individual adopts a role as part of his or her self-concept, this is called an *internalized role*. The role expectations that an individual believes others have of his or her behavior in a given situation constitute a *perceived role*. *Reciprocal roles* define patterns of interaction between two or more related statuses, such as teacher–student, husband–wife, or nurse–client. *Multiple roles* occur when a person has various statuses, or positions, simultaneously at a given time, such as nurse, wife, mother, daughter, friend, and neighbor. A *role set* is a complex of behaviors centering around a particular status, such as the status of nursing supervisor, which involves roles of administrator, teacher, counselor, and consultant. When individuals with different roles switch roles, this is a *role reversal*. For example, a parent may take on the role of child while the child takes on the role of the parent.

Role Theory and Nursing Education

How and why does a person decide to be a nurse? There are many reasons for nurses to become nurses, but very basic is the fact that the nursing student was attracted to some idea about what a nurse does. This is the student's *role perception* of a nurse.

A major task in nursing education is to provide experiences that help the student identify with and internalize the role of a professional nurse, which involves the process of being socialized into the profession. Nursing educators do not provide the only input that influences the socialization process of nursing students. Each student enters nursing school as a unique person and brings a unique cultural complex. Each student's life experience has been different from that of all other students. Each one has had different family, educational, and religious experiences. This helps explain why all graduates of a given nursing program will not solve problems and perform their role as a nurse in exactly the same way, even though they took the same courses, had the same teachers, and used the same books. The students' own value systems and motivations and other factors affect how they perform the role of nurse after graduation.

Nursing educators do, however, have a key responsibility in the socialization of nursing students. There is much interaction between teacher and student, which emphasizes the principle of *role reciprocity* in the teacher–student dyad. The student tries to perform the role based on the *role prescriptions* as defined by the teacher: those behaviors that have been outlined and described. The teacher adjusts to the student's responses, and thus both student and teacher are influenced by the role interaction between the two (Hardy & Conway, 1978). This helps explain why experienced nursing educators say they never teach in exactly the same way in any two semesters.

Figure 4.1 shows the role theory concepts involved in the nursing student's process of socialization into the nursing profession. Nursing faculty members are responsible for *role clarification,* or defining the knowledge base, the methods for performance of skills, and the general behavior appropriate for a nurse. This is accomplished through explanations in lectures, seminar interaction, assigned readings, planned practice laboratory experiences, supervised client care, and other learning experiences. The faculty members clarify what the nursing role is and often alter the students' prior

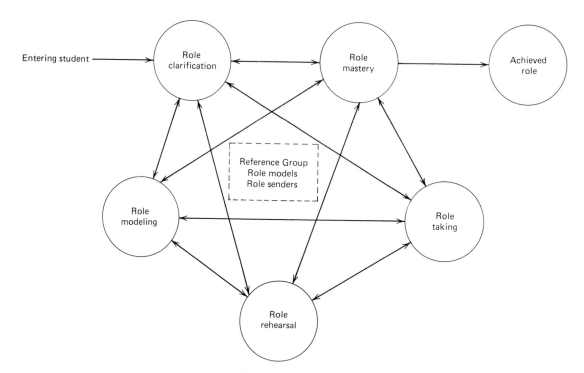

Figure 4.1   Role theory and nursing education.

role perception. The students' previously conceived role perceptions typically were formed by watching television programs or movies, reading books, or perhaps even talking with nurses or other health care professionals. Often these resources do not give a realistic description of the role of the nurse.

Role modeling occurs when the student, after having been exposed to and having observed one or more ways of performing a nursing function, chooses to use an observed pattern. Role models for nursing students include faculty members and other professional nurses with whom they come in contact during their education. By watching role models, students have an opportunity to see a professional at work. Role models act as *role senders* since they are responsible for helping to form the role a student takes as he or she goes forth to establish his or her own role in nursing.

Role rehearsal activities occur when the student performs procedures in the practice laboratory. Students also rehearse roles by role playing in seminars and other classes. Role rehearsal activities prepare the student to perform a role in the expected manner when the opportunity comes. An important activity related to role rehearsal is evaluation of the rehearsal by the student and by faculty members. This provides for both suggestions for improvement and positive reinforcement of the student's performance.

In *role taking*, the student identifies with a role model or with someone in the *reference group*, which includes both role models and role senders, who help prepare the nursing student to function in the real world. The reference group influences the student's formation of values related to nursing practice and is the group whose acceptance the student wants and seeks. The student tries to anticipate how the role model would respond in a given situation

and performs the role in the same manner: the student does what he or she thinks the role model would do. The student's success in role taking depends on the extent of his or her experiences with the role model, the student's acquired knowledge base for decision making, and the extent to which the student paid attention and remembered information regarding observational experiences (Hardy & Conway, 1978).

Role mastery is accomplished when the student successfully performs the role of nurse. The values and behaviors of the student's nursing reference group are internalized, and the student has no difficulty with role taking. When a student has mastered the role of nurse, cognitive and affective responses and psychomotor skills are judged appropriate by members of the reference group.

The *achieved role* is attained when the student meets requirements for graduation, passes the licensing examination, and moves into the professional nurse's role. Attaining this role involves much interaction, role clarification, role modeling, role rehearsal, role taking, and role mastery. Although the role is achieved, it is not static. This makes it necessary for the nurse to continue to learn more about the most appropriate and responsible way to perform the achieved role.

Role Theory and Nursing Practice

Role theory assists the nurse in two basic ways. First, the theory provides a framework for looking at what a nurse does, is qualified to do, or is expected to do. Second, the theory gives the nurse a framework for understanding clients. Role theory helps explain why clients react as they do, why they do or do not comply with prescribed treatment regimens, and why they interact as they do with family members and friends. Since roles give structure to behavior, understanding roles is a key to understanding client behavior.

Nursing practice takes place in many forms and in many different settings. There are nurses prepared at different educational levels, ranging from associate degree to doctorate, each of which provides the foundation for a different role. In addition, the knowledge explosion has led some nurses to specialize their roles to become, for example, intensive care nurses, operating room nurses, school nurses, or nurse-practitioners in various fields. These factors have added complexity to describing the role of nurse. Role theory can provide a framework for understanding what a given nurse does or what nurses in a given job situation do.

In addition to knowledge related to the practice of nursing, there are many other factors affecting the role of a nurse. Some of these include the specific education and socialization experience; factors in the societal environment, such as technological development, political events, and economic conditions and changes; and structure and function of the family as a social institution.

Factors within an agency have a significant impact on the role of nurses who work there. Some of these factors are part of the formal and informal methods for establishing who leads, who follows, who makes the rules, who controls the budget, and who has sanction and other powers. Another important factor determining what a nurse really does is the agency's funding source: federal, state, private, voluntary, or some combination. For example, roles in a private agency differ from those in state or federal agencies, because of different degrees of bureaucratic structure.

Nursing is an *achieved role*, since one works to take on the role of nurse. Once the role is achieved and internalized, the nurse develops some ideas about what it is appropriate to do or say in the nurse role. This is the nurse's *perceived role*, which may or may not differ from what other nurses and nonnurses perceive the nurse role to be. The practicing professional nurse works continually to redefine and refine ideas about the nursing role.

Role conflict occurs for the nurse when he or she is expected to perform two or more incompatible roles in a given situation. This stress, which is experienced in various forms of role conflict, is also referred to as *role strain*. Role conflict can result when the expectations of the nurse are not the same as those of clients, physicians, other members of the health care team, or family members. A discrepancy between what the nurse expects and what others expect can cause stress, because both sets of expectations cannot be met. Thus the nurse may sometimes sacrifice self-satisfaction in order to satisfy the role performance expectations of others.

One cause for role conflict results from the fact that a nurse has a *role set* that centers around a particular status. A nurse who occupies a particular position may be expected to provide care for clients, to teach, to participate in research, to serve as consultant for others, to counsel staff members, and to perform administrative functions. Availability of time and energy may limit the completion of these behaviors. For example, on a given day, the charge nurse may be confronted with a staff shortage, a staff member who needs counseling, the monthly staff assignment schedule that needs to be completed, a staff meeting to attend, and a scheduled teaching session for a group of clients. This situation presents potential for role conflicts when the nurse sets priorities.

Another cause of role conflict for nurses

concerns *multiple roles.* A nurse typically has several roles other than nurse, such as father or mother, son or daughter, husband or wife, neighbor, friend, member of a church or other organizations. All of these roles require time and energy. Some may demand more of the nurse than others, and various roles demand different amounts of time and energy at different times. However, on a given day at work, the nurse may be preparing for a nursing audit or accreditation visit, a child may become ill and need care, and a friend may call about a personal crisis.

Role sets and multiple roles tend to create potential for *role diffusion.* Role diffusion occurs when the nurse's responsibilities as a professional include widely scattered kinds of involvement, and as a result the nurse feels ineffective in most or all roles. The nurse must learn to set priorities and to make efficient use of time. When the nurse can effectively budget time, set priorities, and gain a realistic perspective about time, he or she will experience far less role conflict attributable to complications of role set, multiple roles, or role diffusion.

Role theory serves as a tool in understanding role sets, multiple roles, and role diffusion of clients. They, too, experience the results of maladaptive responses to role conflict, and they often need assistance in dealing with them. For example, the demands a new mother and father feel when adjusting to having a baby can be overwhelming. When their work roles, spousal roles, and home maintenance roles are added, the experience may seem frustrating and impossible. The nurse may need to help the new parents set priorities for the demands of their various roles.

Role theory provides a framework for understanding the community health nurse's clients, whether they are individuals, families, communities, cities, or states. *Network analysis* is a perspective which focuses on relationships between individuals or between individuals and collectivities. A client's social network includes individuals and groups with which the client has some type of significant interaction. This social network frequently includes, for example, family members, friends, and work or recreation groups. Network analysis enhances the application of role theory by determining interaction patterns with a role network. Studying the existing role interaction or lack of interaction helps the nurse better understand situations, which enables the nurse to use the nursing process more effectively.

NURSES AND PHYSICIANS

A nurse does not work independently of all other health care professionals. In any health care setting the nurse is part of a network of professionals, sometimes referred to as the health care system. The nurse interacts with various health care professionals, but one of the most common role interactions occurs between the nurse and the physician. The nurse–physician role interaction is a special one in which the intensity of the shared responsibilities commands a degree of mutual respect and cooperation.

The Doctor–Nurse Game

Stein (1968) describes details of what he calls the "doctor–nurse game." First, he describes the object of the game: the nurse is to be bold, have initiative, and be responsible for making significant recommendations, while at the same time appearing to be passive. The nurse's recommendations must appear to be initiated by the doctor.

Both doctor and nurse must play the game with "the nimbleness of a high wire acrobat" (p. 102). Rules of the game are basic. Open disagreement between doctor and nurse must be avoided. The nurse's recommendations must not appear to be recommendations, and the physician must request a recommendation from the nurse without appearing to do so. Stein continues by describing details of the game. The nurse who successfully plays the game is passive, makes suggestions indirectly, and never embarrasses the physician by having information about clients that the physician does not have.

Stein (1968) explains that the doctor–nurse game arises as a result of the socialization process in medical and nursing schools. He points out that medical students are taught that their decisions are matters of life and death and that they are warriors against death and disease. Since making a mistake seems intolerable, a phobia develops. Medical students, as a defensive maneuver, develop the belief that they are omnipotent and therefore incapable of making mistakes. A paradox develops: medical students, wanting to give their client the best possible care, want input, but they shun advice because of its threatening effect on their omnipotence. The solution is to learn to play the doctor–nurse game.

In the past, nursing students were taught to relate to physicians in a specific way: physicians were to be treated with the utmost respect because of their superior knowledge. For example, nursing students were taught to stand when a physician entered the room. Nursing students were not taught to take independent action, but they were taught a strong sense of responsibility for the care of the client. This resulted in nursing students sometimes being caught in a paradoxical position, and thus they learned to play the doctor–nurse game to

get out of the bind. Another factor influencing the traditional doctor–nurse game is the influence of sexual identity: male dominance in physicians, who are predominately men, and female passivity in nurses, who are predominately women. Stein concludes his discussion of the doctor–nurse game by saying that the major disadvantage of the game is that it is stifling and anti-intellectual because it inhibits open dialogue. He feels that both professions would benefit by changing attitudes that perpetuate the game.

Current Attitudes

The current socialization of nursing students differs from that described by Stein. Nursing students for the past several years have been taught to use the nursing process to think and act independently. Unfortunately, it seems that in an attempt to establish an independent and autonomous role not subservient to the physician, nurses have given up some useful, significant interaction with physicians. In order to regain the close relationship, some physicians and nurses have tried to establish a new form of complementary role interaction. Nurses and physicians who were socialized into their professional roles according to the old doctor–nurse game are finding it difficult to develop a new type of relationship. Overall, the current role interaction between nurses and physicians is changing, but many remnants of the old doctor–nurse game still persist.

Thomstead, Cunningham, and Kaplan (1975) give an account of a physician and nurse who intentionally decided to play the game according to new rules. Their goal was to develop more direct and open communication in their roles as codirectors of an ambulatory pediatric care center. As they discussed new roles for nurses and physicians in this project, they explicitly attempted to reform their own role behaviors and to break out of the old doctor–nurse game. Each grappled with his or her own habits and training as much as with those of the other. Reactions from other professionals were stronger than they had expected when they threatened the old game, system, and players. The assessed benefits of their efforts were improved health care and consumer satisfaction and increased job satisfaction. Only because this physician and nurse were both well-qualified professionals strongly determined to make the new game rules work were they successful. Their experience leads one to believe that further changes in nurse–physician role interaction will not be easy, but it is encouraging to see that efforts are being made to improve role interaction patterns between nurses and physicians. This will surely result in more effective cooperation and teamwork in the future, which should improve the quality of health care.

THE SICK ROLE

The sick role is one of the most common and universally understood roles. Our society has specific expectations for the behavior of an individual who is defined as "sick." Parsons (1951), a sociologist, articulated the most widely accepted description of the sick role. He describes two main rights that a sick person has: (1) the sick person is exempted from the performance of normal social role obligations, and (2) the sick person is exempted from the responsibility for his or her own sickness. In reality, this means that other people view the sick person as having a good reason for not going to work, not performing other tasks, not going to school, or not meeting deadlines. In addition, the sick person is not blamed for being sick, and other people do not view the person as having caused the illness in order to get out of some responsibility. More recently, however, with the increased emphasis on health care and prevention, health care professionals and laypeople are learning more about the relationships between health and life-style. Much illness that was thought to be independent of personal health habits, such as eating habits, rest, and life-style in general, is now being linked to the behavior of the sick person. In the future, people may be held more accountable for their health and illness and therefore not completely exempt from responsibility for their own state of illness.

According to Parsons (1951), the sick role also includes two main obligations: (1) the sick person must be motivated to get well as soon as possible, and (2) the sick person must seek technically competent help and cooperate with medical experts. Health care professionals, family members, friends, and employers all expect the sick person to try to get well. This means that the sick person is expected to go to a physician, to take medications as ordered, and to follow through on other activities to facilitate a speedy recovery, such as staying in bed if needed, exercising appropriately, or staying on a diet. When the sick person does not do these things, the sick role obligations are not met, and other people become frustrated and intolerant of this perceived irresponsible behavior. With more understanding of health and prevention of illness, in the future these two obligations may be viewed as even more important.

Parson's description of the sick role explains a great deal about the interaction that takes place between clients and health professionals both in hospital settings and in community-based health care settings. Clients are expected to be submissive to the health care professional, who, because of professional training, is supposed to know what is best for the client. It is easy for a nurse or physician to become annoyed with a client who will not follow through on prescribed treatments and health care practices. The nurse or physician wants to see success: the client to get well or at least get better. When it seems that the client is not fulfilling the role expectations, the nurse should take a closer look at the client's situation. Other factors related to the client's situation and role network may be influencing the client's sick role behavior. Cultural practices or family problems may be causing the client's noncompliant behavior. If cultural practices, as role determinants, have contributed to noncompliance, an alternate treatment plan can be worked out by the client and the nurse. Sometimes problems arise because communication between the nurse and the client has been unclear, thus creating problems with the reciprocal role interaction between client and nurse.

Conflict can also arise in a family if a sick family member does not follow through with expected obligations or the sick role as defined within the family. In this kind of situation, the nurse can sometimes help by encouraging family members to talk about their expectations and frustrations. This will in some situations help the family in problem solving and finding a workable solution to the conflict. In short, clear communication between nurse and client, as well as between family members, about the sick role is of utmost importance in aiding people who are in the sick role.

DEVELOPMENTAL STAGES

In the play *As You Like It*, William Shakespeare noted that roles are related to a person's age:

All the world's a stage,
And all the men and women merely players:
They have their exits and their entrances;
And one man in his time plays many parts,
His acts being seven ages . . .

When the community health nurse works with families as clients, it is usual that different family members will be in different developmental stages. Individual family members have roles that are largely dependent on their particular developmental stage.

The constellation of persons in the family system constitutes the *family structure*. This structure forms the *family network*, and when the community health nurse needs to learn more about the family roles, network analysis can be effectively used. Each family member has position, or status, in this structure, and each occupant of a position plays culturally and socially defined roles. Cultural forms specify the rights and obligations of family members who occupy particular positions. Within the guidelines for behavior set by their culture, the family members establish variations in role definition and expectations for specific roles. Each family has its own traditions and value system, and each sets its own standards for interaction, both within and without the family (Whaley & Wong, 1979). Individual family members have *ascribed roles*, such as age and sex, and more specifically, "daughter," "son," "mother," and "father." The role activities that belong to ascribed roles are determined by the structure of society. For example, socialization into sex roles begins during infancy. Baby boys are treated differently from baby girls and are given different toys to play with. Differences continue throughout the socialization process in succeeding developmental stages. Individual family members may also have achieved roles such as nurse, teacher, leader, or president. Achieved roles may affect family relationships as well as relationships outside of the family.

A basic concept in role theory is the *complementarity* of roles. In other words, a role does not exist in isolation but is patterned for reciprocal interaction with that of a role partner. For example, the student and teacher roles are complementary roles, as are the husband and wife roles. Society as well as the individual family specifies behaviors for each person in these reciprocal arrangements. Individuals learn role expectations, and each person in the complementary role *dyad* (pair) knows what to do and what kind of behavior to expect from the other. This permits social interaction to be orderly and predictable. A family's equilibrium depends in large part on the complementarity of roles. These well-defined complementary roles ensure coordination of individual behaviors into a meaningful whole. Ill-defined roles can create tension and role conflict and produce disequilibrium (Robischon & Scott, 1969).

The roles of husband and wife are basic to the family network as well as to the structure and function of society. Each couple that gets married works out its own complementary role interaction patterns within the boundaries of what is expected by the larger society. Some of the variables that affect particular role arrangements include whether the wife works, whether the husband works, whether one or both are in school, and the availability of basic resources such as food and shelter. The complementarity of their roles changes over time. The husband and wife role interaction takes on different forms as they progress through the stages of the first year of marriage, beginning parenthood, raising children, being alone again after children leave home, and entering the later adult stage in life. Husbands and wives must decide who is going to work to provide family income, who is going to prepare food, who is going to do housekeeping chores, and who is to keep track of the budget. They must also decide on other role responsibilities, such as who disciplines and counsels children or who gets up with sick children at night, who decides when to seek medical care, who is responsible for arranging family social activites, who takes care of family automobiles, and who makes decisions regarding insurance or investments. The decisions about all of these factors make each husband–wife dyad unique. That is why it is important for the community health nurse working with a family to gather information about the way each couple sees the roles of husband and wife.

Because roles are related to developmental stages, role prescriptions are dynamic, always changing. The nurse must be aware that the roles of family members are continually emerging, being modified, and terminating.

The Eight Stages of Life

Erikson (1963) identified eight developmental stages and described the developmental tasks of each stage. The first is the infant stage, in which the developmental task is to master the conflict between trust and mistrust of others. In the second stage, the toddler deals with the conflict between desire for greater autonomy and feelings of shame and doubt. The preschool-age child faces the conflict between initiative and guilt. The task of the school-age child is to master feelings of inferiority through being industrious. The adolescent faces the problems of identity versus identity confusion, while the young adult must deal with conflicts of intimacy versus isolation. The middle adult is in the stage of generativity versus self-absorption and stagnation. In later adulthood, the task is to establish ego integrity and overcome despair.

The infant has roles as a child, a son or

daughter, a grandchild, and so on. Role expectations for the infant are relatively simple. The infant is expected to be dependent on others for basic care. Expectations regarding role behavior relate to growth and development, as the infant is expected first to watch others, then to respond with smiles, laughter, and gurgling sounds. Sometimes conflict results when parents do not know much about normal growth and development and expect more than an infant is usually capable of doing, such as sleeping all night every night or being toilet trained before 1 year of age. Role expectations in these cases are unrealistic. It is often the responsibility of the community health nurse to clarify role expectations by giving information about the child's developmental stage.

The role expectations for the toddler are that the toddler feeds himself or herself, responds affectionately by hugging and kissing, and explores the environment. Parents and others who interact with toddlers may tolerate such behaviors as temper tantrums, lack of judgment regarding personal safety during exploration, and short attention span. These toddler activities are to be expected but often cause problems when parents have unrealistic role expectations for what a toddler can and should do.

The role expectations for the preschool age child are more complex. For example, the 3-year-old is expected to try to please others, to be aware of and respond to family relationships, and identify with the parent of the same sex. The 4-year-old child is expected to act more independently and to play cooperatively. When the 4-year-old expresses many fears and plays with imaginary playmates, this should be tolerated, as it is normal role behavior for this age. Role expectations for the 5-year-old child are that the child will enjoy playing, like rules, and like following rules.

The role expectations for the school age child are that the child will enjoy making things, will enjoy and be successful in school, and will share ideas and feelings. There should be decreasing dependence upon the family and an increased ability to become a more active and cooperative family participant. The school-age child does not meet role expectations if the child's behavior indicates that the child feels inadequate, is unable to learn or do tasks, is lazy, or is unable to compete, compromise, or cooperate.

The role expectations for the adolescent are that the adolescent will accept the physical changes taking place in his or her body, develop intellectual and social skills of a competent citizen, and develop a workable and responsible philosophy and set of values. Role conflict often results as the adolescent moves toward these role expectations and establishes identity. The adolescent's choice of role behavior may be quite different from that of his or her parents. This can create turbulent family interactions as the adolescent struggles to establish identity. The adolescent fails to meet role expectations when he or she fails to achieve a sense of identity and experiences doubts and confusion about himself or herself and about life roles.

A child at any stage will have more difficulty meeting role requirements if he or she has a physical disability, is mentally retarded, or has a disabling chronic disease. These conditions typically delay the child's growth and development, either mildly or severely. Parents may not understand that these developmental delays are to be expected and therefore that role behaviors are likely not to correspond with those for a healthy child of the same age. This lack of understanding can cause parental frustration as a result of unrealistic role expectations. Even if the parents do have a cognitive understanding of their child's handicap, they may become frustrated and disappointed by the child's role performance in day-to-day activites. Parents of these children need supportive guidance.

The role expectations of the young adult are that he or she will establish independence from parental financial aid, which involves becoming established in a vocation or profession; will establish an intimate bond with another person, either in marriage or friendship; will formulate a meaningful philosophy of life; and will become a responsible citizen.

The role expectations of the middle adult are that he or she will discover new satisfactions in marriage and with friends, help growing children become happy and responsible adults, experience a sense of satisfaction from work or responsibilities as a citizen, accept and adjust to physical changes in the body, and continue to formulate a meaningful philosophy of life. The middle adult who fails to meet these role expectations has a tendency to regress and does not function as a responsible citizen or family member and suffers from feelings of self-absorption and stagnation.

The role expectations of the person in later adulthood are that he or she will decide on a location and meaningful style of life for retirement; continue to cultivate and maintain supportive, close, warm relationships with family members and friends; maintain a maximum level of health; continues to work out a significant philosophy of life; and adjust to the death of a spouse and other loved ones. The older adult who fails to meet these role expectations experiences despair and causes a sense of despair in others. This last developmental stage is the culmination of all previous stages in the life cycle.

The person who has successfully met role expectations of other stages is likely to meet the expectations of this stage. The cultural value that society places on the knowledge and experience of the older adult is an important factor in how the older adult feels about herself or himself. It is unrealistic to assume that any person will ever perfectly meet all role expectations of every stage of life. Therefore, it is reasonable to expect varying degrees of adjustment to the roles of this last stage in life. Most individuals have some difficulty adjusting. Satisfactory achievement of the role expectations for this developmental stage depends on existing support systems and the individual's ability to relate to others in his or her social network. This interaction facilitates the development of integrity as opposed to despair.

Some societies have well-established rites of passage that signify the change from one stage or position in life to another. These rituals help the individual identify with new roles. A lack of such rites may create uncertainty for the individual who is entering a new stage in life (Robischon & Scott, 1969). Although rites of passage in North America are not as well established and uniform as they are in some other societies, there are some social activities and practices that serve this purpose. For example, when a child learns to walk, parents celebrate. They are celebrating symbolically the passage from infancy to toddler. The passage from toddler to preschool age may be marked by the child starting to go to a preschool, sleeping in a bed rather than a crib, and being toilet trained. Family members celebrate these activities. The passage from preschool age to school age is most characteristically marked by starting to go to school. This can be an exciting event for the whole family and is marked in various ways, such as buying school supplies and school clothes, successfully learning a safe way to walk to school or to get on and off a bus, and sharing the activities of the first few days of school with family members.

The passage from school age is more complicated, as various activities occur. For example, the family does not openly celebrate the girl's first menstrual period, but a subtle change in role interaction takes place when the family recognizes her as a young woman. One activity that often serves as a rite of passage is obtaining a driver's license. The adolescent as well as other family members looks forward to this accomplishment. Accompanying this is the freedom as well as responsibility that having access and control of a car brings.

The passage from adolescence to young adulthood may be identified with the graduation from high school or college, with engagement or marriage, or by the young person's move away from the family home. All of these occasions signify a rite of passage to a new role. The passage from young adulthood to middle adulthood also varies in form. It may be associated with children leaving home, achieving a prestigious and worked-for goal in one's profession, or simply a particular birthday. The passage from middle adult to later adult is probably most commonly associated with retirement. Parties are commonly given in honor of individuals who retire. Other life changes commonly occur at this age that affect the individual's role. These changes may include moving to a new residence.

The happy, well-adjusted person is one who learns to accomplish the developmental tasks appropriate to each developmental stage. A crucial way in which a community health nurse can promote health is to help people accomplish developmental tasks so that they can successfully fulfill the roles of the different stages. If nurses could find a way to help our society promote positive recognition and practices of rites of passage, this might improve our society's method for facilitating adequate role performances in all developmental stages.

FUTURE IMPLICATIONS

Numerous factors have affected the changing roles of nurses and clients. Technological developments in transportation mean that supplies and information, as well as nurses and clients, can travel faster. The ongoing explosion of scientific discoveries and technological advances have provided a greater knowledge base for nursing as well as more sophisticated tools for performing nursing functions. Thus the role of the nurse has experienced a continual change, and this will no doubt continue in the future. Daily newspapers as well as professional journals continue to present new information that will cause nurses to modify their roles in the future. Nursing will continue to incorporate new information into nursing practice.

The roles of family members in our society have continued to change over time. No longer do we automatically assume that it is always the mother's role to bring a sick child to seek medical care, nor is it the responsibility of the father alone to provide financial support. Many different divisions of labor are accepted. The family of the future will be more flexible as such changes become accepted as norms of society.

Individuals are now expected to accept greater responsibility for their health status than ever before. As more people become interested in learning about health maintenance and care in illness, the nurse's role will include more teaching about these topics. We are past the days when people relinquished total control over health and illness to the physician. It is an appropriate expansion of the nurse's role to help individuals and families take on more of this responsibility.

SUMMARY

Role theory provides a useful way of viewing the dynamics of a community. The domain of role theory is real-life behavior in given situations. The language of role theory includes a number of concepts used to describe the dynamics of real-life behavior. Role theory, as applied in nursing, incorporates the use of a number of related concepts. The most basic concept is that of *role*, which refers to what an individual really does, the dynamic aspect of behavior.

Role theory is useful for describing the dynamics of nursing education. Concepts related to role theory help to describe the role interaction of students with teachers, clients, the client's family and support network, and other health care professionals. Related concepts include role clarification, role modeling, role rehearsal, role taking, and role mastery.

Role theory provides a framework for understanding what a community health nurse does in a given job situation. This is of value in helping community health nurses juggle their many different roles.

The interaction between nurses and physicians is a unique one. Nurses and physicians have historically worked together to help the client achieve a more healthful state. In the past, much of this interaction was characterized by the traditional dominant male role and the passive female role. Currently this reciprocal role interaction is moving toward a more open communication wherein nurses and physicians recognize each other as professionals who have different kinds of expertise.

Role theory helps describe the dynamics

of behavior at the different developmental life stages. Different kinds of behavior characterize the eight developmental stages described by Erikson (1963). An individual's developmental stage is related to the roles he or she has within the family and in society in general.

Roles of nurses, other health professionals, and clients will continue to change in the future. Whatever forms different roles take in the future, role theory will still provide a valuable framework for understanding dynamics of behavior. Change in our society is an ongoing process, and the community health nurse must continually examine and reassess roles in order to be effective in the practice of nursing.

DISCUSSION TOPICS

1. Discuss ways in which you have used the concept of "role" in the past.

2. Review the terms and concepts related to role theory. Discuss these terms in relation to experiences you have had in nursing.

3. Discuss concepts of role theory related to nursing education and the process of socialization into the nursing profession. Illustrate application of role theory in nursing education.

4. Discuss the doctor–nurse game. Give examples of the doctor–nurse game from your own experience. Plan and discuss strategies for improving current and future nurse–physician reciprocal role interaction.

5. If you are sick, what kind of behavior is expected of you? Discuss ways in which your ideas about the sick influence how you implement the nursing process.

6. Discuss ways in which role theory can

help you understand different developmental stages. Discuss ways in which a knowledge of role theory would help a community health nurse interact with a family whose members included a mother, father, children ages 2, 5, 7, and 10, and a grandmother.

7. Discuss your ideas about what the role of the community health nurse will be in the future.

BIBLIOGRAPHY

Bezold, C.: Health care in the U.S.: Four alternatives. *The Futurist* 16(4), 14–18, 1982.

Biddle, J., & Thomas, E.J.: *Role theory: Concepts and research.* New York: John Wiley & Sons, 1966.

Blumer, H.: *Symbolic interactionism: Perspective and method.* Englewood Cliffs, N.J.: Prentice-Hall, 1969.

Cooley, C.H.: *Human nature and the social order.* New York: Scribner's 1902.

Dewey, J.: *The school and the society.* Chicago: University of Chicago Press, 1899.

Durkheim, E.: *The division of labor in society* (trans. George Simpson). New York: Free Press, 1933.

Erikson, E.H.: *Childhood and society* (2nd ed.). New York: Norton, 1963.

Hancock, T.: Beyond health care: Creating a healthy future. *The Futurist* 16(4), 4–13, 1982.

Hardy, M.E., & Conway, M.E.: *Role theory: Perspectives for health professionals.* New York: Appleton-Century-Crofts, 1978.

Kulbok, P.: Role diversity of nursing administrators: An obstacle to effective leadership? *Nursing and Health Care* 3(4), 199–203, 1982.

Linton, R.: *The study of man.* New York: Appleton-Century-Crofts, 1936.

Mead, G.H.: *Mind, self and society from the standpoint of a social behaviorist.* (ed. C.W. Morris) Chicago: University of Chicago Press, 1934.

Meleis, A.I.: Role insufficiency and role supplementation: Conceptual framework. *Nursing Research* 24(4), 264–271, 1975.

Moreno, J.L. ed: *The sociometry reader.* Glencoe, Ill.: Free Press, 1960a.

Moreno, J.L.: *Who shall survive?* New York: Beacon House, 1960b.

Murray, R., & Zentner, J.P.: *Nursing assessment and health promotion throughout the life span* (2nd ed.). Englewood Cliffs, N.J.: Prentice-Hall, 1979.

Parsons, T.: *The social system.* New York: Free Press, 1951.

Robischon, P., & Scott, D.: Role theory and its application in family nursing. *Nursing Outlook* 17(7), 52–57, 1969.

Ross, E.A.: *Social psychology: An outline and source book.* New York: Macmillan, 1908.

Schuster, C.S., & Ashburn, S.S.: *The process of human development.* Boston: Little, Brown, 1980.

Simmel, G.: Zur philosophie des schauspielers (On the philosophy of the actor). *Logos* 1, 339–362, 1920.

Stein, I.: The doctor–nurse game. *American Journal of Nursing* 68(1), 101–105, 1968.

Sumner, W.G.: *Folkways.* Boston: Ginn, 1906.

Swendsen, L.A., Meleis, A.I., & Jones, D.: Role supplementation for new parents—A role mastery plan. *The American Journal of Maternal Child Nursing* 3(2), 84–91, 1978.

Theodorson, A., & Theodorson, A.G.: *Modern dictionary of sociology.* New York: Crowell, 1969.

Thomstead, B., Cunningham, N., & Kaplan, B.H.: Changing the rules of the doctor–nurse game. *Nursing Outlook* 23(7), 422–427, 1975.

Toffler, A.: *The third wave.* New York: Bantam, 1980.

Whaley, F., & Wong, D.L.: *Nursing care of infants and children.* St. Louis: Mosby, 1979.

Williams, A.: Role considerations in care of the dying patient. *Image* 14(1), 8–11, 1982.

5

Assertiveness and Leadership

Estelle H. Rosenblum

> One's philosophy is not best expressed in words, it is expressed in the choices one makes. . . . In the long run, we shape our lives and we shape ourselves. The process never ends until we die. And the choices we make are ultimately our responsibility.
>
> ELEANOR ROOSEVELT

OBJECTIVES

After reading this chapter, you should be able to:

- ☐ Differentiate among assertive, aggressive, and passive behavior.
- ☐ Describe specific ways in which a community health nurse can be assertive in community settings.
- ☐ Describe how the nurse can teach and model assertive behavior to clients.
- ☐ Identify competencies necessary for effective leadership.

INTRODUCTION

Assertive behavior has been defined as an honest, direct, and appropriate expression of one's feelings, beliefs, and opinions. Assertiveness is a type of interpersonal behavior that enables an individual to act in her or his own best interest without anxiety and to exercise her or his own rights without denying the rights of others. Many people still confuse assertion with aggression.

In contrast with assertiveness, *aggressive behavior* manipulates, dominates, humiliates, and infringes on the rights of others; it is an attack on a person rather than on the person's behavior.

ASSERTIVENESS AND FEMININITY

Being unassertive or exhibiting passive behavior has generally been seen as an asset for women in our society. The typical feminine role in our culture has called for women to be submissive, to minimize their own competence, and always to suppress negative feelings. Traditionally, society has also seen women as existing to care for others. Even today, assertive behavior is sometimes associated with loss of femininity. Nurses who provide nurturance and care have been doubly rewarded for passive, nonassertive behavior. As members of a largely female profession under the domination of male physicians and hospital administrators, nurses who are quiet, obedient followers have frequently been valued, praised, and promoted. Nurses have far too long allowed themselves to be self-effacing and timid in acknowledging the unique contributions they make in meeting the health needs of clients. Assertiveness can be learned, even though for some learning it requires courage and determination. It is an essential part of any nursing curriculum, and it can be taught.

Unfortunately, many faculty members serve as inadequate role models in this regard, since they were educated in an atmosphere in which assertive behavior was not condoned, much less encouraged. It is important to realize that acquiring new behaviors takes time. Nursing students should be socialized early in their professional program to think positively about themselves and their profession.

Moloney (1979) writes about the socialization and resocialization necessary to prepare professional nurses. She states that nurses should be encouraged to be assertive and articulate in expressing their convictions about their contributions to health care. She further states that the social, cultural, economic, and political components of health care problems deserve increasing emphasis in preparatory nursing programs. Baccalaureate and graduate nursing students must understand the art of confronta-

tion, negotiation, conflict resolution, and the politics involved in the present health care delivery system if greater cooperation and collaboration among health team members is to be achieved. Nurses must be highly motivated to change the present health care delivery system and confident in implementing their ideas even if it requires challenging others (Moloney, 1979).

According to Marriner (1982), nurses must overcome many barriers in order to achieve total female sex role socialization:

Women have been expected to be passive, dependent, sensitive, weak, inconsistent, and emotionally unstable, while men are pictured as aggressive, objective, independent, confident, and competitive. The nursing socialization process further complicated the situation as both nursing schools and health agencies have organizational hierarchies with power concentrated at the top. This autocratic atmosphere promotes compliance and conformity. (p. 32)

Nurses have been taught to value sacrifice, humility, and service to others. In the past, women were not expected to express their thoughts and feelings or to become emotionally involved with clients. Nurses were expected to follow doctors' orders without question or challenge. Nurses have been so busy performing these tasks that they have frequently ignored they own rights.

Nurses must also deal with male–female role competition problems and female–female relationship problems. Men are more competitive against women than against other men, and women are more competitive against other women than against men. Consequently, attempts to develop nurse support systems are often unsuccessful. The "queen bee" and "trashing" syndromes have been described by many writers. The *queen bee syndrome* works as follows: a woman leader strongly identifies with men and enjoys her successful position. The queen bee feels superior to other women. She has worked hard to achieve her status and must be cooperative and nonthreatening with men in order to maintain it. To protect her turf, she never makes it easier for other women to succeed.

Coupled with the queen bee syndrome is another very damaging activity, "trashing." *Trashing* is character assassination. Trashing is done to destroy people rather than to expose honest disagreements and try to resolve them. It can be done in public or in private, to one's face or behind one's back. It questions one's motive and stresses one's worthlessness. The victim may be ignored, or anything she says or does may be interpreted negatively. Unrealistic expectations may assure her failure. A student who performs extremely well in a clinical rotation may not win the praise of her peers. Rivalry or jealous feelings may result in disparaging remarks. The person who does the trashing may lie to the victim about what others think of her or may lie to others about the victim. Trashing is manipulative and destructive. Nurses must become aware of what they are doing to each other, commit themselves to supportive instead of destructive responses, learn assertive behavior, and practice peer pressure to change norms.

VALUES AND ASSERTIVENESS

Community health nurses, by the nature of their job functions, find themselves meeting and working with a large variety of people. They are confronted with health problems and value systems that challenge their personal beliefs and attitudes. How the nurse reacts to a given situation will probably have a great impact on its outcome.

Nurses must learn how to relate to persons whose values are quite different from their own. The value orientations of the nurse and the client can play an important part in how creatively and productively each person relates to the other. Furthermore, the success of nursing interventions can be enhanced if congruency of values exists between the people involved. It has been frequently observed that when people's values are congruent, their interaction will be satisfying, but when they are incongruent, the involved parties tend to withdraw and avoid each other.

Physicians and nurses do not always share the same values. A community health nurse who works with families in a wide variety of situations, neighborhoods, and areas often finds that it is difficult to establish a trusting relationship with all of these people. Some of the clients' behaviors may be difficult for the nurse to comprehend or accept. By the same token, clients often are confronted with situations in the community that make for difficult relationships. Both the nurse and the client must be willing to accept each other's values if they are to sustain meaningful relationships.

Determining that assertiveness is "good" for nurses or for clients is a value choice. People whose needs are served by the passivity of others may label assertive behavior as "bad." For example, the word "uppity" was used to label black people and women when they began to be assertive. The use of such a label indicates that those doing the labeling felt threatened by the changing behavior of the formerly passive groups. When one displays assertive behavior in a situation where such behavior is atypical, other people in the situation may feel their values threatened. Therefore it is important for one who is attempting to be assertive to appreciate the potential threat this carries for others and to realize the likelihood of negative responses.

A common negative response in situations such as those described above is to label assertive behavior as aggressive, insensitive, or unfeminine, if the assertive person is a woman. If the assertive person checks his or her behavior against the definition of assertiveness, and the two are congruent, that person can feel confident that his or her behavior is appropriate. The assertive person must understand that his or her behavior may be uncomfortable to the other person and must realize that that does not make the behavior wrong. This assessment of behavior is also necessary for clients to understand, so that they will be willing and able to be assertive in their own behalf.

ASSERTIVENESS IN THE COMMUNITY

The example that follows and the discussion of three possible responses illustrate the choices a nurse often has to make in rendering quality care.

A community health nurse was directing a well-child clinic in a city in the southwest. There were approximately 35 parents and 20 infants and children waiting for the resident physician from a nearby medical center. All physical assessments, nutritional counseling, and activities involving the nurse had been completed. The doctor was to examine the infants based on the initial assessments, prescribe any needed medications and treatments, and approve the giving of immunizations.

The physician had been expected at 10 A.M. but arrived at 1:30 P.M. accompanied by a colleague. The two entered laughing and unconcerned, and the physician began the examinations without any explanation for his tardiness. He completed examining the last child at about 3:30 P.M., when the nurse approached him and asked him what had kept him. He responded with these comments: "They have been waiting. . . . Let them wait. They aren't paying for care. They aren't private patients. The care they are receiving is

free. I worked all morning, and this was an unexpected visit [meaning his colleague]; and you didn't expect me to skip lunch, did you? What's your name? I'm going to report you to your supervisor for your officious behavior."

This was a difficult and threatening situation. The three examples that follow describe three different ways of responding to this situation. The characteristics, interpretation, and consequences of the three styles are summarized in Table 5.1.

PASSIVE BEHAVIOR

The nurse listened and said nothing in response. She completed the health records, packed up the equipment in her car, and started back to the health department. She decided that perhaps she would tell her supervisor about this or perhaps "just let it ride."

AGGRESSIVE BEHAVIOR

The nurse raised her voice and stated, "These people need their lunch, too. Who do you think you are?" She then told the physician about past incidents and other situations that point out how doctors view themselves as gods. She slammed the records on the desk and angrily loaded up her car with the equipment used that day.

ASSERTIVE BEHAVIOR

The nurse responded with, "I know you have a busy schedule and that this clinic is just one extra assignment you have to do. Yes, I understand that you need lunch. If you're going to be late the next time, could you please phone us so we can ask the parents to come back after lunch and not inconvenience them by long delays?"

The passive response neither changes the physician's behavior nor solves the problem. The nurse will still have angry feelings and be dismayed. Her inability to respond appropriately in this interaction will leave her feeling inadequate, fearful, and anxious.

The aggressive response ventilates angry feelings immediately, but they will return,

TABLE 5.1
Comparison of Assertiveness, Aggression, and Passiveness

Communication Style	Characteristics	Interpretation	Consequences
Aggressive Behavior	Either a very loud or a very soft voice. Poor choice of language: Swearing Vulgarity Disparaging remarks Ethnic/racial slurs Physical reactions (slamming things down or raging and stamping feet) Ridiculing or humiliating Embarrassing someone in front of others	Release of anger Poor control over angry feelings Infringes on rights of others Manipulative Attempts to frighten or gain control	Feelings of guilt, anger, dismay, fear, anxiety, inadequacy
Passive Behavior	Retreating from the interaction Silent response or no verbal reaction Blaming self or assuming role of victim Crying or pleading Apologizing for something that is not one's fault	Fear of reprisal or harm Feeling overpowered Submitting rather than confronting Feeling intimidated	Same as above[a]
Assertive Behavior	Assuming natural voice Choosing words carefully Expressing understanding for someone else's point of view Explaining without blaming Trying to be direct and honest	Ability to take risks Attempt to express one's views without infringing on another Tolerance for another's values, beliefs, or feelings Putting oneself up without putting someone else down	Little guilt Much relief of anger or tension Feelings of adequacy Release of fear

Communication Style	Characteristics	Interpretation	Consequences
TABLE 5.1 (*continued*)			
	Trying not to intimidate or to be intimidated		
	Using humor to deflect or disarm if appropriate		

a It is well accepted that both aggression and passivity lead to similar feelings.

along with feelings of inadequacy, fear of retaliation and anxiety about future interactions. There has been no real problem solving or constructive solution, which means that hostilities may continue, covertly or overtly.

The assertive response does not meet anger with anger. It does not challenge the physician's statements, which in this case show selfishness and a lack of concern for the welfare of others. An honest, direct response attempts to be future oriented. It does not focus on blaming or finding blame but instead is productive in looking for a solution that leaves everyone a winner. No interaction should attempt to place blame, find a victim, or identify a scapegoat. The assertive response does not guarantee a successful outcome. However, it does permit people to share value conflicts openly and directly. In the above example, the nurse was able to express her own rights, beliefs, and feelings without infringing on the rights of others. Below is the internal response of the nurse who made the assertive response:

I was that nurse and I learned some valuable lessons that day. First, I added a new word to my vocabulary. When I got home that night, I looked up the word "officious" in the dictionary. Second, I learned how assertiveness and values clarification are inextricably related. I got in touch with my own values and beliefs. This expression of my conviction that these people deserved the same kind of care private clients received was delivered not in a rage of anger but in a statement that was direct and honest. Further, I showed my respect for the doctor's beliefs by waiting until the hall was cleared of people. I did not embarrass or humiliate him in front of others. We had not yet formed any kind of relationship, so I did not attempt to use humor to deflect the seriousness of the situation. Humor is probably one of my most valued strategies now, but it can easily be misinterpreted by someone who doesn't know you well.

Last, I indulged myself in the valuable and uplifting exercise known as risk taking, for which at that time I had no name. This standing up to a physician could have meant losing a job at that time, as it still does today in some places. I did not generalize that all physicians are thoughtless and selfish, just as I don't believe all nurses are noble and selfless.

What was the outcome of this incident? Because the nurse had a sympathetic supervisor, steps were taken to ensure that the physician did not repeat his thoughtless behavior. That outcome was instrumental in shaping the nurse's future attitudes about assertiveness and risk taking. It is possible that such assertive activities could lead to some dire consequences. There are no guarantees that assertiveness will lead to successful outcomes, but it almost always leads to greater peace of mind.

ASSERTIVENESS AND LEADERSHIP

There is a strong relationship between assertive behavior and leadership qualities. In a nursing class, leaders emerge in both formal and informal ways. Some individuals are given the right to lead because they have certain admired qualities in their interpersonal relationships or because of the way they accomplish and complete assignments. Perhaps they have demonstrated nonaggressive or assertive behavior that has won admiration.

The ability to internalize the quality of assertive, nonaggressive behavior patterns is the foundation for providing leadership. Are some nurses better equipped than others to be leaders? Should all nurses be prepared to be leaders? Most nurses have not been prepared for leadership roles and believe they have no responsibility to lead—that leadership is required only of certain "elite" members of the profession. However, many within the profession are strongly urging nurses to assume leadership roles to improve the health care delivery system. Moloney (1979) states that for far too long many nurses have been content to leave the responsibility for improved client care and for improved nursing education to a select few. The belief that nurse leaders can come only from scholars prepared at the doctoral level must be dispelled. Moloney (1979) states that the need for leadership is obvious but that highly visible leaders are not the only persons capable of providing it.

Leadership Competencies

What do we mean by leadership? The whole concept of leadership is spelled out by Warren Bennis (1976), who states:

The concept of leadership embraces five important sets of competencies.

1. Knowledge of large complex systems, their dynamics, and their (tribal) customs.
2. Practical theories of intervening and guiding these systems, theories that encompass methods for seeding, nurturing and integrating individuals in groups.
3. Interpersonal competence—this includes at least three components: a. the sensitivity to understand the effects of one's own behavior on others and how one's personality shapes his or her particular leadership style and value system; b. a capacity to develop adequate methods for valid feedback; c. managing conflict.
4. A set of values and competencies which enables one to know when to confront an attack if necessary and when to support and provide the psychological safety so necessary for growth.
5. An ability to develop and use all types of information systems, including high speed electronic computers. The job of the leader will be to collect, organize, and transmit information. (pp. 126–127)

Leadership, then, is characterized by those attributes or personal characteristics that contribute to influencing others through the leader's observed capabilities. Leadership may also be defined as an interpersonal process of influencing the activities of an individual or group toward goal attainment in a given situation.

Leadership Qualities and Behaviors

Leadership requires that the nurse possess certain qualities, attributes, or personal behaviors, including (1) risk taking, (2) assertiveness, (3) autonomous intervention, and (4) accountability (Mauksch, 1981).

Risk Taking

One takes a risk when one asserts a position that may not be recognized by others. For the nurse, risk taking may be involved in the process of establishing a collegial relationship with physicians and other health professionals, because in the past this relationship did not always exist. According to Mauksch (1981), as the nurse equalizes her or his way of viewing and perceiving physicians, shares observations of the client, and records these and other interventions in the client's record, she or he continually takes risks generally associated with any professional practice but not part of traditional nurse behavior. Recently, nurses took a risk by developing the term "nursing diagnoses." Thirty years ago, a nurse would not dare use the word "diagnose" to describe part of the nursing process. It was only through the risk taking of nurse clinicians and nurse educators who were able to make a conceptual distinction between medical diagnoses and nursing diagnoses that this concept became part of professional nursing practice.

Assertiveness

Assertiveness underlies the presentation of self by the nurse. Assertiveness includes nurses' putting their perspective on client needs or management into the picture, insisting upon having their competence recognized, expressing their perspective of client care priorities, and ceasing to cover up the deficiencies of others. Assertiveness permits an expression of self-worth and allows nurses to validate their own professional thrust rather than having to depend mainly on external validation. Nurses do not have to depend on another person's opinion to define their own self-worth and their own value. Nurses perceive themselves to be valuable and able to perform their professional work based upon their own opinions of themselves. Nurses can reach a point beyond self-esteem where they are, according to Maslow's hierarchy of needs, at a point of self-actualization. Such nurses can reach their own highest potential to reach out to others to perform all that they are capable of doing.

Many nurses suffer from severe isolation from the main current of activity in the health care system, often because educational programs for nurses and other health professionals have offered limited experience in multidisciplinary education. Yet nurses and other health professionals are expected to become active members of the health care team. Developing team relationships with other health professionals requires self-confidence and knowledge of the contribution one has to give to health care, along with an understanding and appreciation of the contributions made by other professionals.

According to Moloney (1979), in order to develop self-confidence, nurses and nursing students must develop a strong self-concept and believe in their own worth as contributing members of the professional health care team. Each member has something unique to bring to the solution of health problems.

Autonomous Intervention

Mauksch (1981) describes *autonomous intervention*, a concept that is essential to achieving assertiveness. How much can a nurse do for a client without a doctor's order? Probably quite a bit. How much of care is independent, nurse directed and managed? *Autonomous intervention* refers to the use of the protocols for assessment and intervention that have been mutually agreed upon and that are contracts between nurses and doctors. The protocols that have been constructed reflect the autonomous independence of each professional involved in the health care team.

Nurses design interventions based on a careful and comprehensive assessment that reflects their own independent nursing judgment. Autonomous intervention currently is still more readily accomplished in ambulatory health care settings than in hospitals.

Accountability

Accountability is one of the cornerstones of all professional practice; it has always been part of nursing behavior but has been applied only to certain segments of the nurse's job, according to Mauksch (1981). *Accountability* means being responsible and answerable for the consequences of one's behavior. Certainly it has always characterized nurses' conduct in the administration of drugs. However, it is often lacking in many other areas of nursing practice, such as when nurses acquiesce to institutional rules and dicta that do not represent the client's best interest. Examples of not being accountable are when nurses enforce impersonal restrictions in intensive care units or accept a physician's directive not to respond to a client's inquiry about his or her condition. These behaviors are gradually becoming less common, and they may soon pass out of existence. It is very difficult to act as an interdependent, autonomous professional when one is restricted by regulations that do not permit achievement of full professional behavior.

In child abuse and neglect cases, for example, the nurse faces the concept of accountability head-on. There are many factors to consider if child abuse is suspected. The welfare of the child is foremost. The family's welfare and the future consequences of intervention must be weighed. Past history of the family and possible predictors of future behavior play a role in the assessment process. If a nurse takes the nec-essary legal steps to remove a child from a dangerous or unhealthy situation, she or he must be accountable for that decision. In some states, failure to act for the removal of a child from a situation where child abuse is suspected constitutes breaking the law. Therefore, accountability includes responsibility for decisions to be inactive as well as active.

ANGER AND ASSERTIVENESS

Assertiveness, risk taking, autonomous intervention, accountability . . . these words may sound like a formula for success in community health nursing. However, everyone becomes involved in some situations that generate angry feelings, and dealing with that discomfort is highly relevant to a discussion of assertiveness. Anger and its consequence, dismay, can lead to alienation. Much assertive behavior is a learned response that represents a conscious choice between responding in an angry or aggressive manner or actively avoiding this communication hazard.

Duldt (1982) reports that

anger is a commonplace, yet little investigated, phenomenon, and, by the same token, angry communications occur frequently, yet have not been systematically examined. An exploratory study suggests that any nurse has a fifty-fifty chance of encountering angry communications during a week at work. The study compared the frequency with which a group of 322 registered nurses—mostly staff nurses—received angry messages over a five-day period to the frequency with which 334 non nurses did so. Among the findings were that only one-fourth of the nurses had received no angry communications in that period, half had received up to three, one-sixth had received between four and seven. (p. 168)

How do nurses cope with such angry moments? Open expressions of anger are socially forbidden to women. Lerner has noted (Duldt, 1982) that women have been denied the direct and open expression of even healthy and realistic anger. Men have not been socialized to this same restriction. Women who express anger openly, directly, or loudly are regarded as unladylike, unfeminine, unmaternal, and unattractive. When women engage in angry confrontations, they display a complex cluster of behaviors and emotions: tears, guilt, anxiety, and sadness. Duldt has labeled this set of responses the anger-dismay syndrome. She notes that this response is common when women nurses receive angry messages from colleagues, especially men.

The *anger-dismay syndrome* is defined as being "perplexed, shocked, and at a loss about how to deal with another's angry expressions to the extent that one feels powerless and overwhelmed, tends to cower and cringe, and is unable to change these responses" (Duldt, 1982, p. 170). The syndrome appears when the colleague who is angry has status or power in relation to the other person and is someone whom the dismayed person must deal with in the future. Many people, both men and women, feel uncomfortable when others express anger toward them. However, some people experience such a severe feeling of discomfort that it is debilitating to their accomplishment of personal and professional goals. These people are experiencing the anger-dismay syndrome.

Some of the characteristics of the anger-dismay syndrome are the following:

1) Having a self-image of a dignified, professional person who does not want to behave in an undignified manner in the presence of colleagues and clients; 2) feeling embarrassed, punished and shamed during the encounter; 3) being unable to look at the angry person or to think of what to say during the interaction; 4) feeling a need to apologize, explain, and defend one's own beliefs or behaviors, yet believing none of these responses are appropriate; 5) feeling put down, foolish, perplexed, helpless, and even guilty after the angry encounter; 6) shying away from future encounters with the angry person and limiting contacts to mere necessities in order to complete tasks; 7) describing the angry person thereafter as being ugly, rude, unprofessional, obnoxious, and the like; 8) feeling very distant and cold toward the angry person; 9) believing the angry person to be untrustworthy and questioning his or her credibility professionally; 10) feeling disgust with one's inability to cope more effectively in the "heat of battle"; and 11) being reluctant to verbalize these feelings and beliefs.

(Duldt, 1982, p. 170)

One method of dealing with an angry communication is to apply the basic steps of the nursing process, which is a problem-solving framework. A nurse who receives an angry communication from a patient who is quite ill and in pain would immediately assess the situation and realize that pain prevents one from behaving in a considerate and thoughtful manner. The nurse would assess the frequency, quality, and quantity of pain and plan for nursing measures to intervene and return the client to a healthy level of functioning.

Even in the absence of a physical or biological disruption, someone who is sending an angry communication is still experiencing pain. The most critical tool at the nurse's disposal is to try to be patient, to listen to the message (both verbal and nonverbal), and then to be sensitive to what is really being communicated. This responsiveness will permit the angry person to ventilate pent-up feelings and the nurse to size up the situation. This first phase is developing sensitivity and awareness to alienating messages.

Mothers of young children soon learn that an "I hate you, Mother" message is delivered out of frustration over blocked goals. Children often react with anger and personal attack when told they cannot do something or have something they want. Adults may attack themselves ("Oh, I can't do that") or direct the attack on others ("Why did you make me do that?"). Whether the angry person is an adult or a child, he or she should be perceived as owning the anger and also as being frightened. With this assessment, one can begin to plan an intervention that requires effective interpersonal communication skills. Will reflection be appropriate? "You're obviously feeling very angry about that. . . ." Is confrontation the most effective way to deal with this problem? "We've been working together a long time. Your attacks on me make me feel. . . . Are you willing to listen to how I feel?"

Humor, if appropriate, can be a disarming and engaging way of permitting someone to ventilate angry feelings, frustration, and pain. It usually works best when a certain amount of trust has been built up. "Did you take too many angry pills today?" Such messages are not delivered to someone in an authority position (teacher, boss, supervisor) but are frequently effective with peers. The style in which any responsive message is delivered conveys whether a person can be trusted to respect another's angry feelings. A well-chosen response encourages communication and preserves the self-concepts of those involved.

Since anger is a consequence of some interactions, what then can community health nurses do to deal with their own anger? First, they can recognize that they are entitled to their anger and that feeling angry is healthy and natural. They can begin to try to submerge the guilt and anxiety that most people have learned from childhood. They can learn to express anger in a healthy manner, as well as learn a new way of coping with the pattern of shock, fear, anger, hurt, sadness, and anxiety evoked by angry encounters. Second, women especially need to recognize other people's anger in order to avoid being the victims of the anger-dismay syndrome. They should learn how to communicate in a manner that will promote cohesive interpersonal relationships and self-confidence rather than alienation and distrust when they face angry people. To be less than assertive with an angry person is to be, in essence, inert.

FOSTERING ASSERTIVENESS

Nursing education must bear some of the responsibility for the nonassertive nurse. Selfless denial, humility, service, and reliance on those in authority have been part of the education of nurses over the years, as has fear of making incorrect decisions. The accountability concept is relatively new to nursing education. If the faculty of schools of nursing and other experienced nurses are teaching students to become dependent, how then can new nurses transmit values of independence, self-care, and autonomous behavior to their clients? Nurses need to examine themselves and nursing education to be sure that they are not transmitting negative values. The transition from dependent student to graduate nurse has been described as traumatic (Kramer, 1974). Nursing education has not been noted for the development of independent and fearless thinkers. In the future, as nursing moves toward expanded roles and more responsibility in client care management and health care delivery, nurses must become aware of the need for assertiveness.

How does one teach the new desired behavior? Short workshops or small-group sessions are one way of teaching assertiveness that can be tailored to meet the needs of nurses or of clients. The goal might be to expunge unwanted behavior that has been learned through experience. Unwanted behavior can be extinguished and new, more adaptive behavior can be substituted.

Behavioral theory focuses on what can be done in the present to change undesirable behaviors, since behaviors are easier to change than attitudes and feelings. Once behavior becomes assertive, the response from others is often favorable and the newly assertive person experiences enhanced self-esteem. This leads to further assertion; thus a positive cycle is established. Assertive behavior tends to be self-rewarding, so that even if agreeable responses do not always result from an assertive exchange, the assertive individual still feels better about herself or himself.

FUTURE IMPLICATIONS

Perhaps one of the consequences in the next 20 to 30 years for nurses who learn assertiveness will be the following leadership activities: (1) More nurses will become involved in active policy making in administration. They will become confident of their own ability and self-worth and of their own opinions and beliefs. (2) Nurses will become better trained in organizational development. They will understand how to propose and implement change processes both within hospitals and in ambulatory care settings as well as in the community with groups and with organizations. (3) Nurses will become acknowledged as key primary care health practitioners within certain health care settings. Their skills will become incorporated as the basic professional skills that will be taught in the future in all educational programs for professional nurses. (4) Technical skills to accompany nursing will involve strategic planning, financial analysis, and marketing. Nurses will become confident of their business and management skills. They will become engaged in evaluative research so that they can measure patient outcomes and make statements about the value and role of professional nursing care. (5) Issues will be discussed on the basis of their merits rather than being sex-role focused. (6) Nursing will become egalitarian.

Community nurse leaders will adapt to what may become the most popular leadership style, participative leadership. Leaders have been strongly urged to include their followers in the decision-making process. Yet many leaders and theorists who support this style differ about what it really means. Some individuals believe that "participatory leadership" refers to mutual goal setting. This is certainly important when one is dealing with families in the community. Others believe that it implies listening more and speaking less. Some writers distinguish between democratic and participative leaders by saying that democratic leaders allow the group to have final authority in decision making, whereas participative leaders retain decision-making authority while seeking input in the process. Participative leadership does not imply majority rule.

The attempt of leaders to be democratic while still maintaining authority and control has produced considerable conflict for them. This same problem is faced by many executives today. Since there are many factors related to the leader, the group, and the situation that affect the leader's style, a single best style for leading is unlikely to be found. Instead, effective leaders seem to be those whose style is contingent on the interaction of leader, group, and situation. For example, although the autocratic leadership style is not always the most effective, emergency situations do call for an autocratic approach. Such an instance requires the expertise of the leader and his or her control of resources in order to provide the most efficient solutions. Other circumstances, such as goal setting and program planning, call for active participation such as is encouraged by a democratic approach. A challenge for the future will be to increase the knowledge and ability of nurses in selecting and using contingency approaches to leadership.

Throughout this discussion, the concepts of assertiveness and leadership have been integrated as they affect the work of the community health nurse. In considering assertiveness, one must take into account varying personalities and situations. Internal and external forces operate both on persons and on situations. In addition to their sex roles and work role focus, nurses must also take into consideration individual versus group norms. Assertiveness is clearly one vital component of leadership. Without assertiveness, there is no leadership.

With the professionalization of nursing, more men are coming into the profession of nursing, and this promotes male–female integration. Nurses are pursuing higher degrees in education, and there is a greater acceptance of professional nurses in the health care system. With current changes in the health care billing structure and the movement toward third-party payment, nurses are gaining acceptance as true professionals who have something to offer in the health care system.

There are now new relationships between nurses and physicians, as Mauksch (1981) has so eloquently stated. Because of the liberation of the 1960s and the realignment of rules and attitudes for women, there are significant changes in today's nurse and tomorrow's future-oriented practitioner. There will be a newly discovered sense of professionalism in tomorrow's practitioners. More than ever, there will be a realization that medical care is only a part of health and illness care. Today's nurse affirms that nursing care is an equal partner to medical care, social work, and the work of other professionals. Tomorrow's nurse must shift from a unilateral power base to a bilateral power base. Nurses are moving from situations in which they were dependent on physicians into situations that offer considerable autonomy in decision making (Mauksch, 1981).

Schlotfeldt states that "leadership requires enough courage and faith in the ability to build a better future, to take reasonable risks, and to go in advance of those who are being led" (Moloney, 1979, p. 6). Nurses who practice in the community have long been leaders in the health care delivery system. These are the nurses who provided adequate housing for the poor, who immunized people, who fought for adequate nutrition for women and children, and who made childbirth safer. Nurses helped to establish safety in hospitals, compassion in nursing homes, and variety in birthing centers. The nurses of the future not only will learn and practice assertiveness and leadership in their own professional lives but also will transmit this skill to the clients they serve. Assertive nurses will promote health care delivery in the community through self-care and through client autonomy and participation and will mitigate the dependency that exists in our medicocentric health care delivery system. The society will evolve into one in which the client is responsible and accountable for his or her own health care.

Community health nurses have long been the assertive leaders who have helped improve and transform society. Let us feel confident of our ability to contribute greatly to an improved health care system and to a better and more humane world.

DISCUSSION TOPICS

1. Darrell Marks is a school nurse in a small district. A child has come to school

with a syringe, a needle, and an unmarked vial. A note with these materials from the child's parent states that this is an "allergy shot" and would the nurse please administer it to the child. The nurse attempts to contact the mother and the child's physician and is unable to do so. He goes to the principal and describes the situation and informs the principal that he will not give the injection because he cannot personally identify the drug or verify that it was prescribed for the child. The principal orders Mr. Marks to give the injection. Describe what Mr. Marks could say to the principal to clarify his role as a nurse assertively.

2. The situation described above happened to Donna Cowles. When she refused to follow the principal's demand that she give the injection, the principal got angry and said, "You stupid woman. Don't you know nurses who want your job are a dime a dozen? You do what I say or you can look for another job!" How could Ms. Cowles respond assertively?

3. Do you recognize assertiveness in certain fellow students? In certain teachers? What do they do particularly that makes you aware of their ability to be assertive? What kinds of feelings and emotions do you experience after an assertive rather than a passive or aggressive interaction?

4. Describe one way to do each of the following assertively:

a. Change your mind.

b. Refuse to offer reasons for your behavior.

c. Acknowledge a mistake.

d. Admit ignorance about something.

5. Keep a log for a week of social and professional interactions. Note the times you are passive when you want to be assertive. Note the times you are too aggressive. Describe your first conscious attempt at shaping assertive behavior and the style that you use. Ask yourself how you can incorporate humor into your assertiveness style. How are you able to refuse requests, change your mind, make a mistake, and admit ignorance of something without feeling guilty? This exercise is planned to look to the future and does not ask you to analyze past behavior.

6. Describe an assertive response to a discussion that is trashing an individual.

7. What leadership qualities and behaviors do you currently possess?

8. What are your personal and professional goals for community health nursing? How will assertiveness and leadership qualities contribute to achieving those goals?

9. Describe how you would present a workshop or class to help people:

a. Become more assertive rather than passive or aggressive.

b. Speak out for their own needs.

c. Achieve what they need without violating the rights of others.

d. Refuse requests from others without feeling guilty.

10. How will health care professionals be affected as consumers become more assertive?

BIBLIOGRAPHY

Baumgart, A.J.: Nursing for a new century: A future framework. *International Nursing Review* 28(5), 139, 142, 153, 1981.

Bennis, W.G.: New patterns for leadership of tomorrow's organizations. In S. Stone, M.S. Berger, D. Elhart, S.C. Firsich, & S.B. Jordan,

Management for nurses: A multidisciplinary approach. St. Louis: Mosby, 1976.

Burke, S.: Sheila Burke urges students to be activists. *American Nurse* 13(9), 4, 8, 1981.

Davidson, R.D.: The future of home health agencies. *Journal of Community Health* 4(1), 55–66, 1978.

Diers, D.: Lessons on leadership. *Image* 11(3), 67–71, 1979.

Donnelly, G.F.: The assertive nurse. *Nursing '78* 8, 65–69, 1978.

Donnelly, G.F.: Assertiveness workbook: How to take your assertiveness home. *R.N.* 42(8), 33–35, 1979.

Donnelly, G.F.: Assertiveness workbook: When it's best not to assert. *R.N.* 42(9), 48–51, 1979.

Donnelly, G.F.: Assertiveness workbook: "You're right, I'm not all that terrific." *R.N.* 42(6), 40–43, 1979.

Donnelly, G.F.: The insubordination game. *R.N.* 43(4), 58–60, 1980.

Duldt, B.W.: Helping nurses to cope with the anger-dismay syndrome. *Nursing Outlook* 30(3), 168–174, 1982.

Edmunds, M.: Non-clinical problems: Assertiveness skills. *Nurse Practitioner* 6(6), 27–31, 39, 1981.

Ferguson, M.: *The aquarian conspiracy.* Los Angeles: J.P. Tarcher, 1980.

Gluck, M., & Charter, R.: Personal qualities of nurses implying need for continuing education to increase interpersonal and leadership effectiveness. *Journal of Continuing Education in Nursing* 2(4), 29–36, 1980.

Greenlaw, J.: Can you be fired for speaking out? *R.N.* 45(8), 71–72, 1982.

Hamm, B.H., & Brodt, D.: Guts: Teaching assertiveness skills by simulation and gaming. *Nursing Research* 31(4), 246–247, 1982.

Hutchings, H., & Colburn, L.: An assertiveness training program for nurses. *Nursing Outlook* 27(6), 394–397, 1979.

Keeler, J.D.: *The future mission of community nursing.* New York: NLN, 1979.

Kramer, M.: *Reality shock: Why nurses leave nursing.* St. Louis: Mosby, 1974.

Mauksch, I.G.: Nurse–physician collaboration: A changing relationship. *Journal of Nursing Administration* 11(6), 35–38, 1981.

Marriner, A.: Action strategies for the 1980's: Overview of current nursing administration issues. *Nursing Leadership* 5(2), 27–33, 1982.

Migut, P.J.: Self-care for nurses: Assertiveness. *Nurse Manager* 13(2), 13–14, 1982.

Moloney, M.M.: *Leadership in nursing: Theory, strategies, action.* St. Louis: Mosby, 1979.

Palmer, M.E., & Deck, E.S.: Teaching assertiveness to seniors. *Nursing Outlook* 29(5), 305–310, 1981.

Toffler, A.: Reflection on the third wave. *National Forum* 61(3), 3–6, 1981.

Whitman, M.: Toward a new psychology for nurses. *Nursing Outlook* 30(1), 48–52, 1982.

Wilson, H.S., & Kneisl, C.R.: *Psychiatric nursing.* Menlo Park, Calif.: Addison-Wesley, 1979.

Ethical Practice

Myrtle P. Matejski

Man is an animal with primary instincts of survival. Consequently, his ingenuity has developed first and his soul afterwards. Thus, the progress of science is far ahead of man's ethical behavior.

CHARLIE CHAPLIN / *My Autobiography*

OBJECTIVES

After reading this chapter, you should be able to:

☐ Define ethics, moral responsibility, and values.
☐ Explain deontological and utilitarian ethical concepts as a basis for selected nursing activities.
☐ Analyze the impact of selected ethical concepts on nursing functions in the community.
☐ Explain the effect of ethical concepts on community health problems.

INTRODUCTION

Most people today recognize that changes are occurring more rapidly than at any time in history. Further, there appears to be little time to prepare for the swift tide of change that engulfs us. Nowhere is this more true than in matters concerning medical and health care.

Science, technology, and research have resulted in the development of machines and surgical techniques that enable health care providers to preserve and extend life beyond what was once thought possible; fetal surgery has been successfully performed. The result is that infants and others now survive health problems and accidents that formerly would have been fatal.

The development of renal dialysis equipment enables many people with renal failure to dialyze themselves at home, allowing them increased personal freedom and more normal lives. Improvements in communication allow both health care recipient and provider to have almost immediate access to new therapies for illness and methods of illness prevention.

Accompanying the new knowledge and skills are new human concerns that until now required little consideration. Some people who are receiving renal dialysis question the quality of their lives. People ask if health care professionals ought to extend life. Clients ask about the extent of their moral responsibilities for the care of family members. To improve their ability to resolve these conflicts, new members— psychologists, sociologists, and ethicists— have been added to the health team.

Community health nurses are often in the forefront of change as they analyze factors that create health problems in a community and identify methods of resolving them. Added to these challenges are the economic realities of the 1980s. Increased unemployment means that fewer people are able to afford health care, and thus it can be hypothesized that unidentified health care needs exist. With less financial support from federal and state governments, health care providers, including nurses, have to set criteria for deciding who will receive health care. This requires using principles of ethics. The purpose of this chapter is to provide nurses in the community with tools for making ethical and moral decisions as they work with the complex maze of care providers and client health problems.

HISTORICAL BACKGROUND

For much of the early twentieth century, health care was directed by physicians, with nurses (usually students) providing most of the care, usually in a hospital. Although health care was viewed as a valued resource and an indicator of individual and social well-being, the emphasis was on cure and medical care. Patients, who were often viewed as helpless, remained in hospitals for prolonged periods of time. When the physician finally discharged them, patients of the middle and upper socioeconomic classes were frequently accompanied to their homes by private duty nurses, usually ones recommended by the physician.

Trained nurses (people who received instruction from nurses and doctors in hospital schools of nursing) gradually entered industry as industrial nurses; some became school nurses; others went to work in voluntary and nonvoluntary public health agencies; still others performed home health nursing paid for by the client's insurance company.

Overall the health care delivery system mirrored, for the most part, the fundamental socioeconomic divisions in American society. While health care problems received attention in 1930s through the 1950s, it was not until the 1960s that public attention was focused on access to health care and equity in quality of care (Reversby & Rosner, 1979).

Health care now is increasingly perceived by the public as a right, and with this perception has emerged a number of ethical issues concerning public health policies—who should pay for care and to what extent. To meet the health needs of the poor and the underclasses, neighborhood health care centers were established, funded largely by federal and state governments. This extended health care benefits to a wide clientele (Reversby & Rosner, 1979). Community health nurses, working in these settings, often found it necessary to acquire new methods of health assessment and an increased knowledge of the public policies that affected health care agencies and their public.

There were other challenges as well.

Feminist leaders declared that the medical profession was sexist. They questioned the overmedicalization of women, contending that such treatment perpetuated the dependency role of women (Ehrenreich & Ehrenreich, 1975). Others questioned the effectiveness of medical and health care generally in reducing mortality and morbidity (Carlson, 1975; Fuchs, 1974; Illich, 1975). These and other events have encouraged people concerned with health and health care issues to reconsider methods of treating clients. Health is a complex personal matter that involves values, customs, and attitudes toward personal responsibility. Nurses, and especially community health nurses, with their emphasis on prevention and concern for the social and environmental factors that influence health, have a particularly important contribution to make.

The current state of the American economy has altered public support for health care agencies. The closing of many neighborhood health care centers, increased unemployment, and economic uncertainty have resulted in a rising demand for fewer available services. Meeting consumer health care needs now and in the decade ahead will require that community health nurses increase their health-promotion and illness-prevention activities. The community health nursing field, then, seems likely to expand, especially given the reluctance of physicians to work in rural or low-income areas. Accompanying this expansion of role are issues of accountability, moral responsibility, and the factors influencing nursing decisions. Studying ethics expands nurses' understanding of the value systems and moral positions of people who enter the health care system and thus increases their awareness of the humanness of nursing.

There are no perfect solutions to the problems community health nurses can ex-

pect to encounter when confronted with consumer demands and expectations on the one hand and fiscal constraints on the other. However, approaching issues and solutions based on ethical and moral choices provides a foundation for solving many difficult problems.

WHAT IS AN ETHICAL DILEMMA?

Community health nurses work with families in community agencies to promote and maintain the health of the people living in a specific geographic area. They accomplish their task by assessing, diagnosing, treating, and evaluating the health care needs of the people they serve. Thus the scope of their activities is broad, including health teaching; planning and promoting well-child clinics; providing follow-up care for the elderly and others discharged from acute care facilities; identifying predisposing, enabling, and reinforcing factors that create health problems; and promoting change where necessary (Green, Kreuter, Deeds, & Partridge, 1980). They may be expected to teach family planning and diet planning and to assume a large share of responsibility for instructing families about immunization and self-care. Community health nurses, then, are expected to assume responsibility for solving health problems efficiently, effectively, and ethically.

The following four situations, which present common community problems, will be used throughout this chapter to illustrate ethical problems and solutions.

SITUATION 1

A community health nurse employed in a health care agency has been assigned to work with a family that includes a husband and wife, two normal children ages 2 and 4, one severely retarded child age 5, and the husband's 75-year-old mother. When the nurse visits the family unit, the parents complain of the stress of caring for the retarded child and the elderly parent, who, they fear, is becoming senile. They also are worried about the two normal children suffering because of their limited time for the total family unit. The parents ask the nurse if placing the retarded child in an institution would be the best solution to the problem. What would the nurse do in a similar situation, they want to know. How should the nurse reply? What ethical concepts might influence the reply?

SITUATION 2

A 13-year-old girl, complaining of nausea and vomiting, reports to the school health nurse. Upon examination the nurse finds the girl to be 20 weeks pregnant. The student says that her parents want her to have an abortion, but she does not want one. What is the nurse's responsibility? What is the nurse's moral obligation to the teenager? To her parents?

SITUATION 3

A new set of laws has been passed that will eliminate federal funding for a local health care agency that provides services for 1,000 families residing in a slum area. The state legislature decides to reduce funding also. As a result, many services will have to be eliminated. Given the health problems common to slum areas and the overall economy, does the community health nurse have any ethical or moral responsibility to those likely to be affected by the decision? If so, on what is that responsibility based? If the nurse is involved in making the decision about what services to eliminate, what ethical considerations should he or she use in determining what services to eliminate?

SITUATION 4

A health clinic in a rural area is scheduled to close because it provides services to only 500 families. The nearest facility is 200 miles away, and there is no public transportation. What is the professional responsibility of the community health nurse in ensuring access to health care? Is this an ethical issue? If it is, what are the nurse's moral obligations? What factors must the nurse consider?

WHAT IS ETHICS?

Ethics has been defined variously as a science of whole man (Bahm, 1974), a branch of philosophy concerned with what is good and bad, and a study of principles of conduct (Moore, 1944). It involves a systematic examination of moral life and conduct that enables people to establish principles to guide behavior (Hill, 1976; Moore, 1944). As a branch of philosophy, ethics is often referred to as moral philosophy. Ethics is concerned with what ought to be (Ladd, 1978). Ethics encourages one to "feel" and to "consider our own personal well being, that of others and of human society as a whole" (Hill, 1976). It demands that people examine and reexamine their judgments and actions. Ethical principles ask nurses to examine the whys of a moral code. What ought one do in a given situation? Aristotle insisted that if one understood the qualities and distinctive functions of human nature, one would know what is good. Presumably then, if a nurse has studied those sciences that explain human behavior (philosophy, psychology, and sociology, for example), there is little need to explore or discuss ethics. Yet increasingly, nurses are faced with situations that require them to take a moral position and to make decisions based on concepts of rights, obligations, and accountability. Frequently nurses find themselves faced with values, beliefs, and moral stances that vary considerably from their own. To respond appropriately in such situations requires one to realize one's own ethics and concept of moral values as well as the values, beliefs, and ethics of others.

Ethics can be differentiated into two categories: normative and nonnormative. *Normative ethics* investigates and analyzes issues according to what one ought to do or how one ought to behave (Dyck, 1977); thus normative ethics asks people to identify moral standards. It provides them with a plausible understanding of moral standards (Dyck, 1977, p. 52) and with enduring rules.

"Ought" questions arise from conflicts between what people want, desire, need or prefer, and what is morally right. In the problem described in Situation 1, for example, the family includes three young children, each with particular needs, wants, and desires; an elderly parent with special needs and demands of her own; and the strain of a mother and father attempting to meet family needs as well as personal needs. How ought they to solve the problems, given the nature of the conflicts? What solutions are best for all family members?

Nonnormative approaches to moral problems involve descriptive ethics and metaethics. *Descriptive ethics* is concerned with investigating moral behavior, beliefs, attitudes, and codes in different societies (Beauchamp & Childress, 1979). The nurse who investigates different beliefs concerning the care of elderly parents, or codes that dictate the treatment of children in the family unit, is involved with descriptive ethics.

Metaethics involves analyzing the meaning of ethical terms such as "right," "obligation," and "responsibility" (Beauchamp & Childress, 1979). Metaethics is also concerned with the logic of moral reasoning and includes "the nature of moral justification" (p. 8). It would be appropriate to analyze Situation 2 from this perspective. Using metaethics, one would address the obligations and responsibilities of the 13-year-old girl to herself, to the fetus, and to her parents, and the logic of moral reasoning that would dictate either continuing the pregnancy or aborting it.

Both descriptive ethics and metaethics attempt to address each situation according to "what is the case": what are the real-

ities of the situation. For the teenager, the questions to be asked are: What is the case with respect to her pregnancy, to herself, and to the life of the fetus? Does she view life as the final value upon which all other values depend? The answer to these questions would clarify what she sees as her responsibility concerning fetal life and the course she will pursue. Nonnormative ethics (descriptive ethics and metaethics) is concerned with what one ought to do and obviously must be considered in discussing ethical solutions to human problems. Nurses ought to be aware of their clients' values of how clients' beliefs concerning family obligations and social constraints affect concepts of health care if they are to provide nursing care that demonstrates respect for human dignity and uniqueness (Dilday, 1978, pp. 10–17).

From the four situations described earlier in the chapter, it can be assumed that nurses must make moral judgments. *Judgments* are decisions, verdicts, or conclusions concerning what one ought or ought not to do in given situations. The decisions are justified by moral rules grounded in principles (Beauchamp & Childress, 1979) or general and fundamental rules concerning moral conduct. In Situation 1, the young couple needs principles to guide them in deciding how to resolve their problems. The nurse needs a knowledge of basic ethical theories (bodies of principles) as a guide in making judgments concerning his or her obligation to the family. *Moral judgments*, then, involve applying ethics (principles) as action guides to concrete situations (Beauchamp & Childress, 1979; Frankena, 1973).

General Rules and Ethics

Rules exist both to guide one's actions and to provide a basis for evaluating the action of others (Solomon, 1978). Rules vary in their force of restrictions, regulations, permissions, or prescriptions (Solomon, 1978). Rules are usually established to ensure the efficient achievement of goals. A decision to close a health care facility is a type of rule. Such a rule can be said to achieve a goal of lowering the cost of health care to the community. However, closing the facility may deny health care to a large segment of the community. Closing a health care facility may also cause people to delay seeking health care until the health problem becomes critical. The result is higher cost to both the individual and to the community. In determining the effect of closing the health care facility, then, one must deal with ultimate results as well as the moral issues of reduced health services. This involves investigating the parameters of the rule as a goal for action.

Ethical Theories and Moral Rules

Ethical theories provide a framework that enables people to determine morally appropriate rules of behavior. There are two major classifications of ethical theories: deontological and teleological or utilitarian theories. For deontological theories there are four basic paradigms: those of Hebrew-Christian theology, the theories of the philosopher Immanual Kant, intuitionists, and contract theorists.

DEONTOLOGICAL THEORIES. The Hebrew-Christian paradigm, the oldest of the group, conceives of the ideal life as one of obedience to God's Will or to a rule or rules that express that Will. Basic to this paradigm is the notion that what one wishes may differ considerably from what is right. However, what is right is that which has been commanded by God and must be obeyed. "Honor thy father and mother" (Exodus 20:12) is a rule that would dictate to the husband and wife in Situation 1 that they must care for the elderly parent. The rule

"Thou shalt not kill" (Exodus 20:13) prohibits compromise so far as killing is concerned. In the situation concerning the pregnant 13-year-old girl, if the girl, the nurse, or the physician accepts the position that the fetus is a human being, and if they oppose killing based on Hebrew-Christian ethics, the rule would preclude participating in abortion.

The New Testament rule that "thou shalt love thy neighbor as thy self" (Matthew 22:38) could, in a broader interpretation, mean that in loving oneself one would desire access to adequate health care; therefore, if one is commanded to love one's neighbor as oneself one would strive to assure that the "neighbors" in Situation 3 have access to health care. The community health nurse, confronted with the removal of health care from a neighborhood, would feel a sense of moral obligation at least to act as a client advocate by trying to change the decision or to locate an alternate source of health care.

The second paradigm, that of Immanual Kant, demands that morality always override other reasons for doing or not doing something (Solomon, 1979). Thus it is duty that decides if an act has moral value. Imperatives of duty (categorical imperatives) must override hypothetical imperatives; that is, people are obligated to submit to duty regardless of their wishes. The husband and wife in Situation 1 would see their duty to their children, parent, and each other as overriding all other imperatives. A nurse who perceives her basic duties as promoting, attaining, and maintaining client health, or ensuring equality of access to care, would do whatever seemed essential to ensure that community citizens in Situation 4 would have health care facilities available. In many aspects, Kant's ethical concepts are similar or parallel to the Hebrew-Christian paradigm.

A major component of Kant's categorical

imperative is that it must be possible to subject the duty to universal law; that is, the duty must hold in all circumstances regardless of human desires. A perceived duty to sustain life would be extended to include all life.

Yet another important feature of Kant's theory is that for people to have a "good life" they must follow moral commitments to others. Thus, if a promise is made, it must be kept. Other significant precepts include the idea that a person should be regarded as an end in himself or herself and not as a means to an end; and all people should have a life in which individual rights, freedom, self-respect, justice, and dignity are maintained (Solomon, 1979).

In Situation 2, one can interpret a moral responsibility in various ways. Faced with a 13-year-old girl who does not wish an abortion and her parents who demand she have one, the nurse who follows Kant's principles has to ask if the ends (aborting the fetus) are justified. Whose ends are being served—the young girl's or her parents'? Whose rights are involved in this situation? Is it just to deny certain rights (the rights of the girl to have the baby and the right of the fetus to life) while granting rights to others (the rights of parental authority over a young teenage daughter)? What is just? While one may argue that Kant's absolute rule does not solve a problem, it does force the nurse to consider important facets of a problem, such as rights and autonomy.

The intuitionists determine the moral rightness or wrongness of an act based on the intrinsic nature of the act. That is, they maintain that one must first consider all the factors that go into making the decision, the "right/wrong-making properties" of the act, and then determine the weights of the right- or wrong-making properties in order to establish the final duty. A nurse who adheres to this third paradigm in Situation 2 would assess the situation in terms of the age of the girl, her physical and emotional state, her socioeconomic status, and her potential support system in this time of need. Likewise, the nurse would have to conduct a total family assessment, including the possible status of the fetus. Included in the assessment would be the issue of rights.

Contract theories are the fourth group of deontological theories. Classical contract theory, as established in the seventeenth and eighteenth centuries by Hobbes, Locke, and Rousseau, was a political concept concerned with how society was bound together by rules (Thompson & Thompson, 1981). The social contract was viewed as an agreement among men, written or unwritten, whereby people renounced the right to do whatever pleased them in favor of an ordered social organization. It bound together citizens as a group and established agreement between them and a governmental agency. However, recent theorists maintain that there are certain irreducible moral principles that must be considered before deciding what ought to be done. These principles are fidelity, beneficence, and justice (Ross, 1970). In determining how to regulate society, people must find the greatest balance of right over wrong. Other ethicists, such as Rawls, maintain that one must address the principles of justice, balancing the values of freedom, autonomy, rights, dignity, and self-respect and the distribution of goods. (Rawls, 1971; Baier, 1978a).

In situations 3 and 4, a nurse adhering to the principles of the social contract would have to weight all elements—dignity, autonomy, freedom of the members of the community, their desire for health care, as well as principles of justice—before determining what course should be taken or what commitment ought to be made to the communities. A question that must be addressed is: what was the contract between the community, the health care facility, and the government?

TELEOLOGICAL OR UTILITARIAN THEORIES. *Utilitarian theory* is associated with the nineteenth century English philosopher John Stuart Mill. It rests primarily on the belief that the right act will bring about the greatest happiness or good for the greatest number; it will result in the best balance of value over disvalue for all persons involved in a situation (Beauchamp & Childress, 1979). Utilitarian theory provides a moral rule or principle that can be accepted without exceptions (Dyck, 1977). Utilitarian theory can be used to decide on a course of action when one is faced with a conflict, such as who should receive health care; it demands that one assess the end result of an act, since results are used to gauge the worth of an action. For example, community health nurses would generally agree that health is good in itself and is necessary to enable people in a community to lead happy, productive lives. Following this belief to its seemingly logical conclusion, then, nurses who practice utilitarian ethics and who are confronted with situations such as the withdrawal of funds to support a health care agency would have to gauge the results of closing the health care centers against health as a value to determine actions to be taken. The principles of utility also include other elements, such as ultimate cost and autonomy, both of which must be included in making an ethical decision.

It now should be apparent that there are few clear-cut distinctions between the two major groups of ethical theories. Therefore, it is important to consider elements of both sets of theories. In including dignity, self-worth, freedom, and autonomy as ethical imperatives, one must address the attitudes of a given society concerning norms, morals, and values. For as social creatures, people conform to the rules and values that their particular culture has determined are moral, and they are influenced by the behavior of other members of their culture, whether the behavior is moral or not.

Morals and Values

Morals are personal rules of conduct. They are reflected in the activities and institutions that societies use to preserve and enhance social order and welfare. They are reflected in each individual's ideas of what is right or wrong, just or unjust. Moral theories serve to guide people to action, enabling them to deal with conflict and to adjust to new knowledge and change as they occur.

Values are the traditional institutions and ideals of a society. Since values generally influence the rules that shape people's behavior, they tend to reflect the ethics and moral dimensions of a society.

However, values change as situations and social conditions change. Furthermore, not all values are equal—some are more important than others. For example, the community health nurse may value teaching prevention of illness or accidents. If people pay a fee to learn about illness prevention, they convey the message that health is important to them. This reinforces the nurse's perception that health is a value. If the nurse and the community share health as a value, the nurse might feel a moral obligation to confront the decision makers if they planned to close a rural health care facility or eliminate services in an urban area.

Both nurse and community might agree that health care is a right. But what is a right? A *right* is something that everyone in a society agrees that everyone should have. Rights also contribute to guidelines for moral activity and provide a framework for resolving disputes (Churchill and Simán, 1982). Rights are based on an individual's sense of self and "indicate the need for a sense of morality in which individual rights and social obligations are seen as mutually critical" (Churchill and Simán, 1982, p. 11). Personal rights and social rights are interdependent. Rights, then, designate relationships among people and relate to both duties and obligations.

In the situation involving the pregnant teenager, one must ask: Does the girl have individual rights? What are her parents' rights? If the young girl bears her child, she has the moral obligation to care for it. In our society, the infant has a right to be cared for. Both mother and child, as members of our society, have a right to expect society to provide the resources to maintain and support them, especially if they reside in an area where laws prevent abortion.

Where health care is deemed a right, both the individual and society share a mutual responsibility to ensure citizens' access to health care. If health care is perceived as a value by the community, the community health nurse has a responsibility to assess the knowledge, attitudes, and beliefs of community members concerning health problems. The nurse needs to identify the base of support, determine the existence of resources and skills for providing health care, and develop a plan to make optimal use of available resources, such as people and money.

Where the nurse is confronted with the family problems described in Situation 1, many rights must be addressed: the right of the retarded child to have loving care, the rights of the two normal children to attention and parental concern for their human needs, the right of an elderly parent to comfort and love, as well as the rights of the young couple for some time for themselves. These rights are not exclusive of society's rights or of the right of the nurse to suggest assistance to the family. The nurse has a moral right to help the young couple realize their personal rights. The nurse might locate a day care center for the elderly and find someone to care for the retarded child, thus enabling the parents to spend time together and with their two normal children. Responsibility, then, entails identifying values, rights, and needs of people.

Autonomy as a Moral Value

Concepts of autonomy are basic to both Kant's and Mill's philosophy and embody both individual will and action. *Autonomy* is freedom to govern oneself and to make choices according to one's own moral principles.

Concepts of autonomy are an important consideration for health care providers. The fact that a client comes to a clinic seeking health care is itself an autonomous act. The young girl in Situation 2 approached the school nurse autonomously. Likewise, the parents in Situation 1 autonomously requested guidance in solving their particular problem. Inherent in these situations, then, is autonomy as a value. The young girl might have approached the nurse because, in her view, "nurse" means someone who is an authority and also someone who is compassionate and understanding. The parents of the retarded child may view the nurse as an equal and also as someone who has special knowledge and skills. While the nurse and the people involved in each of these situations may not share the same moral and ethical values, it is important that the nurse recognize each client as an autonomous agent. As such, the values of each person are equally important. If one accepts Kant's view that each person has inherent worth, then everyone's values and opinions must be respected. Although a client may ask for advice or an opinion, the nurse must recognize that the ultimate decision is the client's.

Quite clearly, then, the nurse's moral obligation includes recognizing and respecting client values, including the client's self-value. If the young couple, for instance, concludes that placing the retarded child in an institution is in the best interests of the family, the nurse's responsibility to assist in this process is well-defined. The nurse has an obligation to assess the situation, to determine when an activity is beneficial (promoting client well-being) and when it is nonmaleficent (inflicting no harm). The nurse has an obligation to be certain that the parents understand the nature of their consent to institutionalize their child. This includes assurance that the parents understand any consent form they must sign. The same obligation holds should the couple ultimately decide to place the elderly parent in a nursing home.

Ethics and Cost/Benefit Analysis

So far the issues discussed have not considered the economics of health care problems. Yet clearly the issue of cost must be addressed. While in each of the situations described here cost is an issue, probably it is most important in the two situations that involve closing facilities and curtailing health services. At issue is cost or risk/benefit analysis as a means of establishing priorities and determining what services to eliminate or reduce.

Utilitarian ethics defines *cost* as the risk or possible future harm that might be caused by a particular act. A *benefit* is something of positive value, and since this chapter is concerned with health and health care, a benefit would be construed as something that promotes health and welfare. When tied to the principle of utility, costs and benefits must be weighed against issues of risk or harm and the greatest possible benefits (Beauchamp & Childress, 1979). The principle assumes that in weighing these values one is obliged to determine the balance of benefits against any possible harm. This does not mean that one ought to sacrifice the rights of one person to the interest of the community, for one must keep in mind the principles of autonomy and justice. When one is faced with complex problems and conflicting solutions, the principles of cost and benefit must be considered both for the overall good of a community and for individual families.

When discussing health care issues, the term "cost" is here interpreted as something that detracts from health and welfare. A "risk" refers to possible harm that may result from a given activity. For example, in Situation 4, closing a rural health center, there is a cost in terms of withdrawing a valued resource from the community. The withdrawal takes away or detracts from the health and welfare of individual community members. There is also a risk that the loss of a health-promoting facility could jeopardize the lives of residents.

In Situation 3, discontinuing health care service in a slum area, there is a cost: a lowering of the overall community health and welfare. The extent of the cost depends largely upon the extent to which the lost services were perceived to benefit members of the community. If the agency staff members are left to determine what services to cut, they may be able to minimize or avoid potential harm. For example, if the largest population served by the agency in Situation 3 is comprised of adolescents and young adults, the community might determine to use available funds for family planning services or to support mental health personnel. Similarly, if the agency's clients were predominantly elderly people, using funds to support activities important to the elderly and eliminating or restricting family planning funds would be the logical course. Obviously, the community health nurse's knowledge of the community in question, the prevalence of health problems, and the factors contributing to these problems are important factors in the decision. Also, the nurse's knowledge of the attitudes, beliefs, and values of the community would be invaluable aids in deciding what costs to cut. The nurse's knowledge of community members' feelings about health would be useful tools to use in opposing cuts in funding for care facilities. Since personal values are inseparably linked with choice of behavior, any information the nurse can obtain to support the thesis that health is a value in the community might help fight the decrease in agency services.

Risk/Benefit Analysis

Another element in decision making is risk to the community. The nurse must identify the population most at risk when services are curtailed and determine the nature of the risks involved. Obviously, where there are diminished services, efforts must be made to achieve a maximum balance of costs, risks, and benefits. The skill with which the nurse as health care provider can accurately assess the community and eliminate problems of overuse or underuse of facilities is critical to improving agency utilization and assuring equitable care to the families and individuals served. Ethics, then, demands that the nurse in Situation 3 assess the risks of curtailed services to the community.

Risk/benefit analysis is also important when the nurse works with individual families. In dealing with the family in Situation

1, for example, the community health nurse has a responsibility to help the parents assess the possible harm or benefit to the other two children as they work with the severely retarded child. Does having a handicapped sibling make the other children more compassionate and understanding? Is there a risk that as the children become older they will feel ostracized from friends or unable to have friends visit the home? Does the continued presence of the retarded child limit a healthy development of self-concept? How much benefit is there to the retarded child who is kept in the home? Do all the benefits balance the risks? These and many other questions concerning costs, risks, and benefits must be addressed. The nurse must explore all facets with the parents to ensure that justice and right have been attained. Clearly, then, it is the moral obligation of the professional nursing staff to ensure that clients (families, individuals, and communities) have enough information to determine the costs or risks and benefits involved in their choices of health promotion, prevention of illness and disability, and care. When there is an unfavorable balance of risk or cost, the nurse has the moral obligation to alert the clients. When the recipients profess a willingness to accept the cost or risk, the decision must be honored, for the recipients are autonomous agents and the final choices are theirs. As far as possible, in all instances, the principle of not inflicting harm should prevail.

Ethics and Personal Concerns

Finally, there is the issue of what to do when the nurse's own ethics, morals, and values conflict with an agency's purpose or its methods of performing care. If the nurses who work in an agency are requested to assist with a procedure that they oppose on moral grounds, they have a moral responsibility to notify the agency. For example, if a nurse's ethics support a belief that the right of a fetus to life should always prevail, the nurse has a right to refrain from participation in abortions. When decisions are made regarding issues of abortion, life support, and life-extending systems, the nurse who expresses moral concern for the sanctity of life has a moral responsibility to consider all sides of an issue before refusing to participate in a given therapy or surgical procedure. Where one's ethics do not permit following a given set of procedures, it is a moral obligation to defer client care to those who can support the consumer's choice. For consumers, as autonomous agents, make the final decision and have a right to the care they seek.

FUTURE IMPLICATIONS

Scientific research over the past two decades has resulted in rapidly developing technology, greatly altering health care and medical and nursing practice. Research has forced health care providers to address such issues as who should receive the benefits of technology, what are the long-term results of life-supporting and life-extending procedures, and what kind of future generations we are preparing. Having addressed these issues, can we say that our decisions are ethical? What will be the ultimate cost in consumer health? What will be the actual cost to society? And where do nursing responsibilities lie?

Modern consumers of health care have added new dimensions to the problem by their changing perceptions of health; their relationships to health care providers; and their ideas concerning their right to know, their right to care, and their right to refuse care recommended by health care professionals. Consumers are vocal about the quality of care they receive. They have come to accept their participation in the health team as a right. They expect to be considered in decisions that affect their lives and health. But where does client autonomy end?

Nurses have become more aware of clients' ethnic origins. Many clients come from social and cultural backgrounds that are quite foreign to the nurses who provide their care. For community health nurses, questions raised are: What is the extent of my professional and moral obligation to learn about a client's cultural background? Does the care I provide reflect my concern for client differences? How do I ensure client autonomy and provide knowledge that is meaningful, given varying values and beliefs?

In addition to changes in the population, there is now the recognition that material and financial resources are finite. There is a growing awareness that preventing illness is, in the long run, less expensive for clients and society than reliance on curative or even maintenance health care. Thus goals for health promotion have become increasingly important to individuals and families. In keeping with this changed philosophy is the idea that responsibility for one's health rests primarily with the individual. However, if clients are to discharge their responsibilities effectively, social policies must provide necessary environmental protection, health information, and access to health care. Nurses who believe they have an ethical and moral responsibility to assure that clients are capable of practicing health promotion will endeavor to learn ways to help clients assume this responsibility. Nurses who are alert to the extent of environmental hazards will feel compelled to help educate and protect the community from such threats.

With limited resources available, all the factors that influence health must be weighed. The community health nurse who can assess communities is in a unique position to assume moral responsibility for improving the environment and health. As the United States becomes more crowded and society becomes more complex, community health nurses will have an increasingly important role as client advocates in influencing health policies. Nurses can promote change if they use their knowledge about nursing and keep abreast of environmental and social factors that affect health. However, to assure appropriate use of time and energy, the nurses of the future will have to be cognizant of the goals of society. Clients and health care providers will have to become interdependent as they pursue mutual objectives and health goals. Clients and health care providers will have to work as partners, sharing responsibilities that, in another era, were assumed by physicians and nurses alone. To ensure the best possible consumer health care in the future, physicians and nurses will have to forge a closer, more collegial relationship. Such a relationship will demand a high order of ethical and professional obligation. If a health care professional feels an ethical responsibility to provide for the health of individuals and communities, he or she will endeavor to meet that end, even if the result means a change in function or status for the health care provider.

The community health nurse of the future will likely be more involved in family practice and may be the principle health care provider in that area. Therefore, skill in the holistic assessment of all family members will become increasingly important. The nurse must therefore assume a moral responsibility for continued learning, for developing new techniques and refining old ones.

Dubos (1968) has noted that marching in a parade is easier than blazing a trail. Community health nurses, by virtue of their interaction with a variety of health care consumers in the community, are in a unique position to blaze trails in preventive health care, health promotion, and health policy. Ethical issues of justice should impel nurses to question health policies and examine health care. Using the tools of ethics (principles of autonomy, rights, obligations), nurses can assess the ethical implications, for the community, of changes in health policy and health care delivery.

Principles of ethics suggest that the nurses of the future will need knowledge of historical precedents concerning public health policies and public health problems and solutions if they are to take advantage of current events and make responsible decisions. Qualitative as well as quantitative research, knowledge of ethical concepts, and moral responsibility for one's learning will enable community health nurses to become a major force for the improvement of health care in the United States. The future will bring many new situations and problems. The most effective way for nurses to face and solve new ethical problems is for them to consciously examine and affirm their personal ethics. Few problems can be solved simply by judging what is right and what is wrong. To practice nursing ethically and to remain comfortable with themselves, nurses will have to be aware of the duties, rights, obligations, costs, and benefits that comprise some of the variables in emerging health care issues.

SUMMARY

Nurses must understand the ethical principles that undergird what they do in the community and what they ought to accomplish. It is also important for nurses to analyze the moral codes under which they function and to determine appropriate ethical and moral responses to the many issues they confront daily.

In many instances, nurses' personal philosophies and ethics differ from those of their clients. A study of ethical concepts and moral obligations and responsibilities to the self and others provides increased awareness of the many moral positions that exist. An awareness of the principles of ethics can help nursing students question the decisions they make and the philosophical basis upon which their moral obligations rest.

DISCUSSION TOPICS

1. Think about your own ethics. Which of the ethical principles discussed in this chapter influence your nursing decisions?

a. What rules govern your nursing actions? Where did you learn these rules?

b. What situations have you already faced that have challenged your ideas of moral nursing practice?

c. What are some of the values that influence how you work with clients?

d. What rights do you believe a client has when working with you? What rights do you have in giving care to clients?

2. A community health agency serves people in a middle-income community. The population is predominantly Polish, Irish, and Italian, and most people are Roman Catholic. The principal of the high school approaches the agency and contracts to have a nurse come to the school once a week to assess student health problems and establish a health-teaching program. On the first visit, the nurse talks with four girls who say they are pregnant and have not told anyone other than their boyfriends. Another girl and boy tell the nurse that they have what they think are venereal diseases.

a. What is the nurse's moral responsibility to each of the students described?

b. What are the rights of the various people involved? These include the students, their parents, and their sexual contacts, as well as the nurse.

c. What steps should the nurse take? How do your values and ethics influence your idea of what the nurse should do?

3. Several older people in a community function quite well in their own homes, but they have problems in arranging for reliable transportation to the community health center.

a. How can their autonomy be maintained?

b. What individuals or groups have a duty to support the autonomy of these people?

c. Which nurses in the community have duties or rights in relation to the needs of these older people?

4. The discovery is made that prolonged periods of weightlessness in space are useful in relieving certain types of pain. Several individuals offer to pay for the cost of including themselves and a few other sufferers of chronic pain on a long-term mission on a space station.

a. Who should decide whether to permit this use of the space station?

b. What ethical principles enter into the decision about whether or not to pursue this proposal?

c. If the proposal were adopted but the number of people permitted to go limited, how should the people be selected to participate? Who should make the decision?

BIBLIOGRAPHY

Baier, K.: Deontological theories. In W.T. Reich, ed., *Encyclopedia of bioethics*. New York: Free Press, 1978a.

Baier, K.: Teleological theories. In W.T. Reich, ed., *Encyclopedia of bioethics*. New York: Free Press, 1978b.

Bahm, A.J.: *Ethics as a behavioral science*. Springfield, Ill.: Charles C. Thomas, 1974.

Beauchamp, T., & Childress, J.F.: *Principles of biomedical ethics*. New York: Oxford University Press, 1979.

Carlson, R.: *The end of medicine*. New York: John Wiley & Sons, 1975.

Churchill, L.R. & Simán, J.J.: Abortion and the rhetoric of individual rights. *The Hastings Center Report* 9, 10–12, 1982.

Dilday, R.C.: The code for nurses: An educational perspective. In American Nurses' Association, *Perspectives on the Code for Nurses*, Kansas City, Mo.: Author, 1978.

Dubos, R.: *So human an animal*. New York: Scribner's, 1968.

Dyck, A.J.: *On human care: An introduction to ethics*. Nashville, Tenn.: Abington, 1977.

Ehrenreich, J., & Ehrenreich, B.: Medicine and social control. In B.R. Mandell, ed., *Welfare in America: Controlling the dangerous classes*. Englewood Cliffs, N.J.: Prentice-Hall, 1975.

Fuchs, V.: *Who shall live: Health, economics and social choice*. New York: Basic Books, 1974.

Frankena, W.K.: *Ethics*. Englewood Cliffs, N.J.: Prentice-Hall, 1973.

Green, L.W., Kreuter, M.W., Deeds, S.G., & Partridge, K.B.: *Health education planning: A diagnostic approach*. Baltimore: Mayfield Publishing, 1980.

Hill, I.: *The ethical bases of economic freedom*. Chapel Hill, N.C.: American Viewpoint, Inc., 1976.

Illich, I.: *Medical nemesis: The expropriation of health*. New York: Pantheon, 1975.

Ladd, J.: Ethics I: The task of ethics. In W.T. Reich, ed., *Encyclopedia of bioethics*. New York: Free Press, 1978.

Matejski, M.P.: Ethical issues, nursing and the health care system. *Nursing Leadership* 27, 33, 1981.

Moore, D.T.V.: *Principles of ethics*. Philadelphia: Lippincott, 1944.

Rawls, J.: *A theory of justice*. Cambridge, Mass.: Belknap Press of Harvard University, 1971.

Reversby, S., & Rosner, D.: *Health care in America: Essays in social history*. Philadelphia: Temple University Press, 1979.

Ross, S.D.: What makes right acts right? In K. Pahel & M. Schiver, eds., *Readings in contemporary ethical theory*. Englewood Cliffs, N.J.: Prentice-Hall, 1970.

Solomon, W.: Rules and principles. In W.T. Reich, ed., *Encyclopedia of bioethics*. New York: Free Press, 1978.

Thompson, J.B. & Thompson, H.V.: *Ethics in nursing*. New York: Macmillan, 1981.

7

The Politics of Nursing

Marilyn M. Bagwell

Politics: who gets what, when, and how.
HAROLD D. LASWELL

OBJECTIVES

After reading this chapter, you will be able to:

- [ ] Identify power strategies applicable to nursing.
- [ ] Define terms relevant to legislation.
- [ ] Identify methods of influencing legislation.
- [ ] Analyze nursing networks, political action committees, and coalitions.
- [ ] Define statutory law.

INTRODUCTION

The various definitions of politics derive from varying frames of reference. According to Weissberg (1974), some scholars define politics as an all-inclusive phenomenon: wherever there is conflict or a choice to be made, there is politics. In this frame, politics happens not only in government but also in the home, in schools, in community agencies, in the hospital, on any job, or wherever else decisions are made. Politics can, however, be defined to include only the behavior of public officials. Used in this way, "politics" is virtually identical with formal government and becomes considerably removed from the realm of daily activity.

Nurses no longer function only at the bedside of the acutely ill person. They function in homes, clinics, and communities as well as in hospitals, and the care they give has changed dramatically. With the changes in technology and political attitudes that have taken place both locally and nationally, nurses are giving primary care, acting as client advocates, and making critical decisions. This expanded role of

103

nursing has actively involved nurses in decisions that directly affect their clients' lives.

Political action in the narrower sense is for nurses a relatively new phenomenon that has evolved over the past 10 to 15 years. According to Deloughery and Gibbie (1975), nurses must expand their knowledge base from the pathophysiological needs of the client to theoretical knowledge in the field of political science and public administration. Such knowledge is essential today, because nurses must function in society in which decisions about health care are frequently made in the local, state, and national political arenas. Consequently, nurses, in conjunction with other health professionals, must work together throughout the political and social systems to achieve desired changes in the health care system.

LEARNING ABOUT POLITICAL ACTION

Few nurses have the time, the means, or the desire to return to school to broaden their knowledge of politics, nor are most nurses aware of the means by which they can obtain this knowledge as individuals or groups. It is clear, however, that the more knowledge about the political system that nurses have, the more opportunity they will have for effective action. Once nurses understand the dynamics of political involvement, they can use their political knowledge to reach their individual nursing goals and those of the profession as a whole. Although there seem to be many ways of experientially learning about political action, in actuality, there is one basic process of developing political effectiveness as individuals or groups. This process includes understanding the power structure and developing adequate factual knowledge and expertise in all levels of government.

Power

First, nurses need to understand the structure of power and the impact of power in relation to political activity. The concept of power generally refers to the ability of an individual or group to influence the behavior and actions of other individuals and groups.

Types of Power

TRADITIONAL POWER.   The power that hospital administrators and doctors hold over nursing action is an example of traditional power. *Traditional power* reflects the established beliefs that have been passed down from generation to generation. It is vested in traditional institutions. This type of power is strong because its persuasiveness makes change difficult. To make changes, nurses would have to clarify their "comfort zones" and articulate the needs of the health care system and of the nursing profession.

LEGITIMATE POWER.   *Legitimate power* is the power derived from authority that is given, accepted, and recognized by the members of an organization or system. The members of an organization or system give the leader the right to exercise authority over them. For example, nursing aides accept the power of registered nurses, who act as their leaders in making decisions about patient care.

EXPERT POWER.   *Expert power* is the power based on individual skills, knowledge, and abilities. Thus a nurse is an expert in nursing procedures and other aspects of health care that affect the client. However, most consumers have difficulty understanding the relation of the nurse's role to society today in light of common notions about nursing education and practice. This lack of comprehension results in nurses being unable to use their capabilities in expanded nursing roles. Hence, nurses' expert power is limited because they are not permitted to function within the full range of their capabilities.

REFERENT POWER. *Referent power* evolves when a particular group or individual serves as a role model for others. This type of power is demonstrated by a group or leader who is charismatic. In a hospital setting, the head nurse of a unit is usually the person other nurses rely on for decisions on patient care. However, in some units, a staff nurse who is willing to give information and to be supportive is sought out by others for help in decision making. This situation exemplifies referent power.

Increasing Power

Many other types of power have an effect on nursing. However, knowledge of traditional, legitimate, expert, and referent power enables nurses to realize the far-reaching effects of power in relation to the nursing profession. In applying this knowledge, nurses must rely on their expert power to enable them to wield legitimate power. For nurses to receive societal acceptance and recognition of their expanded role, they must educate society about nurses' education and skills—their expert power. A means of educating society about nurses' expert power is to increase referent, or charismatic power. Nurses might use the mass media to increase the visibility of the various aspects of their profession. Articles and human interest stories, accompanied by photographs, in magazine supplements of local newspapers and local and national magazines would increase visibility. Designing informative programs for local public television and cable stations would also increase referent and expert power. To apply their increased expert and referent powers, nurses must be aware of the effects of the traditional power of doctors and hos-

pital administrators on nurses individually and on the nursing profession. Such awareness will enable nurses to identify areas in which they can apply referent and expert power to increase their legitimate power. This integrated awareness and application of powers reveals the potential of nursing power. As Chaisson (1979, p. 5) stated, "I believe that the power of nurses, individually or collectively, is not absent but rather dormant." This dormant power can be awakened by political participation.

Barriers to nurses' active participation in the political process derive from lack of knowledge about the political process. Hence effective political participation for nurses requires adequate knowledge of the political system. Nurses first must understand that, as Weissberg (1974) maintained, direct citizen influence is important but it plays only a minor role if unaided by organization. The individual is not all powerful in politics—the power of the average individual is much less than that of the media and large organizations such as corporations and interest groups. Individual efforts are important, but group efforts are more effective:

Politics is basic to policy making and by no means irrelevant to administration. It conditions relations between governor and legislature, between upper and lower legislative houses, between the governor and other executive officials and agencies, between national and state government and between state and local. Private interest groups are a part of the picture, for their influence on the formal holders of governmental power depends very much on the range of public and private interests to which officeholders in the political system must be responsive.

(Fesler, 1967, p. 30)

Individual and group effectiveness derive from analytical thinking. *Analytical thinking* involves the ability to conceptualize, organize, and evaluate political phenomena coherently. Such an ability can foster nurses' ability to think in a politically sophisticated manner. Analytical thinking also involves the capacity to understand the possible consequences of various political options. In these times, nurses evaluate choices not only for good or bad, right or wrong, but also for relative costs and benefits and long-term social implications. Such analysis enhances politically sophisticated thinking, which in turn fosters individual and group effectiveness in the political arena.

POLITICAL ACTION

The political system is made up of conflict between interests, some of which are embodied in social groups. Nurses must analyze the resources available to them and the willingness and capacity of the profession to fight for goals. Once nurses have developed general political knowledge and ability, they can build specific knowledge and application of political processes.

Levels of Government

Nurses must develop a working knowledge of all levels of government if they are to affect the political system. The three levels of government in the United States are federal, state, and local. Each of these levels divides into three branches: executive, legislative, and judicial. However, a fourth branch, the regulatory or administrative agencies, has developed a powerful base over the past several years. Furthermore, the interrelationship of the three original branches and the regulatory agencies has an impact on the nursing profession and individual nurses.

Within this governmental framework, the political power most readily available to nurses is that on the local or state level. National power must be long and carefully nurtured; hence, only a few nurses can ever hope to serve at the national level or in a national office. However, nurses' knowledge of the structure of power, their ability to analyze political phenomena, and their working knowledge of the levels of government make local and state involvement or offices attainable to those nurses who are willing to participate in politics.

Party Politics

First, nurses can participate in political issues by becoming directly involved with a political party. After registering to vote and exercising this right, nurses may become "grass roots" workers and begin to develop basic knowledge about party politics. Such involvement often encourages nurses to campaign for a particular candidate. Nurses can also become involved as a group to support a candidate who favors the health care issues they consider most important.

After such involvement with a political party, nurses might be encouraged to campaign for office. For a nurse to be a credible candidate, experience in community organization is helpful. Working in community groups is an invaluable means of learning local problems, recognizing the community power structure, and meeting potential supporters.

Working with Representatives

Another method of increasing nurses' political awareness is the identification of the federal congressional district and the state legislative districts in which they reside. This knowledge permits identification of the people who represent nurses within their state and in Washington, D.C. There are several resources a citizen can use to identify national and state districts. In most states, the office of the Secretary of State has maps outlining the national and state districts. The offices of the leaders of the house or houses of state legislatures or state assemblies have state maps showing areas of representation. Either the information desk or the public information office at the state capital will have various materials for the public, such as legislative maps, directories with information about each legislator, and lists of legislative committees and their chairpersons. Some states have newspapers that cover legislative action which may be available in local libraries or by subscription. The League of Women Voters is another resource for finding out about legislative districts, registering to vote, or the progress of specific legislation.

Nurses should be aware of their representatives' voting history on legislation related to issues of current concern to them. Many state nurses' associations employ lobbyists or a legislative committee to keep records of the progress of bills related to health care issues and of the activities of legislators. An individual can contact the association for information about his or her representatives, or the association may provide a periodic report.

The nurse should determine whether the legislator has a position on the legislation of concern and what that position is. If the legislator has taken an unfavorable position, the nurse should contact the legislator, either by letter or by appointment, to try to persuade him or her to change the position. If the position is favorable, the contact will be made to express support. If the legislator has not taken a position, the nurse can provide information to clarify the issue for the legislator. Another method of contact is to invite the legislator to a small gathering of nurses and health care professionals to discuss specific issues related to health or the profession. Contact with a legislator fosters mutual understanding between the representative and the constituent. Each contact helps nurses become less hesitant about future contacts on other issues.

A nurse who lives near a state capital may be able to attend sessions of the legislature and committee meetings when health care issues are discussed. However, the majority of nurses need other resources to keep abreast of legislation. One source is a list of current bills before the legislature. The information desk or public information office at the capital will provide information about obtaining such a list. Once the nurse identifies bills that are significant, he or she can keep informed about the progress of the bills by contacting his or her representative or the authors of the bills.

Legislators have staff members to research and summarize information pertinent to the issues they vote on. These staff members analyze issues that are likely to be of interest to constituents. Hence nurses should develop rapport with legislative staff members as a means of providing them with accurate information about health care or nursing issues. Once staff members recognize the nurse as a person who has valuable information, they will use this expertise.

THE LEGISLATIVE PROCESS

Understanding the legislative process includes knowing what kinds of laws there are, understanding the meaning of legislative terminology, understanding how a bill becomes a law (described in Chapter 26), and understanding how to read a bill. Such knowledge will enable nurses to function effectively in the legislative branch of the government.

What Is a Law?

According to Creighton (1975, p. 2) *laws* are "those standards of human conduct established and enforced by the authority of an organized society through its government. Law is not synonymous to custom, although custom plays an important role in creating and enforcing law." Laws originate as bills in the legislature, and upon the chief executive's signature, they become statutory law.

A *statutory law* (or *statute*) is an act of legislative bodies declaring, commanding, or prohibiting something. Statutes are always written, are firmly established, and can only be altered by amendment or repeal. Statutes can concern many things, from the distribution of property to the definition of criminal conduct, and they are limited only by the jurisdiction of the legislative body that enacts them. The nurse-practice acts of each state are examples of statutory law. That these statutory laws are written by legislators who are generally not health professionals makes it imperative for nurses to have input into the process.

Another important type of law is *regulatory law*. Within the administrative branch of government, designated agencies write regulations according to a specific process. These regulations have the full force of law. The board of nursing is an example of a designated state agency. Legislatures mandate programs that require implementation by an administrative agency, which employs people with an understanding of specialized, technical information. Legislatures then delegate authority to make regulations to those agencies with expertise in a particular area. This delegation of power is particularly apparent in the field of health. Hence the most critical part of a government health program can be the regulatory law.

Legislative Terminology

Understanding terminology used in the legislative process is essential for nurses' effective participation in the process. Some key legislative terms are defined in Tables 7.1 and 7.2.

How to Read a Bill

In reading a bill that is before the legislature, nurses need to remember that the laws made by the legislatures are statutory law. Consequently, bills refer to existing statutory law. Words in CAPITAL LETTERS are new language proposed by the bill, and language that is struck-out is existing law that would be deleted, as illustrated in Figure 7.1. The page number of the bill and the line number of the changes provide additional reference. With basic knowledge of law, legislative terminology, how a bill becomes a law (described in Chapter 26), and how to read a bill, nurses can actively support or fight a particular piece of legislation.

Influencing Legislation

Assessing Support

Once individual nurses or nursing organizations have sharpened their political skills, they can attend to bills that have implications for health care and nursing. Two factors will determine nurses' political strategy: legislative support for the bill and its status. To determine the strength of legislative support, nurses can call interested legislators, contact staff members, and contact the nurse lobbyist. Nurses should use all three approaches to obtain a reasonably accurate estimate of support. Nurses can request interested legislators to obtain a

TABLE 7.1
Glossary of Legislative Terminology

Adjournment sine die	Final adjournment of legislative body
Adopt	To accept or approve
Amendment	Changes in pending legislation by adding, deleting, or modifying material
Apportionment	Establishment of legislative districts after every federal Census, based on population with boundaries established by legislature
Bill	Proposal for the enactment of a new law, the amendment or repeal of an existing law, or appropriation of public money. The only vehicle for enactment of a law by the legislature. It may originate in the upper or lower house but must be passed on roll-call vote by both bodies and be approved by the governor to become law. If the governor vetoes the measure, the legislature may override this decision as provided by the constitution of the state
Committee	*Committee of the whole:* informal session of entire membership of one of the legislative houses acting as one committee presided over by chairperson appointed by speaker or president
	Conference committee: joint committee made up of representatives appointed by speaker and senators appointed by president to try to resolve differences in legislative measures. A majority of conferees of each house is required to approve a compromise before submitting it to the entire membership of each house for final approval
	Select committee: created by speaker or president to handle specific matters and usually dissolved when purpose is accomplished.
	Standing committee: members appointed by speaker and president at beginning of legislature. The name of the committee reflects area of jurisdiction, e.g., education, health, welfare, cities and municipalities.
	Subcommittee: small committee appointed by a standing committee chairperson to research and study a bill or problem and to report findings to the entire committee
Constituent	A citizen residing within the district of a legislator
Engrossed bill	A version of a bill that includes all amendments attached to the original measure
Enrolled bill	Final official version containing all necessary signatures
Majority	Group of legislators, usually of the same political party, who have the greatest number of elected members and who control top leadership positions
Minority	Group of legislators, usually of the same political party, that number the fewest members
President	Presiding officer of the upperhouse elected by its members
Quorum	The majority of the membership necessary to conduct business
Rules	The set of regulations and parliamentary procedures adopted separately by each house of the legislature
Speaker	Presiding officer of the lower house elected by its members

SOURCE: Adapted from Arizona House of Representatives: *Arizona Bill*, 1977, by permission.

TABLE 7.2
Provisions for Enactment of Laws

Emergency clause	Statement added to legislation that declares necessity for immediate enactment. Requires two-thirds vote by each house and becomes law immediately upon governor's signature
With effective date	Date given in measure, providing it is at least 90 days after adjournment of legislature
With emergency clause	Date governor signs bill into law
Without emergency clause or effective date	Bill automatically becomes law 90 days after adjournment of legislature

SOURCE: Adapted from Arizona House of Representatives: *Arizona Bill,* 1977, by permission.

vote count. If the legislator is sufficiently interested, the nurse has sufficient influence, or a suffecnt number of nurses make the request, the legislator may consent. After assessing the support or nonsupport of legislators, nurses need to determine the status of the bill. If it is in the early stages of the legislative process, letters or visits are most appropriate. If a vote is imminent, telephone calls or wires will be most effective.

Public Hearings

Another way of using political and professional knowledge is to testify at hearings. Nurses who want to testify should contact their legislators' staff members or the desk clerk of the legislature to determine the procedure for being placed on the agenda. The procedure varies from state to state. The nurse who testifies not only must be

```
 6        Sec. 4.   Section 32-1606, Arizona Revised Statues, is amended to
 7     read:
 8        32-1606.   Powers and duties of board
 9        A.   The board may adopt and revise rules and regulations necessary
10     to carry into effect the provisions of this chapter. The rules and
11     regulations shall be published and copies thereof furnished to any person
12     upon application REQUEST:
13        B.   The board shall:
14        1.   Establish minimum curricula and standards for schools of nursing
15     and courses preparing persons for licensing under this chapter and provide
16     for surveys of schools and courses it deems necessary.
17        2.   Accredit schools and approve courses meeting the requirements of
18     this chapter and of the board.
19        3.   Examine, license and renew the licenses of duly qualified
20     applicants and conduct hearings upon charges calling for suspension on. . . .
```

Figure 7.1 Reading a bill.

well informed about the issues and its alternatives but also must know the procedure that the particular committee follows. A method for becoming comfortable with the committee procedures and correct methods of testifying is to visit several hearings before deciding to testify. Before beginning their testimony, nurses should identify themselves and state whether the testimony is that of an individual or an organization. There are several other helpful points: dress appropriately for the hearing; be brief and articulate on the issue and use nontechnical language; be prepared to think under pressure and not to react emotionally to the comments from the committee members; and be well versed on facts, honest, and willing to say, "I don't know but I will try to get that information to you later." Being accustomed to speaking to a group enhances these points.

Lobbying

Lobbying is attempting to influence legislators to support or oppose a particular piece of legislation. Lobbyists are generally paid representatives of special interest groups; however, there are some unpaid lobbyists who volunteer their time.

Many states have passed laws in the past few years that require professional lobbyists to register and adhere to certain regulations. Few nursing organizations have the benefits of a nurse lobbyist. Any nursing organization or individual nurse interested in hiring or becoming a nurse lobbyist should be aware of what is involved in lobbying. Any lobbyist needs to develop interpersonal relationships with many legislators, because it is of highest priority that legislators know the lobbyist to be trustworthy and reliable.

Lobbyists attempt to influence legislation both directly and indirectly. Direct methods include testifying at hearings or meeting with a legislator. Sometimes, lobbying is effected at lunch, dinner, golf, tennis, boating, or other such activities that enable the lobbyist to provide information to the legislator or to introduce resource people to the legislator in a casual atmosphere. Other direct methods are telephone calls, telegrams, and letters. Indirect methods utilize an intermediary. The intermediary could be a close friend or respected acquaintance of the legislator who might be able to discuss the issues with the legislator on the lobbyist's behalf. For both methods, an effective lobbyist knows "the ways of legislation" and is "often familiar with legislators' personalities and idiosyncrasies." Furthermore, lobbyists "are invaluable in keeping their interest group informed about any pertinent legislation and the problems involved and in aiding the group in effective action (Kelly, 1981, p. 337)." Such aid frequently constitutes their ability to dissect the conflicts that arise in the political arena. They develop expert skills in identifying areas and causes of conflict and in negotiating and comprising.

In negotiating, individuals or representatives of groups confer with each other to reach a compromise on essential issues and concerns. According to Ilich's (1978) theory, every issue has only a few basic areas that will ultimately be negotiated. Hence nurse advocates of a bill must identify those areas on which they will be prepared to yield and those on which they will hold firm. They must also estimate their opposition's needs. There will be areas on which the opposition will not yield. Hence, within the context of specific professional goals, nurses should determine priorities. It may be that yielding on some less-important items is preferable to no success at all. Nurses must be aware that compromise is a key word in the legislative process. Individual nurses or groups who are unwilling to compromise on an issue will be ineffective.

Political Action Committees

Another method of influence is *political action committees* (PACs), which have developed across the United States over the past few years. PACs are special organizations set up to influence Congress and state legislatures through campaign contributions. These contributions affect the public policy legislation that will be voted on in the legislatures and each sponsoring organization hopes that their contributions will be effective in getting their special legislation enacted.

The giving of money has always been a part of a campaign. However, in recent years regulations on political campaign contributions for corporations and organizations have been strengthened. PACs were formed to continue to contribute money and not violate the federal Election Campaign Act. According to the National League for Nursing public policy bulletin of August 1982, the approximately 3,000 PACs were expected to contribute more than $80 million in the 1982 congressional elections.

The major legal requirements of PACs (National League for Nursing, 1982) are:

· The PAC must meet the requirements for tax-exemption under the Internal Revenue Service code;

· The full name of the sponsoring organization must be included when identifying the PAC (a recognizable acronym or abbreviation may be used on letterheads and checks);

· The PAC must register with the Federal Election Commission within 10 days of its formation;

· PAC funds may be used only for campaign contributions and its own administrative costs; a PAC may not engage in general political, educational, or legislative activities if its contributions are to be eligible for tax-exemption;

· The PAC may not receive contributions for candidates from the sponsoring organization, but association funds may be used to establish and administer the PAC;

· The PAC may solicit any individual members of the sponsoring association without restriction, while solicitation of people affiliated with institutional members requires prior written authorization;

· Individual contributions to a PAC may not exceed $5,000 per year, and may be earmarked for a specific candidate rather than for general use by the PAC;

· Association PACs may not contribute more than $1,000 to any candidate in any election (primary and general elections are counted separately) or more than $5,000 if the PAC is qualified as a multicandidate committee;

· Each PAC must adhere to the detailed reporting and auditing requirements of the Federal Election Law and the IRS code.

The American Nurses' Association formed a PAC in 1974, called Nurses' Coalition for Action in Politics (N-CAP). N-CAP is supported by donations from nurses and others interested in promoting health care legislation. Several state nursing organizations have also formed PACs.

Petitioning

Nurses must also realize that alternatives exist if they are unsuccessful in getting state legislation that is supportive of health care consumers and of the nursing profession. One alternative is direct legislation in the form of the initiative or the referendum. An *initiative* is a method by which citizens petition to place a proposed measure on the ballot. A *referendum* is a method by which the legislature or citizens petition to place an already enacted law on the ballot for popular approval or rejection. Both of these methods take a great deal of organization to be effective.

Simulations

Involvement in the legislative process by testifying or participating at any level can generate much anxiety and result in inactivity. One method of lowering such anxiety is to simulate the situation. Some methods of simulation are computer, gameboard, and role playing.

Because role-playing simulation is simple, inexpensive, and effective, a role-playing simulation game was selected for senior nursing students in a professional development course at Arizona State University. These nursing students during their junior year had various class meetings on identifying congressional districts and state legislative districts, knowledge of the legislative process, terminology, and process of a bill becoming law. The professional development course during their senior year was geared to foster greater participation in the legislative process. In the role-playing simulation, the students conducted a mock standing-committee hearing either in the classroom or at the legislature.

At the legislature, the students conducted a mock hearing of the Health Committee in the Arizona House of Representatives committee room. A current bill before the legislature affecting nurses was selected for the hearing.

The Health Committee of the Arizona legislature had 15 members, each of whom represented a different legislative district. Thus, each of the 98 students was assigned to one of the 15 legislative districts. The students met in their respective legislative districts, discussed the pros and cons of the bill, set up their groups to seek further basic facts, and selected their respective legislators. Since the committee's membership was composed of 10 Republicans and 5 Democrats, the student legislators were also divided in this manner. These Republican and Democratic members of the "legislature" then met in their respective political groupings and discussed their stands.

Special interest groups were also active. There were three nonpartisan special interest groups, and the student legislators received advance information about the significance of each such group in their district (very significant, fairly significant, or not significant). Thus each "legislator" could estimate the importance of pressure from each interest group. Finally, those students who were not student legislators decided who would testify at the hearing and whether their group would take a stand for the bill or oppose it.

Chairing the students' health committee was Anne Lindeman, a state senator, who had also been a representative for eight years. She is an RN and a member of the Health Committee of the Senate and was a member of the Health Committee in the State House of Representatives during her tenure there. The usual rules governing the hearings of the legislature applied to this mock hearing. After hearing all the testimony, the student legislators voted on the bill.

The students' comments on this simulation were overwhelmingly positive. Students stated that they learned more this way than in any other way. The smallness of the simulated legislative districts enabled the students to be aware of their group dynamics. Being members of special interest groups made students aware of the potential power of such groups. The students realized that by analyzing the situation they had increased their knowledge, thereby enabling them to control or reduce their emotional responses. They learned about majority control of the committees and the power of the committee chairperson. Those who testified experienced emotions ranging from fright to self-confidence and authority. Finally, the simulation created an enjoyable atmosphere for learning.

Nursing Networks

Since nurses are beginning to recognize the need to make decisions about their role in the health care delivery system and since political decisions are crucial to these decisions, nurses must have input into their local and national legislative processes. Because strong input is essential, it must be presented in a powerful voice by nurses who are united in a common purpose—to promote health care for the consumer. One plan of uniting nurses is to form a *nursing network:* a group of individual nursing organizations that have united as one group.

In January 1978, the Arizona Nursing Network (designed by Marilyn Bagwell) was implemented to help local nurses become aware of and knowledgeable about legislative issues on a state and national level. The distribution of information is reciprocal—from the *Legislative Information Reporter* (LIR), to groups, to individual nurses, and vice versa. An important element of the network is that any nurse as an individual or within any group can give information about legislative issues to the *Legislative Information Reporter.* Other sources of information for the LIR are members of the legislature and lobbyists interested in nursing and health care legislation.

A key factor in the success of the network has been the establishment of communication between legislators and network members. Members have provided legislators with a considerable amount of useful information. The network encourages nurses to become analytical thinkers about decisions and policy, skills necessary for nurses in the current health care industry.

COMPOSITION. The Arizona Nursing Network is composed of nursing groups from a variety of settings as well as clinical specialty groups. The following partial list illustrates the variety of groups that belong to the network: Arizona Association of Nurse Anesthetists; Association of Operating Room Nurses of Phoenix and the Valley; Central Arizona Nurse Practitioners Group; Arizona Federation of Licensed Practical Nurses, Inc.; Arizona Society of Nursing Service Administrators; Arizona Association of Student Nurses; Arizona Health Plan; and Arizona Nurses' Association, Inc. The ex officio members are the State Board of Nursing, the State Department of Health Services, and the nursing lobbyist for the Arizona Nurses' Association, Inc.

The network membership consists of two types: voting and nonvoting. The voting members are those nurses designated by nursing organizations, associations, or services to represent them. Each group has one representative. The nonvoting members are individual nurses who want to be active within the network and support its purposes and functions but who do not represent a nursing group. The voting members participate on committees and pay higher annual dues than nonvoting members.

FUNCTIONS. The Network has four basic functions: to disseminate information and educate nurses about health legislation, to increase the political awareness of nurses, to encourage nurses to participate in the legislative process, and to promote and support the advancement of nursing through the legislative process.

The dissemination of information and education of nurses about health legislation occurs during monthly meetings held from September to June each year. The meetings are usually held at the state capitol complex so that the members have easy access to the bills and legislators during the time the legislature is in session. During meetings, members discuss all bills affecting health and nursing that either have been introduced to the legislature or are pending introduction. New members to the group are given a pamphlet, "How a Bill Becomes Law," and are taken on a tour of the capitol complex so that they will learn how to get information from various sources. Instruction about various aspects of the legislative process occurs during some of the monthly meetings. Workshops are held on topics about the legislative process, key issues that will affect health care and nursing, and any new legislation that affects the nursing profession.

The political awareness of nurses is increased by having the individual nurses in the various organizations identify what legislative districts they live in. Then the representative of each organization helps the individual nurses in the organization make contact with the appropriate legislators.

The Arizona Nursing Network has at least one member in each of the 30 legislative districts in Arizona. This distribution is important when the network is seeking support in the legislature. When the network is seeking support for or fighting against a bill, the chairperson calls five network representatives, each of whom in turn calls four other network representatives. Ultimately, these representatives activate the communication trees of their respective organizations. The method of reaching all the members is demonstrated by the communication tree in Figure 7.2.

Encouraging nurses to participate in the legislative process is accomplished by encouraging individuals and groups to contact their representatives and discuss the network's position on issues. This process, it is hoped, will become increasingly influential and effective as the individuals and

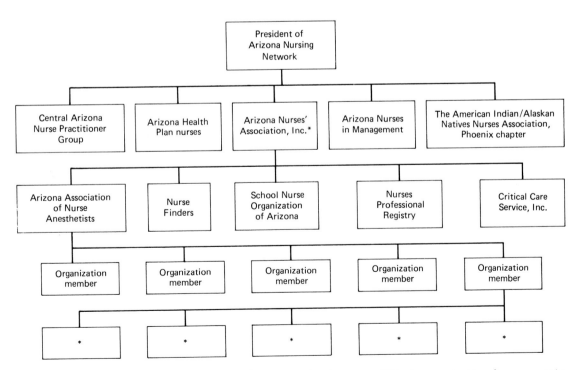

Figure 7.2 The Arizona Nursing Network communication tree. (*Each organization has a certain number of representatives to call; however, space limitations prevent showing each one separately.)

groups increase their experience and knowledge in the legislative process. Because the member organizations in the Arizona Nursing Network represent nurses from all over the state, it is possible for the information the network provides to its members to reach a majority of the members in both the House and Senate.

The final function of the network, to promote and support the advancement of nursing through the legislative process, is accomplished not only by disseminating information and educating nurses but also by planning offensive and defensive strategies to influence legislators. In 1981, the Arizona Nursing Network hired a lobbyist. Furthermore, network members have provided excellent information to legislators at the time bills are in preparation. This is a critical time, since many decisions are made before a bill is introduced into the legislature. Network representatives analyze and interpret data concerning each piece of legislation and distribute a network opinion that ultimately reaches all members of the network. In network meetings, representatives discuss the various proposals and through negotiation and compromise devise strategies for presenting the stand of the network to the legislators via the lobbyist, individual members, and individual groups.

FUTURE IMPLICATIONS

Those who take the initial steps toward involvement with the political process, whether as individuals, groups, or networks, will be the ones who will influence future health care legislation: "Our power is there for the taking. It is free, inherent in nature. By the simplest gesture we can reclaim it" (Ferguson, 1980, p. 239).

In the future, nurses and their organizations might form a coalition with other groups, such as The League of Women Voters, Business and Professional Women, or The Soroptomist. In such a coalition, nursing organizations would support certain legislative issues the other organizations supported in exchange for those organizations' support of nursing issues. Because health care affects everyone, a coalition of this type would exert great pressure on legislative bodies. It would have large financial resources to conduct media campaigns, and its size would attract the media's attention. By combining coalitions, the groups will increase their opportunities to communicate with legislators. The combination of staffs and of information-gathering ability will increase the effectiveness of each group. Finally, a united front helps eliminate the charge that individual groups act only for selfish reasons.

The nursing profession is the largest group of licensed health care providers in the United States. Individual nurses and nursing groups, if they work toward unity in purpose and function, could be extremely influential in health care and policy for themselves and the consumer. This potential nursing power must be channeled into the social and political system. A knowledge of the political system, the power of the political system, the steps in the legislative process, the means of identifying laws that affect nursing, and the technique of networking give the individual nurse and nursing organizations the basic tools for participation.

In this decade nurses must be taught and encouraged to become politically active. Ultimately, it will be individual nurses, operating independently or within various groups, who will foster and facilitate clout for nursing and for the consumer of health care. As individual nurses become better prepared for political participation, they will realize that "our sources and uses of power set our boundaries" and that "personal power defines our politics" (Ferguson, 1980, p. 190). The knowledge that leads to autonomy will lead to useful political coalitions, confident entry into the political arena, and effective use of personal power.

DISCUSSION TOPICS

1. How do networks differ from political action committees? How does their impact on nursing and health care differ?

2. How can an individual nurse become politically active in the support of nursing practice and health care?

3. If your legislature were considering a bill you considered to be detrimental to nursing practice, what could you do to prevent its passage into law?

4. In the nurse-practice act of your state, identify a regulation that needs change to reflect current nursing practice. Design a campaign to effect the change.

BIBLIOGRAPHY

Archer, S.E., & Goehner, P.A.: *Nurses: A political force*. Monterey, Calif.: Wadsworth, 1982.

Arizona House of Representatives: *Arizona Bill*, 1977.

Bagwell, M.: Motivating nurses to be politically aware. *Nursing Leadership* 3(4), 4–6, 1980.

Bagwell, M.: The nursing network—A united front. *Nursing Leadership* 2(2), 5–8, 1980.

Bettingham, E.: *Persuasive communication*. New York: Holt, Reinhart, and Winston, 1968.

Chaisson, G.M.: Nursing's sense of powerlessness. *Arizona Nurse* 32(5), 1979.

Creighton, H.: *Law every nurse should know*. Philadelphia: Saunders, 1975.

Deloughery, G., & Gibbie, K.: *Political dynamics: Impact on nurses and nursing*. St. Louis: Mosby, 1975.

Ferguson, M.: *The aquarian conspiracy—Personal and social transformation in the 1980s*. Los Angeles: J.P. Tarcher, 1980.

Fesler, J.: *The 50 states and their local governments*. New York: Knopf, 1967.

Grissum, M., & Spengler, C.: *Womanpower and healthcare*. Boston: Little, Brown, 1976.

Ilich, J.: *The art and skill of successful negotiation*. Englewood Cliffs, N.J.: Prentice-Hall, 1978.

Kelly, L.: *Dimensions of professional nursing* (4th ed.). New York: Macmillan, 1981.

Mullane, M.F.: Nursing care and the political arena. *Nursing Outlook* 23(11), 699–701, 1975.

National League for Nursing: *Public policy bulletin* 1(4), 1–4, 1982.

Roper, W.: *Winning politics*. Radnor, Pa.: Chilton Book Co., 1978.

Walcott, C., & Walcott, A.: *Simple simulations: A guide to the design and use of simulation/games in teaching political science*. Washington, D.C.: American Political Science Association, 1976.

Weissberg, R.: *Political learning, political choice, and democratic citizenship*. Englewood Cliffs, N.J.: Prentice-Hall, 1974.

8

The Use of Consultation

Victoria Schoolcraft

I am able to enlarge my experience by the experience of others.

R. BUCKMINSTER FULLER

OBJECTIVES

After reading this chapter, you should be able to:

☐ Define consultation.
☐ Describe the consultation process.
☐ Describe the consultant–consultee relationship.
☐ Differentiate between the use of a professional consultant and a peer consultant.
☐ Describe the role of a peer consultant.
☐ Use appropriate skills in peer consultation.

INTRODUCTION

As organizations and systems become more complex, there is a greater need than ever before for outside assistance. Consultation is relatively new as a formal professional endeavor. In nursing and in other professions predominantly comprised of women, the acceptance of consultation has been slow. Nurses are trapped by a feeling that they must be all things to all people. Therefore, they cannot admit a deficit in knowledge or skill that would require a consul-

tant, because they believe that such an admission would imply weakness and incompetence. On the other hand, women have been socialized into female role prescriptions that make them reluctant to recognize and accept their own expertise or the expertise of other women and other nurses (Polk, 1980).

CONSULTATION

Torres (1974, p. 1) defines *consultation* as "a collaborative effort on the part of the consultant and the consultee(s) which utilizes the problem-solving process for the purpose of creating change." There may be change "in the consultee, change in a program, or change in a service delivery system or institution" (Wilson & Underwood, 1980, p. 256). The primary function of a consultant is to share "specialized knowledge and techniques appropriate to the problem" (Wilson & Underwood, 1980, p. 256) and "to facilitate human potential, i.e., to develop the capacity for self-renewal within individuals, group, and the total system" (Lange, 1979, p. 30).

Lange (1979, p. 31) states that the definition of consultation includes the following assumptions:

a) the consultant relationship is a voluntary relationship between

b) a professional helper (consultant) and help-needing system (client)

c) in which the consultant is attempting to give help to the client in the solving of some current or potential problem,

d) and the relationship is perceived as temporary by both parties.

e) Also, the consultant is an "outsider," i.e., is not a part of any hierarchical power system in which the client is located.

Nurse Consultation

Sedgwick (1973, p. 773) has noted that consultation is "essentially an elaboration of the skills and expertise appropriate to nursing." The nurse-consultant has specialized abilities and knowledge gained through advanced education and experience. There are three general types of consultants, differentiated on the basis of area of expertise, skill focus, and the underlying assumptions of their approaches: the expert consultant, the resource consultant, and the process consultant.

The *expert consultant* is someone who has unique skills and expertise in a particular field and who is called upon to deal with a particular problem in a particular situation (Sedgwick, 1973). For example, a generalist community nurse might request consultation from a pediatric nurse-practitioner (PNP) for a problem with a certain child. The consultant would discuss the child with the consultee and might even see the child and the family. The PNP would then make suggestions to the community nurse. The expert consultant is responsible for solving the problem, although the consultee carries out the actions needed for solution.

A *resource consultant* is someone who provides relevant information so that the consultee can make choices from a variety of alternatives (Sedgwick, 1973). The consultee has the necessary ability to select and carry out appropriate interventions but may have insufficient knowledge and experience to recognize what the alternatives are. An example of resource consultation is the following:

Lillian Palmerez called a psychiatric nurse because one of Palmerez's clients had been raped. The psychiatric nurse, Joyce Lynn, had considerable experience in working with rape victims. Palmerez requested information on what she should do for the client and what other resources were available in the community. Lynn knew that Palmerez was competent in crisis intervention and told her that those skills would be useful in helping the client through the aftermath of her attack. Lynn also identified various agencies and professionals that could offer services to rape victims. Palmerez then formulated a plan of action incorporating some combination of the alternatives described by Lynn.

The third type of consultation is *process consultation*. The process consultant "brings about changes in the situation that enable the consultee to make a decision in this particular instance and in future situations" (Sedgwick, 1973, p. 773). In such a relationship, the consultee is in need of assistance in diagnosing the problem but has the ability to solve the problem with the help of the consultant. This kind of consultation is often useful to an organization that includes many people with expertise at various levels.

Frequently, one's competence in nursing is undercut because of an inability to see the larger issues in a situation. The following example demonstrates a situation in which process consultation was useful:

A consultant was contacted by Margie Douglas, a nurse who managed a clinic in the city health department. Ms. Douglas said she thought the problem was that too much time was elapsing between an initial visit to the clinic and some action on the part of a clinic nurse. In investigating the roles of the staff members, the consultant found that the intake nurses did a thorough history and physical assessment on each new client. However, when they referred clients to nurse-practitioners in the clinic, the practitioners would disregard the information obtained by the intake nurses.

Clients complained about having to relate the same information more than once. The intake nurses expressed resentment that their work was ignored. The process consultant worked with all the nurses in the clinic to identify the problems, to investigate strengths and weaknesses in the situation, and to help the nurses to find possible solutions.

Since process consultation is so frequently the appropriate type, it will be discussed at greater length in other sections of this chapter.

DECIDING TO SEEK CONSULTATION

When and Why

Since nurses and other professionals so often feel that they must be entirely self-sufficient, consultation is frequently not initiated until long after it was first needed. As a nurse becomes familiar with the process of using consultation, however, she or he gains skill in identifying the need and in seeking the appropriate consultant.

There are several reasons for seeking consultation (Luskin, 1981; Nuckolls, 1977; Sedgwick, 1973). Some of the reasons are:

1. The consultee feels incompetent in a particular area and the problem requires special knowledge or skill.
2. The nurse is uncertain about his or her ability to solve the problem and seeks validation from an expert.
3. Full-time attention is required for a short time.
4. An independent viewpoint is needed because the consultee lacks objectivity.
5. The problem relates to a disagreeable or difficult client who has generated negative feelings.
6. Staff members are communicating ineffectively or are avoiding the problem.
7. There is a need for legal protection for the nurse or the client.
8. Change can be justified only on the basis of an impartial assessment.
9. There is a need for knowledge, creativity, or imaginativeness to expand the alternatives available.

All these reasons make the prospective consultee feel that things are somehow not right. Many consultees experience growing discomfort for some time before recognizing the need for consultation.

Who

Once the nurse decides that a consultant may be useful, she or he must determine the type of consultant required. If the problem is related to a specific client or type of client, an expert in the clinical area of need is appropriate. Other expert consultants would be those who have competence in areas such as setting up clinics, developing record-keeping systems, designing in-service programs, or writing for publication.

A resource consultant would be sought if the need is for information to enhance what the consultee is already doing. Situations calling for this kind of consultation include selecting optimal health care delivery methods, expanding the use of personnel, finding and linking up with other services in the community, and generating fresh solutions to old problems.

A process consultant is appropriate when the problems are related to relationships, communications, general problem-solving ability, philosophy, or goal setting. This type of person is often the best choice when the consultee is having difficulty diagnosing what is wrong.

Qualifications of Consultants

Great care must be taken in selecting a consultant once the consultee has determined the kind of consultant needed. The consultant should have the following qualifications (Lange, 1979; Nuckolls, 1977):

1. Appropriate formal credentials
2. Broad experience in the area of consultation
3. Competence in the problem area
4. An organized philosophy and theoretical framework about the practice of consultation
5. Ability to function well in new situations
6. Ability to listen
7. Ability to synthesize discussion and ideas accurately

8. Understanding of applicable ethnic, regional, and economic issues
9. Knowledge of whether to be directive or nondirective in the consultation
10. Ability to determine the correct locus of decision making in the given situation.

As this listing indicates, a great deal of attention must be given to reviewing the qualifications of a person who might be chosen for consultation. When these criteria are met, success in the relationship is much more likely.

Professional Consultants and Peer Consultants

A *professional consultant* is a person who earns all or part of his or her living by providing consultation services. This is generally the kind of consultant needed for complex or persistent problems. By and large, this chapter discusses the work of professional consultants.

However, on occasion, it may be appropriate to consult with a peer. *Peer consultation* is a deliberate action to work with a peer to solve a particular client or organizational problem. Many of the same criteria apply in choosing a peer for consultation as in selecting a professional consultant. For example, if the client in question needs information about discontinuing breast feeding, the student or nurse would seek a peer with specific knowledge and experience in this area.

In another situation, the student or nurse might possess the necessary clinical knowledge and experience but have difficulty in figuring out how to use it. She or he would seek out a peer who was good at helping people through the problem-solving process. Peer consultation will be further discussed later in this chapter.

How

Once the potential consultee has determined the type of consultant needed and the qualifications of the person to be selected, the consultee must find the right person to fill the job. Some of the resources that might be used in locating a consultant are:

· Professional associates
· Professional nurses' organizations
· State nurses' associations and the American Nurses' Association
· State leagues and the National League for Nursing
· Specialty nursing organizations
· Nursing networks
· Local or state health departments
· State agencies (such as departments of mental health)
· Schools of nursing
· Directors of nursing
· The American Association of Hospital Consultants
· Journal articles and books
· Speakers or participants at conventions or workshops
· Previously used consultants

It is important to find out as much as possible about the prospective consultant in the initial contact. The qualifications listed earlier can serve as a guide for asking questions or for reviewing résumés. It is helpful to get evaluations from people who have used the consultant's services.

The prospective consultee should also provide information to the consultant about the scope and nature of the problem, the goals or expected outcomes, the projected time parameters, and the resources available.

Usually, the consultant is first contacted by telephone. If the consultant can discuss the problem at that time, the consultee can describe the situation and seek information about the consultant's qualifications. The consultee should follow up the telephone contact with a letter detailing the particulars that were discussed and providing any additional information that was requested. The letter should make it clear whether or not the consultee is offering the job.

The magnitude of the problem and the expense involved will determine the extent of the search process. For example, if the problem is with a single client or type of client, the consultee may simply contact a professor at a local college of nursing with clinical expertise in the applicable area, request an hour of time at the professor's usual rate, and make an appointment. If the problem is complex and a substantial amount of money is available for expenses and fees, the consultee may wish to contact two or three potential consultants to locate one with the most suitable qualifications.

What

Consultation Formats

The formats for consultation may be periodic or episodic. *Periodic consultation* occurs at regular intervals. For example, an expert mental health nurse consultant would be engaged to meet biweekly with a group of staff nurses in a local health department to discuss current problems. Another kind of periodic consultation would involve the consultant in nursing rounds. The consultant meets with staff members as they review clients' cases and participates in the discussion as appropriate (Weinstein, Chapman, & Stallings, 1979).

Episodic consultation occurs at irregular intervals in response to a particular crisis. This kind of consultation requires the services of the consultant for a specific and time-limited purpose. One episodic format is *crisis intervention*. A crisis is a situation in which one's usual problem-solving abilities function inadequately. A consultant may be called in on a one-time or short-term basis to assist a person or group to cope with a crisis. For example:

The director of the nursing department of a local health department was notified by the chief executive officer that her budget was being cut by 15 percent, effective immediately. The director contacted a nurse who had expertise in budgetary management and hired her for one day of consultation with the last $400 in her "miscellaneous" budget. The consultant helped the director reallocate resources in such a way that essential commitments were maintained, no one was laid off, and some nurses were actually given the opportunity to try creative ways of providing service to clients.

Another format for episodic consultation is the one-time or short-term contact, such as a single appointment to discuss a particular client or a two- or three-day visit in which the consultant works with the client to solve a problem and initiate change.

The consultee may have a clear idea of the format for the consultation before contacting the consultant, or the format may be established after the initial discussion with the consultant. When an individual or an agency frequently seeks episodic consultation on the same or similar problems, all those involved might well consider a format of periodic consultation or might decide to engage a different consultant. By the same token, after a consultant has been used on a periodic basis, the consultant and consultee might negotiate a new episodic relationship.

Consultation Foci

Caplan (1969) and others (Larkin & Crowdes, 1976; Robinson, 1974) have dis-tinguished the various foci in the consultation relationship: client-centered, program-centered, or consultee-centered. This is another way in which the consultant's style and experience and the consultee's needs must fit each other.

CLIENT-CENTERED CASE CONSULTATION. In client-centered case consultation, the focus of the consultation is on a problem the consultee has encountered in working with a particular case (Caplan, 1969). The consultee may be having difficulty diagnosing the problem or prescribing appropriate nursing interventions. The purpose of the consultation is to determine client needs (Robinson, 1974). The consultant may have contact with the client as a part of the process.

PROGRAM-CENTERED ADMINISTRATIVE CONSULTATION. Program-centered administrative consultation focuses on current problems with the administration of a program (Caplan, 1969). The example given earlier of the nurse who sought consultation in revising her budget is an example of such a focus.

CONSULTEE-CENTERED CASE CONSULTATION. Consultee-centered case consultation focuses on the nurse's problem in working with a particular client (Caplan, 1969; Robinson, 1974). The consultant helps the nurse discuss and examine her or his own thoughts, feelings, or needs in order to improve the nurse's practice. Caplan (1969, pp. 424–430) named four categories of difficulty that indicate the need for this kind of consultation: lack of understanding, lack of skill, lack of objectivity, and lack of confidence and self-esteem.

CONSULTEE-CENTERED ADMINISTRATIVE CONSULTATION. Consultee-centered administrative consultation focuses on the consultee's problems with administration (Caplan, 1969). The consultant helps the consultee identify and solve problems related to planning and maintenance of programs. The consultee may have difficulties in such areas as establishing and exerting authority, fostering effective communications, dealing with interpersonal relationships, or using resources effectively and efficiently.

THE CONSULTATION PROCESS

Preliminary Phase

When consultant and consultee have gained an initial sense that they are willing to work together, they negotiate the terms of their relationship. A fee is established. If the consultant is a professional, he or she may have a set per-hour or per-day fee. The fee may be higher if the consultant has to travel. A person who is a nationally recognized expert will command a higher fee than a competent but less well-known expert from a local university. The fee is payment not only for the actual time the consultant spends with the consultee but also for the time spent in preparation directly or indirectly connected with the current request (del Bueno, 1978).

In lieu of a fee, the consultee and consultant may negotiate an exchange of services in kind. This means that at a later time the roles will be reversed: the consultee will serve as a consultant or will provide another service of equal value. For example, a nursing instructor may agree to provide consultation to the nurses in a visiting nurses' association in exchange for having one or more of the visiting nurses serve on a course-planning committee at the instructor's school of nursing.

For consultants from outside the area, travel arrangements, living accommodations, and local transportation must be arranged. The consultee pays for these items and makes all arrangements, unless the consultant states a desire to make his or her own plans. These considerations should be taken care of as soon as possible after the consultant agrees to work with the consultee. As soon as the arrangements are made, they should be confirmed in writing.

Other issues that are settled in advance are the amount of time the consultant will spend at the site, postvisit expectations (such as a written report), the format of the report, and a tentative agenda. The consultee should draw up the agenda and the consultant may recommend additions or deletions. If the consultant is to meet with people other than the consultee, this should be specified on the agenda.

Occasionally, since consultants may have reputations within the professional community, other groups, such as schools of nursing or professional organizations, may request some of the consultant's time. It is up to the consultant to determine whether to honor such requests, and the details, including additional fees, must be negotiated separately.

The consultee will furnish the consultant with information about the situation before the beginning of the visit. For example, applicable items include program objectives, description of facilities and other resources, organizational and flow charts indicating communication links and others processes, preliminary assessments of the problem as the consultee sees it, and the consultee's goals.

Data-Gathering Phase

When the consultant enters the situation, he or she begins to collect information. The consultant will probably wish to meet with everyone relevant to the problem situation and hear their viewpoints on the problem and the solutions. If the consultant is working with an individual nurse, such data gathering may be limited to that nurse and his or her records. If the problem pertains to a partnership, clinic, or agency, several meetings with individuals and groups may be required.

During this phase, people may be reluctant to share information with the consultant because they fear that they will be found at fault. On the other hand, some people may use this opportunity to vent anger and dissatisfaction. If the consultant is a psychiatric mental health specialist, members of the organization may attempt to use the consultant as a therapist or may couch observations in psychiatric jargon. An experienced consultant and a knowledgeable consultee can recognize this behavior as an expected part of this phase and treat it accordingly.

The consultant may need to obtain first-hand knowledge of actual facilities involved in the situation. However, tours should be limited to relevant areas. Such activities are time consuming and expensive in terms of the consultant's time.

The consultant will need access to relevant written information as well as a time and place to review such materials. Some direct observation by the consultant may be necessary. For example, in the situation in which there was friction between the generalist nurses and the nurse practitioners, the consultant might follow clients through their clinic visits. This would enable him or her to observe interactions and processes that the participants were unable to articulate.

If direct observation is difficult, audio or video recordings can be made for the consultant. This method was used in working with a nurse who felt he had problems interviewing clients. By viewing several videotapes of the nurse with various clients, the consultant was able to identify verbal and nonverbal aspects of the nurse's style that interfered with communication.

Identifying the Problem and Alternative Solutions

Many experienced consultants have pointed out that the problem as it has been initially described quite frequently is different from the real problem (Ferguson, 1969; Luskin, 1981; Norris, 1977; Nuckolls, 1977; Schien, 1969; Sedgwick, 1973; Wilson & Underwood, 1980). This happens precisely because of one of the reasons a consultant is often sought in the first place: lack of objectivity. Even so, it is important for the consultee to state the problem before consultation. This helps focus attention on the problem and encourages commitment to the need for change.

After the data-collection phase, the consultant, either alone or in collaboration with the client, formulates a new problem statement describing the factors that contribute to the problem. In addition, the consultant may enumerate personal, situational, institutional, or environmental strengths and weaknesses that have a bearing on the problem.

If the consultant is an expert in a specific area, he or she may suggest a particular plan for solving the problem, such as the budgetary expert did in an earlier example. When a resource or process consultant is involved, he or she will describe some general alternatives from which the consultee can select a variety of approaches to deal with the problem. Returning to an earlier example will help illustrate how a consultant determines a new problem statement.

In studying the clinic managed by Margie Douglas, Tim Elliott found that the nurse-practitioners trusted the ability of the intake nurses to do adequate histories and physicals. They stated they usually repeated these activities in order to get better acquainted with new clients. However, they occasionally did arrive at findings different from the intake nurses'. Some of the nurse-practitioners felt uncomfortable about using someone else's data as a basis for action and some felt they were not doing enough for clients if they did not do the history taking and physical assessment.

Mr. Elliott clarified that the problem had to do with self-esteem and trust. Most of the nurses were uncomfortable with their roles. The intake nurses projected this feeling on the nurse-practitioners in arriving at the conclusion that the practitioners distrusted their abilities. On the other hand, the practitioners were so concerned about missing something themselves that they implied distrust of their colleagues.

The nurses had never attempted to agree on a standard format for taking and recording histories and physicals, and few of them ever observed each other's techniques or discussed the process.

The consultant assists the client in planning how to implement the recommended alternatives. This involves examining the possible outcomes of the intervention and verifying that these match the goals of the consultee. The consultant may spend some time giving feedback to everyone involved, allowing them to begin incorporating the new perspectives of the problem before any specific action is taken.

Once a general solution is agreed upon by the consultee, the consultant assists in devising a plan for implementation. Complex problems are sometimes solved by simple changes, but usually some time is necessary and many changes required to accomplish goals. The plan specifies the goal and lists the steps required to reach it. The plan also specifies who is responsible for particular components of the plan. The plan must be as clear and specific as possible.

The following example shows part of the plan formulated for the nurses in the health department clinic managed by Margie Douglas:

Tim Elliott restated the problem as dysfunctional communication among the intake nurses and the nurse practitioners. One goal he and Margie Douglas determined was to eliminate duplication of effort in history taking and physical assessment. To accomplish this, it was decided that:

1. All the nurses would agree on the information that would be obtained by the intake nurses and the form in which it would be recorded.
2. Intake nurses and nurse-practitioners would periodically observe each other's techniques in taking histories and performing physical assessments and discuss the process.
3. All the nurses would agree on a protocol for determining when clients would be seen by the intake nurse only and when clients would be referred to nurse practitioners.
4. When a client is admitted who clearly needs to see a particular nurse-practitioner, he or she would be referred to the practitioner, who would take the history and perform the physical assessment.

During this phase, the consultant can often serve as a catalyst for change by identifying and removing communication blocks. Since the consultant is transient, she or he can put things in a different light or confront people in a way that is impossible to those who are permanent members of the system. For example, a consultant can approach and spell out to an administrator the strengths and needs of others in the organization and help the administrator gain objectivity.

The consultant can also coach the consultee in trying out new behaviors (Schien, 1969). In coaching, the consultant observes the consultee as he or she attempts unfamiliar activities. The consultant gives suggestions and provides feedback as the consultee tries out different responses. The consultant may also provide a role model so that the members of a group can gain skill in coaching each other and in providing useful feedback (Ferguson, 1969).

Evaluation Phase

A consultant who has been engaged for episodic consultation works with the consultee to evaluate the work that has been done: have the goals been accomplished? The agreement with the consultant may entail additional evaluation at a later date, or the consultant may agree to respond to a self-evaluation done by the consultee at a particular time.

Together the consultant and consultee plan for ongoing evaluation. Part of this plan is to specify warning signals that indicate further need for consultation. If the consultant is hired on a periodic basis, the consultant and consultee will establish a plan for regular evaluation of the relationship. It is valuable to verify periodically that progress is being made toward reaching identified goals.

The consultee will also evaluate whether the consultant was effective. The consultant may request specific feedback about particular aspects of the process.

In evaluating what has transpired, the consultee may decide not to take the consultant's advice. There may be many reasons for this. The people in the organization may feel that the consultant is mistaken either about the nature of the problem or about the possible alternatives. Or it may be that the problem is beyond the expertise of the consultant. No matter how impressive their credentials, experiences, or reputations, consultants are sometimes wrong or at least wrong for a particular job. No matter how appropriate and well-designed a consultant's recommendations may be, the consultee may be unwilling or unable to change at the time. In such an event, the consultee should not feel constrained to make ill-timed changes just because much time and money have been invested in the process.

Sometimes a situation improves even though no solution has been identified or implemented. This may occur because of the increased interest of those involved in the situation; they may feel a renewed devotion to the tasks at hand because someone thought they were valuable enough to hire a consultant (Randolph & Bernau, 1977).

PEER CONSULTATION

A *peer* is another nurse in an equal or similar position. Peer consultation includes consultative relationships that are informal or that involve people who are not ordinarily sought for professional consultation. Such people include students, staff nurses, head nurses, or faculty members who consult within their own groups.

Although it may be unstructured and informal, such an effort is a useful way for nursing students or nurses to work together and share their strengths. It is helpful to begin by making expectations explicit, as would be done with a professional consultant. Both consultant and consultee structure the interaction to enhance the likelihood of meeting the goals.

The following dialogue demonstrates how the process might proceed:

Kay Scisc and Ming Chin are staff nurses in a city health department.

KAY: Ming, I have a problem I need some help with. I've been asked to teach some classes to some Vietnamese women in one of my neighborhoods.

MING: That's a great opportunity. What are the classes for?

KAY: The women are limited in using English, and they need to learn how to communicate some common information about symptoms and so forth. (She proceeds to describe her plan and the help she will get from an interpreter.)

MING: So far it sounds like you've got it under control. What's the problem?

KAY: Well, I feel uncomfortable about talking about things pertaining to sexual organs with them.

MING: You mean like discussing menstruation?

KAY: Yes. Is that an acceptable topic culturally, or is it going to be a problem?

MING: I think they'll be very interested and will listen to you because you're the authority. Because you're a nurse, it's acceptable for you to talk about it, and they probably won't be uncomfortable. If you weren't a nurse, they would probably be embarrassed. (Ming goes on to volunteer some information about how to assess the clients' understanding of the information.)

As this interaction shows, the two nurses have proceeded through the steps of gathering data, clarifying the problem, and suggesting a solution. Kay sought out her colleague because of Ming's knowledge of a particular ethnic group. Not only did Ming help answer the original question, she also provided some additional information to assist Kay in her work. The example futher indicates the informality and goal directedness of peer consultation.

Goals of Peer Consultation

The primary goal of any consultation process is to solve the problem at hand. Some people would add that the consultee should learn from the solution in order to be better at solving the same or other kinds of problems in the future. In addition to this goal, there are three general guidelines to help the peer consultant select the behavior and communication that will facilitate the process:

l. Promote the consultee's autonomy and independence.

2. Maintain or improve the consultee's self-esteem and self-confidence.

3. Facilitate open communication.

These guidelines provide a basis for assessing the actions needed to achieve the goal in a professional manner. For example, if the consultant feels inclined to tell the consultee what to do, the consultant is encouraging dependence, implying inferiority, and blocking communication. When the consultant judges, criticizes, or blames the consultee, this also undermines the consultee's sense of autonomy and competence. The approach that is most conducive to meeting the goal is one that conveys respect and understanding of the other person.

Being an Effective Peer Consultant

The skills used in peer consultation are the same as those used in other helping relationships. The first step is to clarify that the person who seems to be seeking help really wants help. There are times when people are not looking for a solution to their problems—they just want a chance to blow off steam. When this occurs, the peer might suggest that at some point the two of them get together to try to solve the problem. For example, Paul Baker calls Mark Corey to say he cannot leave the unit to go on a break with him:

PAUL: (sounding very angry) I'm tired of those nurses on the other shift leaving things undone. Don't they know we're busy, too?

MARK: Have you talked to them about it?

PAUL: Look, they don't care how I feel or what I think.

MARK: It's frustrating when people don't seem to care.

PAUL: It sure is. This place gets more like a zoo everyday. I've got to get back to work.

MARK: I'd be willing to talk with you later to look at ways to improve this situation. You've really helped me work on some problems before, and I'd like to work with you.

PAUL: OK. I've got to cool off first. See you later.

This interaction demonstrates the principle elements for being an effective helper (Adams, 1979, pp. 182–189):

1. *Acceptance.* Mark accepted Paul's view of the situation and Paul's feelings: he did not challenge or judge him.

2. *Empathy.* Mark demonstrated empathy by verbalizing Paul's frustration.

3. *Genuineness.* Mark communicated a real interest in helping Paul cope with the situation.

4. *Reciprocity.* Mark acknowledged that Paul had helped him in the past and that he was willing to return the support.

A fifth element of the helping process is that a helper must be able to experience a degree of *personal fulfillment* outside of the helping relationship. This means that a person should not rely exclusively on such helping opportunities for a sense of satisfaction or personal worth (Adams, 1979). Peer consultation is a service nurses and friends can perform for each other, but just as with other helping activities, it is not healthy for a person always to try to meet other people's needs with no regard for personal needs.

The most crucial factor for the peer consultant is to determine whether he or she is needed as an expert consultant (like Ming Chin) or as a process consultant (like Mark Corey). For example, when Kay Scisc asked Ming Chin for help, it was clear that she did not want help on planning the class. She wanted information to make the class relevant and acceptable to the participants. When Paul Baker began to articulate his problem, he did not want Mark Corey to suggest solutions. Mark responded appropriately by permitting Paul to vent some of his frustrations and to help him begin to perceive the situation as one which he could master.

Encouragement

Encouragement is an especially useful skill in peer consultation and in similar relationships, such as that between teacher and student or nurse and client. The following are characteristics of encouraging people (Dinkmeyer & Losoncy, 1980):

· Effective listening
· Focus on positives
· Cooperative
· Accepting
· Use hope and humor
· Stimulated
· Recognition of effort and improvement
· Interested in feelings
· Base others' worth on just being who they are

Developing these characteristics helps a person become a more effective helper.

Encouragement is different from praise, particularly because praise is given to reinforce responses that meet external standards (Dinkmeyer & Losoncy, 1980). Praise tends to cause one's sense of self-worth to be determined by others' opinions and one's worth to others to be measured by how closely one approaches perfection. Encouragement involves a different process, with the following components (Dinkmeyer & Losoncy, 1980):

· Focus on person's ability to manage life constructively

· Focus on internal evaluation

· Recognition of effort and improvement

· Focus on assets, contributions, and appreciation

· Person acquires the courage to be imperfect and a willingness for self-evaluation

· Person learns to accept efforts of self and others

Perfection seems like a worthwhile goal, and there are certain situations in which nothing less can be tolerated. However, even a person who is able to perform perfectly in given circumstances is still not perfect in every situation, because perfection is often an externally determined ideal. For example, a nursing supervisor may consider her staff to be perfect only when they have completed all their written work. Another may consider his nursing staff perfect if they finish each shift with each client adequately served. When one incorporates strong beliefs about being perfect, this interferes with one's accepting oneself when the standard is not met. This may result in rebellion against the standards or covering-up errors for self-protection. This phenomenon is at the base of why it is frequently difficult for nurses to seek consultation as mentioned earlier in this chapter. It may be particularly difficult to admit to a peer that one needs help.

A nurse who is encouraging gives other peers a sense that they can confide in him or her. The encouraging nurse can serve as a role model and can overtly identify the skills he or she is using so that other nurses can learn them. Ultimately, that nurse can return to his or her colleagues for consultation.

Trust and Confidentiality

As in any helping relationship, trust must be established. The consultee must have enough experience with or knowledge about the peer consultant to believe that that person can help. People are often reluctant to divulge personal information, especially in regard to problems or shortcomings in themselves. However, it is crucial that people learn to trust one another.

Consultive relationships must be characterized by confidentiality. No information disclosed during the consultation should be shared without permission. This means that even though the peer consultant believes that the supervisor should know how the staff nurse feels, only that nurse can decide when to share the information—not the consultant.

FUTURE IMPLICATIONS

Ferguson (1980) has pointed out how rapidly knowlede has been growing. The shape and structure of knowledge are changing. Knowledge has become fragmented, and it is difficult for anyone to keep abreast of current developments in his or her own field, let alone related fields. Many consultants fulfill their role by helping to apply knowledge from one field to another. There is a great need for interdisciplinary collaboration and consultation. For example, if community health nursing continues in a generalist orientation, nurses will need frequent consultation from other disciplines that specialize in public health. There is a danger that community nurses will become such generalists that they will no longer have a discrete role. Consultation can help them integrate and collaborate with nonnurse colleagues in order to continue to be able to make worthwhile contributions to health care.

The future will require increasing use of resource consultants. With so much information stored in diverse locations, nurses and other professionals will rely on people who are able to locate knowledge and facilitate the use of it. These consultants may be nonnurses, but there will also be nurses who will provide a valuable service because of their familiarity both with resources and with nursing situations.

As nursing evolves and becomes publicly acknowledged as a profession based on physical and psychosocial sciences, the preconceptions of potential nurses may be more realistic. That is, the people who enter nursing may be more professional in their approach than humanitarian. A truly professional person recognizes the existence of strengths and weaknesses and knows when he or she needs help. A humanitarian, on the other hand, feels that he or she must give and give and never ask for help. The nurses of the future will accept their own needs and realize that they must continue to grow throughout their professional lives. Some of this growth will be stimulated through work with consultants.

Our culture is also evolving. Many relationships have been perceived as putting one person in a subservient role, such as teacher–student, physician–patient nurse–client, consultant–consultee, counselor–counselee. Our American values have caused us to view those who need help as weak; and when someone has needed help, he or she has been relegated a helpless, powerless role. It is no wonder that people avoid those roles when they can, particularly if they have occupied the powerful, helper role. Things are changing. Students, clients, and others are asserting their rights as well as their needs for independence and

autonomy. Gradually, a new sense of what it means to be in the helper role is developing. People are not willing to abdicate control over their bodies and destinies to the degree they have in the past. This change will enhance the consultant–consultee relationship by minimizing the subordinate, inferior attributions of the consultee's role.

SUMMARY

Consultation is a helping relationship in which the consultant and consultee collaborate to examine and solve a problem. Consultees must have skill in selecting the appropriate consultant. Although the consultant has expertise either in special content, processes, or resources, the burden of choosing and implementing a solution rests with the consultee.

Even though the consultee needs the assistance of an objective person, the consultee possesses knowledge and skill needed to arrive at a resolution. Steele (1975, pp. 148–149) summed up this element of the consultee's contribution in the following way:

The client often has great wisdom (intuitive if not systematic) about many aspects of his own situation, and an overweighting of the vaule placed on the consultant's knowledge may indeed cause poorer choices to be made than if there were a more balanced view of what each can contribute to the situation.

In order to ensure continued effectiveness as nurses, it is valuable for nurses to seek and receive consultation. Although many problems warrant the use of an outside expert, many common problems can be dealt with by means of peer consultation. The elements that contribute to effective peer consultation are essentially the same as those that facilitate a therapeutic relationship between nurse and client.

Consultation is a collaborative relationship in which the person seeking help retains his or her self-esteem and autonomy. Nurses must help to dispel the dysfunctional notion of inferiority belonging to the status of consultee in order to promote their personal as well as professional growth.

DISCUSSION TOPICS

1. Which kind of consultant (expert, resource, or process) would you seek in each of the following situations? Explain your choices.

    a. The client, Ms. Mooten, has eight children with various health needs. She has been visited for brief periods of time by two other nurses. Each transferred her to another nurse because she is described as "obnoxious and incorrigible." You have the same impression but are worried about the plight of the children if service is discontinued.

    b. Mr. Chang is having problems adjusting to behavioral and dietary changes required by his recent cardiovascular problems. Much of the difficulty seems to lie in his traditional Chinese values and life-style.

    c. A new system of record keeping that involves the use of word processors has been adopted by the agency's administration. Some nurses are excited about learning how to use the machines, but most feel they do not have time to learn this system. Those in the latter group feel that valuable time with clients is being robbed.

2. Select one of the situations in topic 1. Describe how you would seek and contact the type of consultant you need. Identify two people you might actually contact if you had the problem described.

3. Describe an incident in which you have sought peer consultation or in which you might have sought peer consultation. What kind of person was appropriate as a peer consultant? Describe what happened or what might have happened in working with a peer consultant.

4. Select a recent problem you had related to a community experience. Choose a peer and seek consultation (even if the problem was solved satisfactorily). Then reverse roles and act as a peer consultant to your peer.

5. Evaluate the process in topic 4 according to the goal and guidelines for peer consultation and the elements of being an effective helper.

6. Name other implications for the future of consultation in community health nursing.

BIBLIOGRAPHY

Adams, L.: *Effectiveness training for women.* New York: Wyden Books, 1979.

Benne, K.D.: Some ethical problems in group and organizational consultation. In W.G. Bennis, K.D. Benne, & R. Chin, eds., *The planning of change* (2nd ed.). New York: Holt, Rinehart & Winston, 1969.

Bennis, W.G.: Theory and method in applying behavioral science to planned organizational change. In W.G. Bennis, K.D. Benne, & R. Chin, eds., *The planning of change* (2nd ed.). New York: Holt, Rinehart & Winston, 1969.

Caplan, G.: Types of mental health consultation. In W.G. Bennis, K.D. Benne, & R. Chin, eds.,

The planning of change (2nd ed.). New York: Holt, Rinehart, & Winston, 1969.

del Bueno, D.J.: No free lunch. *Nursing Outlook* 26(8), 513, 1978.

Dinkmeyer, D., & Losoncy, L.E.: *The encouragement book.* Englewood Cliffs, N.J.: Prentice-Hall, 1980.

Ferguson, C.K.: Concerning the nature of human systems and the consultant's role. In W.G. Bennis, K.D. Benne, & R. Chin, eds., *The planning of change* (2nd ed.). New York: Holt, Rinehart & Winston, 1969.

Ferguson, M.: *The aquarian conspiracy.* Los Angeles: J.P. Tarcher, 1980.

Fine, S., Krell, R., Stephenson, P.S., Freeman, R., & Berlin, I.: Practical application of mental health consultation techniques. *Canadian Psychiatric Association Journal* 19, 569–575, 1974.

Goodstein, L.D.: *Consulting with human service systems.* Reading, Mass.: Addison-Wesley, 1978.

Krauss, J.B., & Slavinsky, A.T.: *The chronically ill psychiatric patient and the community.* Boston: Blackwell, 1982.

Lange, F.M.: The multifaceted role of the nurse consultant. *Journal of Nursing Education* 18(9), 30–34, 1979.

Larkin, M., & Crowdes, N.E.: Nurse consultation: The instilling of hope. *Supervisor Nurse* 7(11), 54, 57–58, 1976.

Luskin, D.: Social controls in consultation. In J.C. McClosky, & H.K. Grace, eds., *Current issues in nursing.* Boston: Blackwell, 1981.

Marcus, J.: Nursing consultation: A clinical specialty. *Journal of Psychosocial Nursing and Mental Health Services* 14(11), 29–31, 1976.

Norris, C.M.: A few notes on consultation in nursing. *Nursing Outlook* 25(12), 756–761, 1977.

Nuckolls, K.B.: The consultation process: A re-

ciprocal relationship. *Maternal Child Nursing* 2(1), 11–12, 14, 16, 1977.

Polk, G.C.: The socialization and utilization of nurse consultants. *Journal of Psychosocial Nursing and Mental Health Services* 18(2), 33–36, 1980.

Randolph, B.M., & Bernau, K.: Dealing with resistance in the nursing care conference. *American Journal of Nursing* 77, 1955–1958, 1977.

Robinson, L.: *Liaison nursing.* Philadelphia: F.A. Davis, 1974.

Schein, E.H.: *Process consultation.* Reading, Mass.: Addison-Wesley, 1969.

Sedgwick, R.: The role of the process consultant. *Nursing Outlook* 21(12), 773–775, 1973.

Steele, F.: *Consulting for organizational change.* Amherst: University of Massachusetts Press, 1975.

Stickey, S.K., Moir, G., & Gardner, E.R.: Psychiatric nurse consultation: Who calls and why. *Journal of Psychosocial Nursing and Mental Health Services* 19(10), 22–26, 1981.

Torres, G.: The consultation process in higher education. Memo to members, Council of Baccalaureate and Higher Degree Programs, National League for Nursing, New York, January 1974.

Watzlawick, P., Weakland, J.H., & Fisch, R.: *Change: Principles of problem formation and problem resolution.* New York: Norton, 1974.

Weinstein, L.J., Chapman, M.M., & Stallings, M.A.: Organizing approaches to psychiatric nurse consultation. *Perspectives in Psychiatric Care* 18(2), 66–77, 1979.

Wilson, H.S., & Underwood, P.R.: A consultation analysis of learned helplessness at "City Hospital." *Perspectives in Psychiatric Care* 18(6), 256–260, 1980.

Zaltman, G., & Duncan, R.: *Strategies for planned change.* New York: John Wiley & Sons, 1977.

9

Standards for Practice

Victoria Schoolcraft

Look for the ideal, but put it into the actual. Not by vague
exhortations, but by striving to turn beliefs into energies that
would work in all the details of health.
FLORENCE NIGHTINGALE

OBJECTIVES

After reading this chapter, you should be able to:

☐ Identify the American Nurses' Association Standards for Community Health
Nursing Practice.
☐ Give the rationale for each ANA standard and describe how each can be
assessed.
☐ Discuss the process of implementing the ANA standards.
☐ Develop practical means for evaluating community health nursing in a variety of settings.

INTRODUCTION

One of the determinants of a profession is
that the members of the profession adopt
standards for the practice of their calling,
establish criteria by which conformance to
the standards will be measured, and have
the primary responsibility for seeing that
the standards are enforced. If the professional group abdicates its responsibilities,
the public may step in and set standards for
it. When the system is functioning optimally, the profession and agents for the
public collaborate to establish whatever
laws or legal processes are necessary for the
designation and application of standards.

In the profession of nursing, the group
that has been responsible for devising and
publishing standards has been the American Nurses' Association. Various units of
this professional organization have studied
the general and specialty areas of practice
within nursing and have established standards for the practice of professional nurs-

ing. These standards are published in a variety of documents and have been given wide distribution. They are the best resource within the profession for the study of the use of standards.

Standards should be easily understood and readily available so that they may be integrated into the planning and implementation of nursing care. They should be general enough to include various aspects of practice. At the same time, standards should be specific enough to be measured in meaningful ways. This chapter describes standards and gives the student a framework within which to practice responsibly.

WHAT IS A STANDARD?

A *standard* is a means of determining what something should be. In the case of nursing practice, standards are the established criteria for the practice of nursing. Standards are statements that are widely recognized as describing nursing practice and are seen as having permanent value. Generally, standards specify what is necessary for high-quality practice (ANA, 1973). Such statements go beyond what is included on the National Council Licensure Examination. The purpose of that instrument is to determine whether a candidate meets the minimum requirements of a safe, competent beginning practitioner. The standards that are adopted by the profession describe what the best nursing practice should be.

Ethics are different from standards (see Chapter 6). Ethics describe the rules that direct individual behavior "by stating that certain actions should (or should not) be performed because they are right (or wrong)" (Fry, 1982, p. 365). Such statements guide what each practitioner does within the practice of nursing. A standard describes what the practice of nursing itself is when carried out on a high level (ANA, 1973). Both ethics and standards are determined by the members of the profession, and both describe the commitments of nurses to basic beliefs about what the profession and its practitioners are obligated to do in relation to the public.

Nursing has come a long way as a profession since the days when Florence Nightingale established basic standards for the education of nurses. The standards she set emphasized the importance of nurses understanding the rationale for their actions. She designed a curriculum that included classroom time and study as well as the practice students engaged in on the wards. Her innovations clearly indicated that she believed in the value of education for practicing nursing rather than in the mere repetition of certain behaviors, often without supervision.

In 1893, Lystra E. Gretter led a committee of nurses in the development of "The Florence Nightingale Pledge" (Kalisch & Kalisch, 1978). This was an effort to identify a set of ethical behaviors by which nurses could be judged. One passage within it states, "I will do all within my power to maintain and elevate the standard of my profession. . . ." However, the standard for the profession was not defined at that time, and a clear and objective establishment of standards was not attempted until much later. It was not until the 1960s and 1970s that the American Nurses' Association began developing standards for nursing practice in general and for the various specialties.

The concern for standards was further enhanced by the interest in and development of various quality-assurance activities. Nurses and other agency personnel began to determine methods and measures of quality care for consumers. This movement began in the 1970s, and a great deal of work remains to be done. Standards for nursing practice establish the basis for the assessment of the quality of care given by nursing staff. In addition, standards help in the evaluation of the practice of professional nursing by independent caregivers.

The challenge for the nurses who practice in the community of the future will be to continue the work on the development of relevant standards and the increased precision of measurement. As they are now written, the American Nurses' Association Standards are based on the nursing process. These are likely to serve well for a long time. More work must be done, however, on the assessment of practice according to these standards. Each nurse must become familiar with the standards, and practitioners must incorporate the standards into their practice.

STANDARDS FOR COMMUNITY HEALTH NURSING PRACTICE

The following standards for community health nursing were published in 1973 by the American Nurses' Association (ANA, 1973).*

Standard I.   The collection of data about the health status of the consumer is systematic and continuous. The data are accessible, communicated and recorded.

Standard II.   Nursing diagnoses are derived from health status data.

Standard III.   Plans for nursing service include goals derived from nursing diagnoses.

---

* Extensive quotations from *Standards of Community Health Nursing Practice* have been used with the permission of the American Nurses' Association.

Standard IV.   Plans for nursing service include priorities and nursing approaches or measures to achieve the goals derived from nursing diagnoses.

Standard V.   Nursing actions provide for consumer participation in health promotion, maintenance and restoration.

Standard VI.   Nursing actions assist consumers to maximize health potential.

Standard VII.   The consumer's progress toward goal achievement is determined by the consumer and the nurse.

Standard VIII.   Nursing actions involve ongoing reassessment, reordering of priorities, new goal setting and revision of the nursing plan.

The standards proceed in the same order, with some elaboration, as the nursing process. The standards also reflect some assumptions and ideals about nursing in the community, such as the involvement of the client in the planning and evaluation of nursing care. Each of the standards will be discussed, with some examples of the processes involved in meeting them.

Standard I

The nursing process always begins with the systematic collection of data. The nurse may have lengthy relationships of months or even years with clients in the community. To continue to give effective service, the nurse must continuously bring the data base up to date. Aspects of clients' lives that have been in control may become problematic with the passage of time. By the same token, as individuals grow and change, they learn new ways of coping that may solve problems.

In order to provide for comprehensive care by a number of professionals and for the orderly transfer of care, the data pertaining to a client must be readily available, easily understood, and accurately recorded. There are four assessment factors identified for Standard I (ANA, 1973). These are the content of the data, the sources for the data, the methods for obtaining the data, and the considerations for the data collection methods. The *content of the data* must be comprehensive and must include all the information necessary and relevant to giving care to the client, whether an individual, a family, or a larger group such as a community. The factors listed for the assessment of individuals and families are:

Growth and development

Biophysical status

Emotional status

Cultural, religious, socioeconomic, and occupational background

Performance of activities of daily living

Patterns of coping

Interaction patterns, family dynamics

Consumer's perception of and satisfaction with his or her health status

Consumer's health status

Relevant codes, statutes, regulations, contracts, and agreements

Environment (physical, social, emotional, ecological)

Available and accessible human and material resources

The factors listed for assessing groups and communities are:

Community dynamics

Power structures (legislative, political, decision making)

Economic and cultural considerations, values

Demographic data

Information derived from current local, national, and international studies of disease surveillance

These lists provide a framework for the accumulation of data which will serve the nurse well in beginning to plan care for the client.

The *sources for data* are the individual consumers, the family and significant others, health care providers, individuals and groups within the immediate environment and the community, and relevant scientific literature and studies. The *methods for obtaining the data* include interviews, examinations, observation, surveys, and reading reports, records, and other documents. The *considerations for the data collection methods* include expectations that they will provide for systematic collection, completeness, frequent updating of changes in the health status, retrievability, and confidentiality, when appropriate.

These four assessment factors give a basis by which data collection can be planned and implemented. The final category provides the criteria by which one's data and methods can be evaluated when applying the standard. These factors provide guidelines for people learning about nursing in the community, as well as for those who are establishing new areas of practice. For example, if a group of nurses were establishing a private corporation to offer home health care to consumers, they could determine the kinds of support systems they might use to meet the standard. They might select an appropriate computer system that would allow the recording and recall of the data. In addition, they might arrange to have the computer data bank periodically updated with new data in the areas of community regulations or laws or relevant demographic statistics.

This standard provides the basis for the

development of data-collection tools and for the design of evaluation instruments to be used by nurses in their practice. By consulting the factors listed, nurses can verify whether they have exhausted all the sources appropriate to obtaining data for a given client or group of clients. Even though health needs change for individuals and for the society as time goes by, this format will stand the test of time. The content may vary greatly in the next hundred years, but the outline for the content and the process of data collection will continue to be useful and highly adaptive.

Standard II

A nursing diagnosis is a "description of the effect of . . . symptoms and pathology on the activities and style of living, now and in the future" (Little & Carnevali, 1976, p. 6). It is the "identification of a patient's unmet needs and the determination of associated nursing problems" (Luckman & Sorensen, 1980, p. 16). The community health nurse uses data on many aspects of the client's or group's health status to arrive at a diagnosis or diagnoses appropriate to the client or group.

The ANA (1973) identifies the following assessment factors for Standard II:

Health status evaluation is based on the identification of health needs.

Health status evaluation includes the availability of resources and the patterns of delivery of health care.

Potentials and limitations are identified.

The health status data are analyzed and selectively applied in arriving at a diagnosis.

These factors provide checkpoints for evaluating the nursing diagnoses for the clients,

families, and groups. In order to meet all the factors, more than one diagnosis based on the data collection may be necessary. For example, the following diagnoses were set for a family after a nutritional assessment:

1. Family members suffer from chronic anemia due to inadequate intake of iron.
2. Ms. Danberry prepares nutritionally inadequate meals because of lack of information on proper nutrition.
3. Ms. Danberry is willing to learn about nutrition, because she is concerned for the well-being of her family.

The preceding diagnoses give a comprehensive summation of the family's iron-intake problem. They also indicate the role of the nurse in teaching and the potential of the family member most involved in meal preparation to learn and implement the necessary information. The assessment factors allow the nurse to verify that she or he is making diagnoses that relate to real needs and to determine the causes of those needs. The process of arriving at nursing diagnoses is described in Chapter 11.

Standard III

The next step in the nursing process is the identification of goals that grow out of the nursing diagnoses. Goals provide the foundation for the remainder of the nursing process and serve as indicators of our relative success in nursing. The assessment factors identified are (ANA, 1973):

Goals are mutually set with consumers and relevant others.

Goals are congruent with other planned approaches.

Goals are stated in realistic and measurable terms.

Goals are assigned a time period for achievement.

Goals are consistent with human and material resources.

These five factors give an excellent guide for evaluating goals set for any purpose. They portray the values set forth for holistic, comprehensive care of clients and families. Some examples of goals that meet these criteria follow.

1. Ms. Danberry will be able to prepare nutritionally balanced, affordable meals for her family. She will do this after reading some pamphlets and discussing them with the nurse. This will be completed in three weeks.

In this goal statement, three sentences are used to convey all the necessary information, but the goal is clear. A nurse's note on the client's record would indicate that the client and the nurse collaborated in setting this goal. A review of the client's record would also demonstrate that this was consistent with other approaches planned for the individual and the family. The goal is measurable: at the end of the teaching sessions, Ms. Danberry could write out planned menus, present a diary of meals she actually prepared, or demonstrate the preparation of a meal to the nurse. The goal statement specifies that the family's income will be taken into account in meal planning and includes a time by which the client will achieve the goal.

2. After one month, Mr. Markey will engage in two exercise periods every day, doing exercises that will promote heart action.

This goal statement is briefer, but not necessarily better. The statement itself includes the information by which achievement can be measured and states the time period allowed to accomplish the goal. Notes elsewhere in the record would state whether the goal was mutually set, its consistency with the overall plan for Mr. Markey, an indication of whether it is realistic for the client, and how it falls within the personal resources of Mr. Markey.

The goals for both Ms. Danberry and Mr. Markey would be compared to their respective nursing diagnoses for assessment of the relevance of the goals to the diagnoses. This is another step in the process of ensuring that the nurse will systematically move from one step to another in the nursing process.

Standard IV

In the evaluation of nursing service plans, the next step is to see that priorities have been appropriately defined and that the nursing interventions to be used will help to achieve the goals that have been set. The accurate assessment of Standard IV requires a thorough investigation of the factors that contribute to meeting this standard. The assessment factors for this standard are (ANA, 1973):

Primary, secondary, and tertiary measures are planned to meet specific consumer needs and are related to nursing diagnoses and goals of service.

Teaching–learning principles are incorporated into the plan of care. Objectives for learning are stated in behavioral terms; reinforcement is planned; readiness is considered; and the content is at the learner's level.

Approaches are specified for orientation of groups and communities to changing roles and life styles and patterns of health care delivery.

The plan includes the utilization of available and appropriate human and material resources.

The plan is flexible and includes an ordered sequence of nursing actions.

Nursing approaches are planned on the basis of current scientific knowledge.

To assess these factors, one would look at the nurse's and agency's records of service to clients. It is helpful to set up the ongoing care plan as a self-contained document so that it can be reviewed quickly and easily. Since many of these factors are related to the process as well as the content of working with clients, it is helpful to date entries so that the nurse can crosscheck them with other notes in the client's record and thus validate factors that may not appear in the care plan. For example, in order to incorporate teaching–learning principles, the nurse would include a teaching plan within the care plan. However, she or he would date the goals so that anyone who evaluated the plan of care could refer back to the notes to see whether they reflected collaboration with the client as well as the client's readiness and learning level.

Each nurse or each agency may adopt its own format for keeping track of nursing care plans, but the format should be consistent among the clients assigned to a specific nurse. Dating entries and following a given format helps demonstrate the orderly sequence of developing and implementing a plan. Retaining original entries as well as the actions that were actually taken shows that the plan is flexible. This type of recording shows what has worked with the client and what has not. Notes in the record would provide explanations of why certain interventions were planned and not implemented.

Generally, client records do not include detailed references or explanations such as those students are required to record when they are first learning the nursing process. However, the nurse may occasionally include a note about a particularly useful reference to allow another person to assess the appropriateness of the intervention. The selection of nursing actions should reflect the nurse's awareness of current scientific knowledge in relevant areas. For example, if the nurse is working with a client with herpes genitalis, the direct and indirect interventions should be reported. This would include notes on the teaching done by the nurse to help the client understand the disease, as well as records of the required reporting, since this is a communicable disease. The content of the teaching and the manner of reporting would demonstrate the nurse's knowledge of the current information available on the control and treatment of this disease.

Standard V

This standard emphasizes the importance of the consumer's participation in promoting, maintaining, and restoring his or her own health. It can be assessed by examining the nature of the nursing interventions that have been planned and implemented, which should include the active involvement of the client and family members. The nurse's notes should also reflect the level of involvement by the client and the family at various points during the implementation of the plan.

The assessment factors for Standard V concern three general points: the kind of information that should be shared; the kinds of decisions the consumer should make; and the support the consumer is given by the nurse in becoming as independent as possible in making decisions (ANA, 1973). The specific factors within these broad areas are:

The consumer and nurse share information about:

· Current health status.
· Changes in health status.
· Total health care plan.
· Nursing care plan.
· Roles of health care personnel.
· Health care resources.

The consumer is provided with the data needed to make informed decisions about:

· Promoting, maintaining, and restoring health.
· Seeking and utilizing appropriate health care services.
· Maintaining and using health care resources.

The consumer is supported in making independent judgments and decisions, implementing plans and seeking assistance when needed.

These factors show that the role of the nurse is as a collaborator with the client. The relationship of the client and nurse, when carried out in this way, helps promote the highest level of wellness consonant with the client's health status. The nurse works with the client to promote increased independence and resourcefulness. As indicated in Chapter 1, our society is currently in an information age. Nurses are key people in the gathering and transmitting of information about health. This standard shows that this definition of the nurse's role fits with the ideals of professionals practicing in the community. The inventiveness and creativity of nurses in this area will have a great deal to do with determining the future practice of nursing. Consumers are coming to expect that those

who have information, whether related to health or not, will share it rather than guard it.

Standard VI

This standard clearly grows out of the previous one. It emphasizes the ultimate goal of the information-sharing and collaborative relationship between nurses and their clients: the goal of all the actions taken by nurses with their clients is to maximize their health potential (ANA, 1973). The assessment of this standard takes into account the level of health and wellness of the client in every aspect—physiological, psychological, and social.

The assessment factors are all statements about nursing actions (ANA, 1973). They state that nursing actions:

· are consistent with the nursing plan.
· are based on scientific principles.
· are individualized to the specific situation.
· promote a safe, healthful and therapeutic environment.
· provide opportunities for consumer learning and participation.
· utilize appropriate resources.
· influence consumers' physiological, psychological and social behaviors that maximize health potential.
· are directed in order to influence community actions as well as the behaviors of individuals.

These factors can be incorporated into the criteria that should be used to evaluate the plan of care and the nursing interventions selected and implemented. If these criteria are met, then the standard will be met.

Standard VII

Given the collaborative nature of the relationship between the client and the nurse, both should participate in evaluating progress toward achieving the goals they have set together. "The effectiveness of nursing service depends on comprehensive and intelligent determination of the impact of nursing on the health status of consumers" (ANA, 1973). Any nurse or nursing student is by now familiar with the universality of the evaluation step in any application of the nursing process. Without evaluation, a nurse cannot judge the value of his or her work with clients. The client's involvement in the evaluation process helps the client learn the difference between useful and worthless expenditures of time, effort, and money for health care.

The factors used in the assessment of this standard are (ANA, 1973):

Baseline and current data about the consumer are used in measuring progress toward goal achievement.

Nursing and consumer actions are mutually analyzed and evaluated for their effectiveness toward goal achievement.

The first factor shows the importance of the initial data base. It is meaningless to judge the results if one cannot determine the starting point before the nurse's intervention. By assessing the progress from the beginning to the present, both the client and the nurse can make decisions about their work together. In some situations, a small amount of change may represent a great deal of progress. For example, a nurse who worked with a client with a life-long problem in controlling her weight might be satisfied if the client lost a pound a week consistently for several months: the consistency of the weight loss would be an improvement over the client's previous pattern. On the other hand, another client who is attempting to lose weight might have a life-long history of normal weight previous to a recent weight gain. He might lose a large amount of weight each week by crash dieting. Although this would be progress toward the goal of losing weight, it would be in opposition to a goal of promoting the client's general level of wellness, since he would not be consuming a nutritionally complete diet. As these two examples show, in the application of the standard one must take into account many aspects of the client's history and current behavior.

In working with clients, the nurse must be concerned not only with the client's progress toward goals but also with the effectiveness of the nurse's and client's actions toward the goal. A client asked a nurse for some advice in developing a daily exercise regime. In the course of accomplishing this goal, the nurse gave the client a great deal of written material about the rationale for daily exercise. In evaluating the nurse's interventions, the client and nurse concluded that all that technical information was inappropriate, since the client already valued the institution of a daily exercise plan. Although the information was interesting, all the client wanted and needed were suggestions for specific kinds of exercises and some resources for learning the exercises.

Standard VIII

As long as the nurse has a relationship with a client, the nursing care plan continues to change. As nursing interventions are evaluated and as goals are achieved, new goals with additional interventions are established. Priorities change as new needs arise and as current needs are met. Lack of progress also requires changes in the care plan.

This standard is assessed by the following factors (ANA, 1973):

Reassessment is an ongoing process in evaluating goal achievement or lack of goal achievement.

New priorities and goals are determined by the nurse and consumer.

Alternative actions are identified and mutually initiated.

Termination of service is based on reassessment and evaluation.

Provision is made for follow-up of particular consumers, groups and communities to determine the long-term effects of nursing service.

By examining the care plan itself and the nurse's notes, one can validate most of these criteria. When a client relationship is terminated, the nurse's notes should document the rationale for such a decision as well as related information about whether the client was referred to some other health care giver. Long-term follow-up of clients assists the nurse in determining whether the changes made during the relationship persisted. This measures the real impact of nursing on a client, family, or community. In order for the philosophical goals of nursing in the community to be accomplished, positive changes in health status must persist over time. This does not mean that the client will never again have a health problem or need to seek the nurse's assistance. What it does mean is that the client will be able to continue a healthy life-style independently and to seek nursing intervention if his or her life situation changes enough to warrant it.

EVALUATING OUTCOMES

There are several general concerns that can assist the nurse in applying these standards. The standards should be used as a guideline for planning and implementing care. They can provide a basis for the development of policies, procedures, and record-keeping materials. When the nurse is working with a client, she or he can use the standards to provide direction in systematically applying the nursing process.

In order to be able to evaluate nursing care in terms of the standards, all client-related records must be systematically organized in the same way for all the clients a nurse works with. Provision should be made for easy retrieval of any aspect of the care plan. In the discussion of several of the standards, it was suggested that dates be used for cross-referencing interrelated material that appears in different parts of the client record. The actual entries should be concise and explicit. Key words can be underlined or highlighted. The sections of a client's care plan and the client's record shown in Figures 9.1 and 9.2 demonstrate how such cross-referencing helps facilitate evaluation of nursing care.

The nurse should periodically review all client records to assess the level at which the standards are being met. In addition, the agency, may periodically evaluate nurses' records to maintain the integrity of the agency or to evaluate the nurses. This evaluation may be done by nurse colleagues within the agency, by nurses from outside the agency, or by consultants in other health care fields. In order for the standards to have meaning, they must be used as a standard of evaluation.

FUTURE IMPLICATIONS

The standards, as they are now stated, should serve the community nursing profession for some time to come. They follow the nursing process, which is likely to remain the cornerstone of nursing practice in the foreseeable future. The content of goals and interventions may well change as

CARE PLAN FOR Ms. Danberry
DATA: (See Danberry Nutritional Assessment, 11/1/83, in client file)
NURSING DIAGNOSES: (11/1/83)

1. Family members suffer from chronic anemia attributable to inadequate intake of iron.
2. Ms. D. prepares nutritionally inadequate meals because of lack of information on proper nutrition.
3. Ms. D. is willing to learn about nutrition, because she is concerned about the well-being of her family.

GOAL: (11/1/83)
Ms. Danberry will be able to prepare affordable, nutritionally balanced meals for her family. She will do this after reading some pamphlets and discussing them with the nurse. This will be completed in three weeks.

INTERVENTIONS:
1. Provide pamphlet about food groups and a list of foods especially high in iron. (11/1/83)
2. Ms. D. will attend a meal preparation class at the YWCA. (See note on 11/15/83)
3. Discuss pamphlet and YWCA class and plan three different meals. (11/15/83)
4. Ms. D. will plan meals and keep a food diary for assessment on 11/22/83.
5. Identify additional sources for basic food groups and iron. (11/22/83)

Figure 9.1   Cross-referencing information in the client's care plan.

health care needs become more complex or as consumers become more independent. The standards tend to promote this kind of growth.

The precision with which nurses record the information used in planning and implementing care is likely to improve as they become more familiar with technology. Nurses will begin to invent systems that will enable them to be more efficient at recording, organizing, and recalling information. This will increase their efficiency and release them from much of the time-consuming aspects of maintaining and evaluating records. Although permanent copies of client records will be maintained for legal purposes, records will be produced by word-processing systems rather than by hand.

Those clients who have their own com-puter systems or word processors can maintain a copy of their own records. This will aid their efforts to be as independent as possible in promoting, maintaining, and restoring their own health status. They will be able to maintain their own reference files to provide a display of data when new problems develop. Their records will become their own possessions, and they will not have to rely on agencies or bureaucracies to keep accounts of their personal health information.

The retention of client information in computer banks will make it simpler for new health care providers to sort through information. For example, if a nurse were to take over another nurse's caseload, the new nurse could quickly review all the client records by calling only for data relevant to the current health status of each client.

CLIENT RECORD FOR Ms. Danberry and Danberry family

11/1/83 Discussed nutritional assessment and nursing diagnoses with Ms. D. She and I set goals for her to accomplish. Gave her pamphlet and list of iron-rich foods. Gave her information to enroll in YWCA food preparation class. She is eager to learn.

11/15/83 Ms. D. did not attend YWCA class, because her car broke down. We discussed pamphlet and list; planned breakfast, lunch and dinner menus for two days. She understood pamphlet and the menu-planning process.

11/22/83 Evaluated her menu plans and food diary. She and I thought she met her goal but needs more information to provide for more variety. I will bring that next week.

Figure 9.2 Cross-referencing information in the client's record.

This would save hours that might be spent going over handwritten records on each client. Nurses who study particular health care problems will be able to prepare computer programs to provide them with a list of all clients within the data base who have a certain kind of problem or other variable. For example, a nurse might wish to investigate long-term effects of living in an area with a certain level of air pollution. The computer could be asked to print out the names and addresses of all clients living in relevant areas.

SUMMARY

The definition of a profession includes the responsibility of its practitioners to evaluate their practice. As the nursing practice has become more sophisticated, practitioners have adopted standards to guide and evaluate nursing care. In the future, we will develop increasingly more effective means of using the standards, although the standards themselves may stand for many years.

DISCUSSION TOPICS

1. Using the American Nurses' Association Standards for Community Health Nursing Practice, evaluate a client record and client care plan.

2. Discuss the advantages and disadvantages of the formats of the record and care plan you used in Topic 1 in terms of the ANA Standards.

3. Design a record-keeping format based on the ANA Standards that would facilitate the planning and evaluating of nursing care.

4. Select any one of the ANA Standards and develop one additional assessment factor that might be included based on some future development in nursing practice.

BIBLIOGRAPHY

American Nurses' Association: *Standards of community health nursing practice.* Kansas City, Mo.: Author, 1973.

American Nurses' Association: *A conceptual model of community health nursing.* Kansas City, Mo.: Author, 1980a.

American Nurses' Association: *Nursing: A social policy statement.* Kansas City, Mo.: Author, 1980b.

Flynn, B.C., & Ray, D.W.: Quality assurance in community health nursing. *Nursing Outlook* 27(10), 650–653, 1979.

Fry, S.F.: Ethical principles in nursing education and practice. *Nursing and Health Care* 3(7), 363–368, 1982.

Kalisch, P.A., & Kalisch, B.J.: *The advance of modern nursing.* Boston: Little, Brown, 1978.

Little, D.E., & Carnevali, D.L.: *Nursing care planning* (2nd ed.). New York: Lippincott, 1976.

Luckman, J., & Sorensen, K.C.: *Medical-surgical nursing* (2nd ed.). Philadelphia: Saunders, 1980.

Smitherman, C.: *Nursing actions for health promotion.* Philadelphia: F.A. Davis, 1981.

10

Effective and Creative Thinking

Victoria Schoolcraft

Without . . . playing with fantasy no creative work has ever
yet come to birth. The debt we owe to the play of imagination
is incalculable.

CARL GUSTAV JUNG

OBJECTIVES

After reading this chapter, you should be able to:

☐ Describe the states of thinking and the behavior typical of each state.
☐ Define creativity and describe creative behavior.
☐ Identify blocks to effective and creative thinking.
☐ Describe ways to overcome blocks to thinking.
☐ Describe and use strategies for fostering effective and creative thinking in one's self and in others.
☐ Apply strategies for improving planning and problem solving in groups.

INTRODUCTION

In order to make the best use of one's experiences and education, one must be able to think effectively, efficiently, and creatively. In our information society, everyone is in the business of gathering, using, and transmitting information. With more content available every day, and with increasingly sophisticated processes with which to use content, the ability to think has an ever-expanding role in achievement in any field.

Our attempts to augment the human brain's information-handling capacities through the use of computers has increased our appreciation of the versatility and complexity of human intelligence. People are only now beginning to appreciate the capability that human beings have for changing and bettering the large systems of which they are a part. R. Buckminster Fuller in his book *Critical Path* (1981, p. 47), has stated the relationship of human thinking and its potential for enormous impacts:

Fortunately the unrealistic thinking of humans has had little effect on Universe and evolution whereas realistic thinking has cosmic effectiveness in pure principle. Realistic, comprehensively responsible, omnisystem-considerate, unselfish thinking on the part of humans does absolutely affect human destiny. If the realistic thinking can conceive of technically feasible options facilitating satisfactorily effective human fulfillment of its designed functioning as local Universe information inventorying and local Universe problem-solving in support of the integrity of eternally regenerative Universe, then the accomplishment of that realistic conceptioning is realistically effective in satisfying Universe that human mind is accomplishing its designed evolutionary role.

The foregoing quotation must be read two or three times for its value to be appreciated. It probably must be read a few more times before one can begin to understand its implications for each of us. Fuller is emphasizing the development of more complex mind in human beings and the potential for this higher order of mind to accomplish things on the grandest scale of all—the universe.

Even though we may begin improving our thinking skills as single individuals, we eventually must consider the use of our intelligence and abilities on larger and larger scales. One can have a greater impact on individuals by striving to address the needs of large groups. Fuller, who as a futurist has made a nearly life-long commitment to bettering the lives of all inhabitants of "Spaceship Earth," has elegantly stated the outcome of his commitment (1981, pp. 250–251):

The larger the number of humans I undertook to serve, the more effective I became, wherefore I concluded that if I committed myself to serving everyone, I would be optimally effective . . . . To be optimally effective, undertake at the outset the most comprehensive task in the most comprehensive and incisively detailed manner . . . . Undertake the greatest task with thorough commitment of attention to every detail.

THINKING

Thinking is to form or to have something in one's mind. Other definitions of thinking include: to reflect on, ponder, or consider; to call to mind; to center one's thoughts on; to form a mental picture; to subject something to the processes of logical thought; to exercise the powers of judgment, conception, or inference; to reason; to engage the mind in reflection or meditation; to have a view or opinion; and to have concern. The dictionary lists synonyms that include conceive, imagine, realize, envisage, and envision. The common element of meaning is forming something in the mind.

A great deal of the brain research that is receiving attention in the professional literature as well as in the popular press is the investigation of the specialized functions of the two sides of the brain. Table 10.1 com-

TABLE 10.1
Comparison of Left-Brain and Right-Brain Modes of Thinking

Left Mode	Right Mode
Verbal: Uses words	*Nonverbal:* Awareness without words
Analytic: Step-by-step problem solving	*Synthetic:* Forms wholes from parts
Symbolic: Represents things with signs and pictures	*Concrete:* Relates to things as they are
Abstract: Represents the whole with a piece of information about it	*Analogic:* Sees likenesses among things; understands metaphors
Temporal: Keeps track of time; sequences things	*Nontemporal:* Without a sense of time

TABLE 10.1 (continued)	
Left Mode	*Right Mode*
Rational: Uses reason and facts to draw conclusions	*Nonrational:* Not requiring reason or facts; suspends judgment
Digital: Uses numbers	*Spatial:* Sees things in relation to other things and how the parts form a whole
Logical: Draws conclusions based on logic	*Intuitive:* Makes leaps of insight based on hunches, feelings
Linear: Thinks in terms of linked ideas, leading to a convergent conclusion	*Holistic:* Sees whole things all at once; perceives overall patterns leading to divergent conclusions
Other terms: secondary, propositional, sequential, objective, successive	*Other terms:* primary, imaginative, multiple, subjective, simultaneous

From Edwards, B.: *Drawing on the right side of the brain;* and Bogen, J.E.: Some educational aspects of hemisphere specialization.

pares the thinking modes attributed to the two sides of the brain. Although researchers are continuing to pursue this direction of studying the brain, David Bohm and Karl Pribram proposed that the brain does not function in the totally dichotomized way described by the "split-brain theory." What they have proposed is that the brain functions holographically (Dossey, 1982, pp. 102–114; Ferguson, 1980, pp. 177–187). A *hologram* is a picture of something, any piece of which will reconstruct the entire image. Photographically, this picture is taken on a special plate using a laser beam.

A three-dimensional likeness of the original object can be projected into space using the plate and laser beams. If the plate is shattered, each piece seems to contain the entire image and can in fact be used to project the same three-dimensional representation as the original intact plate.

Bohm and Pribram have advocated the notion that each hemisphere of the brain encodes all the information available to the brain. They believe that every brain cell contains all the information stored in the total organism. This model of looking at the brain is only a part of their larger model as it applies to the entire universe. This model may help to explain some of the mystical experiences of many people, such as extrasensory perception. The so-called holographic super theory states that "our brains mathematically construct 'hard' reality by interpreting frequencies from a dimension transcending time and space. The brain is a hologram, interpreting a holographic universe" (Ferguson, 1981, p. 182).

These approaches to looking at the brain are not necessarily contradictory. Even though further research may support the holographic model, there are still some parts of the brain that seem to specialize in certain processes, although other parts of the brain can take over these processes under certain circumstances, such as after brain injury. Furthermore, even though the processes carried on by each side of the brain seem to differ, it seems to be advantageous to cultivate the functioning and interaction of the thinking modes of each hemisphere.

The modes common to the left hemisphere, analytical, rational, and logical thinking, have been highly valued and even have been given a masculine connotation. The qualities of the right hemisphere, nontemporal, nonrational, intuitive, and holistic thinking, have been devalued and often attributed to feminine thinking styles. Some investigators are pursuing the seeming gender-linked preferences for the utilization of one hemisphere or the other, but no conclusive evidence has been produced to provide a biochemical explanation for the link of one hemisphere to a particular gender.

Although many people still think that men and women think differently and that the male way of thinking is better, there is more and more evidence that both sexes are capable of thinking in the same ways. Researchers may eventually discover that there is some sex-linked preference for the thinking mode a person uses most, but there is already much evidence that people can and do learn to use both types of thinking. The trend is toward unifying our ideas about the functioning of the brain, in accord with the trend toward unifying concepts about the functioning of the body, mind, and spirit. Models like the holographic idea support the concept of unity among human organisms, the environment, and the universe.

Thinking about thinking increases our effectiveness in using that process and therefore increases our effectiveness as nurses. The remainder of this chapter explores some ideas about thinking more effectively in narrowly circumscribed areas and examines ways of using our thinking capacities to grapple with complex global issues.

States of Thinking

Steele and Maraviglia (1981, pp. 4–6) have identified four states of thinking:

1. *Vertical.* Thinking in expected ways. It is logical and progressive; steps are in sequence.

2. *Lateral.* Thinking in unexpected ways; not sequential. Enhances the possibility of discovering new and different solutions to a problem.

3. *Creative.* More advanced than vertical and lateral thinking. Goes beyond past experiences; innovative and imaginative.

4. *The 4th Dimension.* Thinking that is "cosmic," holistic, intuitive.

Vertical thinking parallels left-brain thinking, while the other three states can be included in right-brain thinking. Each state is useful and valuable. One can develop one's ability to think in all of these states and be able to determine which state is appropriate in a given situation. For example, think of the mundane things one does everyday: getting up and going to the bathroom, driving to work or school, or going from the parking lot to the building. Usually, vertical thinking is not only appropriate to such activities but also helpful. By going about routine tasks in sequential, logical ways, a person can do them automatically and at the same time use his or her intellect for things that are more meaningful. Beyond basic daily activities, there are many situations in which the problem-solving process warrants a logical, vertical approach. Using a lateral, nonsequential approach may be frustrating and time consuming and may not produce better results.

Since vertical thinking is so useful and since it is the process most people have been taught, people tend to rely on it and forget that there are other ways of approaching old and new problems. Occasionally, it may be helpful to apply lateral thinking to common situations. For example, what if you approached a mundane task with a lateral state of thinking. What if you took a different route to work or to school? You might find that you were much more aware of your surroundings than you were following the old route. The same thing might happen when more significant changes must be made. Frequently you become so accustomed to doing things in a certain way that you have not examined whether that is the most effective or efficient way to accomplish a goal.

In busy, full lives, people infrequently step back, reexamine, and plan new ways of doing the same things they have been doing. Planning that is *proactive,* or brought about by internal motivation, is usually much more effective and satisfying than a reactive response. Naisbitt (1982) has identified several trends that indicate that our society is becoming less crisis oriented and more interested in long-term planning. He has also noted our new tendency to think of ourselves as world citizens rather than merely as citizens of this nation. People are choosing to become more involved in governance and more insistent on self-determination. All of these changes require versatile thinking.

Becoming a Versatile Thinker

The first step in becoming a versatile thinker is to be willing to acknowledge that there are different ways of thinking and that all of these ways have value. The next step is to develop skill in thinking in different states, from vertical through fourth-dimension thinking. Finally, it is necessary to learn when it is appropriate to use each state of thinking.

Vertical Thinking

Vertical thinking is logical, sequential, and progressive. The scientific method and the nursing process are examples of this kind of thinking. The first step in vertical thinking is gathering data and organizing it in some meaningful way. Next, the data is analyzed and conclusions are drawn about what requires action and in what order action must be taken. Goals and objectives are set. Actions are planned, based on goals, and priorities are assigned. Then action is implemented and evaluation, based on the objectives, is undertaken. The qualities of the left-brain mode of thinking described in Table 10.1 fit the nursing process accurately.

Even the novice nurse can see, however, left-brain thinking is not all that takes place. For instance, many times a nurse "knows" something is wrong with a client without knowing how she or he knows. A nurse may sometimes do exactly the right thing for a client based strictly on a hunch. Some of the difficulty in learning and teaching nursing is inherent in the difficulties of integrating left- and right-brain modes of thinking. It is difficult for nursing students to learn how to be sequential and logical in planning client care and also to be holistic in their approaches. It is also difficult for the teachers of nursing to teach the whole nursing process by focusing on the parts. Everything is linked to everything else.

Lateral thinking, creative thinking, and 4th Dimension thinking are characterized as nonsequential, unexpected, innovative, imaginative, holistic, and intuitive, all qualities of the right-brain mode of thinking. Some writers include all these kinds of thinking under the same category, creativity. These states will be considered here as increasingly higher levels of right-brain thinking.

Lateral Thinking

Lateral thinking is being able to come up with solutions that are unrelated to previous ways of solving a problem. For example, economic restrictions and resulting personnel decreases may necessitate changes in how a city health department provides immunization services to children. Thinking vertically, one would assess what resources were available and reallocate them so that the same number of children could be immunized at centralized clinics as at satellite clinics in the past. Thinking laterally, one might set community nurses up in booths in shopping centers, where overhead costs would be assumed by the shopkeepers and clients would not have to make an extra trip for the service.

Creative Thinking

To be considered creative, thinking must be novel. It must solve a problem, fit a situation, or accomplish a goal; and it involves sustaining and elaborating an idea to its fullest (MacKinnon, 1965). Some thinking that is novel in a particular situation or for a particular person may not be considered creative, because it is not truly innovative. For example, a beginning nursing student is assigned to a client who speaks a different language from the student. The student makes flash cards with common phrases and words to enable her to communicate with the client quickly about typical daily needs and activities. Since she was new to the field, the student was probably unaware that this is a relatively common solution to the problem. However, it was a fresh approach, if not novel, and would be an example of lateral thinking. Creativity often springs from a thorough knowledge of a field. That is, once a person knows what is already common practice, that individual is better prepared to go beyond previous solutions and develop innovative approaches. Therefore, once that same nurs-

ing student became more knowledgeable about nursing, she was in a position to solve the same problem in a genuinely unique way.

Guilford (1959) identified several traits that characterized creative behavior. Successive research has tended to confirm these traits as definitive of the creative thinker. The traits are:

1. *Problem awareness.* Ability to find, describe, and state a problem.
2. *Fluency.* Ability to generate many ideas.
3. *Flexibility.* Ability to generate a variety of ideas.
4. *Originality.* Ability to produce novel responses.
5. *Elaboration.* Ability to develop an idea from a simple to a complex form.
6. *Problem solving.* Ability to analyze a situation and produce an answer.
7. *Tolerance of ambiguity.* Ability to be flexible in categorizing or classifying.
8. *Convergent thinking.* Ability to deduce a correct solution to a problem.
9. *Divergent thinking.* Ability to search for alternative solutions to a problem.

Note that these traits represent both left- and right-brain thinking. A creative person is versatile in the thinking modes he or she uses.

4th Dimension Thinking

4th Dimension thinking is thinking that transcends space and time. The model described earlier of a holographic universe is an example of a holistic, cosmic leap in conceptualizing the universe and everything within it. This is probably the most difficult type of thinking to cultivate, because it requires such a high degree of freedom from one's usual way of functioning. It requires an openness and a willingness to explore uncharted territory that is as threatening as it is exciting.

BLOCKS TO EFFECTIVE THINKING

Certain things tend to get in the way when you try to solve problems, especially if you are moving to a new level of thinking. Adams (1979) classified these as perceptual, emotional, cultural, environmental, intellectual, and expressive *blocks*. By being aware of these influences, it is possible to confront them and to become more productive in solving problems.

Perceptual Blocks

Perceptual blocks are those that interfere with the problem solver's ability to perceive the problem itself or the information needed to solve the problem. Some common examples of perceptual blocks are:

· Seeing what one expects to see.
· Having difficulty isolating the problem.
· Defining the problem too narrowly.
· Being unable to see the problem from more than one viewpoint.
· Saturation: being so familiar with something that one cannot describe it.
· Failing to utilize all sensory inputs: relying only on visual perceptions and ignoring auditory or olfactory data.

Emotional Blocks

Emotional factors intervene when an individual's personal problems are counterpro-

ductive to solving problems or when an individual's needs are threatened by the problem or by the problem-solving process. Some examples of emotional blocks are:

· Fear of taking a risk.
· Inability to tolerate ambiguity; strong desire for security and order.
· Preference for judging ideas rather than generating them.
· Inability to relax and let ideas incubate.
· Lack of challenge or interest in the problem.
· Excessive zeal and desire to succeed quickly.
· Lack of imaginative thinking.
· Inability to control the imagination.
· Inability to distinguish fantasy from reality.

Cultural and Environmental Blocks

Cultural and environmental restrictions to imagination are learned from significant others and from life experiences. Cultural restrictions may be based on beliefs such as the following:

· Fantasy and reflection are lazy.
· Playfulness is only for children.
· Problem solving is serious business and humor is not appropriate.
· Reason, logic, numbers, utility, and practicality are good; feeling, intuition, qualitative judgments, and pleasure are bad.
· Tradition is preferable to innovation.
· Any problem can be solved given scientific thinking and plenty of money.
· Taboo subjects are not to be thought about.

Environmental blocks include the following:

· Lack of cooperation and trust among colleagues.
· Autocratic bosses, leaders, or teachers who value their own ideas and do not reward others.
· Distractions, such as telephone calls and other intrusions.
· Lack of support to bring ideas into action.

Intellectual and Expressive Blocks

Intellectual blocks result from inefficient ways of thinking about a problem or from inadequate intellectual power. Expressive hindrances are difficulties in communicating ideas effectively. Examples of these difficulties are:

· Thinking about things vertically rather than laterally or creatively.
· Lack of or incorrect information.
· Using the incorrect language for the problem: for example, using mathematical approaches when visualization would be more efficient.
· Inflexible or inadequate use of intellectual problem-solving methods.
· Inadequate language skill to express and record ideas.

By being aware of some of the common blocks to effective thinking, people can analyze their own approaches and identify ways in which they can become proficient at tactics other than those they currently use. The following example shows how these blocks can diminish one's problem-solving ability:

A nursing student was assigned to a young woman who had four children under 5 years of age. The client was afraid of becoming pregnant again, as she already felt overwhelmed by her children. The student immediately accumulated literature on various conception control methods and explained several methods to the client in the course of one home visit. The woman had a sixth-grade education, and she seemed to learn very little from the student's well-meant presentation. Several weeks later, the student reviewed the woman's clinic record and discovered that an intrauterine device (IUD) had been inserted during the client's first clinic visit after delivery of her last child. When the client was seen a few days before the student read the record, the IUD was still in place.

The student relied on vertical thinking. In addition, her information was inadequate, not only about the client's history but also about appropriate teaching-learning methods. These are indications of problems in the intellectual area. Some examples of perceptual blocks are the student's definition of the client's problem as a need for information on conception-control methods and her difficulty in determining exactly what the problem was before she tried to solve it. The student's apparent need to succeed quickly indicates an emotional block. This situation shows how easily a well-motivated, intelligent person can still get off on the wrong track by not thinking a problem through.

DEVELOPING THINKING SKILLS

Much useful literature on increasing one's ability to think effectively deals specifically with creativity. However, many exercises are just as useful for promoting vertical and lateral thinking. There are several resources included in the reference list at the end of this chapter, but four of the best ones are James L. Adams, *Conceptual Blockbusting;* Edward deBono, *Lateral Thinking;*

George M. Prince, *The Practice of Creativity*; and Shirley M. Steele and Frank L. Maraviglia, *Creativity in Nursing*.

The methods used to increase effective problem solving are usually designed to promote problem awareness, fluency, flexibility, originality, elaboration, tolerance for ambiguity, and convergent and divergent thinking. The following sections describe factors and activities that enhance effective thinking.

Making Expectations Explicit

To facilitate effective and creative thinking, one's expectations about the eventual outcome must be made explicit. Making expectations explicit means describing required limits completely, clearly, and inclusively. Occasionally, the process of clarifying and identifying expectations helps solve a problem. Sometimes, something has been defined as a problem only because people's expectations are unclear. For example:

Some members of a nurse's association expressed concern that the organization had not been more productive in getting legislation passed. Discussions were held to identify ways of being more productive. The nurse leading the discussions first suggested that the group clarify what degree of effort or success would be considered the target level of productivity. Finally, it became clear that the group members were looking only at the numbers of bills passed without considering association priorities and resources. Once they compared the effort expended with the priorities that had been established by the general membership, the group realized that the legislative efforts had been very effective.

By clarifying expectations, the people in this situation were able to value the work being done and avoid fruitless hours of trying to figure out how to accomplish the vague goal of "becoming more productive."

In other situations that require problem solving, setting expectations helps one weed out unsatisfactory solutions. Seemingly wonderful ideas either may not be realistic or may have untenable consequences. Some solutions are useless, trivial, or even dangerous. On the other hand, some solutions that at first seem strange may fit the expectations quite well. It is helpful to list all the possible outcomes of the favored solutions in order to evaluate them. If the person or group that selects the solution is fearful about possible consequences, they should dwell on the most catastrophic possibilities. This will demonstrate that it is relatively difficult to do real damage; it will also help them avoid such problems or to cope with them if they do arise.

Risking and Persevering

In five minutes, list as many unusual uses as possible for a common object, such as a brick. Evaluate your performance on the basis of the number of different uses listed (fluency), the number of different kinds of uses (i.e., if three different uses were related to propping something up, together they comprise one kind of use—flexibility), the average number of words used to describe each response (elaboration), and, compared to other people, the frequency or infrequency of given responses (originality). If this kind of exercise piques your interest, Reid J. Daitzman's book *Mental Jogging* has one for each day of the year.

The unusual-uses type of problem encourages two valuable strategies for thinking more effectively: *risking* and *persevering*. People who quit before they start or who quit too soon are not as productive as those who risk trying and who persevere. Puzzles are good ways to try out thinking strategies in controlled, nonthreatening circumstances. People who work puzzles may become more flexible, fluent, elaborative, and original.

Whether or not you attempted to solve the brick exercise may reveal something about your current interest and ability in thinking. Many people enjoy such mental exercises, and probably they immediately grabbed a piece of paper and began jotting down ideas. Others might have felt that it was a frivolous suggestion to find in a textbook; while others skimmed over the exercise, assuming that they would be unsuccessful even if they attempted to produce such a list. The second group is responding to the culturally inculcated belief that playfulness is appropriate only in certain situations and that learning is definitely not one of them. The third group is giving in to the emotional factors of fearing risks and lacking imagination. (Of course, there are other reasons, such as a feeling that one has to get through the material that is assigned reading for class!)

The people who tend to respond to opportunities to solve puzzles and to take challenges are probably more successful the longer they stay with the task. It is not too difficult to come up with several ideas immediately, but the people who stick with such activities tend to come up with the best ideas. Recent studies by Sternberg and Davidson (1982) have demonstrated that the people who are most successful at this type of task are those who are willing to spend the necessary amount of time on it.

Expanding Perceptions

Expanding your perceptions will help you to conquer many of the perceptual blocks to creative thinking. It will increase your ability to define a problem, to use all your senses, and to see what is really there rather than what you expect to see. With the problem with the brick, your responses might have been limited because of an inability to conceive of the object as anything but a brick. Listing the qualities of a brick will help you see it as a more versatile article. Some of its qualities are: heaviness, roughness, three-dimensionality, and capacity to store heat. Looking at a brick as a receptable of heat may lead to some familiar uses, such as bed warmer, as well as other uses, such as food warmer, water heater, wax melter, wrinkle presser, and plastic bonder. Another expansion of the perception of the brick is to think of it in other forms rather than only in the present form. For example, pulverize the brick and use the particles in an hour glass; chip pieces off to use as ground cover in a terrarium; or break it in half and bang the pieces together for a noisemaker.

Some other activities to expand your perceptions are: from memory, draw the dial or push bottoms on a telephone, with the numbers and letters; draw the face of your watch; draw the dashboard of your car. Sometimes it it surprising to realize how little you can remember of things you see everyday.

Challenging Assumptions

A common block to problem solving is making unwarranted assumptions. A useful exercise is one that causes you to challenge your assumptions. An example of an assumption would be having assumed that you were not really expected to respond to the brick problem. Sometimes people assume limitations that are not implicit in an assignment, such as assuming that the brick had to remain intact. A classic problem demonstrating how people may be limited by assumptions is shown in Figure 10.1. In the figure, there are nine dots. Cross all the dots using only four straight lines

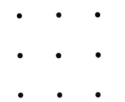

Figure 10.1 Nine-dot problem.

and without lifting your pencil from the paper.

Even though you have been prepared to realize that the secret to solving this puzzle lies in challenging assumptions, you may still limit yourself. The most common assumption that people make is that the lines have to be within the rectangle formed by the dots. Other common assumptions are that the lines have to go through the midpoints of the dots; the paper has to stay flat; the lines cannot go beyond the confines of the page; and the paper has to stay intact. The only limits, all of which are explicit, are: all the dots must be crossed; there are to be four straight lines; and you may not lift your pencil from the paper until all the lines are drawn. Making the limits explicit may help those who have not already solved the problem. Some inventive people have solved it using only three lines or only one line. How might the problem be solved with fewer lines? (Solutions are at the end of this chapter.)

Suspending Judgment

A common emotional block to effective thinking and problem solving is premature judgment. This can affect one's own ability to generate solutions; this kind of behavior limits one's ability to support others in solving problems. It is useful to suspend judgment until after there has been a reasonable amount of time spent in generating ideas. The amount of time that is reasonable depends on the nature of the problem. For example, in the unusual-uses exercise, 10 minutes would be a useful time span. For a more significant problem, several hours at different times might be appropriate. Evaluating every idea as it occurs limits people from ever coming up with an unusual solution that might actually work. Sometimes people do not follow through on ideas because they believe the ideas are too obvious or too ordinary. People also are reluctant to share ideas that seem outlandish.

The following exercise illustrates the value of suspending judgment (Adams, 1979, p. 54):

Assume that a steel pipe is imbedded in the concrete floor of a bare room. The inside diameter of the pipe is .06″ larger than the diameter of the ping pong ball (1.50″) that is resting at the bottom of the pipe. The pipe protrudes 4″ above the floor. You have only the following objects with you in the room: 100′ of clothesline; a carpenter's hammer; a chisel; a box of corn flakes; a file; a wire coat hanger; a monkey wrench; and a light bulb. List as many ways you can think of in five minutes to get the ping pong ball out of the pipe without damaging the ball, the pipe, or the floor.

In this exercise, fluency and flexibility as well as originality and elaboration are required. Assess your propensity to judge by noting if you kept yourself from thinking about any possible solutions because the idea seemed silly, weird, or difficult to implement. Adams gives an example of how people confronted with this problem keep themselves from voicing a particular solution. That solution is that one could urinate into the pipe raising the ball to a level where it could be retrieved. People may be embarrassed to mention urination and thus prejudge this solution as impossible. Judging ideas too quickly may cause you to rule out entire groups of solutions.

Fostering Self-Esteem

People who feel good about themselves are usually more willing and able to submit their ideas for the consideration of others. They are able to laugh at themselves and not take themselves too seriously. However, most people have some difficulties with self-esteem in situations that remind them of unpleasant experienes. One way of building and protecting self-esteem in problem-solving situations is to deliberately set up opportunities to work on problems in an atmosphere designed to protect your self-esteem. Working on nonthreatening activities with supportive groups can build your willingness to work with other groups of people on problems of greater consequence. Later in this chapter there is a section on working in groups.

Being Patient

Another problem related to emotional factors is the felt need to hurry to a solution. Be patient. People often undercut their own abilities by trying to produce a quick solution. People often implement their first idea or preliminary plan, as if that were the only possible choice. It is much more useful to let an idea incubate. Develop the habit of writing down your ideas, developing them for a while, and then leaving them for a while. When you come back to them, the situation may look entirely different. Commonly when an idea is percolating in your mind, you will be more aware of and receptive to related information. This helps you sharpen and develop ideas or perhaps discard them for better ones.

Tolerating Ambiguity and Chaos

Tolerance for ambiguity and chaos enhances productivity. *Ambiguity* is the state of being uncertain or obscure in meaning.

Chaos is a state of confusion. Since ambiguity and chaos are uncomfortable, most people will do almost anything to force clarity or to enforce order. Whenever possible, it helps to let the disorder persist until a good solution develops. Hasty solutions are seldom the best ones when they are motivated chiefly by the desire to relieve anxiety.

In an ambiguous situation the nurse may be uncertain about what is actually happening because she or he receives so many stimuli simultaneously. For example, when an individual, a group, or an organization is in the process of change, the situation becomes ambiguous because it is unclear how much of the old will persist and how much newness will be introduced. People who attempt to function in an ambiguous situation should take every opportunity to clarify their roles and expectations, but they must also try to tolerate the uncertainty and obscurity, which may persist for a time.

Chaos is more obviously disruptive than ambiguity. Chaos is sometimes the result of prolonged ambiguity; that is, conditions are uncertain and unclear for long enough that extreme confusion and disorganization result. A premature push to establish order may promote chaos. For example:

The waiting room of a maternity clinic was always noisy with the sounds of clients' children. The children were sometimes poorly supervised by their parents and troublesome. The nurses at first decided to require parents to keep their children quiet while in the waiting room area. This seemed to have little effect, and some of the clients were openly resentful of this request. Some clients discontinued their association with the clinic.

Finally, the nurses decided to convert part of the waiting room into a play area. It was enclosed with sound-deadening walls and had unbreakable windows on the side facing the rest of the room. Soft toys, blocks, picture books, and other play materials suitable for young children were put in the room. No one was required to use the room, but frequently mothers as well as children waited there. Some children were old enough to be together in the playroom while their parents visited with one another in sight through the windows.

In this example, the nurses recognized the needs of the parents and children for a suitable place to wait. By tolerating some of the confusion inherent in serving parents with small children, the nurses provided a less chaotic atmosphere that was more pleasant for clients, their children, and the nurses.

APPLYING THINKING SKILLS

The following situation demonstrates the application of the activities for developing thinking skills in working with a client:

Jennifer Bryant told Martha Miller, a registered nurse, that her 18-month-old son, Robin, would not stay in bed alone when she put him there at 8:00 P.M. To get him to stay in bed and go to sleep, Ms. Bryant would lie down with him. Robin still would not go to sleep until after 10:00. Ms. Bryant said that she was frustrated because she had no time in the evening to get anything done.

Ms. Miller talked with Ms. Bryant about what her expectations were in the situation. Ms. Bryant wanted to be able to get things done in the evening, and she wanted Robin to get as much sleep as he needed. Then they brainstormed and generated several possible alternatives:

· Have Mr. Bryant take a turn on alternate nights
· Lock Robin in his room
· Make Robin stay in bed and ignore his crying
· Give him a sedative
· Don't let him take a nap during the day
· Spank him
· Put him to bed at 10:00
· Let him stay up as late as he wants
· Make him stay up later than 10:00

Ms. Bryant had assumed that Robin needed 12 hours of sleep, but realized he was not getting

that much and still seemed fine. At first she thought making him stay up even later than he wanted to was silly, but Ms. Miller encouraged her to try the idea. Then Ms. Bryant said she was not sure what he would do if he stayed up. She finally decided that she would keep him up until half an hour after he first asked to go to bed or until 11:00, whichever came first, and that she would spend one hour with him doing whatever he wanted to do from 7:00 to 8:00. After that, he would play by himself or be with Ms. Bryant while she did what she needed to do.

When Ms. Miller followed up on how Ms. Bryant was doing, she found that things had worked out well. At first, Robin tried to get Ms. Bryant to come to his room later than 8:00 P.M. Then he would say he was ready to go "night-night." He would say this until the half hour was over and she put him to bed. Then, two nights in a row, she found him asleep on the floor in the living room at 11:00. After that, when he asked to go to bed, she spent 10 minutes with him; he usually fell asleep in that time. If he pleaded with her to stay with him, she got him up until he decided to go back to bed.

Ms. Bryant felt that her expectations had been met, and she felt better about herself as a mother. She expressed surprise that the plan had worked, but once it did, she thought of additional ideas on her own for dealing with Robin. She felt that solving this problem had enriched her relationship with her son.

This example demonstrates Ms. Bryant's abilities to become more versatile in her thinking because of the stimulation provided by the nurse. Ms. Bryant was willing to suspend her initial judgment on the problem-solving approach. She expanded her perception of the situation by recognizing that her logical approach to putting Robin to bed was not working. She was willing to risk trying what seemed an absurd solution, and she kept working at it and elaborating the solution to fit her situation. She was patient, knowing that the pattern of Robin's behavior had been established over time and that it would take time to change it. She also was willing to tolerate the paradox of trying to get her son to go to bed by keeping him up late.

The nurse, Ms. Miller, promoted and encouraged the planning process, but she let Ms. Bryant decide on the action that would be taken. In this instance, the choice was workable and the client carried it out effectively. Sometimes a client makes a choice that he or she is not able to carry out. In such a situation, the nurse can help the client go through the problem-solving process again to find a workable course of action.

THINKING IN GROUPS

Although many people work well and productively when they try to plan or to solve problems alone, a group can often be more productive than an individual. The most significant effect of a group working together is synergy. Fuller defines *synergy* as "behavior of whole systems unpredicted by the behavior of their parts taken separately" (1982, p. 3). When groups of people work together in planning and problem-solving situations, their combined efforts are often more effective than the sum of their individual efforts might have been. This is an example of synergy.

Understanding

There are two aspect to a group's working together. The first is understanding. Each person in the group must understand the assignment or mission of the group: everyone must be working toward the same end. If the situation has limits, these must be clarified. Everyone must understand who is responsible for generating, elaborating, and implementing ideas. The group's authority must also be delineated. For example, the group's ideas may serve as advice to someone in authority or as direction. Whichever it is to be, the members of the group must understand this from the outset.

The process of clarifying a group's mission sometimes helps demonstrate that those who are trying to explain the mission do not understand it themselves. No group should try to plan or problem-solve without agreeing on a statement of what is to be accomplished. If the task has been assigned by someone outside the group, it will help to have that person either appear before the group or send a written statement of the group mission.

Planning or Solving

The second aspect of the group's working together is the work phase, planning or solving. There are three principles that promote effective group work (Prince, 1970):

1. Everyone in the group should have the right to protect his or her self-image.
2. Aggression in the group should be directed toward the problem, not toward group members.
3. Effective group work results in everyone winning.

In group planning or problem solving, the focus is on the mission, not on the individuals. The way to generate and maintain the momentum of the group is for all members to respect each other and value each other's contributions. Competition is not productive among group members, nor is aggression. Positive interaction among group members will promote effective planning and problem solving.

The activities listed earlier in the chapter for promoting effective thinking all apply to group work: making expectations explicit, risking and persevering, expanding perceptions, challenging assumptions, suspending judgment, fostering self-esteem, being patient, and tolerating chaos. Four other behaviors are particularly important in group thinking. First, when a member wishes to express a feeling or idea, stating it in the first person is best: "I feel uncomfortable with this idea," rather than "The group seems uncomfortable with this idea." This is related to risking: the group member should be direct about what he or she thinks or feels.

Second, don't ask questions when it is more appropriate to make statements. Frequently, we ask questions to help us avoid revealing our thoughts or feelings. Unless asking a question is really the best way to draw out additional information, making a statement is better, because it is less threatening. For example, instead of asking, "What would you do about people earning too much overtime with this plan?" one might state, "It looks like people would earn too much overtime with this plan. That bothers me."

The third behavior is listening. When someone expresses ideas or feelings, listen to what he or she says as well as the manner in which it is said. One of the most common interferences to listening is that we tend to hear just enough of what another person says to formulate a response or opinion. Really attending to what the other person says and encouraging elaboration shows people that their contribution is important.

Sometimes in group sessions, everyone is generating ideas and people quickly pick up on each other's thoughts and declare their own slants on them. This tends to be productive, even though it may appear that people are not listening to each other carefully. This heightened productivity comes about when people build on each other's ideas. Building on ideas must be balanced with listening, so that no one's contributions are ignored. If some people are reluc-

tant to join in, other group members can encourage them by reiterating earlier ideas those quiet people contributed.

Brainstorming

When people are building on one another's ideas and elaborating on the newly developed ideas, synergy is taking place. People think of things they would never have thought of alone, or they remember things they have forgotten. This process has been given the name "brainstorming." *Brainstorming* is a technique for encouraging spontaneous contributions from members of a group. The ground rules for brainstorming are (Pfeiffer & Jones, 1971, p. 19):

1. No criticism of ideas is allowed during the brainstorming phase.
2. Far-out ideas are encouraged, since they may trigger other, more practical ideas for someone else.
3. Quantity of ideas is desirable.

Brainstorming exercises may be done on simple, nonthreatening problems in order to practice playing by the rules. For example, the group may be asked to think of as many uses as possible for a brick, a safety pin, a pop bottle, or a ball of string. Pfeiffer and Jones (1971) suggest the following problem:

Imagine you are cast ashore nude on a desert island with nothing but a leather belt. What can be done with the object? The group has ten minutes to generate ideas. (p. 20)

This assignment always yields many suggestions. Groups are usually amazed at how many ideas they come up with, as well as how members stimulate each other.

Once a group appreciates the effectiveness of brainstorming, they can utilize it for planning and solving in more significant areas. For example:

After doing the exercise above, a group of nursing students told the faculty member that they wanted to apply the process to an issue they were interested in. The issue: How can we get as many students as possible from our school to the National Student Nurses' Association Convention? The outcome was that all 30 students who wanted to go to the convention went, mostly supported by funds raised in activities suggested in the brainstorming session.

The fourth thing that must take place during group thinking is deciding. At some point, the group must rank ideas, discard some, and begin to determine what is useful as well as how to use it. This part of the process should include stating and listening behaviors. The group that works effectively will come up with collaborative plans and solutions—solutions that contain some of everyone's input but that represent unique constructs devised by the group as a whole. All of the suggestions given here for individual and group thinking will promote collaboration.

There is another stimulant for promoting thinking in groups and in individuals: laughter. Humor often livens things up and reduces tension. The important consideration is that one not laugh at another person. However, many ideas are humorous, and laughing at them is fine. It is also acceptable to laugh at oneself. Some people are good at introducing humor intentionally at the appropriate moments. Other people are good at unintentionally generating hilarious ideas that loosen up a group. Even if the topic under discussion is serious (maybe especially if the topic is serious), humor is valuable.

FUTURE IMPLICATIONS

Ferguson (1980) states that survival skills for the twenty-first century include synthe-sis and pattern seeing. These thinking processess represent whole-brain functioning. The right side contributes innovation, sensing, and dreaming, and the left side provides analysis, ordering, and validating. New information based on experience and research is supplanting what students of a generation ago learned. To confront this continous upheaval, people must recognize that all so-called facts are contingent on present knowledge. Therefore, new facts may emerge as knowledge advances. Thus knowledge itself is ambiguous—we learn things we are sure to have to correct later as new knowledge and new ways of handling information emerge.

Eventually, there will be answers to many of today's questions about how the brain functions, how people think, and how people know. But then there will be more questions—questions at present unimaginable because we have not discovered the answers to the intervening questions. A seventeenth-century Pilgrim would not have wondered about problems such as how to develop public transportation systems for cities with a million or more citizens. By the same token, we of the late twentieth century cannot imagine what questions will demand the attention of people ten generations in the future. As sophisticated, inventive, and clever as we seem to be, we will appear fairly naive to inhabitants of earth in the twenty-third century.

Loye (1982) has begun to investigate the relationship of the brain areas to success in forecasting future events. Loye's preliminary research indicates that those who balanced their use of the two sides of the brain tend to be better predictors than those who rely more one one side or the other. Further investigation may yield more information about how people learn not only how to think more effectively but also how to become better predictors and planners.

Einstein, as well as other physicists, used thought experiments to test models and theories that were untestable in any other way. A thought experiment involves testing a plan or hypothesis in your imagination and projecting the possible outcomes. This is a useful method for thinking in any field. It is a blending of innovation and analysis that nurses can use to solve today's problems as well as to formulate plans for the future.

Future research in thinking may extend into areas concerning perception of other people's thoughts or thought transference. Some people speculate that such extrasensory abilities are within any person's capacity. Although some of us may be skeptical, the future of nursing may be affected by discoveries about direct communication of thoughts. Perhaps technological devices will be invented to make this possible between people or between people and machines.

Computers are already being used in planning and problem solving. As technology develops and as we expand our ability to use it, we will make even better use of computers for conceptualizing, analyzing, and synthesizing. Possible solutions to a problem can be tested in a computer simulation that carries some of the emotional impact of a real-life situation but does not endanger people. As nurses become more familiar with computers, they will enhance the learning and the practicing of nursing. Computers will be used to guide and challenge nurses as they go through the planning and problem-solving processes.

SUMMARY

Many of the tools a nurse uses change rapidly. New medications are produced; new technology replaces the old; physical assessment becomes more thorough;

knowledge of the community population becomes more specific; communications systems become more diversified. With all this change, the nurse's consistent tool is his or her mind and the ability to use it. Research about the brain is already improving its use and will undoubtedly continue to do so.

There are techniques for improving and enhancing thinking processes that can promote more effective nursing practice. As nurses participate more in promoting the health of individuals and of populations, they will need to be good thinkers, both alone and in groups of colleagues and consumers.

Thinking and nursing are often limited only by the bonds put on them by the thinker or the nurse. To promote both processes, it is up to each nurse to loosen those bonds and fly. Ferguson (1980, p. 293) quotes a poem by Guillaume Apollinaire:

Come to the edge, he said.
They said: We are afraid.
Come to the edge, he said.
They came.
He pushed them . . . and they flew.

DISCUSSION TOPICS

1. Would you characterize yourself as a right-brain thinker, a left-brain thinker, or an equal combination of both? Give two examples to support your answer.

2. Give an example of your own thinking for each of the four states of thinking: vertical, lateral, creative, and 4th Dimension.

3. Interpret the word or phrase implied by each of the following:

Examples:

$$\frac{glass}{pheasant} = \text{pheasant under glass}$$

$$nommag = \text{backgammon}$$

a. /r/e/a/d/i/n/g/
b. stand
   ‾I‾
c. r
   r o a d
       a
       d
d. ‾o‾
   bsn
   msn
   dns
e. he's/himself
f. ecnalg
g. sympho
h. carthorse
i. cycle
   cycle
   cycle
j. m e
   l a

Answers are at the end of this chapter.

4. What do the puzzles in topic 4 have to do with improving thinking? How did you figure them out? If you had trouble figuring them out, how can you improve your ability to solve these puzzles?

5. Generate several solutions for the following situation by brainstorming in a group. Use the ground rules given in this chapter.

Ms. Tooker has a fracture of her leg. She is 48 and lives alone. She has been unable to master crutch walking. She can use a walker and will be relying on that and a wheelchair for mobility. The most accessible entrance to her home has four narrow, steep steps. (The steps are not as wide or as deep as the base of the walker legs.) How can Ms. Tooker get in and out of her house?

6. What would it be like if thoughts could be directly transmitted from one brain to another?

BIBLIOGRAPHY

Adams, J.L.: *Conceptual blockbusting* (2nd ed.). New York: Norton, 1979.

Bogen, J.E.: Some educational aspects of hemisphere specialization. *UCLA Educator* 17, 24–32, 1975.

Daitzman, R.J.: *Mental jogging*. New York: Richard Marek, 1980.

deBono, E.: *Lateral thinking: Creativity step by step*. New York: Harper & Row, 1970.

Dossey, L.: *Space, time and medicine*. Boulder, Col.: Shambhala Publications, 1982.

Edwards, B.: *Drawing on the right side of the brain*. Los Angeles: J.P. Tarcher, 1979.

Ferguson, M.: *The aquarian conspiracy*. Los Angeles: J.P. Tarcher, 1980.

Fuller, R.B.: *Critical path*. New York: St. Martin's, 1981.

Fuller, R.B.: *Synergetics*. New York: Macmillan, 1982.

Guilford, J.P.: Traits of creativity. In H.H. Anderson, ed., *Creativity and its cultivation*. New York: Harper & Row, 1959.

Loye, D.: The brain and the future. *The Futurist* 16(5), 15–19, 1982.

MacKinnon, D.W.: Personality correlates of creativity. In M.J. Aschner & C.E. Bish, eds., *Productive thinking in education*. New York: National Educational Association and the Carnegie Corporation, 1965.

Naisbitt, J.: *Megatrends*. New York: Warner Books, 1982.

Pfeiffer, J.W., & Jones, J.E.: *A handbook of structured experiences for human relations training*. Iowa City: University Associates Press, 1971.

Pfeiffer, R.S.: The scientific concept of creativity. *Educational Theory* 29, 129–137, 1979.

Prince, G.M.: *The Practice of Creativity*. New York: Collier Books, 1970.

Steele, S.M., & Maraviglia, F.L.: *Creativity in

Nursing. Thorofare, N.J.: Charles B. Slack, 1981.

Sternberg, R.J., & Davidson, J.E.: The mind of the puzzler. *Psychology Today* 16(6), 37–44, 1982.

Other Resources

Aichlmayer, R.H.: A need to identify and develop the creative student. *Journal of Nursing Education* 8(4), 19–21, 24–27, 1969.

Bailey, J.T., McDonald, F.J., & Claus, K.E.: Evaluation of the development of creative behavior in an experimental nursing program. *Nursing Research* 19, 100–108, 1970.

Cole, K.C.: On imagining the unseeable. *Discover* 3(12), 70, 72, 1982.

Cox, R.S.: Rewarding instructions vs. brainstorming in creativity test scores of college students. *Psychological Reports* 41, 951–954, 1977.

Givens, P.R.: Identifying and encouraging creative processes. *Journal of Higher Education* 33, 295–301, 1962.

Glover, J.A.: A creativity-training workshop: Short-term, long-term, and transfer effects. *Journal of Genetic Psychology* 136, 3–16, 1980.

Hofstadter, D.R.: *Gödel Escher, Bach: An eternal golden braid.* New York: Vintage Books, 1980.

Hofstadter, D.R., & Dennett, D.C., eds.: *The mind's I.* New York: Bantam, 1981.

Klimoski, R.J., & Karol, B.L.: The impact of trust on creative problem solving groups. *Journal of Applied Psychology* 61, 630–633, 1976.

MacKinnon, D.W.: Educating for creativity: A modern myth? In P. Heist, ed., *The creative college student: An unmet challenge.* San Francisco: Jossey-Bass, 1968.

MacKinnon, D.W.: The nature and nurture of creative talent. *American Psychologist* 17, 484–494, 1962.

Olmo, B.: Can creativity be taught? Yes. *Social Education* 41, 648–654, 1977.

Olson, R.W.: *The art of creative thinking.* New York: Barnes & Noble, 1980.

Osborn, A.F.: *Applied imagination* (3rd ed..). New York: Scribner's, 1963.

Stafford, L.: On promoting creativity. *Journal of Nursing Education* 20(7), 27–30, 1981.

Torrance, E.P.: Creativity and futurism in education: Retooling. *Education* 100(4), 298–311, 1980.

Torrance, E.P.: *Torrance tests of creative thinking.* Lexington, Mass.: Ginn, 1974.

SOLUTIONS

Nine-Dot Problem

a. Four-line solution to nine-dot problem.

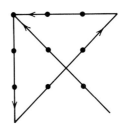

b. Three-line solution to nine-dot problem: The dots were made thicker and the lines did not have to go through the centers of the dots.

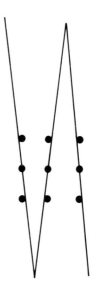

c. One-line solutions have been suggested which include placing the paper on a globe and drawing completely around the globe twice.

Discussion Topic 3

3.a. Reading between the lines
 b. I understand
 c. Crossroads
 d. 3 degrees below zero
 e. He's beside himself
 f. Backward glance
 g. Unfinished symphony
 h. Putting the cart before the horse
 i. Tricycle
 j. Square meal

11

Nursing in the Community

Victoria Schoolcraft

No system can endure that does not march. Are we walking to the future or to the past? Are we progressing or are we stereotyping? There is still so much to do.

FLORENCE NIGHTINGALE

OBJECTIVES

After reading this chapter, you should be able to:

☐ Define the concept of "client" as contrasted to the concept of "patient."
☐ Differentiate between public health nursing and community health nursing.
☐ Describe the American Nurses' Association Conceptual Model of Community Health Nursing.
☐ Define roles of nurses within the community.

INTRODUCTION

As we move through the last part of this century, our society is experiencing many changes that will affect the practice of nursing. Some of these changes have special implications for the practice of nursing in the community. For example, our society is becoming an information society (Naisbitt, 1982), and nurses are among those involved in gathering and relaying information. Clients are coming to expect professionals to teach them what they need to know and to promote their independence rather than

take care of them. This is evidenced in the trend toward primary prevention and the conservation of health. Clients want professionals to keep them well as well as to treat them when they are ill. This new paradigm of health contrasts sharply with the old paradigm of medicine (Ferguson, 1980). The new paradigm emphasizes the interrelationships of mind, body, and spirit that are vital to maintaining wellness. The individual is responsible for attaining this holistic functioning; professionals are involved in health care as "therapeutic partners" (Ferguson, 1980, p. 247).

Advances in technology have made the treatment of illness more aggressive and expensive than ever before. Acute care centers, such as hospitals, have become highly specialized in their complex response to severe illness and traumatic injury. Many conditions that formerly resulted in hospitalization are now treated outside hospitals. For instance, in the first half of this century, pneumonia was nearly always treated in a hospital. It was a life-threatening disease, and its complications were often fatal. With the advent of new pharmacological agents, this disease is now easily managed outside the hospital.

There will always be a need for hospitals for the treatment of severely ill people who are unable to care for themselves. Traumatic injuries will nearly always require hospitalization in order to repair and stabilize the injured person. However, many conditions that now require hospitalization will be treated outside the acute care setting in the future. An area that is already in flux is the treatment of women in childbirth. Since early in this century, this event has been defined as an acute care situation requiring medical intervention in order to promote the health and well-being of the mother and infant. Since the medical paradigm was applied to this event, research and intervention have treated pregnancy and birth as a disease rather than as a normal process. Now there is a trend to put the process more within the control of the client and her family. Hospitals, physicians, and nurses have worked together and independently to establish alternatives to the medical paradigm for the pregnancy and birth experience. Women who proceed normally through their pregnancies have many options for where their pregnancies will end. Nurses, in collaboration with physicians, provide service during normal pregnancies and may even assist the women in delivering in a nonhospital setting. If a woman develops complications, she is referred to the nurse's medical colleagues for appropriate treatment. Physicians and hospitals have established birthing centers, which deemphasize medical intervention and emphasize the family group. Although there are still many physicians, nurses, and others who resist this trend and see it as somehow aberrant, the wish of women and their families to have these options will cause them to persist.

As clients become more sophisticated about health care, they will increasingly demand a variety of health care givers who can truly meet their needs. Clients will be willing to pay nurses reasonable fees to help them maintain their health, and thus there will be more nurses who are either based in the community or who can move comfortably into the community from a base in an acute care setting. As clients grow to value health, they will also increasingly value those who help them promote and maintain health. Nursing has always promoted health, and nurses who wish to make this their primary focus within the community will find an eager clientele.

The promotion of health for whole communities and the identification of populations at risk are traditional public health foci that are experiencing a resurgence. Such broad-based approaches to improve the health of the community at large result in improved health for individuals within the community. A redefinition of nursing in the community is also taking place. In the past, nursing has been a service within the realm of public health and has focused on the whole population. As nursing evolves and practice becomes more diverse, more nursing service is being rendered outside of acute care settings. Such practice has frequently focused on the care of a specific group of clients (the nurse's caseload) rather than on the population as a whole. Many nurses who are involved in public health have become concerned about the lack of precision in defining the practice of nursing within the community. This chapter defines nursing in the community and describes an appropriate role for the practitioner who has been prepared at the undergraduate level.

CLIENTS AND PATIENTS

In the past, people who received service from physicians, nurses, and other health care professionals, especially in a hospital, have been called "patients." Someone who receives service in some other setting is now commonly called a "client." The distinction between these terms is somewhat philosophical, but it is important. A *patient* is generally a person who is under medical care, one who is acted upon. The term often implies passivity: the patient becomes an "object 'to whom' or 'for whom' something is done" (Dossey, 1982, p. 145). Lydia Hall states that "what *characterizes* a patient . . . is his lack of full self-awareness and self control" (Stevens, 1979, p. 24). "A person who does not have control of his own fate is a patient" (Stevens, 1979, p. 25). This term is acceptable for people who are hospitalized with complex diseases or traumatic injuries.

In the new paradigm based on health and wellness, the traditional term for an individual who seeks and needs services is inaccurate. People are now expressing the desire to be independent and are more self-directed than ever before in taking care of their health. The term "client" connotes different behaviors than does the word "patient." A *client* is a person who engages the professional services of another person or agency. Even though a patient certainly can be a client, a client is not always a patient. A client has an independent role. He or she makes decisions about health promotion as well as about care in the case of disease. Perhaps the most important aspect of the use of the term "client" is that it implies use of the client's judgment about whether to engage a given professional in the first place. Once a client has contracted for certain services, she or he can decide whether to follow the advice given, as well as when to terminate the relationship. Health professionals have often spoken about and to "patients" as if the "patients" were obliged to do as they were told. This attitude is inappropriate not only for self-directed adults but also for children, adolescents, and adults who are limited in their abilities, such as retarded people. Even when people are limited in judgment, whether because of age or disability, they are not the property of those responsible for their health or illness care.

Often when clients or patients fail to comply with medical or nursing advice, it is because of the underlying assumptions of the physician or nurse involved. If a health professional regards a patient as dependent, he or she is unlikely to give the patient reasons for the recommendations given. Other physicians and nurses consider the people they work with to be clients who are able to make their own decisions and with whom they should collaborate. They will provide appropriate information and guidance to enable the client to make a wise decision. The nurse or physician who feels responsible for his or her "patients" and who tries to make decisions for them will become frustrated and angry when they do not follow advice. Those who recognize that the clients themselves must decide what to do will be able to evaluate failures in compliance much more realistically. Frequently, problems in compliance are associated with information or communication problems within the client–professional relationship.

If professionals put themselves in authority over dependent clients, they run the risk of forcing the clients to respond in childlike ways. Considering those he or she works with as clients enables the nurse to avoid re-creating interactions typical of parent–child relationships. By treating the client as a competent, self-directed individual, the nurse will create a context in which the two can work most effectively.

Although the definition of a client is based on the fee-for-service principle, many clients do not actually pay the nurse or the agency that employs the nurse. This should not alter the context that the nurse establishes with clients. The essential factors are the same: the nurse works with the client and promotes independent functioning. The nurse's actual contact with clients in the community is quite limited, and the client can terminate the relationship at any time. For these reasons, the nurse must foster an interdependent, collaborative relationship when promoting the client's health status.

An additional advantage of the use of the term "client" is that this term lends itself well to a family, group, or entire population as the focus of nursing service. It is not unusual for a family or community to be referred to as the client in the practice of nursing in the community (Eigsti, Stein, & Fortune, 1982; Young, 1982). This concept will be discussed at length in other parts of this book.

PUBLIC HEALTH NURSING

Originally, the practice of nursing within the community was identified with public health (Barkauskas, 1982). For that reason, a definition of public health will be helpful:

Public health is the science and art of preventing disease, prolonging life, and promoting physical and mental health and efficiency through organized community efforts toward a sanitary environment; the control of community infections; the education of the individual in principles of personal hygiene; the organization of medical and nursing service for the early diagnosis and treatment of disease; and the development of the social machinery which will ensure to every individual in the community a standard of living adequate for the maintenance of health. (Winslow, 1952, p. 30)

Kark (1974, p. 319) further emphasizes that the focus of public health is on "the health of population groups such as the community" as opposed to the individual client.

The Public Health Nursing Section of the American Public Health Association defined *public health nursing* in a position paper adopted in 1981 (APHA, 1982). Part of the definition is as follows:

Public health nursing synthesizes the body of knowledge from the public health sciences and professional nursing theories for the purpose of improving the health of the entire community. This goal lies at the heart of primary prevention and health promotion and is the foundation for public health nursing practice. To accomplish this goal, public health nurses work with groups, families and individuals as well as in multidisciplinary teams and programs. Identifying subgroups (aggregates) within the population which are at high risk of illness, disability, or premature death, and directing resources toward these groups, is the most effective approach for accomplishing the goal of PHN. Success in reducing the risk and in improving the health of the community depend on the involvement of consumers, especially groups experiencing health risks, and others in the community, in health planning, and in self-help activities. (APHA, 1982, p. 210)

The further definition of public health nursing practice denotes the activities within each phase of the nursing process as follows (APHA, 1982, p. 211):

Assessment of health needs:

1. Nurses identify groups within the population at increased risk of illness, disability, or premature death; and
2. consider environmental, psychological, social, and personal health factors.

Planning for health care:

Nurses may be working with the family or individual, as well as the group, but the emphasis is for the community as a whole and the interrelationships between the individual, family, and community rather than for the individual. The plan

1. includes community and consumer involvement in health planning, self-help, and individual responsibility for personal health habits which promote health and a safe environment;
2. is consistent with community needs and expectations;
3. focuses on prevention at the most appropriate level; and
4. coordinates planning with other services and organizations in the community to maximize resources.

Implementation of the plan:

To accomplish the goal of effective, efficient, and equitable intervention, public health nursing

1. provides nursing care that incorporates health promotion and disease prevention;
2. works with groups, families, and individuals who have increased risk of illness, disability, or premature death;
3. exhibits concern for those who do not present themselves for care through casefinding;
4. functions in multi-disciplinary teams and programs;
5. refers to other agencies in order to ensure comprehensive health and welfare services needed to support health care; and
6. works with and through community leaders, health-related groups, and relevant social action programs to advocate and develop programs of health promotion and disease prevention.

Evaluation of public health nursing practice:

Evaluation is based on

1. identification of measurable service program and patient care objectives; and
2. outcome criteria to determine changes, following intervention, in the health status of groups to which programs have been directed.

COMMUNITY HEALTH NURSING

Community health nursing is defined by the context in which it is practiced more than by its content. The American Nurses' Association has defined community health nursing as follows (ANA, 1973):

[Community health nursing] is a synthesis of nursing practice and public health practice applied to promoting and preserving the health of populations. The nature of this practice is general and comprehensive. It is not limited to a particular age or diagnostic group. It is continuing, not episodic. The dominant responsibility is to the population as a whole. Therefore, nursing directed to individuals, families or groups contributes to the health of the total population. Health promotion, health maintenance, health education, coordination and continuity of care are utilized in a holistic approach to the family, group and community. The nurse's actions acknowledge the need for comprehensive health planning, recognize the influences of social and ecological issues, give attention to populations at risk and utilize the dynamic forces which influence change.

Community health nursing requires the integration of many general areas within nursing, such as the use of the nursing process, interpersonal skills, and leadership principles. It further necessitates the use of specific content from other practice areas, such as medical-surgical, pediatric, and psychiatric nursing. There is also a specialized body of knowledge pertaining to such areas as public health science, health policy, and community dynamics. The discussion that follows on the American Nurses' Association conceptual model will elaborate on these areas.

Nursing in the community, which is the title of this chapter, implies a somewhat broader concept than community health nursing. The premise on which this chapter and this entire book are based is that although there is a role for generalists and specialists as community health nurses, there is also an important role for all nurses to take in their respective communities. Even nurses who are primarily hospital or institutional nurses have an ever-growing need to be involved in the larger communities in which they work and live.

If we have a holistic view of individuals, we must accept that everything that happens to a person affects that person. By the same token, if we view the community and the world at large as systems, we must conclude that everything that affects the system also affects its components. If nurses are to fulfill their roles as health care professionals, they must be concerned with the health and well-being of everyone within the community, regardless of whether or not they have personal contact with each individual. Every nurse lives in the community. As we face the oncoming century, we must promote nursing in the community, as well.

A CONCEPTUAL MODEL

A *conceptual model* is an abstraction that helps us describe and define a given thing. Many models have been constructed to describe nursing in general and various aspects of nursing practice in particular. The Executive Committee of the American Nurses' Association Division on Community Health Nursing Practice appointed a task force in 1978 to develop a conceptual model for community health nursing. This group included nurses involved in practice, education, and research in community health nursing. With review and advice from many other nurses, the task force developed the document called *A Conceptual Model of Community Health Nursing**** (ANA, 1980a). The purpose of the model is to provide direction in the development of nursing curricula and in the practice of community health nursing.

Assumptions

An *assumption* is something that is taken for granted. The assumptions which are part of the model are about the existing health care system and the practice of nursing within that system. Identifying assumptions that underlie a model make clear the basis from which all other components were developed.

Assumption 1: The health care system is complex.

The complexity of a system is determined by the number and complexity of its components as well as the complexity of the communication processes among the components. A system that is composed of subsystems that are in turn made up of other subsystems is quite complex. The health care system is just such a system. Any change in a part of the system affects the system as a whole and the other subsystems. For example, if nursing practice changes, this will affect medical practice as well as economic aspects of the component parts. The task force made the point that

---

* Extensive quotations from *A Conceptual Model of Community Health Nursing* are used with the permission of the American Nurses' Association.

the health care system must be cost effective in order to remain functional in our competitive society (ANA, 1980a, p. 3).

Assumption 2: Primary, secondary, and tertiary health care are components of the health care system.

Primary care serves the majority of people in our population. *Primary care "is continuous, community-based, and is generally provided apart from and prior to inpatient care"* (ANA, 1980a, p. 3). *Secondary care* services are those that require more sophisticated, continuous treatment from professionals, such as those services given in hospitals (ANA, 1980a, p. 3). *Tertiary care* is that provided to people who have rare or complex conditions that require specialized care such as that received in intensive care units and the like (ANA, 1980a, p. 3).

Assumption 2 concerns the provision of services by professionals who care for illness. This is a different perspective than the levels of prevention. In this context, the reference is to the nature of the care given rather than to primary, secondary, and tertiary prevention of disability.

Assumption 3: Nursing, as a subsystem of the health care system, is the product of education and practice based upon research.

As nursing evolves, the profession is developing, through research, a scientific basis for practice. As practice is influenced by research, so is education. In order to be wholly functional as a profession, nursing must continue to expand the scientific principles on which nurses base their practice. This means that nursing theory continually changes as new studies are conducted and new findings are published and distributed. The education of a nurse is never complete. He or she must continue learning in order merely to stay even with current knowledge. Accountability is maintained through legislation and through peer review (ANA, 1980a, p. 4).

Assumption 4: The provision of primary care predominates in community health nursing practice, with lesser involvement in secondary and tertiary care.

"Primary health care is more often continuous care than episodic and is principally provided in community settings rather than in acute care facilities" (ANA, 1980a, p. 4). The nurse who works with clients in the community is involved in the promotion of health and the prevention of disease. When a client suffers an acute illness, the nurse is most likely to refer the client to an institution for assistance. Nurses in the community also supervise the long-term care of clients with chronic illnesses, such as diabetes, in order to assist them in attaining and maintaining the highest possible level of wellness. Community health nurses may become involved with the acute care of clients at the point at which clients enter or leave the part of the health care system responsible for treating such individuals. Some examples of involvement of community health nurses in tertiary care would include disasters, serious emergencies, and work with the terminally ill (ANA, 1980a, p. 4).

Assumption 5: Community health nursing occurs principally in primary health care settings.

Community health nursing is practiced in a myriad of settings. These include all the places where people normally congregate for work, play, and school (ANA, 1980a, p.

4). The agencies with which community health nurses are associated are as numerous as they are varied: homes, occupational settings, community mental health centers, family clinics. (Many of these settings are described in later chapters.) Even though they practice in the community, nurses may also serve as consultants or liaisons with hospitals and other acute care settings (ANA, 1980a, p. 4).

Beliefs

A *belief* is a principle held to be true by a person or a group. The beliefs listed here are the ideas of the task force about how the practice of community health nursing will affect the health care system. These are the values that underlie the priorities and foci for all nurses in the community.

Belief 1: Health care should be available, accessible, and acceptable to all persons.

Health care should be comprehensive and available to all, regardless of socioeconomic status. The quality of health care should not depend on the socioeconomic level of the clients. Political and economic interests should not determine the care that is received by any consumer (ANA, 1980a, p. 5). Increased access to nurses and to decentralized health care facilities are options that will ensure that all clients have access to care and services that are appropriate to their needs (ANA, 1980a, p. 5).

Belief 2: Recipients of health care services should participate in the making of health policy.

If community health services are to be responsive to the needs of clients, those clients must have a role in determining their own needs and the services they require. The professionals involved are responsible for helping community members find relevant and accurate data with which to make decisions, but it is the citizens of the community who must determine policy (ANA, 1980a, p. 6). Nurses play a part in policy making by contributing information. Within their own communities, nurses do help determine policy because they themselves are the consumers. Nurses also assist their fellow consumers by acquainting them with the process and by encouraging their involvement in policy making.

Belief 3: The nurse as a provider and the client as a consumer of health care services can form a conjoint relationship to advocate and effect change in health policies and services.

Consumers and nurses are more aware than ever before of the effectiveness of activism in influencing change. The community health nurse can directly influence progress in the health care system by participating in local, state, and national policy making. Indirectly, the nurse can influence advances in the health care system by educating and encouraging colleagues and clients (ANA, 1980a, p. 6).

Belief 4: The environment affects the health of populations, groups, families, and individuals.

In considering the environments within which each client functions, the nurse regards the physical, social, and personal environments of each person, family, group, and community. The nurse can influence the client to manage a personal and social environment which is conducive to meeting needs. Furthermore, the nurse can influence community members in general to consider the impact of the environment on the health of all community members. Lack of concern for the quality of our environment has led to present hazards that, if left uncontrolled, will eventually become severe threats to life. The nurse must be informed about such dangers and take appropriate actions directed toward whatever individuals or groups can most effectively confront them.

Belief 5: Prevention of illness is essential to promoting health.

The three levels of prevention are the major components of primary health care. These are *primary prevention,* with an emphasis on health promotion and health teaching with well people. *Secondary prevention* is early diagnosis and treatment in order to limit disability. *Tertiary prevention* is aimed at preventing further disability in those who already have an acute or chronic illness (ANA, 1980a, p. 7).

Belief 6: A health axis intersects with the life span axis.

The health axis is an abstraction that indicates the degree to which a person's state of being is affected by his or her relative level of wellness or illness. Throughout a person's life, the health axis intersects with the life span axis and indicates the relative well-being of the individual. When there is an overabundance of negative aspects on the health axis, this necessitates intervention of a different character than that when the person's health axis predominates with strengths (ANA, 1980a, p. 7).

Belief 7: The client is the only constant member of the health care team.

The team of health care providers involved with a client varies according to the client's needs. The leadership of the team is determined by the client's priorities. When any given health care professional has rendered the appropriate service, he or she concludes the relationship with the client (ANA, 1980a, p. 8). The client must be well informed by the other team members in order to be able to ask for and receive appropriate services.

Belief 8: Individuals within a community are ultimately responsible for their own health and must be encouraged and taught to be active participants in their own health care.

This statement has the most significant future implications. Individuals are unable to control all the factors that affect their health, but there are many things within a person's control that contribute to high level wellness (ANA, 1980a, p. 8). With the trend for people to promote and maintain their own health, it is becoming increasingly important for the nurse in the community to provide health education.

Nurses must have an excellent understanding of teaching–learning principles as well as other skills that promote communication about health-related issues. In this trend toward self-help and self-care there is the potential for all citizens to be more responsible for their own health status and for that of their communities. Nurses can be important promoters of the skills necessary for accomplishing these goals.

Nurses in Community Health

The ANA recognizes the preparation of both generalists and specialists within the various fields of nursing. A *generalist* is a practitioner who has basic preparation in professional nursing and can apply the content areas included in the basic curriculum to a certain area of practice. A *specialist* is one who has received advanced education in order to provide breadth and depth of knowledge in a specific field.

Generalists in Community Health Nursing

The minimum basic preparation for practice in community health is the baccalaureate degree in nursing. Such a curriculum prepares nurses for the future because of the emphasis on processes as well as content within nursing practice. Only baccalaureate programs include sufficient introductory material in community health to enable a practitioner to function in a community setting. Collegiate programs include studies in the behavioral and physical sciences as well as focusing on individuals, families, and groups. Other areas identified by the Division of Community Health Nursing that are necessary to community health nursing and are typically included in baccalaureate programs are (ANA, 1980a, p. 9):

1. General systems theory
2. Introductory epidemiology
3. Statistics
4. Community assessment
5. History, principles, and practice of public health and community health
6. Laws pertaining to public health
7. Environmental health and safety

In addition, the student in an undergraduate program learns to apply the nursing process not only to individuals but also to families, groups, and communities. Such opportunities are usually not available in shorter programs based in institutions other than senior colleges. The baccalaureate program offers the student experience in use of community resources, including working with other health care providers. These experiences teach the student to deliver nursing care to clients in many different settings (ANA, 1980a, p. 9).

Basic nursing education on the baccalaureate level prepares graduates for entry into community nursing. Such graduates are prepared to perform a variety of activities in many different settings. They are also prepared to supervise others in the community who have other types of nursing education. In order to advance and be able to take more responsibility in planning, evaluating, and supervising, the graduate needs additional preparation.

Specialists in Community Health Nursing

To be considered a specialist in community health nursing, the nurse must undertake additional academic studies. Merely accumulating years of experience does not make one a specialist (ANA, 1980a, p. 9). The advanced educational experiences provided at the graduate level give the nurse the necessary breadth and depth of knowledge for dealing with more complex issues in nursing practice. Some of the areas of content included in such a graduate program would be (ANA, 1980a, p. 9):

1. Community health nursing theory
2. Public health science
3. Leadership and management
4. Interdisciplinary collaboration
5. Research and evaluation processes
6. Health policy and planning
7. Community organization
8. Dynamics of health politics and economics

A nurse specializing in community health nursing might also increase his or her knowledge in a given clinical area, such as adult health, child health, or community mental health. Furthermore, the specialist might concentrate on a functional role, such as administration, research, education, or consultation (ANA, 1980a, p. 10). This training prepares the specialist to function in a more advanced manner than the generalist, thereby providing a leader and a role model in the field.

As nurses become more active in the community, and as consumers have increasingly more complex and sophisticated needs that they wish to meet without entering an institutionalized care setting, nurses will require even more advanced education on the doctoral level. Such nurses will be ready to embark on studies that will prepare them to improve the health care of individuals and of communities. They will develop theory that will be useful in the continued practice of nursing within the community, and they will investigate the impact of nursing on specific health problems (ANA, 1980a, p. 10).

Scope of Practice

Scope of practice in the community includes the focus, major thrust, highest priority, objectives, and modes of delivery of care. These components determine the education necessary as well as the activities to be included in nursing done in the community.

The focus of nursing practice in the community is on the prevention of illness and the promotion and maintenance of health. This determines the major thrust of practice, which is the provision of primary health care, with less emphasis on secondary and tertiary levels of health care. The highest priority in giving primary health care is the independence of the client in health promotion and in self-care. These

components lead logically to the major objectives of community nursing practice, which are the "preservation and improvement of the health of the community" (ANA, 1980a, p. 11). All of these aspects determine the modes or roles in which nurses will actually deliver health care.

Modes of Delivery

Mode of delivery is determined by the client's needs and the pattern that nursing care takes in meeting those needs. The first mode is direct care to individuals, families, and groups in a certain community. This mode is directed to the concerns of a particular person or group. The pattern of care is well described by the ANA Division on Community Health Nursing (ANA, 1980a, p. 12):

The community health nurse works directly with clients to attain optimum health, prevent disease and injury, apply therapeutic modalities to help to maintain a high level of wellness, restore health of the ill to a maximal state, manage common illness and stabilize chronic conditions, and refer complex client care to appropriate experts.

The second mode of nursing within the community is delivery of service to the community as a whole. Such services ultimately affect the health of individuals and groups within the community, but the pattern of practice involves the nurse at a level beyond direct client care to individual persons and groups. The mode is described as follows (ANA, 1980a, p. 12):

[The nurse works] with the community and its subgroups to identify health needs and to motivate self-help in a group(s), increase utilization and development of resources, set priorities of community health problems, measure the effect of existing nursing practice on the community, determine distribution of nurses by level and specialty in order to adequately meet the health requirements, and develop mechanisms and process for identifying internal and external factors affecting health of the community.

Primary Health Care

Although all nursing practice is concerned with the promotion of health, the characteristic of nursing in the community that distinguishes it from all other nursing practice is its emphasis on primary health care. *Primary health care* is "the prevention of illness and promotion in maintaining and restoring maximum health" (ANA, 1980a, p. 13). Community health nursing has been in the forefront of health care because of its emphasis on health as a state that can be achieved and maintained at a higher level than merely the absence of disease.

Although attention is given to preventing disease, there is much emphasis on promoting healthy functioning. *Health promotion* assumes that "clients have a higher potential of health than they presently realize" (ANA, 1980a, p. 13). Nurses in the community work with many clients who are well but need to improve or maintain their level of wellness. *Maintenance* health care involves the thorough and continuous assessment of both community and of individuals to ensure that they will continue to function at the same level. *Restoration* activities that contribute to primary health care are those that permit a client to attain the highest level of health functioning given a certain limitation, such as a handicap. Finally, the nurse in the community supports *rehabilitation* by facilitating the return of a client to his or her original state of health after some disruption, such as an illness (ANA, 1980a, p. 13).

Nurses in the community facilitate primary health care by providing direct service to clients as well as by serving as administrators, coordinators, educators, and consultants. The manner in which a given nurse contributes to the health of individuals, groups, or communities depends on his or her educational background and the specific level of knowledge attained.

Implications of the Model

The model described by the ANA Division on Community Health Nursing permits a dynamic practice of nursing that can grow and change as society and its health needs change. The hallmark of a profession is the ability and the commitment to change as knowledge develops and conditions change. A group will cease to exist if it fails to respond to new developments and problems. Nurses in the community must be aware of many issues that influence health, from popular trends to health legislation to environmental changes. This will have a significant influence on ever-changing community health nursing curricula. Furthermore, it will result in the increased needs of community health nurses for continuing education.

Imperatives

The ANA Division on Community Health Nursing identified several imperatives that grow out of the model they designed. These are subsumed under the topics of education, practice, and research (ANA, 1980a, pp. 14–15):

Education imperatives—initiation and continuing development of:

1. Community health nursing core at the graduate level for nurses preparing for practice in community health settings.
2. Courses in environmental and epidemiological sciences that consider the effects on humans in their home, work place, and community.
3. Continuing education to update and upgrade knowledge and skills previously acquired.

4. Increased opportunities for education in administration, leadership, and consultation.

5. Integration of nursing research into all phases of nursing education.

Practice imperatives:

1. Cost-effective services and programs aimed at prevention of illness and injury and promotion of health.

2. Quality assurance measures of health care.

3. Participation of nurses in peer review.

4. Direct client access to and nursing control of community health nursing practice.

5. Alternative health care projects initiated by and directed by nurses.

Research imperatives—investigation of:

1. New and existing methods of educational preparation and clinical practice.

2. Roles, functions, and competence of nurses in practice.

3. Unmet needs of individuals, families, and groups and the capability of communities to meet those needs.

4. The need for primary prevention using health status indicators.

5. Cost-effectiveness of prevention.

6. Cost-effective methods to stimulate self-direction toward health by consumers.

With the statement of these imperatives, the need for a model of practice becomes obvious. A model is a framework within which nursing practice in the community can be learned, carried out, and researched. The model provides direction to ensure consistency among the people who practice nursing in the community.

COMMUNITY HEALTH NURSING AND PUBLIC HEALTH NURSING

The way a profession defines itself determines the scope and nature of its practice,

educational qualifications, research imperatives, and relationships with other groups. As the ANA Conceptual Model for Community Health Nursing indicates, the practice defined as public health nursing is to some extent subsumed under the broad classification of community health nursing. However, the practice of public health nursing has traditionally focused on the health of populations. Within public health, planning and interventions are directed toward groups, by means of such techniques as programmatic planning. Currently most people who consider themselves to be community health nurses function in primary care settings such as homes, clinics, schools, and industry.

Scope and Nature of Practice

Community health nursing emphasizes work with individuals, families, and small groups to promote health and prevent disease. Public health nursing, on the other hand, promotes health and prevents disease by assessing populations and developing programs to meet the needs of populations at risk.

Educational Qualifications

The person educated in a collegiate nursing program with general knowledge of health and illness has been well prepared to apply the nursing process in working with individuals and families as a community health nurse. In order to participate in the broader-based assessments and programmatic planning required in public health, a nurse needs a broader educational experience than that usually included in an undergraduate program. Graduate education is required to prepare nurses to assess and plan for groups as large as communities, cities, states, and nations. Although some related material, such as introductory epidemiology, community assessment, and environmental health, are part of an undergraduate curriculum, undergraduate preparation is only sufficient to make the new practitioner an effective team member in public health nursing. Such concepts are introduced at the undergraduate level in order to make students aware of the complexities that influence primary nursing practice. By the same token, in order to be able to plan programs effectively the advanced practitioner must have knowledge of and experience in working with individuals and families in primary care activities.

Research Imperatives

It is important for those involved in the primary care needs of individuals and families, such as community health nurses, to study health care needs and patterns of care. The research of those engaged in public health nursing focuses on identifying needs of populations and investigating ways in which nursing with a community-wide scope can influence the health of the populations studied. Both kinds of research are important. However, sweeping interventions aimed at whole populations can be more effective in remedying individual health problems than small-scale research limited to community health nurses' caseloads.

Relationships with Other Groups

The nurse with a public health focus is often better able to communicate health care needs to those responsible for health care funding. For example, a nurse whose data base is limited to a caseload from a single area of the community will not have a comprehensive view of health needs in the community as a whole. This parochial perspective will limit the nurse's influence in dealing with legislators. A nurse who is involved in community-wide assessments and who can effectively present data about community needs may be able to influence the decisions made at city, state, and perhaps national levels. For example:

A community health nurse noticed that several of the families in her caseload had daughters who became pregnant in their midteens. She was concerned about the girls and their families but was aware that there were no city services designed to help them. A public health nurse obtained the same information by doing a city-wide survey of prenatal care. However, he also was able to describe the problem as it affected the whole population: one in five adolescent girls became pregnant by age 16. He used this information in various efforts to influence the legislature, clinics, and obstetricians in decisions about educational programs and prenatal care for this age group.

Choice of Focus

Public health nursing requires a high level of skill and involves such advanced areas as epidemiology and statistical analysis. By contrast, primary care is more familiar to graduates of basic educational programs. Working directly with individuals and families is more gratifying to many people than working with other professionals and dry statistics. Therefore, there has been a trend away from public health nursing and toward community health nursing. Unfortunately, this concentration of interest has not promoted the achievement of the goal that community health nurses and public health nurses hold in common: promoting the health of populations.

Nurses have been systematically excluded from decision making in many institutions and agencies. This has contributed to a feeling of helplessness that nurses may inadvertently communicate to clients. For example, Dreher (1982) has pointed out how community health nurses are taught and are expected to practice in a way that will help the individual or family negotiate the difficult and complex health care system. They are not taught to work on an organizational level to make the health care system more accessible and responsive to the needs of the people it is supposed to serve. There is a need for nurses who will choose to forego the immediate gratification of working closely with individuals and families in order to take the risks entailed in redesigning and reorganizing health care systems. This is the role of the public health nurse.

FUTURE IMPLICATIONS

In the near future, there will be an even greater need for nurses who can function with aggregates. Even if our population remains relatively stable, it is already too large for the health care system to render timely and meaningful health care services that can truly attain the goal of promoting health. Continuing to focus on individuals and families is like assigning a lot of little boys and girls to put their fingers in the holes in the dikes. If no one plans how to repair the dikes and follows through in an effective way, the dikes will burst, and the boys and girls making their brave, sincere, but insufficient efforts will be the first ones to drown.

Students and practitioners in the community today are in a crucial position. Students must learn how to function as community health nurses, but they must also begin to prepare themselves for the leap to the level of public health nursing. It is likely that before the turn of the century, the content of today's community health nursing will be considered basic, and

nurses graduating from collegiate programs will be expected to function as public health nurses. In the past, when the pattern for public health practice was set, the populations studied and the problems within the reach of nursing were smaller and less complex. With the passage of time, populations have grown, subpopulations have proliferated, and health promotion has become at once more attainable and more difficult to provide.

The nurses who function in the community, whether they define their practice as community health or public health, have just begun to define what comprises their fields of work. Students who study nursing today will have to refine those definitions of practice and fulfill their challenges. This may require a different commitment on the part of nurses who wish to function in the community. Regardless of how we define our goals, we usually do pretty much what we want to do. Therefore, for example, even though those who call themselves community nurses and those who call themselves public health nurses describe basically the same goal, their willingness to examine how best to achieve that goal varies from one professional to another. Many people who practice nursing in the community merely wish to provide service for a circumscribed group of clients with limited supervision. They are essentially doing a job rather than practicing a profession. On the other hand, those who see the deficits within the system that interfere with their goals for the health of the population will determine ways in which they can change their practice to overcome those barriers. These practitioners are professionals.

In the future there will be an increase in professionalism among nurses; nurses will define their goals and plan ways to implement solutions that will entail risks and determine nursing practice. Nurses must be willing to accept the benefits of working for the collective good as opposed to functioning as individualists. Nurses may be required to forego some of the gratifications of current community health nursing practice in order to develop skills to make themselves better observers of group data, better planners of programs, and better evaluators of group outcomes. Although this future scenario implies self-sacrifice, the long-term rewards of such behavior are considerable. Weigh the satisfaction you might get from improving the health status of 10 families against the satisfaction of helping to institute a health education program that betters the lives of 1,000 families.

Community health nursing in the future will be better defined, as will be its various components, such as primary care and aggregate care. There will continue to be roles for nurses in each area, but there will be an increasing emphasis on applying the nursing process to the needs of entire populations and subpopulations. This is yet another area in which the future must bring consensus on the definition of nursing practice in the community. To ensure that nursing will be a strong and influential part of health care in the community, our most immediate task is to resolve the continuing conflict that has been engendered by misguided efforts at individualism.

SUMMARY

Nursing in the community includes all those aspects of nursing that influence and are influenced by the environment in which nurses function. This is the broadest and most inclusive definition, recognizing that every aspect of nursing, whether in or out of an acute care setting, is influenced by factors beyond the immediate setting. Community health nursing focuses on working with people in the community to promote their healthy functioning. Public health nursing concentrates on health care promotion within populations.

The goal espoused both by those who consider themselves to be community health nurses and those who consider themselves to be public health nurses is to promote the health of populations. Whether the focus of practice is directed toward primary care or toward aggregates, nursing is important in attaining this goal. In the future it may be necessary for more nurses to work in health care planning and implementation with aggregates. Commitment to the goal of promoting health will lead nurses to prepare themselves to benefit the population as a whole. By being willing to make personal goals subservient to professional goals, professional nurses will reach new heights of personal and professional gratification.

DISCUSSION TOPICS

1. What is the difference between referring to a person as a patient and as a client? Give some reasons in favor of using the term "patient" regardless of the situation or setting. Give some reasons in favor of using the term "client" regardless of the situation of setting. Which designation do you prefer. Why?

2. What is the main distinction between public health nursing and community health nursing? Describe the nature of the practice of each that is implied by the difference you identified.

3. Eight beliefs are included in the ANA Conceptual Model of Community Health Nursing. Select one of these beliefs and describe how it would influence your practice as a nurse in the community.

4. Which beliefs are related to the difference in thrust of community health nursing and public health nursing?

5. How would extraterrestrial travel affect the differentiation between community health nursing and public health nursing?

6. Imagine that you are working in the community 20 years from now. What is the community like? What are some of the health problems that might warrant study and intervention?

BIBLIOGRAPHY

American Nurses' Association: *Standards of community health nursing practice.* Kansas City, Mo.: Author, 1973.

American Nurses' Association: *A conceptual model of community health nursing.* Kansas City, Mo.: Author, 1980a.

American Nurses' Association: *Nursing: A social policy statement.* Kansas City, Mo.: Author, 1980b.

American Public Health Association. Public Health Nursing Section: The definition and role of public health nursing practice in the delivery of health care. *American Journal of Public Health* 72(2), 210–212, 1982.

Barkauskas, V.H.: Public health nursing practice—An educator's view. *Nursing Outlook* 30(7), 384–389, 1982.

Cordes, S.M.: Assessing health care needs: Elements and processes. *Family and Community Health* 1(2), 1–16, 1978.

Doeppinger, J., Lassiter, P.G., & Wilcox, B.: Community health is community competence. *Nursing Outlook* 30(8), 464–467, 1982.

Dossey, L.: *Space, time and medicine.* Boulder, Col.: Shambhala Publications, 1982.

Dreher, M.C.: The conflict of conservatism in public health nursing education. *Nursing Outlook* 30(9), 504–509, 1982.

Eigsti, D.G., Stein, K.Z., & Fortune, M.: The community as client in planning for continuity of care. *Nursing and Health Care* 3(5), 251–253, 1982.

Ervin, N.: Public health nursing practice—An administrator's view. *Nursing Outlook* 30(7), 390–394, 1982.

Ferguson, M.: *The aquarian conspiracy.* Los Angeles: J.P. Tarcher, 1980.

Kalisch, P.A., & Kalisch, B.J.: *The advance of American nursing.* Boston: Little, Brown, 1978.

Kark, S.L.: *Epidemiology and community medicine.* New York: Appleton-Century-Crofts, 1974.

Kurtzman, C., Block-Ben Ibgui, D., Pogrund, R., & Monin, S.: Nursing process at the aggregate level. *Nursing Outlook* 28(12), 737–739, 1980.

Leininger, M.: Health care delivery systems for tomorrow: Possibilities and guidelines. Proceedings, *Health of the Nation—5*, University of Minnesota Hospitals, 1973.

Naisbitt, J.: *Megatrends.* New York: Warner, 1982.

Newman, O.: *Community of interest.* Garden City, N.Y.: Anchor Books, 1981.

Reinhardt, A.M., & Chatlin, E.D.: Assessment of health needs in a community: The basis for program planning. In A.M. Reinhardt & M.D. Quinn, eds., *Current practice in family-centered community nursing* (Vol. 4). St. Louis: Mosby, 1977.

Ruybal, S.E.: Community health planning. *Family and Community Health* 1(1), 9–18, 1978.

Schodde, G., Deay, M.A., & Stetson, L.: Extended/expanded role in nursing. In J.B. Walter, G.B. Pardee & D.M. Molbo, eds., *Dynamics of problem-oriented approaches.* Philadelphia: Lippincott, 1976.

Seymer, L.R., ed.: *Selected writing of FLorence Nightingale*, New York: Macmillan, 1954.

Simmons, D.A.: *A classification scheme for client problems in community health nursing.* DHHS Pub. No. HRA 80-16, Washington D.C.: U.S. Government Printing Office, 1980.

Smith, G.R.: Nursing beyond the crossroads. *Nursing Outlook* 28(9), 540–545, 1980.

Smitherman, C.: *Nursing actions for health promotion*. Philadelphia: F.A. Davis, 1981.

Stanton, M., Paul, C., & Reeves, J.S.: An overview of the nursing process. In Nursing Theories Conference Group, *Nursing theories*. Englewood Cliffs, N.J.: Prentice-Hall, 1980.

Stevens, B.J.: *Nursing theory: Analysis, application, evaluation*. Boston, Little, Brown, 1979.

Thurston, H.I.: Education for episodic and distributive care. *Nursing Outlook* 20(8), 519–523, 1972.

White, C., Knollmueler, R., & Yaksich, S.: Preparation for community health nursing. *Nursing Outlook* 28(10), 617–623, 1980.

White, M.S.: Construct for public health nursing. *Nursing Outlook* 30(9), 527–530, 1982.

Williams, C.A.: Community health nursing—What is it? *Nursing Outlook* 25(4), 250–254, 1977.

Williams, C.A., & Heighriter, M.E.: Community health nursing, population focus and evaluation. *Public Health Reviews* 7(3–4), 197–221, 1978.

Winslow, O.E.: *Man and epidemics*. Princeton, N.J.: Princeton University Press, 1952.

Young, R.K.: *Community nursing workbook: Family as client*. Norwalk, Conn.: Appleton-Century-Crofts, 1982.

PART II
NURSING WITH INDIVIDUALS AND SMALL GROUPS

One way to conceptualize nursing in the community is to look at the recipients of nursing service. Nurses often work directly with individuals and groups. Part II describes some of the particular groups of people who may be clients and examines particular aspects of client service. Several of the chapters describe the settings and the ways in which nurses practice.

Part II begins with a discussion of how specific characteristics of clients affect nursing. Chapter 12 focuses on the special aspects of working with children and adolescents, and Chapter 13 describes work with the elderly. Chapters 14 and 15 explore the cultural and spiritual dimensions of working with clients.

The next three chapters focus on the dynamics of the nurse–client relationship and describe what the nurse can do to foster effective communication and successful interaction. Chapter 16 introduces the process of developing contracts with clients as a way of facilitating collaboration. Chapter 17 discusses teaching and learning principles and applies them to a variety of situations. Chapter 18 illustrates how knowledge of group process can be useful to nurses in the community.

Chapters 19 and 20 provide a foundation for understanding and implementing nursing in any setting in which a nurse works with clients. Chapter 19 gives an overview of the many settings of nursing practice and describes some of the specifics of nursing in each. Visiting clients in their homes is the subject of Chapter 20; although not as common today as in the past, home visits are frequently a useful component of nursing process.

The remaining chapters in Part II discuss how nurses apply certain useful theories and principles to nursing practice. Chapters 21 and 22 examine the application of mental health theory and crisis theory to clients in the community. Principles of assessing and promoting health are covered in Chapters 23, and Chapter 24 describes the use of network analysis in understanding and working with individuals and families in the community.

12

Children and Adolescents

Mary Ann McClellan

There is always one moment in childhood when the door opens and lets the future in.

GRAHAM GREENE

OBJECTIVES

After reading this chapter, you should be able to:

☐ Identify current trends in societal relations and health problems of children and adolescents that affect community nursing services.

☐ Explain current trends in terms of historical factors.

☐ Predict possible alternative future roles for community health nurses involved with children and adolescents.

☐ Define the nurse's role under changing practice conditions.

INTRODUCTION

Community health nurses have focused on groups in identifying health needs and in providing nursing service. Some of these groups have included the family and populations in such environments as child-care centers, schools, and work settings. Other groups toward which services can be directed include those based upon age, sex, particular health deficits, ethnic background, or any combination of these.

COMMUNICABLE DISEASES

Before the development of adequate immunizations, nurses caring for children in the community saw "diphtheria cases by the dozens every fall, measles epidemics every two years in the late winter, whooping cough every spring all spring, and polio almost every summer . . . year in and year out" (Smith, 1979, p. 1059). Such factors as immunization practices, disease surveillance, the development of antibiotics, and

187

the increased number of children in day-care centers have had profound effects upon current trends in communicable, or infectious, disease among children in this country. Nurses who provide care for children, who are the population group hardest hit by infections, must continue to update their knowledge about infectious diseases and their effects upon individuals and groups.

Examples of Control Efforts in the U.S.

Measles

Now that smallpox has been eradicated, a major effort is taking place in this country to eradicate indigenous measles, "a measles case that occurs within the United States and cannot be related to an imported case or a measles case that occurs more than two generations after the imported case to which it is epidemiologically linked." ("Elimination of indigenous measles," 1982, p. 517). Approaches include early response to outbreaks and suspected cases by identifying those who are susceptible to the disease, providing vaccinations, and excluding those who are susceptible from school. This effort has required involvement of all levels of government, many professional organizations, private agencies, parents, teachers, and children. As of October 1, 1982, the number of reported measles cases during the first 37 weeks of the year in the United States had dropped from 53,023 in 1977 to 1,230 in 1982.

Rubella

Rubella, also known as three-day or German measles, commonly occurred in epidemics every six to nine years before the licensing of an effective vaccine in 1969 ("Rubella," 1982). Early vaccination efforts were directed toward children ages 5 to 9. This focus resulted in a change in the susceptible population. Since 1976, more than 70 percent of those with rubella have been over 15 years of age. Although epidemics of rubella have not occurred since 1969, it is endemic among adolescents and young adults. Eliminating congenital rubella syndrome may require vaccinating susceptible members of those groups as well as younger children ("Rubella prevention," 1981).

Children in Day Care Centers and in Schools

In 1979, more than 1.2 million children in this country spent more than 30 hours each week in child-care settings outside their homes (Silva, 1980). Over half of U.S. mothers with children under the age of 18 work outside the home, including 28.4 million mothers of households in which both parents work (Silva, 1980). Thus school-age children, as well as preschoolers and infants, may be in child-care settings at least part of each day.

Children who spend these amounts of time in group settings are at risk for acquiring a variety of communicable diseases and for transmitting them to their families. Recently, infestations of head lice and scabies have been significant problems in school settings (Foutes, Spencer, Tucker, & Hoff, 1981; Juranek, 1977). Streptococcal infections, airborne viral infections, and gastrointestinal infections continue to occur in outbreaks in schools (Markowitz, 1979).

A current and significant problem has been the control of communicable diseases in day-care centers. Reports of such outbreaks have included *Haemophilus influenzae* Type B, giardiasis, shigellosis, and multiply resistant pneumococci infections causing meningitis (Black, Dykes, Sinclair, & Wells, 1977; Ginsburg, McCracken, Rae, & Parke, 1977; Radetsky, Johanaen, Laner, Istre, Parmelee, Wiesenthal, & Glode, 1981; Ward, Gorman, Phillips, & Fraser, 1978). In addition, day-care centers have been identified as being a major source of cases of hepatitis A in this country (Silva, 1980).

Several authors have written about the problem of hepatitis A in day-care centers. (Benenson, Takafuji, Bancroft, Lemm, Callahan, & Leach, 1980; Hadler, Erben, Francis, Webster, & Maynard, 1982; Hadler, Webster, Erben, Swanson, & Maynard, 1980; Hammack, Ochoa, Henderson, Fullilove & Fondren, 1982; Panoui, 1979; Silva, 1980; Storch, 1979; Vernon, Schable, & Francis, 1982). Epidemiological studies reported by these writers have indicated that day-care centers that are at risk for a hepatitis A outbreak are those that care for non-toilet-trained children under the age of 2 years and that care for more than 50 children (Hadler et al., 1980; Hadler et al., 1982; Silva, 1980; Storch, 1979; Vernon et al., 1982). Other centers at risk are those that are open more than 15 hours a day and those that are operated for profit (Hadler et al., 1982). Moreover, adults and older siblings in families that have non-toilet-trained children who are 2 years old or younger and who spend 40 or more hours a week in a day-care center are at increased risk for hepatitis A (Silva, 1980; Storch, 1979). One study indicated greater risk to household contacts when children attending the affected day-care center did not receive human immune globulin (HIG) during the three-week period after initial exposure (Hammack et al., 1982). Day-care-center employees who cared for children 2 years old or younger were those at greatest risk in a center. These younger children seem to transmit this infection more often

than do older children, probably because they are asymptomatic or have nonspecific symptoms and their hygiene habits are undeveloped (Hadler et al., 1980).

CONTROL MEASURES. Control measures include immunizing susceptible people with human immune globulin when an outbreak has been identified; closing an affected center to new admissions during an outbreak; and emphasizing personal hygiene, especially careful handwashing, by everyone in the center. Closing an affected day-care center completely or transferring children to another setting is not recommended, since children who were incubating the disease could then spread it further. It is important to remember that the exact mechanism of transmission of hepatitis A is not yet understood (Benenson et al., 1980; Hadler et al., 1980; Hammack et al., 1982; Storch, 1979; Vernon et al., 1982).

The Role of the Nurse

The nurse who is dealing with prevention and control of communicable diseases in children has several responsibilities, including counseling parents about their own general hygiene practices with their children and teaching children about these habits. The nurse may also counsel working parents about selecting an appropriate day-care setting for their children. The nurse may administer immunizations to infants and children and interpret the importance of such programs to parents and to the community. The nurse may inspect day-care facilities and hold training sessions for directors and staff members about ways to prevent transmission of diseases. Some staff members may not understand the benefits of washing their hands with warm water instead of cold water, for example.

NUTRITION

The nutritional status of children is an on-going concern for the community health nurse and for parents. There are many nutritional problems for which nurses assess children. Some of these problems vary with specific groups. For example, Mexican-American children in California and Colorado have been identified as having low niacin intakes. Children of low-income families are more likely to receive inadequate amounts of vitamin C than middle- and upper-income children (Pipes, 1981). There are also particular nutritional concerns for children with specific handicaps, for children in sports, and for children in vegetarian families.

Assessment tools available to the nurse to help determine the nutritional status of children include 24-hour recall diet histories, growth charts, physical assessment, and, in some settings, the children's hemoglobins and/or hematocrits (Rowe, 1980; Zerfas, Shorr, & Neumann, 1977).

The most common nutritional deficiency in this country and in the world is iron deficiency anemia (Woodruff, 1977). Another major community health concern is obesity, which affects at least 25 percent of the children in this country (Bowers, Faulkner, & Michel, 1979).

Iron Deficiency Anemia

Iron deficiency anemia exists when hemoglobin levels are less than 11.0 gm/100 ml and hematocrits are less than 33% (Pearson, 1977; Pipes, 1981). Other laboratory tests can be used to confirm the diagnosis and to rule out other causes of anemia (Woodruff, 1977). In infants and children, four factors determine adequate iron stores in the body: the amount of iron present at birth, growth velocity, loss of blood, and the ingestion and absorption of iron (Woodruff, 1977). Therefore, those at risk are small-for-gestational-age infants, premature infants whose growth is catching up, 4- to 24-month-old infants, adolescent boys, and adolescent girls who are trying to lose weight. Enteric blood loss can result from infants ingesting homogenized, not evaporated, milk. Children from low-income families are at greatest risk for iron deficiency anemia.

The Nurse's Role

The nurse can emphasize the need for dietary iron supplement for premature infants by 2 months of age and full-term infants by 4 months of age. Postponing ingestion of homogenized milk until after at least 6 months of age is recommended as well. In counseling, the nurse can relate an infant's rapid growth to the need for iron. Counseling about dietary sources of iron as the child grows older is important. Adolescents need counseling about their rapid growth and iron needs. Adolescent girls need to be aware of the effects that the onset of menses and limited-calorie diets can have on iron levels.

Obesity

Obesity is usually defined as an accumulation of body fat that exceeds 15 to 20 percent of the person's ideal weight. Skinfold thicknesses of more than 15 mm in boys and 25 mm in girls also indicate obesity (Humphrey, 1979). Obesity may begin in infancy, especially with bottle-fed male infants, or in later childhood or adolescence. Overweight children may be at greater risk for being overweight as adults (Epstein, Wing, Steranchak, Dickson, & Michelson,

1980). Obesity in children may result from genetic factors, family and personal eating patterns, sedentary life-style, or disturbed psychosocial functioning of the family. This dysfunctional pattern has been called *enmeshment:* extreme proximity and intensity of interactions, overprotectiveness, rigidity, lack of conflict resolution, and the significance of the child's obesity in maintaining the family system (Bowers et al., 1979).

Obesity can seriously intefere with development of a child's self-esteem and social skills. Disease hazards seem to predominate in those who are very obese (Weil, 1977).

The Nurse's Role

Providing parents with information on the benefits of breast feeding infants, which include lack of excessive weight gain, can be helpful. Parents of bottle-fed infants may not realize that every cry is not a hunger cry and may overfeed the infant. For older children, one nurse used behavior modification to have children bring nutritious snacks from home. She spent several sessions with the children until they could identify nutritious snacks, then gave gold stars for appropriate snacks. Follow-up evaluation indicated that the children maintained the habit (Pearson, 1977). Behavior modification, as opposed to nutrition education alone, appears to be an effective approach to dealing with childhood and adolescent obesity (Epstein et al., 1980; Jonides, 1982). This approach may be used with groups of adolescents who provide peer support for each other (Langford, 1981; Schlechter, 1981; Zakus, Chin, Cooper, Makovsky, & Merrill, 1981). In a school setting, the nurse can encourage the installation of vending machines with nutritious food rather than junk foods.

LATCHKEY CHILDREN

As many as 10 million elementary school children in this country may be *latchkey children,*

a term that generally defines children who are left to take care of themselves, left to use group recreational programs, play in the street, stay home alone, join a gang, or in general supervise themselves, or for whom the care arrangements are so loosely made as to be virtually ineffective. (Long & Long, 1982, p. 1)

The numbers of these children are increasing every year.

Causes and Effects

The increase in the number of single-parent families, two-thirds of them single-mother families, and in two-parent families in which both parents work, has contributed to this problem. The lack of available extended-family members for child care, because of families' geographic mobility, and the lack of after-school care programs planned for these children are also important factors (McElhinney, 1982; Scherer, 1982; Sklar, 1982).

Long and Long (1982) found that children left at home alone after school felt significantly more isolated, lonely, and fearful than children supervised by adults. These children had considerably less contact with peers after school, since they could not have friends visit them. More research needs to be done to determine if these children are at greater risk for accidents, illnesses, nutritional and dental problems, developmental problems, substance abuse, early and out-of-wedlock pregnancy, and juvenile delinquency. Long-term effects of self-care after school need to be studied as well.

For older children who have been well

prepared to care for themselves after school and who feel that their parents listen to and are available to them, the latchkey experience can be a positive one. Such children master many self-help skills and become more mature and responsible (Long & Long, 1982).

The Nurse's Role

The nurse can assist latchkey children and their parents by early counseling with parents, while children are preschoolers, about selection of appropriate after-school care. The nurse can support the establishment of developmentally appropriate care programs in the community. ("School age day care," 1980). The nurse can provide a "survival skills" course that includes such topics as preparing simple, nutritious snacks, first aid and safety, and answering the telephone appropriately. The nurse might assist in setting up a telephone hotline for latchkey children and help children learn to monitor their own health states more consistently and responsibly. The nurse also needs to be involved in research to determine the effects the latchkey experience has on children and the implications it has for children's health problems and nursing needs.

TRAUMA IN CHILDREN

Accidents

Vehicular Accidents

Beyond the age of 1 year, accidents are the major cause of death in children in this country. Vehicular accidents constitute most of these; they are the biggest killer of children (Avery, 1980). During the first year of life, children are at greatest risk of accidents as car passengers. After that, they are

at risk as pedestrians starting as toddlers, then as cyclists as young school children. As adolescents, of course, they become vulnerable as automobile drivers and as motorcycle riders (Avery, 1980). As passengers or drivers, children suffer injuries and death from sudden deceleration in accidents. These can be prevented by installing and using appropriate restraints for the child's size and developmental level. Legislation mandating the use of restraints for children has been effective in reducing deaths and injuries in some states (Avery, 1980).

As pedestrians or cyclists, children may be the victims of high- or low-velocity injuries when struck or run over by a vehicle. In high-velocity accidents, sudden transmission of force to the child creates characteristic injuries. In low-velocity accidents, which often involve children under 3 who are hit by slowly backing cars, the injuries result from a slow crushing force and may be occult (for example, liver or kidney contusion) (Bell, Ternberg, & Bower, 1980). For bicyclists and motorcyclists, the use of helmets significantly reduces fatalities and serious injuries.

Other Accidents

Other common potentially serious or fatal accidents in children include falls, drownings, burns, and poisonings (Tyrrell, 1981):

After motor vehicle and fall deaths, drownings are the third leading cause of unintentional injury deaths, and for ages 5 to 24 rank second only to motor vehicle deaths. Data show that death rates from drowning are more than five times greater for males than females and nearly three times greater for blacks than whites. ("Aquatic deaths and injuries," 1982, p. 417)

Ornamental ponds, bathtubs, and home swimming pools are major sites of drownings of children. The increased installation of hot tubs and spas in homes are potential threats to children. Moreover, the target group for preventing the annual 700 serious aquatic-accident spinal cord injuries in this country is the teenage diver. ("Aquatic deaths," 1982).

According to Lalor (1981), this country "faces an epidemic increase in serious burn injuries," as many as 75% of which can be prevented (p. 79). In one instance, an educational program for junior high school students was developed based on a profile of burn victims in the local hospitals. This group was selected as the target group because 8–14-year-olds were one of the greatest risk groups for flame burns, which increase hospital stay and the likelihood of serious scarring. The students' fire education was significantly increased by this selective approach (Lalor, 1981).

The Nurse's Role

The nurse can provide parents and other caregivers with guidance about safety hazards related to the child's level of development and to the environments. For example, parents may not have considered the possibility that an infant or toddler can drown in the toilet if the lid is not closed. Families with home swimming pools can install fences and self-latching gates ("Aquatic deaths," 1982). Burns are best prevented by adequate supervision. Sources of fire, such as matches, should be inaccessible to children. Using smoke alarms and practicing a family fire escape plan with an outside rendezvous point are important in reducing deaths from house fires. Accidents are most likely to occur when adults or children are fatigued and inattentive to their environment.

The nurse can also support and participate in community education projects for the use of child auto seat restraints, for example (Duncan, 1979). Other nurses have involved parents as well as teachers in bicycle-safety education for children. Along with information about rules for the road and the meaning of road signs, parents were instructed to observe their children's bicycle-riding practices, to practice safe behaviors, and to correct unsafe behaviors (Miller & Hammer, 1979). Nurses in Sweden are required periodically to review safety checklists when counseling parents about their children (Avery, 1980).

Homicide

Homicide is now one of the five leading causes of death in this country of children aged 1 to 17. From 1925 to 1979 there was a sixfold increase for children aged 1 to 4 and a twofold increase for those aged 5 to 14. Under the age of 12 years, there are no sex-correlated homicide rates. However, homicide is primarily a male victim/male offender situation after the age of 12. Twenty-nine percent of these homicides are committed by the victim's parent or stepparent, 35 percent by an acquaintance, and 10 percent by strangers. Twenty-six percent of the killers are never identified. The precipitating events were poorly described in most cases, especially in intrafamily homicides. Although guns were used in more than 40 percent of these killings, a blunt object or bodily force was used most often when the victim was under 9 years of age ("Child homicide," 1982). In addition, deaths of children that seem to be accidents may be homicides caused by neglect, such as drowning in a bath tub or overdose of medication.

There are two peak age groups in which homicides occur. Under the age of 3, child homicide usually results from violence in the family; death occurs by bodily force, such as battering or strangling, and the circumstances are poorly defined. Over the age of 12, extrafamilial violence is involved, and guns and knives are used. Death usually results from an argument or the killer's criminal behavior. Children between the ages of 3 and 12 are homicide victims in a mixture of these patterns ("Child homicide," 1982).

Other than a focus on parental child abuse, there has been little in the nursing literature about child homicide. Fatal parental child abuse may be prevented by means of family-stress reduction and support systems for parents. Sibling and other caretaker abuse needs greater investigation. Long and Long (1982) suspect that latchkey children are at greater risk for child abuse, including sexual abuse, by siblings than are other children. The relationship of lack of parental supervision and perhaps neglect by society to the homicides of older children needs to be investigated. Risk factors for children need to be accurately established.

FUTURE TRENDS

Societal Trends

Working within the community as a nurse has become more difficult with the breakdown of communities and the increased alienation of adolescents (and to a lesser extent, of children) from adult influence. Peer-group socialization has removed older children and adolescents from the influence of the adults in their immediate environment. Because they are subject to a wide range of value choices, older children and adolescents may independently view health care and its practitioners in ways unlike those of their parents and relatives. Thus a wide range of health care attitudes and values potentially exists.

Trends and Issues

Historical trends have encouraged greater autonomy for both children and adults. The most significant trends are the rise in divorce rates resulting in single-parent homes and stepparenting, and the greater mobility of the American populace, both geographically and in terms of occupations and relationships. Economic and social trends have encouraged mothers to enter or to remain in the work force and place their children in day-care centers, at friends' homes, or on their own. The community health nurse has been aware of the consequences for many children: rising drug use, alcoholism, early smoking, malnutrition, and emotional illness at younger ages and with greater severity. Too often, access to health care has depended upon parental initiative. This initiative may be lacking because of other family problems, lack of awareness, or the child's own unwillingness to obtain care. If independent practitioners of nursing are not directly available to children and adolescents, their newfound freedom may not be exercised in the health area.

The issues raised by recent trends fully challenge the resources of the nursing profession. First, how can nurses take advantage of the greater autonomy of children and adolescents? Second, how will the "responsible adult" be defined for legal permission to treat children and adolescents? Third, how can confidentiality be maintained so that children and adolescents will freely seek care from community health nurses? What are the legal and ethical implications of minor children seeking health care without the knowledge of their parents? Fourth, to what extent will children and adolescents use their own financial resources to obtain health care services? Fifth, if some children will be treated for health care and others for illness, how will community health nurses accommodate this bifurcation? Sixth, what independent community base will be available to nurses: schools, storefronts, community centers, homes, or offices?

To answer these questions, fictitious cases will be presented that address these issues. The following overview defines concepts relevant to recent trends and future directions for community health nursing of children and adolescents.

A CONTEXT FOR NURSING CHILDREN AND ADOLESCENTS IN THE COMMUNITY OF THE FUTURE

Narcissism in American Culture

Perhaps the aspect of American culture that has the greatest effect on attitudes toward children and adolescents is narcissism. Contemporary narcissism is characterized by feelings of emptiness and difficulties with self-esteem:

Narcissism appears realistically to represent the best way of coping with the tensions and anxieties of modern life, and the prevailing conditions therefore tend to bring out narcissistic traits that are present, in varying degrees, in everyone. These conditions have also transformed the family, which in turn shapes the underlying structure of personality. A society that fears it has no future is not likely to give much attention to the needs of the next generation, and the ever present sense of historical discontinuity—the blight of our society—falls with devastating effect on the family. The modern parent's attempt to make children feel loved and wanted does not conceal an underlying coolness—the remoteness of those who have little to pass on to the next generation and who in any case give priority to their own right to self-fulfillment.

(Lasch, 1979, 101–102)

Parents are held "only marginally accountable" in a society in which child rearing has been usurped by specialists of all sorts, resulting in what Lasch calls "the socialization of reproduction," where "helping professions" relieve parents of their burdens. Yet the shift of health and welfare concerns away from families and onto communities and specialists has not resulted in improvements in children's life-styles.

Perhaps the impact of future shock has reinforced narcissistic trends in our society. *Future shock* refers to an overwhelming rate of societal change, resulting in transience, novelty, and diversity impelled primarily by the effects of technology (Toffler, 1978). Future shock strains the limits of peoples' adaptability and challenges them to find coping strategies for survival. Emotional and physical illness increase greatly under stimulus overload of information and sensory impressions and the need to make decisions. Under these circumstances, children and adolescents are affected most. They have less control over their lives than adults do, and they are more vulnerable to events because, at their developmental stages, they lack the ability to conceptualize about the influences upon them.

Effects of Future Shock

Love, marriage, sex, and divorce have become problematic under conditions of future shock, affecting children and adolescents both in general and in terms of health needs. A futurist in this field, Jonathan Gathorne-Hardy (1981) speculates about the future of family life. His predictions are relevant to community health nursing for children and adolescents. Gathorne-Hardy expects therapists of all sorts to continue to support marriage and family life. More efficient birth control methods and smaller families will continue to be trends. With high divorce rates, all manner of consensual unions will exist. Women will probably continue to work through most of their lives. "Marriage for life" is unlikely to be a norm, but second marriages will probably be more stable. The trend in marriage is still toward broad individual exploration, with each person following his or her own vision as freely as possible. Such values should continue the trend toward greater self-care by children and adolescents.

A different prediction entirely is made by Alvin Toffler in *The Third Wave* (1981), one based upon new cohesion as a consequence of technology. Toffler suggests that the computer will revolutionize family life, drawing family members together in work and play, with home-based employment rapidly becoming common. Toffler's scenario includes the rapid, systematic availability of new knowledge to a broader public, with distinctions between producer and consumer blurring considerably. Toffler envisions greater emphasis on families, with economic and social benefits and a more integrated life replacing the estrangement of the present.

Other Influencing Factors

Generational characteristics clearly affect the type of health care people desire and their inclination toward or away from the health/illness system. For example, the baby-boom generation became oriented toward health care during the so-called Me Decade (the 1970s) and was at the forefront of a health movement away from traditional practitioners. Exercise physiologists, health-food advocates, and fitness-center directors dominated, with dietitians and physical therapists as support staff.

Historical accident, great expectations,

childhood and adolescence during economic boom, the Vietnam war, and awareness of the threat of nuclear war and environmental pollution have all combined to affect beliefs about health. Raised in an era of reduced danger of childhood infectious diseases and accustomed to progress against the afflictions of aging (heart disease, strokes, and cancer), this generation, now raising fewer children of their own, expects and plans for a longer and healthier life span. Their children, affected by a health and fitness ideology, will have different expectations of the health care system than previous generations did.

Health Care and the "Aquarian Conspiracy"

Optimism about the future of the family still exists. Marilyn Ferguson's often-quoted book, *The Aquarian Conspiracy*, states that "our pathology is our opportunity" (1980, p. 25). Health care is discussed in terms of its great expense. Ferguson believes that little advance has been made against chronic and catastrophic illness and that care is delivered in impersonal, intrusive settings. Hopeful signs include greater emphasis on the effects of stress, society, family life, diet, and emotions on health. Hospitals are trying to humanize care. Consumers are demanding holistic health. Health care is the third largest industry in the country, accounting for 9 percent of the gross national product; and runaway costs, iatrogenic illness, and declining faith in physicians have contributed to a search for new ways to provide health care.

The new paradigm for health Ferguson describes emphasizes the caring component, a search for patterns and causes and patient autonomy based on a desire for maximum wellness. Qualitative information provided by the patient is regarded as important. Prevention is significant and viewed in relation to the client's entire lifestyle. Flexibility, adaptability, and specific stress-reduction activities are encouraging developments that are as applicable to children and adolescents as they are to adults.

Coping with Change

Productive ways of dealing with inevitable change have received broad circulation in our society. *Shifting Gears*, (O'Neill & O'Neill, 1980) reaffirms the need for commitment within a "crisis culture." The authors perceive people in our society to be adrift as a consequence of "too many options, too much stimulus and no guidelines on how to manage them" (O'Neill & O'Neill, 1980, p. 25). Positive coping requires inner security as a substitute for the stabilizer of the past—societal structures. Crises are viewed as opportunities for growth, despite societal teachings that foster crisis avoidance, which is impossible. Negative coping mechanisms include such physical reassurance during crisis as alcohol, drugs, and cigarettes. Psychosomatic illness may also occur as a release for emotions. Community health nurses, in order to teach children and adolescents how to cope, will have to provide information about the societal conditions that affect health and illness and about means of dealing with widespread substance abuse by minors with normal developmental difficulties.

The Influence of the Community Health Nurse

What can the community health nurse do to affect the health status of children and adolescents? By establishing a direct, significant, and continuous relationship with children and adolescents, the nurse may socialize some individuals toward health and illness care. *Socialization* (Danziger, 1978) is concerned with the long-term influences upon those of formative ages by significant others who are selected as role models. Many factors affect socialization, including age, sex, parental relationships, social attachments, extrafamilial contacts, culture, and social class. Children tend to assimilate new stimuli, to imitate or accommodate new people and activities, and to model others viewed as successful.

The community health nurse can become a socializing agent under certain circumstances. Children and adolescents are more impressionable than the adults in their lives, whose values are already formed. The last section of this chapter presents three alternative scenarios for child and adolescent relationships with community health nurses. In each instance, socialization processes are at work. Under conditions of future shock, in a narcissistic culture where love, marriage, and sexual relationships are unstable and unpredictable, the community health nurse in each case significantly influences the health status of the child. Generational issues, the new paradigm for health care, and knowledge about stress management will make the community health nurse of the future a more potent member of the child's or adolescent's reference group.

THE NURSING PROCESS

Data Collection and Dynamics

As the scenarios indicate, utilization of the nursing process by the community health nurse will change greatly in the future. The nurse must continue formal and informal learning in areas applicable to health care of children and adolescents and must increase his or her breadth of knowledge about economic and social factors that affect provision of nursing care. Increasing use of computers will assist the nurse in obtaining current information and in managing home care. Since a nursing diagnosis results from theory and data collection, an accurate and current theory base is essential for the nurse. This will require more study in the future. In addition, as the nurse's theory base changes with updated information, the framework and format the nurse uses for data collection will also change dramatically and unpredictably.

Since health care consumers—children, adolescents, and their parents or guardians—will make the ultimate decisions about their own health care and status, the nurse will continue to share updated information with clients in a way that they can comprehend and use. Children and adolescents, for example, will need to be much better informed than they now are about their own usual growth and development and about the effects these have on physical, emotional, and social health. Access to such information will not be limited to individual counseling or to teaching a few classes in hygiene. Consumerism is developing rapidly and is growing to include children and adolescents as well as adults. Clients must to be able to learn about themselves at times that are significant to them. Health care hot lines will be expanded to include general health topics as well as specific pathologies. Community or neighborhood computer centers will also supply such information.

Nursing Diagnosis and Objectives

Establishing a nursing diagnosis with an informed client who is buying health or illness care means stating problems in a way that is accurate and valid for the client as well as for the nurse. Until a problem is stated in comprehensible terms, it cannot be solved. The nurse can reach a decision with a young client with such simple statements as "Tell me why you need to see me"; "What do you want me to do for you?" "What do you want to happen, or to be able to do?"

Interventions and Evaluation

Selection of appropriate interventions with the young client is also increasingly important, since credibility issues increase along with media-generated sophistication. The nurse must assess the child's past experiences, successes, and difficulties with self-care. "What have you done about this problem before?" "How did that work?" "How did you know you were getting better?" "What would you do if that didn't work?" All these questions can help determine the child's ability to identify and evaluate interventions. Such questions also raise the child's consciousness about what is important and about how to collect and report personal data.

When the parent is directly involved with the child in the nursing process, several questions should be asked. Some of these are: "How does your child let you know when he has a health problem or need?" "How does she monitor changes in her health status?" "What decisions are you willing to let him make about his health care?" "What sources of information for health care/illness care does she use?" Reaching an agreement about evaluative criteria with the parent or guardian is also vital. Such questions as "When would you decide that this specific treatment is no longer needed?" or "How would you decide that this problem has been solved?" "Who makes these decisions if you are at work and unavailable to make them?" can help the nurse determine the parents' understanding of the appropriate termination of care and enable the nurse to clarify areas of confusion. Further, they indicate the nurse's recognition that the locus of control for use of nursing services rests with the client, in consultation with the nurse, whose functions include education, facilitation, and care.

Parental influences vary in the cases presented here. The common thread is the community health nurse's and the child's freedom to confront each other directly and independently.

A MODEL FOR CHILD/ADOLESCENT USE OF COMMUNITY HEALTH NURSING IN THE FUTURE

Stages of Development

Each of the scenarios poses a different set of circumstances and a unique role for the community health nurse. In each case, the stages of development lead to a positive outcome for the client. These stages constitute a model for the use of community health nursing by children and adolescents. Stage 1 (see Table 12.1) is that of knowledge of the health care system. Knowledge involves awareness of the types of practitioners available and negotiated relationships that can be activated if needed. In Stage 1 the client is aware of cost factors, the range of services, and access routes.

Definition of need, Stage 2, involves an awareness that a health or illness problem requires attention, some weighing of alternative methods or types of care to seek, and an assessment of the chronic or acute nature of the difficulty. Convenience (availability and accessibility) is a factor in se-

lecting where to go and whom to consult once the need is defined.

Stage 3, formation of a relationship, is the period in which the client focuses on one practitioner in a specific location with established frequency or regularity of contact. The parent or guardian's role is clarified. The parent or guardian's health/illness assessment has resulted in selection of a practitioner, a treatment modality, and referrals if they are indicated.

Stage 4, consolidation, is directed toward attainment of optimum health status and is characterized by information absorption, system usage, and new and expanded definitions of health/illness care. It is hoped that the nurse will be defined as the primary health/illness practitioner in the community health settings of the future for the care of children and adolescents.

IMPACT OF CRISIS AND CHANGE ON CHILDREN AND ADOLESCENTS

Crisis theory and change theory are particularly relevant to nursing care of children and adolescents in the community.

Crisis Theory

In crisis theory, a *crisis* is an individual's response to an obstacle that results because his or her usual problem-solving strategies are ineffective. The crisis is the person's response, not the event that precipitates it. An inaccurate perception of the precipitating event, a lack of adequate situational support, or inadequate coping mechanisms can cause an individual to reach a crisis (Aguilera & Messick, 1978). Successful resolution of the problem, with enhancement of the client's coping skills, is possible with effective nursing intervention in the client's

TABLE 12.1
A Model for Child/Adolescent Use of Community Health Nursing in the Future

STAGE 1 *Knowledge of Health Care System*	STAGE 2 *Definition of Need*	STAGE 3 *Formation of Relationships*	STAGE 4 *Consolidation*
1. Types of practitioners 2. Confidentiality 3. Negotiated relationships 4. Cost 5. Range of services 6. Access routes	1. Health or illness problem 2. Alternative methods/types of care available 3. Convenience factor 4. Chronic or acute difficulty	1. Health/illness assessment 2. Selection of practitioner/treatment modality 3. Cost 4. Location 5. Frequency 6. Referrals 7. Determination of legal status (parent/guardian role)	1. Information absorption 2. System use 3. New definitions of health/illness 4. Optimum health status

areas of deficit. Peer counseling and support groups of adolescents and older children are examples of sources of ongoing situational support. Such support must be planned for by those who care for children to compensate for the loss of institutions and guidelines in our society that in the past legitimated and stabilized standards and solutions to common problems.

Preschoolers and young school-age children are excellent observers, but they are poor interpreters of events. Consequently, their perceptions of what adults consider to be commonplace events can be quite distorted and threatening. Their developmentally normal egocentrism leads them to believe that external events over which they have no control or that are not specifically directed toward them are somehow their fault. Therefore, these children can be in

crisis over benign events: for example, because they, or a friend, failed a vision screening test at school.

Effects of Change

In our society, unplanned, rapid change has been identified as a cause of many individuals' crisis states. Even change that is well planned can be threatening to an individual, since change, by definition, "results in an alteration of the object of change" (Smith, 1982, p. 360). With young children especially, health care providers and parents and guardians have traditionally used power or coercive strategies to force compliance with their demands. Increasingly, as children are seen as health/illness care consumers who are responsible for their own care, they will become more involved in the process of planned change. Nursing interventions cannot otherwise be effective.

Developmental Implications

The principle of involving the child in the change process in a manner appropriate for his or her health status and developmental level is vital. For example, toddlers in the process of toilet training can be given the choice of wearing their "big boy" (training) pants before or after their nap. Preparation for change is especially important for children who are at stages critical to their identities, such as toddlers and adolescents. Again, in toilet training, the parent or guardian should be encouraged to talk about this activity with the child before it is initiated (Haber, Leach, Schudy, & Sideleau, 1982). For example, the parent may say, "You told me you were wet so I could give you a dry diaper. That's good! One of these days you'll know *before* your diaper is wet, and you can start to use the potty." It is sometimes difficult for parents to remember to do this with a child with normally limited expressive language. Parents should be reminded that children's receptive language is much more developed than their expressive language and that communication about change is very important to young children.

In working with children and adolescents, nurses need to remember that struggles for autonomy or a sense of internal chaos from developmental or situational crises can result in automatic resistance even to changes that will benefit or reward the child. For example, an adolescent girl who was somewhat overweight as a prepubertal child may insist on dieting to the point of anemia in spite of the nurse's attempts to help her maintain a balanced diet.

SCENARIOS: HEALTH AND ILLNESS CARE OF CHILDREN AND ADOLESCENTS IN THE COMMUNITY OF THE FUTURE

GAIL JONES: A PHYSICAL-FITNESS ORIENTATION

Gail Jones is a 16-year-old who lives with her mother in a rural community within 20 minutes travel time of a large southwestern city. Gail's mother travels extensively as part of her job. Although Gail is in excellent health, she has had occasional sore throats, acne, and viruses. Gail's friends or a college student frequently stay with her when her mother is out of town.

Susan Jones, Gail's mother, was delighted when a nurse-practitioner moved to their area and set up a clinic. Susan gave the nurse-practitioner power of attorney to treat Gail or to refer her to physicians as needed. This arrangement worked out well. Gail knows that she can call and get an appointment or a prescription refill or have a confidential discussion with Joan Davis, the nurse-practitioner, upon request. The cost is reasonable, Joan is always available for emergencies, and she has arranged for Gail to see specialists when necessary (for acne, for example, when the condition worsened and did not respond to usual remedies). The nurse-practitioner's availability and referral capabilities help prevent minor health problems from progressing to a crisis.

Gail has a part-time job and receives an allowance. She has become used to taking good care of her health, because her mother is careful about quality in foods. Furthermore, Gail pays for some of her health care, such as optional extras and care required if she has not made good health decisions at a specific point in time. Now Gail has asked the nurse-practitioner, Joan, for a referral to a physical-fitness assessment center, because she is concerned about a recent weight gain of 10 pounds. On assessment, the nurse-practitioner has determined that Gail's weight gain occurred as a result of overeating caused by stress during the last school semester. Gail feels she has control over some of the physical changes that are occurring during adolescence.

Joan sends Gail to a health and fitness center, where a nurse evaluates Gail's health records and refers her to the exercise physiologist for testing and to the dietitian for counseling. When Gail's mother returns home, she is pleased with the referral. Gail has a sensible exercise plan and a diet that will help her lose those extra 10 pounds.

BILL WILTON: A SUBSTANCE-FREE PROGRAM

Bill Wilton lives in an inner-city area, alternately with one or the other of his divorced parents, who both work. He is 15 and in the ninth grade. He now attends school regularly, after a long period of truancy problems. Bill has struck up a friendship with John Clayton, the nurse who maintains a privately funded store-front clinic in the neighborhood. Bill visits John with some frequency. They met because John coaches the junior high basketball team.

Bill has been using drugs for three years and has been using alcohol heavily for a year. Bill's perceptions of the situation were distorted by substance abuse, resulting in a crisis state for him after arrest for reckless driving while under the influence. This substance abuse also interferes with his basketball. John thinks Bill has a great future as a player if he can lick his substance-abuse problems, and he was able to interest Bill in the drug and alcohol withdrawal program. Bill now attends two group therapy sessions each week and helps clean the center on Saturdays. John has permission from Bill's father to treat him. Therapy has progressed so that Bill is now involved in recruiting other substance abusers into the program. John grew up in the same neighborhood, and he knows that lots of kids like Bill need health care along with therapy and a role model. Bill's program includes nutritional assessment, an exercise program, and work contribution by clients to the center. The program's approach fosters a positive vision of the future.

ALLEN BARTON: A SERIOUS ILLNESS TREATED AT HOME

Allen Barton is 6 years old. He has cystic fibrosis and is cared for at home by his parents, who monitor his medication, prepare a special diet, and perform nursing procedures. Their community health nurse is paid by insurance provided by Computer Technology, Inc., Allen's parents' employer.

Ruth and Peter Barton are computer programmers. Their computer terminal is located at home, allowing them to work at their own pace provided that weekly task schedules are met. Allen's health assessment information is fed into the computer several times daily, reading out medication dosages, procedures to be performed, and health care personnel to be activated on occasion.

The community health nurse, Sharon Wise, is glad she minored in computer programming. Her special program for Allen's case and her teaching of Allen's parents make it possible for him to remain at home. Care is more economical at home. Besides, Allen can learn about his illness and about the computer at the same time. Eventually, it will be a tool for his own self-care. The management of Computer Technology, Inc., is glad that health care costs are held down. Also, they are thinking about marketing Sharon's computer programs for child health care to parents who need such help and who have computers.

The Future of Community Health Nursing

What can we expect to occur in community health nursing of children and adolescents in the future? Societal conditions (see Table 12.2) will result in changes in the health care system that will have profound effects on the nursing profession. Specifically, children and adolescents will exercise greater autonomy in seeking health care. Because of time and work pressures and the potentially earlier maturity levels of adolescents, parents will be more willing to delegate their responsibility. Determining who is the adult responsible for a child becomes more difficult with divorce and geographic mobility so prevalent. Children and adolescents will become consumers of health or sickness care, depending on their physical status, subculture values, and parental attitudes.

Health care system adaptations will include a greater number and variety of community health center bases, such as in schools, storefronts, corporations, and com-

TABLE 12.2
Societal Conditions, Health Care Adaptations, and Effects on the Nursing Profession

Societal Conditions	Health Care System Adaptations	Effect on the Nursing Profession
Greater autonomy of children and adolescents in seeking health care.	Creation of more independent and varied community health care bases.	Increased autonomy and organizational control for nurses.
Willingness of parents to delegate health care responsibilities.	Home health care expansion in relation to family work situation.	Greater visibility of nurses in health care.
Problems in defining the adult responsible for children and adolescents.	More use of own income by adolescents for health care.	Nurses serving as referral sources for children and adolescents.
Differentiation between sickness care and health care.	New standards for confidentiality affecting children and adolescents.	

munity centers. Home health care will expand because it costs less than institutional health care and because more families will work at home. Adolescents, a population with potential for a high disposable income, are likely to use this income for health care. Health care will be viewed as an integral part of a physically active lifestyle. New standards for confidentiality will be developed to accommodate shifts in responsibility for health care and the movement toward self-care. Self-care may be viewed as a response to consumerism in the health care industry.

The nursing profession will change. Increased autonomy and organizational control by nurses will be facilitated by the expansion of care in the community, the greater visibility of nurses in health care, and further likelihood of nurses functioning as referral sources for children and adolescents.

Nurses with various areas of expertise may establish group practices with other health care providers. Such groups may contract with agencies to provide health care for children in schools, a condominium association, or a particular business or industry.

FUTURE IMPLICATIONS

Elucidation of Alternatives for the Future

As the scenarios indicate, there are several issues related to the future role of the nurse in caring for children and adolescents in the community.

The Settings for Nursing Practice

The setting of the nurse's practice is significant, for it will affect how nursing practice is controlled and how accessible nursing care is to clients. Traditional settings for the community health nurse have included health departments and schools, with salaried nurses functioning under the supervision of other nurses or physicians. In such circumstances, it has been difficult for nurses to define their own practices. Nurses who have the freedom and the responsibility to contract with clients on a fee-for-service basis will have a greater opportunity to select the settings in which they practice and to move from one setting to another with the client as client needs and the nurse's skills allow. The demand for such services from such practitioners will come from consumers, parents, and children who want adaptable health and illness care providers.

Community-based nurses who want to work with children and adolescents will reach them by means of geographical proximity in community health agencies, by being available at times that are convenient for young people, such as immediately after school, or through referrals from other traditional and nontraditional health care providers. Other sources might include parents' support groups and referrals from child clients themselves. The expertise of nurses could come to the attention of consumers who use computer programs on health/illness-related topics developed by and credited to a particular nurse or group of nurses in practice together.

Client Relationships

The effectiveness of the nurse's role with children and adolescents will be greatly affected by how the young clients and their significant others view the nurse. They need to see that the nurse values and respects them and has confidence in their abilities to manage appropriate aspects of their care. They also need to feel that the nurse continues to be interested in them and available for support even when the nurse be-

comes less directly involved in their care. The nurse must acknowledge their ability to function autonomously in meeting their health needs. Nurses' behavior must be congruent with their advice and stated beliefs if they are to have credibility with their clients. Children are especially aware and critical of discrepancies between adults' stated beliefs and behavior. Congruence is particularly necessary in advice given to promote health, because in this area the stimulus of changing behavior to avoid the immediate discomfort of current illness or injury is missing. Young clients also need to see the nurse as someone who can provide appropriate access to other competent, knowledgeable health care providers. Such clients need to view the nurse as having current knowledge about their health care problems and concerns. When nurses have such knowledge, they are not only more effective in providing care to clients but also are better role models for continued learning about health and illness.

Legal Implications

When children and adolescents assume a major role in selecting their own health care providers, several questions about legal aspects of health care arise. Currently, many emergency room physicians refuse to treat a child brought to them by anyone who is not the child's parent or legal guardian unless the child has written, dated, signed permission from the parent or guardian. How can long-term care be selected by children with their parents' permission? Nurses need to be sure that the parent or guardian who gives permission to care for a child has the right to do so, and they must document that they asked this question of the parent or guardian. One method of solving the problem of delegating health care is for the parent or guardian to grant power of attorney to another adult who is caring for the child or to the nurse who is providing health care to the child. Such decisions as whether the child can even be seen by the nurse, as well as decisions about management of health needs or illness, can then be made quickly as necessary for the child's best interests. Decisions about what information to share with others, such as health care providers and teachers, could then also be made by the nurse. The issue of confidentiality in relation to the parents' access to information about the child could be dealt with in the same way. Confidentiality is especially important to adolescents. Children and adolescents who seek their own health care providers and who pay for their services are likely to want to control the dissemination of information about their health status.

The Use of Computers

Many people predict that home and neighborhood computers will soon become readily available and increasingly sophisticated. The potential effects of the immediate access to other people and to wide sources of information that computers provide are far-reaching. Nurses who work with children and adolescents could receive immediate assistance from other health care providers and specialists about a specific problem. The community-based nurse could then continue to function, even with acceleration of knowledge and technology, as a generalist health care provider for children of all ages, with a variety of conditions and in different settings. The nurse would become the logical person to assist the child or adolescent in determining the information needed. Computers could also allow the nurse to monitor selected aspects of a client's health status in order to reduce the frequency of more expensive office or home visits. Children and adolescents could use computers to monitor their health status compared to what is optimal for them, thus assuring individualized assessment and care. These are only a few of the many ways in which health care providers and their clients will use computers in the future to prevent illness and to promote health.

SUMMARY

The relationships of children and adolescents to community health nurses in the future will be affected by changing health/illness problems, changing technology, greater autonomy and self-care, and changes in family structure and availability of adults. Nurses can best respond to these changes by assuming greater accountability and adaptability in their practices. Such practices might include a group of other nurses or health care providers or might be solo practices. Practices must, however, be community based, because that is where the client's health needs and illness problems exist. Adapting to such changes will not always be easy for nurses. At times, the nurse may feel like Alice at the Mad Hatter's tea party: nothing seems to make much sense, but it's too exciting to go to sleep!

DISCUSSION TOPICS

The following discussion questions apply to the community health nursing care situations following question eight.

1. How will future community health nurses be viewed by others who are not in health care, such as children, adolescents, parents and guardians, teachers and ad-

ministrators, and members of community organizations?

2. How will community health nurses function in relation to other health care providers, such as physicians, psychotherapists, physical therapists, exercise physiologists, and clinical dietitians?

3. How will legal responsibility for the health/illness care of children and adolescents be managed in the future?

4. How will expanded health care roles for community health nurses who work with children and adolescents be validated in the future and by whom?

5. How will community health nurses develop and use computer technology in the health care of children and adolescents?

6. How will community health nurses develop meaningful and expanded relationships with autonomous children and adolescents?

7. What beliefs, values, and educational experiences will nurses need to be focal referral sources in the health (vs. sickness) care system?

8. Will the community health nurse of the future be required to have more or different interpersonal and technical skills than he or she does today? What will these skills be?

SITUATION 1

A friend who is a counselor in a 300-student junior high school asks a nurse to assist with an ongoing problem in the school population. Many of the students live in "reconstituted" or step families in which incest taboos may break down. The counselor has become aware of several cases of stepfather–stepdaughter incest in this school population. She is concerned about the mental and physical health of these children.

SITUATION 2

A peer support group of elementary school children who have insulin-dependent diabetes requests assistance from a nurse. The group members want to learn individualized monitoring of their health status. They also want sources of information that they can understand about their diabetes and its effects on their lives as well as ongoing group counseling. They have been learning how to use computers at their respective schools, but none has a home computer.

SITUATION 3

The staff of a neighborhood child development center is interested in continued learning about health problems and growth and development of infants and children. They also want immediate access to information and advice about emergencies and illness of the children in their center. There is a computer in the center, and the parents of most of the children have home computers. The child development center's director wants to contract with a nurse for her services in relation to their needs.

BIBLIOGRAPHY

Aguilera, D., & Messick, J.: *Crisis intervention: Theory and methodology* (3rd ed.). St. Louis: C.V. Mosby, 1978.

Aquatic deaths and injuries—United States. *Morbidity and Mortality Weekly Report* 31, 417–419, 1982.

Avery, J.G.: The safety of children in cars. *Practitioner* 224, 816–821, 1980.

Bell, M.J., Ternberg, J.L., & Bower, R.J.: Low velocity vehicular injuries in children—Run-over accidents. *Pediatrics* 66, 628–631, 1980.

Benenson, M.W., Takafuji, E.T., Bancroft, W.H., et al: A military community outbreak of hepatitis type A related to transmission in a child care facility. *American Journal of Epidemiology* 112, 471–481, 1980.

Black, R.E., Dykes, A.C., Sinclair, S.P., et al: Giardiasis in day-care centers: Evidence of person-to-person transmission. *Pediatrics* 60, 486–491, 1977.

Bowers, J.E., Faulkner, B., & Michel, S.: Obesity in children: An ecological approach. *The Journal of Continuing Education in Nursing* 10, 40–49, 1979.

Child homicide—United States. *Morbidity and Mortality Weekly Report* 31, 292–294, 1982.

Danziger, K.: *Socialization.* New York: Penguin Books, 1978.

Duncan, D.R., & Ennis, A.: The Monroe County Childsafe project: Community education on the need for child auto seat restraints. *Health Values* 3, 107–109, 1979.

Elimination of indigenous measles—United States. *Morbidity and Mortality Weekly Report* 31, 517–519, 1982.

Epstein, L.H., Wing, R.R., Steranchak, L., et al: Comparison of family-based behavior modifications and nutrition education for childhood obesity. *Journal of Pediatric Psychology* 5, 25–36, 1980.

Ferguson, M.: *The aquarian conspiracy.* Los Angeles: J.P. Tarcher, 1980.

Foutes, J.A., Spencer, S., Tucker, J., et al: Policy decisions in scabies control. *Journal of School Health* 51, 673–675, 1981.

Gathorne-Hardy, J.: *Marriage, love, sex and divorce.* New York: Summit, 1981.

Ginsburg, C.M., McCracken, G.H., Rae, S., et al: *Haemophilus influenzae* type B incidence in a day-care center. *Journal of American Medical Association* 238, 604–607, 1977.

Haber, J., Leach, A.M., Schudy, S.M., et al.: *Comprehensive psychiatric nursing* (2nd ed.). New York: McGraw-Hill, 1982.

Hadler, S.C., Erben, J.J., Francis, D.P., et al: Risk factors for hepatitis A in day-care centers. *Journal of Infectious Diseases* 145, 255–261, 1982.

Hadler, S.C., Webster, H.M., Erben, J.J., et al: Hepatitis A in a day-care center. *New England Journal of Medicine* 30, 1222–1227, 1980.

Hammack, C., Ochoa, A., Henderson, C., et al: Hepatitis A outbreak related to a day care center in Forrest County, Mississippi. *Journal of Mississippi State Medical Association* 23, 40–43, 1982.

Humphrey, P.: Height/weight disproportion in elementary school children. *Journal of School Health* 49, 25–29, 1979.

Jones, L.Y.: *Great expectations: America and the baby boom generation.* New York: Ballantine, 1980.

Jonides, L.: Childhood obesity: A treatment approach for private practice. *Pediatric Nursing* 8, 320–322, 1982.

Juranek, D.D.: Epidemiology of lice. *Journal of School Health* 47, 352–355, 1977.

Lalor, W.R.: Development of a preventive fire education program based on a profile of the hospitalized burn victim. *Journal of School Health* 51, 80–84, 1981.

Langford, R.W.: Teenagers and obesity. *American Journal of Nursing* 81, 556–559, 1981.

Lasch, C.: *The culture of narcissism: American life in an age of diminishing expectations.* New York: Warner, 1979.

Long, L., & Long, T.J.: The unspoken fears of latchkey kids. *Working Mother* 76, 88, 90, 1982.

Long, T.J., & Long, L.: Latchkey children: The child's view of self. U.S. Educational Resources Information Center, ERIC Document No. ED 214 666, 1982.

Markowitz, M.: Streptococcal infections, rheumatic fever and school health services. *Journal of School Health* 49, 202–204, 1979.

McElhinney, S.T.: The lonely life of latchkey children, say two experts, is a national disgrace. *People*, September 20, 1982, pp. 83–84, 87–88.

Miller, J.R., & Hammer, S.L.: Parent involvement in child bicycle safety education. *Health Values* 3, 113–116, 1979.

O'Neill, N., & O'Neill, G.: *Shifting gears.* New York: Avon, 1980.

Pearson, G.A.: Nutrition in the middle years of childhood. *Maternal and Child Nursing* 2, 378–384, 1977.

Pipes, P.L.: *Nutrition in infancy and childhood* (2nd ed.). St. Louis: C.V. Mosby, 1981.

Radetsky, M.S., Johansen, T.L., Laner, B.A., et al: Multiply resistant pneumococcus causing meningitis: Its epidemiology in a day-care center. *Lancet*, October 10, 1981, pp. 771–773.

Riley, R.L.: Prevention and control of airborne infection in the community. *Annals of the New York Academy of Science* 353, 331–339, 1980.

Rowe, N.R.: Childhood obesity: Growth charts vs. calipers. *Pediatric Nursing* 6, 24–28, 1980.

Rubella prevention. *Morbidity and Mortality Weekly Report* 30, 37–42, 1981.

Rubella. *Public Health Currents* 22, 19–22, 1982.

Scherer, M.: The loneliness of the latchkey child. *Instructor* May 1982, pp. 38–41.

Schlechter, F.: An experiment in group adolescent weight loss guidance. *Journal of School Health* 51, 123–124, 1981.

School age day care: Developing a responsive curriculum. *Child Care Information Exchange* January 1980, pp. 17–20.

Silva, R.J.: Hepatitis and the need for adequate standards in federally supported day care. *Child Welfare* 59, 387–400, 1980.

Sklar, K.K.: Who is minding the children? *Graduate Woman* 76, 12–13, 1982.

Smith, M.: Group and organizational theory. In J. Haber, et al.: *Comprehensive psychiatric nursing* (2nd ed.). New York: McGraw-Hill, 1982.

Smith, M.H.D.: Infectious disease: An overview. *American Journal of Diseases of Children* 33, 1058–1060, 1979.

Storch, G.: Viral hepatitis associated with day-care centers. *Journal of the American Medical Association* 242, 1514–1518, 1979.

Toffler, A.: *Future shock.* New York: Bantam, 1978.

Toffler, A.: *The third wave.* New York: Bantam, 1981.

Tyrrell, S.: Accidents will happen. *Health and Social Science Journal* 91, 263–265, 1981.

Vernon, A.A., Schable, C., & Francis, D.: A large outbreak of hepatitis in a day-care center. *American Journal of Epidemiology* 115, 325–331, 1982.

Ward, J.I., Gorman, G., Phillips, C., et al: *Hemophilus influenzae* type B disease in a day-care center. *Journal of Pediatrics* 92, 713–717, 1978.

Weil, W.B.: Current controversies in childhood obesity. *Journal of Pediatrics* 91, 175–187, 1977.

Woodruff, C.W.: Iron deficiency in infancy and childhood. *Pediatric Clinics of North America* 24, 85–94, 1977.

Zakus, G., Chin, M.L., Cooper, H., et al: Treating adolescent obesity: A pilot project in a school. *Journal of School Health* 51, 663–666, 1981.

Zerfas, A.J., Shorr, I.J., & Neumann, C.G.: Office assessment of nutritional status. *Pediatric Clinics of North America* 24, 253–272, 1977.

13

Elderly Clients

Elsie Maxwell Hamm

Youth, large, lusty, loving—
　Full of grace, force, fascination,
Do you know that old age may come after you
　With equal grace, force, fascination?
　　　　WALT WHITMAN / *Leaves of Grass*

OBJECTIVES

After reading this chapter, you should be able to:

- [ ] Describe the aging process.
- [ ] Identify the specific needs of elderly people.
- [ ] Determine ways of answering the needs of elderly people.
- [ ] Evaluate services for the elderly.
- [ ] Identify future trends for an aging population and those who are responsible for their health care.

INTRODUCTION

Clare Booth Luce has said that at its best, long life has developed its full human potential and has fulfilled its dreams; at its worst, it "has resembled shipwreck with one thing after another going overboard" (Blyth, 1979). Between these extremes, there are many variations of aging, most of them culturally defined. Three twentieth-century phenomena prevail: (1) rapid increase in numbers of people who are 60 years old and over, (2) intensified interest in gerontology, and (3) evidence of ageism.

Increase in Numbers of Elderly People

In the past, few people lived to old age, but the twentieth century has been characterized by a marked increase both in number and proportion of aged people. In the United States the elderly population grew from 4.9 million in 1900 to 32.8 million in

1977, nearly a sevenfold increase. Between 1930 and 1977 the number doubled, and it is projected to redouble by the year 2035 (Fowles, 1978). Moreover, the proportion of people in the 60–69 age group became smaller, while the 75+ age group experienced a tenfold increase and the 85+ age group multiplied 17 times. Thus the whole elderly population became older. The 1980 United States census revealed that people over age 65 constitute 11.3 percent of the population.

The sex composition of the elderly has also changed dramatically (Fowles, 1975). During the nineteenth century a preponderance of men among immigrants to the United States, plus high mortality among women during childbearing years, produced a surplus of men in older age groups (97 women to 100 men). In recent years this trend has reversed, and 134 elderly women are present for every 100 men. The ratio ranges from 114 women to 100 men in the 60–64 age group to over 200 women for every 100 men in the 85+ age group.

Constituting the fastest growing minority and the fastest growing poverty group in the country (Butler, 1975), the elderly form one of the most "information poor" groups as well (Childers & Post, 1975). From all demographic indications, aging people in the United States seem almost predisposed to debilitation. The onus of becoming poorer as they become older can only work to their disadvantage.

The economically poorest group of Americans, according to the 1980 United States census, is single women over age 65 who live alone, and increasing numbers of elderly people (most of them women) are choosing to live alone. A new type of nuclear family, the mature (often single-person) family is developing, with unexplored consequences for society (Riley, Johnson, & Foner, 1968).

Havighurst stated in 1949 that aging is a particularly American problem:

The United States with its accent on youth and growth and speed, tends neither to revere nor to reject but rather to ignore old age—to suppose that it is only a state of mind which can be banished if one keeps busy. (p. 298)

No longer can old age be ignored, however. Burgeoning numbers of elderly consumers have forced an awareness that people should be better prepared for being old. There is also an unprecedented interest in a new field of study, gerontology

Gerontology

The field of *gerontology* began as an inquiry into the characteristics of long-lived people (Birren & Clayton, 1975). Biologists, physicians, and psychologists published papers during the 1920s claiming genetics, diet, or mental attitude as the determining factors of a long life. Their hypotheses were incomplete, however, in light of later findings that the main feature of aging was multiple determination. The 1930s saw a rise in the ecological perspective: that aging was an interactive process between biological disposition and the external environment, as Birren and Clayton point out.

Gerontologists held that studies in human aging must take into account all aspects of the life span. The ecological approach, which relates human beings to their environment, resources, and social and cultural patterns, focuses on human adaptability and studies the aging process free of negative connotations associated with chronological age (Bruhn, 1971).

These diverse views may illustrate the claim that there is no such thing as a "true gerontologist," only members of other professions who are interested in the concerns of aging. Historically, decisions about what to do with old people were based on circumstances: the amount of food available and the individual's productivity, biological capability, and physical or mental health. In some cultures the belief prevailed that old people possessed magic powers and were to be feared (Mead, 1977).

Despite information to the contrary, myths persist today even among professional providers of health and social services (Kent, 1956). For example:

Myth	Fact
1. "The golden past"	Many elderly people lived and died in poorhouses.
2. Three-generation family	Because of migration and short life expectancy, extended families living together were rare.
3. Independence as a basic goal	Aged people tend to seek security.
4. Homogeneity of the aged	Aged people are heterogeneous and more individualistic than young people.
5. Value of retirement villages	Not for everybody.
6. Old age means illness and senility	Only 21 percent of American elderly people report poor health; senility affects only a few; many forms of senility are treatable and preventable.
7. Old age begins at age 65	Aging is highly individualized; some people are old at 40 while others are young at 90; different organ systems age differently, too.
8. Old employees are less capable than young employees	Old employees have less absenteeism and fewer accidents and show less stress than young employees.
9. Old people are sexless	Sexual vigor continues well into old age.
10. Learning ability declines with age	Conceptual and vocabulary skills often grow after age 60.
11. Old people are set in their ways	Old people show remarkable adaptability; it is a secret of their survival.

Seldom mentioned is the fact that fewer than 5 percent of America's elderly population is confined to institutions, which means that 95 percent reside elsewhere, a point stressed by Eisdorfer and Wilke (1976, p. 418):

Much of the early research in behavioral aspects of aging has been with institutionalized people. There is, however, a growing recognition that to investigate the "normal" aging process there is a need to work with healthy and intellectually intact people who can still function in the community.

Paul (1956) challenged social scientists, and in particular public health professionals, by learning to work understandingly and productively with older people, doing less and less to them, and more and more with them. Locus of care has shifted from home, to institution, to overcrowded institution. Now it is moving back to alternate types of care and even back to the home or to surrogate homes in the community.

Undoubtedly the proportion of elderly people in the population will become even higher, and those elderly people who suffer most from poor health, low income, and social isolation (women, blacks, and the very old) will become an even larger proportion of the aged. What are the prevailing attitudes about this demographic trend?

Despite conflicting evidence, stereotypic ideas about the aging process persist at all levels of society. As diverse perceptions of needs cloud the issues, gerontologists generally discern two kinds of problems: the problems that older people actually have, and the problems that the experts think they have (Rosow, 1967). While the two may have common factors, they do not always correspond. Furthermore, programs based on the experts' perceptions have produced myths about the aged as well as a pluralistic and fragmented array of services.

Like public health, services to the aged have not had a strong conceptual base nor a lifetime perspective (Rudd, 1951). As a result, various fads have prevailed: getting people out of mental hospitals, establishing information and referral services, activity centers, protective services, meals on wheels, congregate meal centers, home health care. In only a few localities does a single entry system exist: a single agency through which an elderly person's needs are determined and appropriate services rendered and monitored.

Ageism

Systematic stereotyping of people because they are old has brought a new word to our vocabulary: *ageism*. Dr. Robert N. Butler, a psychiatrist and gerontologist, coined the word in 1968 to describe the profound bias against the elderly that he observed (1975). Ageism refers to discrimination based on age—to the idea that people who have lived for many years are inferior to people who are young.

The 1975 Harris study (Harris and Associates, 1976) sponsored by the National Council on Aging was the most extensive study ever conducted on America's elderly. While it disproved some myths about aging, it acknowledged the wide range of problems faced by older people. The two problems respondents found to be most serious were fear of crime and poor health. Less serious but still causing concern were not having enough money, loneliness, not having enough education, and not feeling needed.

In addition to surveying the experiences of elderly people themselves, the Harris study measured younger people's expectations of old age, and it found wide discrepancies between the two. For example, 21 percent of the respondents over age 65 reported poor health, whereas 51 percent of the general public cited poor health as a prime problem of old age; 12 percent of the elderly respondents reported loneliness, while 60 percent of the general public said that loneliness was a major problem among the aged. For every one of 12 problems studied, major differences existed between the problems experienced by the elderly and those attributed to them.

Few people who work with the aged have had any gerontological training, so it is reasonable to expect that their attitudes about aging will correspond to those found in the general public. In addition, work with the elderly is not held in high esteem nor is it financially rewarding. This picture is changing, however, as providers of services and the elderly themselves take more responsibility for improving conditions and quality of life.

Implications for Nurses

Over the years a strong association has existed in most people's minds between old age and illness. To many people the terms are synonymous. This is as true of professional caregivers as it is of the general public. No matter that the vast majority (95 percent) of elderly people live outside of institutions, that 81 percent of America's elderly people are self-sufficient, and that 80 percent of care given to the frail elderly is given by family members in the home. The myths persist that the aged are sick and cared for by strangers in long-term-care facilities.

A basic need exists for an attitudinal change toward old people. Studies have shown that people who have close association with the elderly tend to ascribe fewer negative characteristics to them than do those who have less association with them (Bekker & Taylor, 1966). Service providers who see only hospitalized aged people with serious illnesses need to become acquainted with the physically and intellectually intact elderly who are still active in the community. Many stereotypical notions are brought into question in such situations, as when medical students are required to work in community-based programs with active and productive elderly people (Birenbaum, Aronson, & Seiffer, 1979).

A California study among nurses employed in extended care facilities revealed overwhelmingly negative attitudes toward people with hearing impairment (Magit, Torbit, & Willis, 1981). Since nurses were trying daily to communicate with those aged people, their attitudes necessarily influenced the clients, the effectiveness of their care, and even the nurses' own job satisfaction. The study demonstrated the need for inservice education in caring for hearing impaired elderly clients.

In contrast, a recent study among nursing students (Olsen, 1982) showed a generally positive set of attitudes toward the aged in the test sample. However, it was easier for the students to accept aging in others than in themselves. This may point to the root cause of negative attitudes toward the elderly: caregivers see not only the wrinkles and gray hair of their elderly clients but also reflections of themselves. Robert Louis Stevenson said it well: "Old and young, we are all on our last cruise." The National Council on Aging adds, "and in the same boat."

Olsen notes that the traits in the elderly most admired by the student nurses were wisdom, patience, and individuality; the least admired were dependence, self-pity, rigidity, and demanding attention. Apparently the aged person is expected to work out a balance between leaning on others and standing up for personal rights. This is difficult at any age, Olsen claims, and she charges nurses to explore their own aging, creative uses of dependency, and the therapeutic role of positive expectations in the healing process.

By all demographic indications, the population aged 65 and over has doubled during the twentieth century and will redouble by the year 2035. Elderly citizens may soon require most of the nation's health care resources. If old age is to be a human triumph rather than an insoluble problem, then the physical and social environments must support it. The helping professions can lead the way by preparing people for long life and by providing community-based services to keep the elderly secure and independent in their own surroundings.

Each year a better-educated cohort enters old age; therefore, the principle of self-determination could become better utilized. The best goals may be to offer the aged stronger defenses against the pitfalls of long life, plus more options in living arrangements and other resources.

Definition of Terms

Ageism. Systematic stereotyping of people because they are old. The term implies that people who are old are inferior to people who are young.

Community-based setting. A place in or near the home where older people voluntarily participate in activities or receive services (*Training Materials Guide*, 1981).

Continuum of care. Comprehensive range of programs and services developed and coordinated to meet physical, social, emotional, financial, intellectual, and spiritual needs (*Long Term Care for the Elderly*, 1980).

Chronic disease. Illness that lasts more than three months, or "illness as comprising all impairments or deviations from normal which have one or more of the following characteristics: are permanent, leave residual disability, are caused by irreversible pathological alteration, require long period of supervision, observation or care" (Katz, Halstead, & Wierenga, 1975).

Frail elderly. Those persons whose physical or mental capabilities or support systems are reduced to the extent that the individual becomes unable to maintain a household or social contacts without continuing assistance from others.

Geriatrics. The specialized branch of medicine that deals with the problems and diseases of old age and aging people.

Geriatric (or adult) day care. Supervised day care in an institutional setting; restorative, maintenance, or social models provide from 8 to 10 hours of supervision per day, 5 days per week for frail elderly people who live alone or whose family members work during the day.

Geriatric day hospital. Inpatient care from Monday morning until Friday evening; allows frail people to spend weekends with family members and thus supports the family unit.

Gerontology. (from *geron, gerontos*, the Greek words meaning "old age" or "old man") the study of aging; particularly, the study of old age.

Health. A process and state of equilibrium within and with the external physical, psychological, and social environments in which the individual functions best, enjoys most, and damages and wastes the least.

High-level wellness. This includes giving good care to your physical self, using your mind constructively, expressing your emotions effectively, being creatively involved with those around you, being concerned about your physical, psychological, and social environments, and becoming aware of other levels of consciousness (Travis, 1977).

Hospice care. A sheltering institution or visiting team of helpers designed to control and relieve the emotional and physical suffering of the terminally ill and their families. Hospice care aims to enable the client to live as fully as possible and makes the family the unit of care.

Network. A pattern or system; a group of people (usually family, friends, neighbors) who maintain an important ongoing relationship with one another

(Rueveni, 1979); or a resource-locating and resource-matching vehicle for helping people (Sarason, Carroll, Morton, Cohen, & Lorentz, 1977).

Protective services for the elderly. Those legal services necessary to maintain an elderly person's well-being in the least restrictive way. In particular, use of a conservator or guardian in cases of allegations of abuse, neglect, or exploitation.

Respite care. Temporary institutionalization to afford the client and the home caregiver a rest from one another, or to give the family vacation time.

CONCEPTS ABOUT WORKING WITH ELDERLY PEOPLE

Gerontological nursing is a specialized field of service. According to the National Institute on Aging (U.S. Department of Health and Human Services) in a statement prepared for the 1981 White House Conference on Aging, the aim of gerontological nursing is to use knowledge of the aging process to design nursing care and services that aid elderly people in achieving health, longevity, and independence.

Based on an understanding of the aging process, gerontological nursing includes assessment of the health needs of older adults, planning and implementing health care to meet these needs, and evaluating the effectiveness of such care. Elderly adults should be actively involved to the fullest extent possible in all decision making that influences the quality of their everyday lives. These are the elements of case management, but community-based care also entails an interdisciplinary approach that appreciates and uses the knowledge and services of other professional and paraprofessional care givers.

The Aging Process

That human bodies deteriorate with time is no secret, but commonly ignored are the facts that individuals age at different rates and that separate organ systems within each individual age at different rates. Viewed holistically, aging is extremely complex. Whether body chemistry or a genetic time clock or some other theoretical system influences aging is still a matter of research and controversy.

Disease, not the passage of time, emerges as the apparent villain of the aging process. The human life span of approximately 85 years has been fixed for 100,000 years; it is not changing now. The *life span* is the length of time which the average person lives, barring accidents or disease (Fries & Crapo, 1981). *Life expectancy* is the expected death age based on mortality rates. The average life expectancy in the United States was 74.1 years in 1981, and it is expected to rise.

Physical Changes

Among the various aspects of aging, *physical changes* usually are noted first. This corresponds with Maslow's hierarchy of needs (1968), which cites physical needs before all others. The cause of physical change is the failure of some cells to replicate themselves, resulting in a reduced number of cells in the body. The barrier to indefinite replication of cells is called the Hayflick limit (Hayflick & Moorhead, 1961). Some organs are more directly affected by this change than others, and the body's defense against the onslaught of disease is lessened.

Briefly, chronological aging affects the anatomical systems as follows:

Skeletal. A loss of bone tissue, resulting in changed structure and posture and a loss of height; osteoarthritis, affecting mobility and causing swollen joints; osteoporosis (particularly in postmenopausal women), predisposing the individual to risk of fractures; loss of teeth.

Muscular. Loss of muscle tissue with concomitant loss of muscle strength. Even regular exercise does not compensate for tissue reduction.

Nervous. Slowed reaction time; greater ability to recall long-past events than recent events; sensory diminution.

Vascular. Reduced circulatory and cardiac efficiency; possible increase in blood pressure.

Excretory. Kidneys decrease in size; loss of muscle tissue, resulting in problems of continence; slowing of digestive process, resulting in constipation; drying and wrinkling of skin and reduced ability to perspire.

Digestive. Smaller appetite; slowing of digestive process; reduced secretion of digestive enzymes.

Endocrine. Alteration in functions of endocrine glands and of hormonal secretion.

Reproductive. Thinning of vaginal walls; reduction in size of uterus and cervix; reduction in size of testicles.

Respiratory. Shallower breathing and reduced lung capacity.

Along with normal anatomical changes, which are not pathological illnesses, come physiological changes that alter health behavior and habits of daily living. Life-long habits of diet and exercise usually prevail in the later years, but if the reduction in caloric need is recognized, the elderly person will eat less; if not, weight gain is inevitable. Good nutrition is important at any age, but equally important are exercise and rest. For some, exercise and rest may even be more important than diet.

If a person is accustomed to regular vigorous exercise (and that energetic type contributes to the highest level of wellness), then the habit of physical exercise will continue. Sedentary people continue to be sedentary, and they do so at their peril.

The only health behavior that shows considerable involuntary change is the pattern of sleep. Older people tend to sleep for fewer hours per night then younger people. Rather than reaching for a sleeping pill, an aging person should realize that four to six hours of sleep at night with a nap during the day constitutes sufficient rest in the later years.

Adequate diet continues to require daily portions of the four main food groups. Older people have reduced needs for calories, carbohydrates, fats, and sodium. Elderly people do not need more vitamins than young people. Each person is unique in assimilation and therefore must be treated on an individual basis. Food and drug tolerances change, because aging affects absorption, distribution, metabolism, and excretion.

In drug administration, doses of medication must be individually adjusted. Drug dosage in pediatrics can be calculated by body weight, but this is not true in geriatrics because of the highly individualistic nature of assimilation. Because of the marked reduction in organ reserve that accompanies normal aging, careful attention has to be given to medication dosage. In general, elderly people should receive smaller doses over a longer period of time.

New aspects of old illnesses appear in old age, as well as new illnesses, such as hypothermia. Older people take an average of twice as long to recover. Too often, caregivers give up on an elderly person who is not responding to treatment, but that is exactly the time when perseverance is needed.

Psychological Changes

Psychological changes of normal aging include:

Loss of self-esteem

Acceptance or nonacceptance of physical changes

Stress caused by change of residence, fear of crime, or personal losses

Coping with personal losses

Slower processing of information

Possible depression

Sartre observed that "we tend to become the people other people think we are." Psychological changes are often caused by expectations, both of elderly people themselves and of those around them. An aged person will often ask: "Who am I?" "What is happening to me?" "What does it mean to act my age?" "To whom am I important?" "Do I like the place where I live?" Both disengagement (Cumming & Henry, 1961) and activity (Havighurst, Neugarten, & Tobin, 1968) are evident among the aged. Some older people revel in participation and new-found freedom, whereas others withdraw into solitude. Those who fare best seem to be the active participants. An antidote for loss is replacement, and old age is, in Dr. Eric Pfeiffer's words (1982), "a season of loss." Caregivers would do well to remember that elderly clients might very well have lost everything and everyone in life that held any meaning for them.

A sense of desolation cannot always be avoided: therefore, depression is not uncommon among the elderly. Some people have many reasons to be depressed at any age, but a marked danger of depression in old age is that it will be ignored and go untreated. "Oh, she's just old!" can be an excuse for not doing anything, as though old people do not count, or as if it would be hopeless to extend aid. Depression at any age is usually treatable.

Considering that 11.3 percent of the population (those over age 65) account for 25 percent of suicides in the United States, and acknowledging that most suicides are preceded by periods of depression, the importance of treating depression in old people is undeniable. Sadly, too, many depressions are physical in origin: malnutrition, too much medication, a harmful combination of medications, and so forth. Acute brain syndrome, often beginning with depression, necessitates prompt attention before it becomes irreversible as chronic brain syndrome. Only a small percentage of the elderly are victims of Alzheimer's disease, a subject of considerable current research. Realistically, caregivers and others can stop using the blanket term "senility" as though it were a disease in itself or an inevitable result of living too long.

Sociological Changes

While these physical and psychological changes are occurring, other changes are taking place in the external social environment and in the older person's relationship to society as a whole. Some of the sociological changes that come with long life are:

Reduced income

Change in life-style

Change of residence or neighborhood

Inability to change residence

Widowhood

Loss of other family members, neighbors, and friends

Social isolation

Isolation from services and activities

Victimization by criminals

Observing all the upheaval that accompanies the transition from middle to old age, one has to marvel at the monumental adaptations most people make. Eighty-one percent of America's elderly people are self-sufficient, despite reduced income, chronic disease, and, in many instances, social isolation. Not only do they manage to survive, they also manage to thrive.

Spiritual Changes

If wellsprings of life are spiritual, then an ecological view of the aging process includes a look at this aspect of the human organism. Generally people carry their values with them into extreme old age; illness and death can hold deep meaning for people of religious faith, and they derive comfort from their beliefs.

Noted spiritual changes are both internal and external. Religious fervor and piety may increase; attendance at religious services may decline for many reasons (disability, lack of transportation, moving away from the familiar congregation). Moberg (1965, p. 508) reports that

research to date seems to indicate fairly conclusively that ritualistic behavior outside the home tends to diminish with increasing age, while religious attitudes and feelings apparently increase among people who have an acknowledged religion.

For those who are devout, inability to join in religious activities is a painful loss. Some denominations recognize this need for continuous association and offer special ministries to home-bound or elderly people. Conversely, older people, having more time than they ever had before, can assist their congregations in outreach services as well as other volunteer projects.

Assessment of Health Needs

Health in old age is measured by functional ability. If chronic disorders are under control and do not result in disability, then an acceptable level of wellness is maintained. While physical health cannot be viewed separately from psychological health or social well-being, some norms are necessary to help nurses determine service needs.

Are self health ratings valid? Friedsam and Martin (1963) compared self and physicians' health ratings in a group of older Texans and showed a positive relationship between the two sets of ratings. Self health ratings proved to be a simple and sensitive barometer of self-image. Similarly, a longitudinal study in self-assessment of health status (Maddox, 1964) showed that two out of three elderly subjects presented a realistic evaluation of their own health that agreed with physicians' assessments.

A nurse with sharpened skills of observation can begin a health assessment with what is seen and proceed by actively listening to the client's own subjective evaluation. Agencies usually develop systematic questionnaires for health histories, or nurses can develop their own. The Older American Resources and Services methodology (OARS), developed and copyrighted by Duke University in the 1970s, is one example of a highly refined instrument with over 25,000 documented uses (Pfeiffer, 1978). Use of this questionnaire requires approximately one hour, which some agencies find too time-consuming, but the advantages of a comprehensive assessment such as the OARS are that such a test:

1. Includes assessment of social and economic resources, mental and physical health, and ability to deal with activities of daily living.
2. Is reliable and valid in the hands of both professionals and nonprofessionals.

3. Yields a cumulative score that points up the client's areas of need.

Admittedly, such an instrument assesses more than physical health status. Experience has shown that older people with supposedly a single problem usually have several problems and that it can be wasteful and ineffective to consider only one small area when other needs abound. A social worker might interview a client for financial assistance but not recommend needed health services. Conversely, a nurse might arrange for specific health services but never look beyond to the client's economic hardship, which might have contributed to the health problems. Anything less than a holistic approach can fall short of answering needs.

Planning and Implementing Care

After a holistic assessment of needs, the nurse develops a care plan in concert with other service providers, giving the client as great a part in decision making as possible. Other family members deserve consideration as well. Eighty percent of the physical care given to the aged in the United States is given by family members. For every person in a nursing home, two or more people of comparable disability are being cared for at home.

Overwhelming evidence supports the economy and advisability of maintaining an elderly person at home in familiar surroundings as long as possible. A point can be reached, however, when that arrangement is no longer cost effective or humanly possible. That point is usually marked by the need for 24-hour skilled nursing care. Before such a crisis is reached, supportive community services should be utilized, two of which are respite care and geriatric day care. Some hospitals and nursing homes are reserving a few rooms for respite care, a temporary institutionalization that accommodates the elderly and their families to give them a rest from one another or to allow a hard-pressed family to have vacation time.

Geriatric or adult day care is growing rapidly in North America. In 1972, only six adult day-care centers were known; in 1982 the National Council on Aging documented 680. These centers range from restorative care to maintenance or simply social supervision. Elderly people who live alone or who live with working people come to the centers for eight or nine hours a day, five days a week, to receive services.

When respite or day care is no longer practical and the client becomes homebound, a new array of possible services is considered. Emphasis is placed on a multidisciplinary approach. When needs for nursing care have been determined, the nurse stands back to take a larger, ecological view to determine what other services could be added to supplement nursing's contribution to this patient. At this point, a working knowledge of community resources is fundamental. Other services the client might use are:

Podiatry
Physical therapy
Speech therapy
Occupational therapy
Meals on wheels
Home health aide
Housekeeping service
Library service
Visual services
Low-cost dental care
Outpatient clinic
Chore service (yard work, laundry)
Home repair
Pest control

Escort service (help with shopping)

Transportation

Friendly visiting

Telephone reassurance

Full- or part-time senior companion

Medical supplies or equipment

Congregate housing

Supervised housing

Nutrition site (congregate meals)

Health screening

Educational programs

Recreational programs

Legal counseling

Part-time employment

Religious ministries

Protective services

Senior citizen discounts (including generic drugs and food)

Financial aid (food stamps, Supplemental Security Income, Medicaid, state old age assistance, Medicare, Social Security)

Agencies providing assistance are found in both the public and private sector (see the list at the end of this chapter). Contingent on the availability of services, a plan of care is written and short-term and long-term goals are developed. Such a plan also includes a time limit, which ensures monitoring and a reassessment of needs. Since change is inherent in life, the original assessment and care plan are valid only for a short time after they are written. Conditions could change drastically in an hour or a day.

Networking of resources and establishing a continuum of services may be the responsibility of a social agency, or they may fall within the responsibility of the nurse's health agency. Formal networks usually involve resources such as those listed at the end of this chapter. Informal networks can involve family members, friends, neighbors, and associates in religious or other organizations. Anyone who has a sincere interest in the client can be part of a support system. Linkage of services from whatever source, preventing duplication, and encouraging cooperation and coordination would be the responsibility of the principle caregiver.

If an elderly client lives alone or has no close relatives or friends, then the service providers are the support system. When family members are involved, the nurse usually teaches them elements of care that is needed between the nurse's home visits. Some frail elderly people are under guardianship or conservatorship, a complex legal situation in which caregivers work with and through the appointed responsible parties.

A close working relationship with the client, family members, and other supportive helpers allows the nurse to observe the results of the care plan, monitor success or failure of a particular regimen, and to suggest changes in services as new needs arise.

Follow-up is indicated at least two weeks after initiation of services; complete reassessment should be undertaken within six months. Have short-term or long-term goals been reached? Have the client's needs changed? Should some services be discontinued or others initiated?

If services are to be terminated, an interview is needed to evaluate the results of services and the condition of the client and also to assure that client that the door is always open for resumption of services if needed. For a frail elderly person living alone, continued follow-up is almost invariably indicated.

COMMUNICATION. There is a relationship between communication and health care, but few studies explore that link. The success of a care plan may well depend on how clearly the message sender and the message receiver understand one another. The elderly cannot take communication for granted. Because of the physiological changes that take place within the individual plus the technological and sociological changes that are taking place in the external environment, an elderly person can easily be cut off from all information.

One observation aged people often make is that the older they get, the younger their caregivers are. Bettinghaus and Bettinghaus (1976) point out two problems arising from this age difference: (1) difference in language (slang, technical terms); and (2) difference in status between an aging person and a care provider.

Language grows and changes continuously, but older people who are not accustomed to an age-heterogeneous environment may not understand modern slang. Neither is it helpful to use highly technical terms in explanations. Such practices widen the gulf between message senders and message receivers and hasten the learned dependency that plagues old age.

An older person accustomed to a position of respect who suddenly must take orders from a younger person might be uncooperative. If the youthful care provider also condescends and talks down to the client, communication may break down.

Getting messages through can be difficult. Hearing impairment is common among the elderly and is one of the most serious hindrances to open communication. Since most information from caregivers to clients is transmitted orally, if messages are not received or are only partially understood, the whole care plan might be in jeopardy. Moreover, unthinking care providers have at times treated hearing-impaired clients as though they were without all their mental faculties. This is guaranteed to ruin a relationship.

CARING. Perhaps the most important component of care is a caring relationship. Human beings with their highly attuned senses can tell by sound, sight, touch, and feel whether a care provider is truly interested in them. Even frail elderly people who exhibit sensory diminution can readily respond to an outgoing, personable caregiver. All people need someone to be concerned about and to have someone be concerned about them in return. Perhaps, next to family members, nurses are the people best qualified to provide warm, human contact. Witness the welcome that usually awaits a nurse at the time of a home visit.

The process of nursing, i.e. everything the nurse does for and with the recipient, is designed to help the individual or family in coping with or bearing the stress of illness and suffering, and to find meaning in the experiences.

(Travelbee, 1971, p. 10)

This process can ensue from the nurse's first visit if trust is built. It may take a little extra time, but clients and their families respond best when they are assured of a caring relationship on the part of the care provider.

Case Studies

Mrs. Albert is an alert 70-year-old widow referred by the social services department of the local hospital after colostomy surgery. She lives alone but has a sister and niece who live next door. Her income is adequate but not large. Although she is physically weak, she is determined to complete her convalescence at home. Ostomy care bewilders her, and she is having difficulty adjusting to the idea of coping with this new arrangement for the rest of her life.

GOALS

To provide health supervision and instruction in ostomy care; to give moral support; to coordinate formal and informal networks to cover 24-hour needs.

PLAN

Demonstration of ostomy care to client and sister; later, observation of client self-care; checking medications and appliances and methods of administration or use; plan of regular follow-up care by nurse.

The nurse consults with the nearby family members and the client about use of supplemental community services (temporary use of meals on wheels, homemaker services, visit from outreach worker from local ostomy organization) to reassure the client about her capabilities and encourages the family members to stay with the client at night until she feels confident and secure.

Mr. Fine is an 80-year-old widower referred by his daughter. He lives with his daughter and son-in-law, both of whom work during the day. Mr. Fine's only income is Social Security. He is a diabetic who takes insulin; he also takes medications for high blood pressure and arthritis pain. Lately he has been disoriented as to time and place. The concerned family members worry that he will wander from home in their absence and get lost in the neighborhood.

GOALS

Reassessment of diabetic condition and use of medications; reorientation and possible remotivation of the client; part-time supervision for client; respite for family but keeping the family unit intact.

PLAN

Immediate in-home check on diabetes and insulin administration; check on amounts and kinds of other medications; communication with physician about health examination; assistance for family in applying to adult day care center for parttime supervision during family's working hours.

Mr. Carter is an 86-year-old retired farmer referred by his doctor for follow-up care after orthopedic surgery (hip replacement). Mrs. Carter is an energetic 75-year old woman who is blind

in one eye. She is apprehensive about her ability to give adequate care to her disabled husband. A vast array of medications is evident on the dresser: prescriptions from more than one physician plus over-the-counter drugs.

During preliminary assessment, the couple reveals that their total monthly income is $172.00, well below poverty level. Their home is modest and paid for; an extra lot next door is cultivated as a well-kept fruit and vegetable garden. When the question arises about asking for supplemental income, both client and spouse state that they tried but nothing came of it. They have been drawing on their savings to pay current bills, and on the day of the nurse's visit the savings have dwindled to $16.00.

GOALS

Instruction in postoperative care; plan of regular home visits by nurse; drug education to avoid overuse, misuse, or possible abuse of drugs; assistance in stabilizing financial condition; arranging for prescribed physical therapy.

PLAN

Outline of care by nurse and instruction for wife and client; transportation for wife to store (subsidized taxi service); escort service to Social Security office and county office of human services to apply for financial assistance (Supplemental Security Income, Medicaid, food stamps, state old age assistance) and to physical therapist.

Mrs. Jarvis is a 75-year-old bedridden arthritic whose total income is Social Security and public assistance. Her only relative is a 47-year-old son. Mrs. Jarvis is referred by the director of nurses at a local nursing home because the son had Mrs. Jarvis released to his care, assuring the staff that he had arranged for adequate care at home. Mrs. Jarvis was submissive, but the nursing staff is skeptical and requests a home visit.

The nurse is admitted to a small, unkempt, lower-middle-class home that is in a state of disarray. Mrs. Jarvis is in obvious need of general care, and she weeps when she sees the nurse. The son is apparently intoxicated, and nurse learns that he is an alcoholic. Mrs. Jarvis states that she wishes she was back in her bed at the nursing home.

GOALS

Institute emergency service for helpless, neglected client; give supportive care during interim; try to control unpredictable son.

PLAN

Call 911 (or other local emergency telephone number) for police protection from son; after arrival of police place emergency call to office of human services to report abuse and neglect of elderly person; await arrival of team of social workers to arrange for readmission of Mrs. Jarvis to the nursing home; subsequently establish guardianship of Mrs. Jarvis to protect her person and property.

Evaluation

A review of short-term and long-term goals forms the basis for evaluation. Short-term goals are easily measured, and they usually lead in a step-by-step order to long-term goals, which may cover many years. Inquiries cover such questions as:

Were the short-term goals realistic? Did they serve the client's needs?

Did they contribute to attainment of long-term goals?

Is the client's condition improved, much the same, or worse?

Were the services appropriate, timely, and cost effective?

Did the services improve the quality of life for the client?

For a specific example, in the rehabilitation of Mr. Carter, who had a hip replacement, the care provider would need to know:

Were all phases of treatment continued?

Was the plan for services adequate?

Are there gaps in services that need to be filled by adding new services or per-

haps by using informal volunteer resources?

How is the morale of the client and the client's family?

Is there evidence of family burnout?

Is consultation with other service providers indicated?

As a matter of quality control, some agencies conduct a "client satisfaction survey" separately from the routine evaluation. This adds another dimension to the client's history. Such a questionnaire can be administered by mail, telephone, or personal visit. The last is the most expensive and time consuming, but it probably produces the most comprehensive results.

Checking goals leads to a rating of a client's health status, which is measured in old age by functional ability. Correcting and preventing disability are prime long-term goals, and care providers should concentrate on positive aspects of health care—health promotion and health education. Health education is needed at all ages, but it is often neglected for elderly clients because of the false notions that people of advanced years are habit prone or unable to learn.

Attaining High-Level Wellness

While nursing procedures may be concentrated on the correction of defects, opportunities abound to teach the client and the client's family how to prevent future disabling conditions. The aim is to help the client achieve the highest level of wellness. As Travis (1977, Introduction) explains, wellness is not a static state. It results when people begin to see themselves as growing, changing beings. High-level wellness at any age means:

giving good care to your physical self, using your mind constructively, expressing your emotions effectively, being creatively involved with those around you, being concerned about your physical and psychological environment, and becoming aware of other levels of consciousness.

Attaining all facets of high-level wellness is difficult for some frail elderly people, but an ideal can serve as something to work toward even though it may not be fully realized.

FUTURE IMPLICATIONS

What does the future hold? Demographic trends observed in the late twentieth century promise to accelerate dramatically toward the year 2000 and beyond. Age distribution will shift toward higher ages, and sex distribution will show an even higher number and proportion of women. Early in this century fewer than one out of every five persons was over age 55; by 1974 that figure became one out of four; by the year 2000 it is projected to become one out of three. While women over age 75 constituted one-tenth of that age group in 1974, they will constitute one-fifth of that population segment in 2000 (Fowles, 1975).

However, each year a healthier, better-nourished, better-educated cohort comes into old age, a vital group that can be depended upon to make its voice heard politically. These able and alert elderly people will be needed to voice concern for that segment of the older population that suffer most from poor health, low income, and social isolation: women, blacks, and the very oldest. In addition to the increase in the number of disadvantaged elderly people there is the prospect of a decrease in resources and services. Government programs threaten to shrink or disappear, and private agencies complain of diminishing support.

How can these challenges be met? Efforts could be made in education, preparation for retirement, abolishment of mandatory retirement, alternate living arrangements, and innovative support systems.

Education

Most people are ill prepared for growing old, nor are they able to distinguish between aging, disability, and disease. Starting in preschool, defensive measures could be taught in health education to protect what is most critically needed during long life, sturdy good health. More than anything else, personal responsibility is important in health protection, as Wildansky (1976) points out:

Medicine is only partially and imperfectly related to health. . . . Health is a product of who we are—our genetic inheritance—and how we live, the air we breathe, the food we eat, the exercise we don't get—and not how often we see the doctor. [It] is a product of innumerable decisions made on a daily basis.

Eight rules should be stressed throughout life (Clemons, 1982, p. 21; Graham, 1977):

1. Don't smoke.
2. Eat breakfast.
3. Exercise vigorously every day.
4. Eat a balanced diet.
5. Keep weight within 15 percent of normal for your body build.
6. If you must drink, limit alcohol intake to two ounces per day.
7. Rest until rested every 24 hours.
8. Do not take yourself or your job too seriously.

Elderly people who continue to abide by these simple rules are apt to be in better condition than young people who observe only half or fewer of the rules.

Another educational aid for healthy living is awareness of one's family health history. To determine genetic health inheritance, trace a family tree through the blood line. Going back as far as possible, record every known illness or disability for each person as well as direct and contributing causes of death. Often in such a chart a pattern develops that informs the current generation about family health traits and what tendencies or specific health problems exist.

A life-long health maintenance plan is an added educational tool that details preventive measures taken daily, weekly, monthly, annually, or biannually. Regular health habits are noted as well, for example: (for women) monthly self-examination of breasts; semiannual dental examinations; vision and hearing tests; (particularly for elderly) regular health screening for hypertension, glaucoma, and diabetes. Putting such plans in writing helps an individual be more health conscious and realize that good health does not just happen. Maintaining vigor and functional ability takes protective measures and considerable personal effort. Equally important is working for a healthier external environment, and preparing for the economic reality of old age.

Retirement

Despite changes in the mandatory retirement age, a national trend toward early retirement continues in the United States. For those who do not wish to retire, the seventieth birthday may loom as doomsday, because an employer can impose retirement on a 70-year-old employee. Because chronological aging is a complex and highly individualized process, it should not be used as the only criterion for a person's capability and worth. Job performance is determined by many variables. The government is gradually accepting this idea, but much work remains to be done to abolish mandatory retirement at any age.

Along with preparation for old age, better preretirement planning is a critical need. Too many working people begin their retirement years without foresight or adequate plans to meet their financial needs. Social Security was never intended to be anything but a supplement to retirement income, yet many elderly people are left below the poverty level with only that monthly stipend. Under the sponsorship of schools, colleges, banks, businesses, or industries, classes are being offered in many areas to help middle-aged people study their options and make serious decisions about long life.

Alternative Living Arrangements

Most elderly people continue to live alone in their own homes. For some this is desirable, but for others it is economically disastrous and physically dangerous, to say nothing of the impact on a society in which housing is in great demand. Sheltered (or supervised) housing has developed in recent years. Congregate housing and shared housing are growing in popularity. "Granny flats" are being added to many single-family dwellings. For elderly people who live alone or with family members who work, adult day care offers an outlet and supervision. England has demonstrated the value of day hospitals for infirm elderly people, who check in on Monday morning and check out on Friday night to spend their weekend with their working family. Foster care for frail elderly people is gaining recognition. It requires a family willing to accept an elderly person for full-time care.

Innovative Support Systems

Who will be the primary caregivers if physicians are not available? Will "physician extenders" make home visits? Will these caregivers be general nurse-practitioners or physician's assistants?

If formal networks do not expand to meet needs, informal networks may be pressed into service. Peer-group networks are developing among able-bodied elderly people. Advocacy groups with members of all ages are answering new needs. Crisis intervention assistance is available in most urban communities, while neighborhood associations and networks are effective in checking on elderly people who live alone. Religious organizations have special ministries to the elderly. Service, fraternal, and civic organizations provide specific services. Some areawide aging agencies, hospitals, and nursing homes are developing outreach programs to locate and serve infirm aged people. Hospice programs are invaluable in assisting the terminally ill. More home-based services are bound to develop as people decide to remain at home as long as possible.

SUMMARY

Rapidly increasing numbers and proportions of older people present a demographic trend that will probably continue well into the twenty-first century. Health care and social service resources are not adequate to meet current or future needs of this age group. Moreover, ageism perpetuates myths about elderly people that hamper realistic attitudes; positive aspects of long life are lost in the face of such negativism. Apparently professional caregivers are as susceptible to these myths as the general public.

While most elderly people (81 percent) are self-sufficient, those who need assistance can be suffering acutely. A majority of aged people prefer to remain in their own surroundings as long as possible, and this preference changes health care administration from an institution base to a community or home base.

The complex aging process involves anatomical, physiological, social, and spiritual changes. Individuals age at different rates, and separate organ systems within individuals age at different rates. Manifestations of change should not be confused with pathology. "Old age" and "illness" are not synonymous. Many illnesses of late life can be prevented or satisfactorily controlled, and "senility" is not a disease in itself nor an inevitable result of living too long.

In old age health is measured by functional ability. Beginning with an elderly person's self health rating, nurses can use skills of observation along with evaluative written instruments to assess a client's needs. Viewed holistically, a plan of care involves many care providers, since an elderly person with one problem usually has several problems. Planning and implementation of a continuum of services requires monitoring and evaluation. Who will be the primary caregivers to the elderly of the future?

Americans are not prepared for old age or retirement. Education for long life needs to begin in the early years, teaching children that the best equipment they can carry into old age is sturdy good health and then showing them a life-style that is conducive to that end. Equally important are working for a healthier external environment and preparing for the economic reality of old age.

New living arrangements can be developed, as can innovative formal and informal support systems that will reach out to clients wherever they live. Since whole generations now survive to old age, plans are needed to accompany the elderly population with caring relationships throughout the life span.

DISCUSSION TOPICS

1. Who is responsible for the frail elderly?

2. Is competition developing between youth and old age for the use of national resources?

3. What new policies are needed to cope with the burgeoning numbers of old people in the industrialized societies?

4. What differences can be expected between today's elderly and the new cohorts coming into old age?

5. What implications does the preponderance of women in older age groups carry for the future of health care or social services?

6. How can elderly people be protected from exploitation, neglect, and abuse?

7. What relationship exists between communication and health care?

8. How can bureaucracies be humanized and personalized to answer the needs of the elderly?

9. How can elderly people be involved in the solution of their own problems?

10. How can future elderly people be adequately prepared for old age?

COMMUNITY RESOURCES

Public

Federal

Social Security Administration
   Medicare, Medicaid, Supplemental Security Income, literature, talks for groups

Housing and Urban Development
   Congregate housing
Community action programs
   Home repair, weatherization, multipurpose centers, friendly visitors, employment, garden seeds
Internal Revenue Service
   Tax assistance
Bureau of Indian Affairs
   Indian Health Service, tribal governments
U.S. Congress
   Information, action on problems
Legal Aid
   Assistance for people with low income
National Park Service
   Golden Age Passport for older citizens
Health Systems Agency
Farmers Home Administration
   Housing construction and remodeling
Green Thumb and Foster Grandparents
   Employment programs
Retired Senior Volunteer Program
Arts and Humanities Council

State

State unit on aging
Areawide agency on aging
   Information and referral service
State department of health
   Information hotline, poison control center, communicable disease control, eldercare projects
State department of mental health
   Community mental health centers, drug and alcohol programs, self-help groups
State department of human services
   Food stamps, casework, income assistance, nontechnical medical aid, visual services, vocational rehabilitation, protective services, emergency assistance
State library for the blind and physically handicapped

Volunteer visitors, books in braille and on tape or discs mailed postage free

State insurance commission
Receives complaints, provides information

Employment office

Tax commission
Information about tax exemptions

State universities
Community services, gerontology centers, extension programs, literature, research projects, possible tuition-free classes for elderly citizens, continuing education, elderhostel program, health professions students.

Arts and humanities council

State legislature
Assistance with problems through legislation

Governor's hotline
Quick information on many subjects

State commission on aging
Usually appointed by governor; advisory group to state government

State parks and recreation
Reduced park fees, free fishing licenses

Silverhaired legislature
Elderly citizens make their needs known

Housing financing
Rental assistance

County

Health department
Health screening, immunizations, guidance and counseling, vital statistics, public health inspections, nursing home surveys, environmental protection services, home health visits

County commissioners
Revenue-sharing funds, sponsorship of programs

Department of human services
All services of state agency dispensed at local level

Housing authority
Rent subsidy

City

Special services for frail elderly

Discounts on public utilities

Police and fire protection
Direct services, education, talks to groups about crime and fire prevention

Public transportation
Reduced rates for elderly

Operation ID
Marking personal property

Senior citizen centers
Recreational programs, classes, transportation, and escort service

Center for victims of domestic violence

Center for displaced homemakers

Library
Large-print books and periodicals, mobile book units

Nutrition sites
Congregate meals, recreation programs, home-delivered meals

Commission on aging
Citizen board to screen and act on problems of the elderly

Private

Organizations listed are either independent local groups or branches of state or national organizations.

Health Organizations

Cancer
Heart
Lung

Mental health
Arthritis
Kidney
Hospice
Visiting nurse
Home health agency

Civic Clubs

Special projects (e.g.: Lions Club Eye Bank, Lead Dogs for the Blind)
Chore or repair service

Professional Organizations

American Nurses' Association
National League for Nursing
American Medical Association
American Dental Association
American Public Health Association

Ethnic Groups

National Association for the Advancement of Colored People
Urban League
Hispanic clubs

Asian-American clubs
Urban Indian centers

Service Organizations

Meals-on-Wheels
Boy Scouts
Girl Scouts
Camp Fire Girls
YMCA
YWCA
American Association of Retired Persons
National Retired Teachers' Association
National Association of Mature Persons
National Association of Federal Retired Employees
Organizations of Blind and Disabled
Traveler's Aid
Telephone reassurance groups
Crisis hotlines
Neighborhood watch groups
Neighborhood associations
Arts Councils
special programs, free or discount tickets
National Council of Senior Citizens
Gray Panthers
Religious groups

BIBLIOGRAPHY

Bekker, L.D., & Taylor, C.: Attitudes towards the aged in a multi-generational sample. *Journal of Gerontology* 21, 115–118, 1966.

Bettinghaus, C.O., & Bettinhaus, E.P.: Communications considerations in the health care of the aging. In H.J. Oyer & E.J. Oyer, eds., *Aging and communication*. Baltimore: University Park Press, 1976.

Birenbaum, A., Aronson, M., & Seiffer, S.: Training medical students to appreciate the special problems of the elderly. *The Gerontologist* 19(6), 575–579, 1979.

Birren, J.E., & Clayton, V.: History of gerontology. In D.S. Woodruff & J.E. Birren, eds., *Ag-*

ing: Scientific perspectives and social issues. New York: D. Van Nostrand, 1975.

Blyth, M.: An interview with Clare Booth Luce. *Family Circle*, June 5, 1979, p. 24.

Bruhn, J.G.: An ecological perspective of aging. *The Gerontologist* 11(4), 318–321, 1971.

Butler, R.N.: *Why survive? Being old in America.* New York: Harper & Row, 1975.

Childers, R., & Post, J.A.: *The information-poor in America.* Metuchen, N.J.: Scarecrow Press, 1975.

Clemons, B.L.: Teaching longevity. *Friendly Exchange* 3(1), 21, 1982.

Cumming, E., & Henry, W.E.: *Growing old: The process of disengagement.* New York: Basic Books, 1961.

Eisdorfer, E., & Wilke, F.: Research in aging. In A.M. Hoffman, ed., *Daily needs and interests of older people.* Springfield, Ill.: Charles C Thomas, 1976.

Fowles, D.G.: *Estimates of the size and characteristics of the older population in 1974 and projections to the year 2000.* Statistical Memo No. 31. DHEW Publications No. (OHD) 75-20013, May 1975, Washington, D.C.

Fowles, D.G.: Some prospects for the future elderly population. *Statistical reports on older Americans,* Washington, D.C., DHEW Office of Human Development, National Clearinghouse, on Aging, January 1978.

Friedsam, H.J., & Martin, H.W.: A comparison of self and physicians' health ratings in an older population. *Journal of Health and Human Behavior* 4, 179–183, 1963.

Fries, J.F., & Crapo, L.M.: *Vitality and aging: Implications of the rectangular curve.* San Francisco: W.H. Freeman, 1981.

Graham, R.: Regional initiatives in education for health care. Address to the second annual governor's conference on health manpower, Oklahoma City, September 15, 1977.

Harris, L. and Associates: *The myth and reality of aging in America.* Washington, D.C.: National Council on Aging, 1976.

Havighurst, R.J.: Old age—An American problem. *Journal of Gerontology* 4, 298–304, 1949.

Havighurst, R.J., Neugarten, B., & Tobin, S.: Personality and patterns of aging. In B. Neugarten, ed., *Middle age and aging.* Chicago: University of Chicago Press, 1968.

Hayflick, L., & Moorhead, P.S.: The serial cultivation of human diploid cells strains. *Experimental Cell Research* 25, 585, 1961.

Kane, R.A., & Kane, R.L.: *Assessing the elderly.* Lexington, Mass.: Lexington Books, 1981.

Katz, S., Halstead, L., & Wierenga, M.: A medical perspective of team care. In S. Sherwood, ed., *Long term care.* New York: Spectrum, 1975.

Kent, D.P.: Aging—Fact and fancy. *The Gerontologist* 5, 51–66, 1965.

Long term care for the elderly: A voluntary perspective. Washington, D.C., NCOA/VOILA, 1980.

Maddox, G.L.: Self-assessment of health status: A longitudinal study of selected elderly subjects. *Journal of Chronic Diseases* 17, 449–460, 1964.

Magit, J., Torbit, J., & Willis, S.: *Nurses' attitudes toward the hard-of-hearing elderly.* Paper presented at The Thirty-fourth Annual Scientific Meeting of the Gerontological Society of America, Toronto, Ontario, November, 1981.

Maslow, A.H.: *Toward a psychology of being,* Princeton, N.J.: D. Van Nostrand, 1968.

Mead, M.: Growing old in America. *Family Circle,* July 26, 1977, pp. 27–32.

Moberg, D.O.: Religiosity in old age. *The Gerontologist* 5, 2, 1965. (Reprinted in B. Neugarten, ed., *Middle age and aging.* Chicago: University of Chicago Press, 1975.)

Multidimensional functional assessment: The OARS methodology (2nd ed.). Durham, N.C.: Duke University, 1978.

Olsen, I.A.: Attitudes of nursing students toward aging and the aged. *Gerontology and Geriatrics Education* 2(3), 233–236, 1982.

Paul, B.D.: Social science in public health. *American Journal of Public Health* 46(11), 1390–1396, 1956.

Pfeiffer, E., ed.: *Multidimensional functional assessment: The OARS methodology* (2nd ed). Durham, N.C.: Duke University Center for Study of Aging and Human Development, 1978.

Pfeiffer, E.: *Values of aging: Achieving high level wellness.* Keynote speech, the Fourth Annual Ward Symposium, Lamar University, Beaumont, Texas, March 1982.

Riley, M.W., Johnson, M., & Foner, A., eds.: *Aging and society.* Vol. 1: *An inventory of research findings.* New York: Russell Sage Foundation, 1968.

Rosow, I.: *Social integration of the aged.* New York: Free Press, 1967.

Rudd, T.N.: The medical care of the elderly. *Lancet* 1, 101–102, January 13, 1951.

Rueveni, U.: *Networking families in crisis.* New York: Human Sciences Press, 1979.

Sarason, S.B., Carroll, C.F., Morton, K., Cohen, S., & Lorentz, E.: *Human services and resources networks.* San Francisco: Jossey-Bass, 1977.

Schrock, N.M.: *Holistic assessment of the healthy aged.* New York: John Wiley & Sons, 1980.

Training materials guide: Community care for the aging. Washington, D.C.: The Washington School of psychiatry, Special Projects Division, 1981.

Travelbee, J.: *Interpersonal aspects of nursing* (2nd ed.). Philadelphia: F.A. Davis, 1972.

Travis, J.W.: *Wellness workbook.* Mill Valley, Calif.: Wellness Resource Center, 1977.

Wildansky, A.: *Can health be planned?* The 1976 Michael W. Davis Lecture, The University of Chicago, Center for Health Administration Studies, 1976.

14

Cultural Implications in Client Services

Martha Primeaux

From the moment of his birth the customs into which an individual is born shape his experience and behavior. By the time he can talk, he is the little creature of his culture.

RUTH FULTON BENEDICT

OBJECTIVES

After reading this chapter, you should be able to:

☐ Define key concepts that provide a theoretical basis for understanding ethnicity and its relation to nursing.

☐ Describe a framework that enables nurses to identify cultural cues in different clients during the assessment process.

☐ Use knowledge of ethnic characteristics in the nursing process to enhance the client's health care experiences.

INTRODUCTION

Historically, America has been a melting pot, a land settled by immigrants from a wide variety of ethnic groups who consciously submerged their heterogeneity in order to assimilate as rapidly as possible into the American mainstream. Education in the public schools was viewed as the vehicle for economic, social, and cultural advancement. The melting-pot concept was questioned in the mid 1960s with an upsurge of interest in ethnic identity and a group consciousness. The history of ethnic groups is a history of resistance to assimilating forces.

The black identity movement created a new awareness of the diverse nature of American society and legitimized the public display of ethnicity. The melting-pot concept was further shattered by Asians, Mexican-Americans, and native Americans. According to Steinberg (1981), this "ethnic fever" soon spread to those of European ancestry (Jewish, Irish, Italian, and Polish) who sought to promote their own ethnic pride and to assert their rights to a separate identity within a pluralistic nation (Steinberg, 1981).

This reawakening of ethnic identification, and more recently the women's movement, clearly demonstrate that America is a society of individuals within identifiable groups. If these movements are not viewed as threats, they can be utilized as channels through which one can give services more effectively. The message of the 1960s was one of basic issues of individual needs and group identity. Further, it became clear that institutions were not meeting the real needs of ethnic groups.

There are numerous problems involved in describing the ethnic identities that have replaced the melting-pot concept. Either stereotyping occurs, which is offensive to members of all groups, or self-aggrandizement occurs on the part of group members. As a result, a variety of ethnic groups now have public relations arms to safeguard their representation by the media.

Ethnic self-consciousness often discourages descriptions of ethnicity. There appears to be considerable variance in attitudes and behaviors toward individual ethnic characteristics and on the values group members themselves place on particular characteristics. For the health practitioner, then, hard-and-fast ethnic descriptions may too loosely fit clients or may result in misconceptions about individuals. This chapter provides a description of variables that health care personnel can utilize to understand a member of whatever ethnic group they encounter.

Certain questions can be posed. What cultural signals must nurses be aware of to work with members of any ethnic group? How does the nurse collect this information and use it in practice? How should the nurse understand life-styles and values that differ both among and within ethnic groups? How can the nurse appreciate differences without imposing values on different life-styles? How does the nurse legitimize and accommodate group differences?

DEFINITION OF TERMS

Many studies of ethnicity have focused on prejudice, stereotyping, social distance, and race relations.

Giordano (1973) contends that the phenomenon of ethnicity is much deeper than a means of political exploitation, a convenience in organization. Rather it is a search for identity, sense of belonging, and self-esteem. Tumin's (1964) derivation of the term *ethnicity* is a combination of the Greek words *ethnos*, tribe, race, or nation, and *ethos*, meaning customs or patterns. Therefore, the term denotes social characteristics as well as biological origins.

Ethnicity can be defined in the context of culture and subculture. *Ethnic groups* are more or less cohesive subgroups in a broader and more diverse cultural setting. Ethnic group identification exists to varying degrees. Values, norms, and customs influence both attitudes and behavior. Health care attitudes and values are of particular interest here.

Culture affects the way an individual regards health and illness and further dictates which measures he or she will utilize for treatment or prevention of illness. Certainly, health and illness are defined differently among different ethnic groups and among the poor. We know, for example, that in health measures, as in other human behavior, individuals and groups are highly influenced by their social identities.

ETHNIC IDENTITY

A genuine concern for the human element in health care services requires that health providers be aware of the specific values, beliefs, and practices of those they serve. Recognition that subcultures function as a focal point for identity and community is paramount (Steinberg, 1981).

Ethnic identity is fundamental to the health care practitioner's understanding of the client, because this identity orients the group member toward or away from usage of the health care system. The extent of ethnic identity is a function of socialization. Socialization occurs throughout the life cycle, but it is usually most powerful in childhood when values are internalized and behavior patterns learned from the significant others in the child's life.

Life experiences may reinforce or undermine prior socialization. Passages or transitions are especially vulnerable periods when prior experiences may be reinterpreted, resulting in new behaviors. Societal acceptance or rejection of ethnic identity affects willingness to move into the mainstream, in which the health care system is centrally located. Thus the individual from an ethnic group or subgroup with marginal status may be reluctant to seek health care services, especially if they are provided in an impersonal environment. There is substantial evidence that various ethnic groups utilize health services differently.

Conflict often surrounds ethnic identity because other equally important identities must be juggled: those relating to work, school, community, sex role, and age group. These roles are also internalized. The values associated with divergent roles are each

applied in appropriate situations. This makes it difficult for the health care provider to predict the behavior that will be evoked in the treatment setting. The care provider must rapidly assess the client's perceived role. To establish a supportive, collaborative relationship with the client, the health professional must understand the common aspects of cultural and ethnic differences.

Life-style is such a broad term that one hesitates to use it. Yet there is no precise way to describe the *gestalt* or fabric of an individual's life. This fabric always includes ethnic components that affect decisions. For example, one chooses an urban, rural, or suburban existence. One's social life may be isolated or integrated with that of one or more groups. The basis for identity is also heavily biased by socioeconomic status, work roles, and time usage, as expressed in hobbies and other leisure-time pursuits.

Work situations may have a greater or lesser impact on ethnicity, depending on the significance of work to the person. Furthermore, education and past experience also affect an individual's willingness to use health care services. A variety of attitudes and values come into play as well, such as dependence–independence or the acceptance of help from family and ethnic group members versus impersonal outsiders.

For the health care provider, determining which ethnic factors and cultural differences are pivotal and which are peripheral is an important task. It would be impossible to understand the cultures of all ethnic groups, especially since many are changing rapidly. For the purposes of nursing practice, it is necessary, however, to have a model for ethnic awareness. A model suggests what variables should be noted for all clients. The model aids the nurse in establishing rapport with the client, so that full and complete information can be exchanged. This will help motivate the client to invest in the relationship and follow through with the entire treatment cycle.

A Model

A model should include the why and what of a specific group's health practices (Henderson & Primeaux, 1981). A brief history of the group is vital. Knowledge of kinship patterns and the traditional family structure will give the practitioner vital information. What is the group's orientation to time? What is the form of expression of pain (or lack of expression)? What kind of folk healers are utilized and at what stage of the illness? What are the social control mechanisms, and how are they used?

Use of such a model enables the care provider to become more alert to ethnic cues so that the client is more inclined to trust the provider. For example, in a rural area of a southwestern state, nurse administrators who functioned as management consultants to hospitals discovered that the quality of information they obtained from the communities was vastly improved if they arrived in the towns early and learned the community speech patterns. The question "Who is your physician?" was rarely answered fully, but the question "Who do you doctor with?" elicited complete replies. It is the simple, highly visible, and often overlooked word or gesture that allows the health care provider to calibrate his or her behavior to the needs and expectations of the client.

For example, the native Americans may not ask any questions during a health teaching session. Most often, they sit with arms folded and make no eye contact, which often projects that they do not understand or care. However, the individual does indeed understand. The lack of eye contact shows respect to the health care provider. Furthermore, it is the native American's belief that the provider has presented him or her with all necessary information: the health care provider is the expert. Native Americans feel that providers will not withhold necessary and important information and will do their best to care for them as clients.

It is advisable for the provider to divulge information about himself or herself during the intake interview or initial history. Members of some ethnic group interpret questions of a personal nature as interrogation that is unrelated to their illness. Sharing of information will elicit responses that may be vital for the initial history. This is especially true with many native Americans.

Understanding the external and internal forces that affect groups is vital to understanding the health behaviors of the people in the group. For example, socioeconomic variables have a powerful influence on health beliefs and practices. However, poor health practices cannot be solely attributed to lack of knowledge or deprived economic situations. One has to look at structural differences among groups and within groups, such as family, tribes, and communities. These structural differences produce differences in attitudes and values. For example, the native American's identity arises from the tribal structure. First there is the family, then the clan, and then the tribe. Native American families often extend over three generations on vertical and horizontal lines. Knowledge that a dependent child may have more than one "mother" is crucial. Grandmothers, sisters and aunts are considered as much the "mother" as the biological mother.

For the Mexican-American, the race (la raza) is important. Knowledge of Spanish culture or knowing that a client speaks Spanish may be inadequate, because of subcultural differences and different dialects (Henderson & Primeaux, 1981). Second to religion, the family is the most important institution for the Mexican-American. Respect and wisdom are accorded the oldest male in a household. In many instances, it is he who makes decisions relating to health.

CULTURAL IMPLICATIONS

The health care provider must recognize a group's ethnicity and their future goals, recognizing intracultural and intercultural diversity. (Leininger, 1976). Culture is a dominant force in determining health and illness behavior.

Being sensitive to client needs includes understanding culturally defined beliefs about health and illness behaviors. The following examples demonstrate the variety of behaviors that can be observed:

A Puerto Rican individual may not seek Western medical treatment for a symptom such as increased temperature because he believes that it is due to an imbalance in the natural condition of the body. Illnesses are classified as hot and cold and remedies are classified accordingly.

(Scott, 1974, p. 532)

A client with any ailment might believe that an injection is the only satisfactory treatment. If he does not receive one, in all likelihood he will continue to see other health care providers until he gets his "shot."

Many native Americans are stereotyped as being stoical. This is seen in many instances when they do not want to bother the nurse or be seen as a nuisance. Therefore, the native American client will endure pain unnecessarily. She thinks, "If the nurse thought I should have something for pain, she would give it to me. She is the expert, and she will do her best for me."

When working with most ethnic groups, understanding the dynamics of the family is crucial. The family is usually the basic unit of health care. The health care provider's manner and personal characteristics will always elicit some reaction from clients. This affects their later relationship. If the provider portrays indifference or insensitivity to folk therapies, the client will not share information in subsequent visits and may choose not to return to this particular setting. According to Leininger (1977), a serious problem facing the health care provider is *cultural imposition*. This term refers to the way in which an outsider imposes his or her own values, beliefs, and practices upon others. An example of cultural imposition is the insistence by health care providers that Western scientific medicine has all the answers to illness or that illnesses are caused by germs. These providers have failed to learn about ethnic health practices, beliefs about the causes of illness, or the treatment other ethnic groups consider to be appropriate.

What the health care provider can do for clients must be sold to the community. One approach that the community health nurse learns is to use more effectively the helping network that exists in the community. This approach involves using family members and the formal and informal networks of the community, such as religious, educational, and social groups. Involvement of individuals of cultural groups in decision making is essential. Knowing the family structure—who makes decisions regarding health care—allows the community health nurse to be more effective. Deciding when to go beyond the family and community folk medicine to seek Western health care involves more than just the client in many ethnic populations.

Knowledge of the importance that male members serve in family life of the Mexican-American client will help the nurse to sell a health care package to a community. Similarly, in the black American family, the oldest female often serves a similar role. Many native American tribes are matriarchal.

One of the fundamental tenets of democracy is that citizens have a right to participate in decisions that affect their lives. This kind of participation requires that sufficient information be made available about programs, policies, problems, and choices. This is no easy task. Overcoming the social distance between clients and health care providers can be difficult if both groups ascribe to different sets of values. Scott (1974, p. 526) describes a "cultural misfit" when two or more cultures are dissimilar in crucial ways that make it impossible for one system to accept certain health-related beliefs and behaviors of the other. This always results in dissatisfaction for both the client and the provider. Leininger (1977) urges that health professionals systematically and critically study health and illness patterns of caring and curing within different cultures. This can best be done through a systematic educational process featuring the ethnoscientific method, which uses indigenous peoples' views of their health care systems (Leininger, 1977). Understanding the health and illness patterns of a particular culture, including the values and goals of health care, will shorten the social distance between client and care provider and establish a better cultural fit.

A specific example indicates how cultural consideration affects health care delivery:

Acceptance or rejection of the health care providers in northern New Mexico communities was heavily influenced by the after-hours activities of the health care personnel. The prospective clients felt that it was especially important that they be "invested" in the community: live in the community, engage in local activities, and spend free time there, and that they closely approximate local standards for sexual behavior and clothing.

As the example illustrates, a nurse who came from outside such an integrated, closely knit, isolated community would probably have an assimilation problem. Even though ethnic group norms were easy to detect, it might be difficult for the nurse to comply with them.

Ethnic groups will continue to influence health care practices in the future. This is an outcome of government contributions toward health care expenses and the political power base of many ethnic groups. The willingness to be treated by the female nurse versus the male physician frequently reflects the ethnic group's attitudes toward sex role identity in the work world. For example, native American women are extremely modest and prefer to have a female nurse or doctor perform a vaginal exam instead of a male health care provider. Many native Americans believe that it is not appropriate for an "outside male" to touch a female body. Such activity is viewed as "women's activity."

With clients from many ethnic groups and clients from mixed ethnic ancestry, the nurse must be able to use a multivariate, descriptive/analytic approach to establishing and maintaining relationships with clients. This complexity is seen in Mexican history (Henderson & Primeaux, 1980). The wealthy Spanish conquerors intermarried with Mexican Indians and later with the blacks brought into Mexico during the colonial period. Mexican-Americans and native Americans thus hold similar cultural beliefs. Usually geographical location determines the major cultural component (a predominately native-American village or a Mexican village). The Kickapoo Indians of Oklahoma, for example, make a yearly trek to Mexico to visit and work with relatives. While in Oklahoma, they receive services and are treated as native Americans.

There are no clear-cut formulas for recognizing ethnic components of character in isolation from the client's total situation. By appearing in the health care setting, the client has acknowledged a need that he or she will act upon, at least initially. The client has admitted that he or she needs assistance for a specific problem. However, this does not mean that the client will comply with the health care provider's advice or prescriptions. The health care provider can act upon information gleaned from the client's history, but the client may not follow instructions after leaving the health care setting. The client may feel better after one day's medication and not take the remainder, or the community healer may not agree with what the client has been given and offer a substitute. Therefore, the client's total environment comes into play, and the health care provider must try to determine whether the client will follow through with the recommended treatment.

THE NURSING PROCESS AND CLIENT ETHNICITY

The nursing process must be related to ethnicity within a theoretical framework to guide the care of clients. Table 14.1 presents the cues related to ethnicity that nurses can observe and build on in assessment, planning, implementation, and evaluation. As Table 14.1 suggests, it is possible to describe the interaction of the nursing process with ethnicity at each stage. The sensitive nurse can then interpret cues for members of any ethnic group. She or he knows what to look for and has narrowed down the field of vision to avoid being overwhelmed by differences.

The variables included in the guidelines are:

1. Mode of expression of behavior.
2. Relationship to the health care system.
3. Family and ethnic group support network.
4. Cultural beliefs that affect use of the health care system.
5. Relationship to the cultural mainstream.
6. Provider–client compatibility.
7. Biographical characteristics.

Assessment

During assessment, the nurse observes the verbal and nonverbal behavior of the client with special attention to the interpretation of cues. For example, native Americans show respect by not making eye contact, but a nurse from another cultural group may misinterpret this as avoidance. Folded arms by native Americans reflect an unhurried attitude and comfort with a situation, not standoffishness or indifference. Past experience with the health care system, which will be evident in the case history, will allow the nurse to determine the extent of exclusion or inclusion the client has experienced in the past. Cultural beliefs about health care can be solicited by asking the client questions: "How do you feel about hospitalization?" "What do you think we should do about your health problem?" "Do you use home remedies such as teas, poultices, or herbal mixes?" "Do you go to the folk healer (medicine man) in your community?"

If an adult client tells the nurse that he cannot be hospitalized now because he needs to take care of other business, he may be referring to getting the proper sanctions from appropriate family members. If a cli-

TABLE 14.1
The Nursing Process and Client Ethnicity

Assessment	Planning	Implementation	Evaluation
Verbal and nonverbal behavior.	Verbal and nonverbal communication.	Verbal and nonverbal communication of activities to be performed.	Evaluation of communication process for building health care attitudes and behaviors.
Inclusion or exclusion from the health care system.	Inclusion through specific stages and methods into the health care system.	Use of health care system facilities for extensive involvement.	Evaluation of willingness to use the health care system.
Extended family or ethnic support network.	Collaboration with key members of the extended family or ethnic support network.	Care provided by extended family or ethnic support network as much as possible.	Extended family or ethnic support network's assessment of the health care system intervention.
Cultural beliefs that encourage or discourage receiving health care.	Building upon cultural beliefs that would encourage openness to receiving health care.	Reinforcement of health care activities consistent with ethnicity.	Congruence of cultural beliefs with health care system usage.
Extent of assimilation into the cultural mainstream.	Consistency with extent of assimilation.	Encouragement of assimilation into the cultural mainstream through treatment and referrals.	Extent of assimilation into the health care client role as a consequence of exposure.
Provider characteristics in relation to client characteristics.	Emphasis on commonality of client–provider characteristics.	Client–provider interaction based on commonality of characteristics and goals.	Client–provider congruence validated.
Biographical characteristics (age, sex, socioeconomic status, education, ethnicity).	Realistic analysis of biographical characteristics: age, sex, socioeconomic status, education, ethnicity.	Use of biographical characteristics: motivating the client to follow through and individualizing interventions.	Biographical characteristics correlated with success or failure of the intervention.

ent states that she has involved the local healer in health care, the provider should ask what the healer has done and if the client took any medicines. If the client is reluctant to answer some questions and keeps looking at an older family member, perhaps it is the older family member who gives approval, even if the client is an adult.

Extent of assimilation into the cultural mainstream is often indicated by geographical location, work roles, and time usage in daily life. For many native Americans, assimilation through marriage and education into the mainstream has had a profound effect on the way they interact with older people. Some native Americans will appear on time for clinic appointments and will be assertive about asking appropriate questions. The health care provider might think, stereotypically, that such individuals would not seek out a medicine man or might disregard their ethnicity altogether. Seemingly atypical behaviors do not connote total adoption of the majority culture.

The provider and client characteristics that can form a basis for compatibility may be situational or biographical. If a provider has lived in an ethnic community, sharing this information may lead to mutual sharing of events or acquaintances. Perhaps the client and provider are of the same generation, or have children of the same age or sex, or are married to cousins. This sharing on the part of the provider will often break communication barriers by making the provider seem less like an outsider.

Age, sex, socioeconomic status, and ethnicity give further clues concerning the client's responsiveness to health care planning and implementation activities. With most ethnic groups, the older the client, the less responsive the client will be, simply because of a lack of experience with the health care settings of the majority culture.

Among native Americans, Mexican-American, and some Asian groups, older clients may not speak or understand English. An interpreter does not necessarily solve language problems. On occasion, translators misinterpret, especially in relation to anatomy. Older native American women will not confide in a male interpreter that they are having pain in the pelvic area, but will describe the pain as being in the stomach. Likewise, in some native American languages there are some words that only males speak and some words that only females speak.

Within ethnic groups, socioeconomic status is usually a good indicator of ease with the health care system. Health care is still a service commodity to be purchased on the market. Members of most ethnic groups fall into the poverty category. It is the exceptional individuals of different ethnic groups who have similar economic resources as members of the majority culture.

Planning

Planning involves negotiating a relationship that recognizes the role and responsibility of both the client and the care provider. The stages of implementation are agreed upon and the interactions appropriate to each are discussed. Key members of the extended family or ethnic support network are included in the planning effort. Cultural beliefs that facilitate acceptance of health care responsibility are reinforced.

Planning should be consistent with the extent of the client's assimilation into the mainstream culture. The nurse should expect neither too much nor too little of the client and his or her significant others. A realistic view of the client's life history suggests the degree to which the client will participate in the planning process.

Implementation

Implementation results in the interaction of nurse and client in the concrete realities of care. Client involvement is extensive. More members of the family and the ethnic support network must be coordinated. Treatment and referrals assist in the client's assimilation into the cultural mainstream. The nurse–client relationship should be firmly established. The nurse uses knowledge of the client's history to motivate follow through. For example, "If you follow the care plan, you'll be able to attend the corn dance in July" could be used for a person not assimilated to a great extent into the cultural mainstream. For a client who is highly assimilated and concerned about education, the direction might be, "If you follow the care plan, you'll be able to attend school in the fall."

Evaluation

Evaluation takes place continuously. Ideally, many factors should be considered, including the effects of the communication process on general health care attitudes and behavior and especially on willingness to use the health care system in the future. For example, will the client return for a follow-up appointment? The provider needs to determine that whoever brings the client to the clinic will know about follow-up. It might be a family member or an indigenous community worker who facilitates this. The extended family or ethnic support network's evaluation of the intervention should be obtained. Perception of the congruence of cultural beliefs and health care system usage can be measured. The effect of exposure on the client's assimilation into the health care consumer role and the cultural mainstream is usually apparent in in-formal conversation. Biographical characteristics are correlated with success or failure of interventions in many instances; these can be collected easily for purposes of evaluation.

FUTURE IMPLICATIONS

The largest single problem related to ethnicity which will face the nurse in the community of the future is the enormity of ethnic and cultural differences. The nurse must develop observational and communication skills. Rapport will be essential for obtaining full and accurate information and active collaboration in the treatment process.

To predict the future is risky at best. Naisbitt (1982) has postulated that we are moving from an industrial society to an information society. Bezold (1982) has stated that the future will be shaped by both large societal trends and individual choices. If this is the case, it will be important for nurses to communicate more effectively in order to help ethnic groups make choices about effective health care measures. Should the client continue to utilize folk medicine and healers when surgery in a hospital is in his or her best interest? More emphasis will be placed on teaching self-care and prevention. There will be a need for more participating, planning, and decision making, which will require more dialogue from those who offer health services and those who receive their services. Individuals from different groups will need assistance in coping with change and increased complexity of choices. Nurses will have to provide and disseminate information creatively and effectively.

The census of 1980 revealed that the number of individuals who now identify with different ethnic groups has increased. With ease of travel and the recent immigration of Asian groups to America, all future nurses will care for members of one or more ethnic groups. For nurses who have been educated about cultural diversity, certain client characteristics will help them work with individuals with a strong ethnic identity: (1) type and degree of verbalization; (2) perception of inclusion or exclusion from the health care system; (3) sufficiency of the extended family or ethnic network; (4) cultural beliefs that support or conflict with participation in the health care system; and (5) degree of assimilation into the cultural mainstream.

Nurses must find ways to foster development of a partnership of professional and nonprofessional groups in matters of health care politics. Nonethnic nurses can serve on boards that govern policies of clinics, such as urban Indian clinics and neighborhood service organization clinics. They can facilitate attention to ethnic differences in agencies that offer home care for diverse cultural groups. Ethnic and nonethnic nurses can share information in seminar or workshop format with indigenous workers in the community.

Nursing as a helping profession is in a prime position to shape the future provision of care to diverse cultural groups. All members of the nursing profession should lobby on state and national levels to include the needs of culturally different people in health care legislation. Local nursing groups can be instrumental in setting up clinics to offer free or minimal-cost services to the ethnic groups that cannot afford health care. Nurses who practice holopathic care (reflexology, herbs, and so forth) will fit into the ethnic communities with little difficulty. Rarely is there a single answer or a single interpretation for any one situation. Nursing's history of helping

can continue to provide the opportunity for groups to choose.

SUMMARY

Ethnic groups often ask for assistance in finding their own solutions. One must not forget that help is help only when it is perceived as such. Helping ethnic groups means understanding cultural norms and values, lest we intervene inappropriately.

Aeschliman (1973, p. 662) has stated that "trying to change people's attitudes is usually less productive than changing the circumstances around them." As health care providers, we need to identify the goals and priorities of the cultural group and assist the group in selecting methods to reach their own goals. No one group is all-knowing about the future. The initiative for defining and creating the future will come from groups that acknowledge their responsibility. Nursing can meet this challenge.

DISCUSSION TOPICS

1. How can the perceptive nurse determine the client's ethnic identity and its intensity before treatment?

2. What are the effects of the nurse's ethnic sensitivity on the client during the different stages of the nursing process?

3. How are ethnic group values, norms, and behaviors used by the nurse to secure client participation in the treatment cycle?

4. How is nonverbal behavior important in treating ethnic group members who are relatively unassimilated and feel excluded from the health care system?

5. What can you predict about the effect of heterogeneity of ethnic groups on nursing practice in the future?

BIBLIOGRAPHY

Aeschliman, D.: Guidelines for a cross-cultural health program. *Nursing Outlook* 21(10), 660–663, 1973.

Bezold, C.: Health care in the U.S.: Four alternatives. *The Futurist* 16(8), 14–18, 1982.

Clark, A.L.: *Culture: Childbearing health professionals.* Philadelphia: F.A. Davis, 1978.

Giordano, J.: *Ethnicity and mental health.* New York: Institute on Pluralism and Group Identity, 1973.

Henderson, G., & Primeaux, M.: *Transcultural health care.* Menlo Park, Calif.: Addison-Wesley, 1981.

Leininger, M.: *Transcultural health care issues and conditions.* Philadelphia: F.A. Davis, 1976.

Leininger, M.: Transcultural nursing: A promising subfield of study for nurses. In A. Reinhardt & M. Quinn, eds., *Current practice in family centered community nursing.* St. Louis: Mosby, 1977.

Morey, S.M., & Gillian, O.L.: *Respect for life: The traditional upbringing of American Indian children.* Garden City, N.Y.: Waldorf Press, 1974.

Naisbitt, J.: *Megatrends: Ten new directions transforming our lives.* New York: Warner, 1982.

Orque, M.S.: Health care and minority clients. *Nursing Outlook* 24, 313–316, 1976.

Scott, C.S.: Health and healing practices of five ethnic groups in Miami, Florida. *Public Health Reports* 89(6), 524–532, 1974.

Spector, R.E.: *Cultural diversity in health and illness.* New York: Appleton-Century-Crofts, 1979.

Steinberg, S.: *The ethnic myth.* Boston: Beacon Press, 1981.

Tumin, E.: Ethnic groups. In J. Gould & W. Kolb, eds., *A dictionary of social science.* New York: Free Press, 1964.

Vogel, G.: *American Indian medicine.* New York: Ballantine, 1973.

15

Spiritual Needs: An Opportunity for Nursing

Thomas S. Allen and Victoria Schoolcraft

> In the past we have had a light which flickered, in the present we have a light which flames, and in the future there will be a light which shines over all the land and sea.
> GILBERT KEITH CHESTERTON

OBJECTIVES

After reading this chapter, you should be able to:

☐ Distinguish between spiritual needs and religious forms.
☐ Relate historical spiritual trends to our world today.
☐ Discuss ways in which nurses can support clients in relation to their spiritual needs.
☐ Discuss the nursing implications of renewed interest in spiritual pursuits.
☐ Discuss possible future changes in the way people treat their spiritual lives and the resulting effects on nursing practice.

INTRODUCTION

Regardless of what he or she believes, every nurse can support the health status of every client by including in the nursing assessment the client's search for purpose and meaning in life.

The authors of this chapter hope that readers will use the ideas, concepts, and techniques presented herein to expand their own practice of nursing into the realms of the spiritual as client needs dictate. This chapter will enable the reader to examine his or her own beliefs and the impact those beliefs have on clients. The reader will then be better able to care for all clients of any faith or persuasion without prejudice and with real concern for spiritual needs. In order to be better helpers to their clients, nurses must understand how spiritual motivations and religious loyalties affect the balance of health.

One way of being of service is to expand other people's views and to explore their perceptions with them in order to expand our own spiritual experiences. However, one does not need to be motivated by a choice to serve God in order to appreciate and respond to the spiritual needs of others. Those who are atheists or agnostics can enrich their clients' nursing care by understanding and accepting the clients' spiritual orientation. By the same token, those who are motivated to lead a God-centered life should try to understand and sympathetically respond to the spiritual needs of those who have different belief systems.

ORIGINS AND HISTORY

Western civilization has emerged from the church-dominated middle ages, when health and illness were conceived to be strictly under the control of a deity. An individual felt little control over his or her own life during those dark times. The scientific attitude had not yet developed, and mankind generally gave up hope of making the world a healthier place to live. All things were under the control of God; therefore, what could an individual human do? The profession of nursing had not yet emerged.

Slowly but surely, the evolution of thought broke the bonds of the church, and people began to realize that indeed human measures could be taken to promote health. The Industrial Revolution unfolded, and modern nursing began to develop under the guidance of Florence Nightingale. Nightingale was a religious and spiritual woman whose decision to become a nurse was based upon her conviction that God's Will was for her to spend her life serving Him. She believed that the finest way to do that was to serve her fellow men and women on this planet. She had a strong and open acceptance of other people's religions. For example, when she was asked to become the superintendent of the Institution for the Care of Sick Gentlewomen in Distressed Circumstances, she insisted that they do away with their policy of admitting only members of the Church of England. The hospital board consented to do so but made her responsible for accompanying clergymen of other sects when they visited their parishioners (Huxley, 1975).

Nightingale usually chose as her nurses women who were members of religious orders or other women who were strong in their own faiths. She appreciated that those who had deep religious convictions, regardless of their form, would be the best co-workers in her various activities. Her written work and the stories about Nightingale reflect her life-long commitment to serve God, and the genuine tenderness she always showed to the people she served shows her true belief in each person's worth as another child of God.

With the beginnings of the Industrial Revolution and the general acceptance of the scientific method, Western society became decidedly secular and humanistic. As nursing grew as a profession, the leaders espoused the philosophy of treating the whole person—body, mind, and spirit. These ideas have grown and expanded as experience and study have shown each of us how important the interrelationship among these facets of our being is. A holistic philosophy has become predominant within nursing. In general, many people have come to accept readily the interplay of the body and mind. Since the middle of this century, our society has been experiencing a reawakening of religious and spiritual beliefs. Now more and more people are also coming to recognize the reality of the holistic approach to understanding and working with all people.

The reawakening of spiritual and religious pursuits began at about the same time that our society began the transformation from the industrial society of the past to a new information society (Ferguson, 1980; Naisbitt, 1982). The country experienced the last great religious awakening in the mid-1700s, at the time of the transition from an agricultural society to an industrial society (Naisbitt, 1982). In times of great societal transformations, people develop new ideas about how society should evolve. Today many people advocate a more personal religion than that of the past. This, in conjunction with the many other changes in society, has threatened people who hold traditional values. Anthony C. W. Wallace referred to these people as "nativists." Nativists are those who cling to the old culture. In regard to spiritual expression, they are the people who value the structured and accepted patterns of religious style (Ferguson, 1980).

In times of great change, many people seek the security of basic and traditional patterns of behavior. They feel that society becomes disorganized when traditional ways break down. There comes a return to traditional activities, and people leave the groups that have become too progressive. For example, Naisbitt (1982) cites the growth of the strict and demanding American churches, such as the Southern Baptists church and the "native grown fundamentalist faiths." The other old, well-established denominations, such as the Methodists and Episcopalians, are losing members because they have become more liberal and less structured.

Many people feel that spiritual values will soon take on new importance in our daily lives. Whether this will come about through the fundamentalistic point of view or through the growth of the personal spiritual orientation, it is clear that there is a greater openness about spiritual ideas and discussions.

Many early settlers came to the American continent to escape religious persecution. They wanted to worship as they chose. Ironically, many of the sects that have developed in this country have sought to institutionalize their versions of the appropriate way to express religious beliefs. While great value was originally placed on the separation of church and state, there is now a movement on many fronts to enforce certain religious values through legislative action. Some of the bitterest confrontations in our various legislative bodies today concern laws growing out of religious convictions. For example, many opponents of the Equal Rights Amendment believed that it was against the Will of God. On the other hand, religious proponents saw this amendment as fulfilling the appropriate place of women as God intended.

Muller (1974) has identified three possibilities for religion in the distant future: there might eventually be a universal faith that would retain the best of all the spiritual beliefs inherent in the many forms now practiced; or there might be continuing diversity of forms and beliefs but a greater overarching tolerance; or there might be a humanistic system that rejects God and elevates human beings as the center and masters of the world. Regardless of the eventual outcome, there is little doubt that the impact and importance of spiritual needs on the health and well-being of people has been well established. Nurses and other health care professionals are increasing their understanding of the spiritual component of health problems and of the solutions to these problems. Furthermore, nurses are beginning to assess and document spiritual expressions as an integral part of their clients' health. Many nurses are still treating this area with some caution, because it is so highly charged emotionally. It will be an adventure for all nurses to expand their repertoire of interventions to include attention to spiritual concerns of clients.

SPIRITUALITY AND RELIGION

The concepts of spirituality and religion are related but different. Dickinson (1975, p. 1,790) defines the *spirit* as the "animating but intangible principle that gives liveliness to the physical organism as well as the literal breath of life." The term *spiritual* describes those motivations and loyalties that intangibly direct the lives of those persons who exercise faith in their reach for supreme values. Such a definition does not necessarily involve the concept of a personal God. *Spiritual needs* include striving to find some value in oneself; trying to discover meaning in one's existence; searching for some sense in suffering and other life experiences; and seeking comfort and inner peace (McGilloway & Donnelly, 1977). A person who is interested in spiritual development searches for meaning and value in life. This includes and transcends conventional definitions of religion. However, religion is often the expression of the quest.

Religion is a personal set or institutionalized system of religious attitudes, beliefs, and practices. As such, a religion can be devised and practiced by a single individual or by millions. We have usually considered a religion to be any of the established sects that include followers of like beliefs who worship in the same way and whose lives are directed to some extent by the common beliefs of the denomination. A religious activity is one characterized by zeal that motivates one to seek and practice concepts of supreme value. With this definition, it is clear that any value held as supreme by any individual can be termed "religious."

A religion need not include God or any other power higher than the individual. A religion need not even incorporate the value of an individual, but may exalt the state or some other concept. A devotee of Communism is pursuing a religious activity. *Humanism*, the idea that human life is the highest value, is a nontheistic religion. Democracy has been called a "humanistic faith" because it proclaims itself to be the protector of the "rights of man" (Muller, 1974, p. 140).

It may be helpful to elaborate further on the concept of humanism, because it is often misunderstood. Humanism is a religion without God that places human beings at the center of the system of values. A humanist is concerned about and considerate of other humans because they are sentient beings, not because they were created by a higher power. Often humanism is confused with *humanitarianism*, which is the promotion of human welfare and social reform. Humanitarianism may be practiced by humanists as well as by theists. Many people, even those who believe in God, use the term "humanistic" to describe their pursuits, which are really "humanitarian": pursuits motivated by the goal of serving one's fellows in order to serve God.

Although there is value in understanding the various forms in which people practice their faiths, the remainder of this chapter discusses the broader concept of spirituality. There are many excellent resources within nursing literature that describe the beliefs and concerns of the religious groups represented in this country. The authors have included some of these in the Bibliography at the end of this chapter.

SELF-AWARENESS

There are three vital prerequisites to spiritual assessment. First, the nurse must become aware of what beliefs, motivations, and values influence his or her own thoughts and actions. The nurse must make a conscious effort to become comfortable with these beliefs and to develop a philosophy of life that promotes a tolerant attitude toward any religious or spiritual belief. A tolerant, nonjudgmental attitude can go a long way in gaining a client's confidence in the nurse, so that the client's real emotional and spiritual needs can be met. Next, the nurse must be educated about the many forms of religious beliefs and varieties of rituals. The nurse must confront any attitudes or biases she or he holds about these forms, practices, and beliefs that might impede efforts to work with clients. Third, the nurse must truly care about the client's search to reach a spiritual goal. Without these three prerequisites, the nurse will be deficient in caring for clients with spiritual needs.

If the nurse is atheistic or agnostic, she or he must acknowledge the impact of this on spiritual interventions. Will these feelings cause the nurse indirectly to belittle or underrate the client's spiritual pursuits? Certainly, there are atheists and agnostics who are sensitive and responsive to the beliefs of others. On the other hand, there are people who have deep religious convictions but are unable to be effective in helping others in this area.

SPIRITUAL ASSESSMENT

It is useful for the nurse to follow a logical format in gathering data pertaining to a cli-

ent's spiritual dimension. The depth to which one pursues these questions will depend on the client's desire to share such information. As a part of the original data base, the nurse can ask some questions to help determine the relationship of spiritual concerns to the client's life. At various points during nurse–client relationship, the nurse can develop some of these areas in order to better respond to client needs.

Initial Assessment

When beginning to assess the client's spiritual interests, the nurse should do more than merely note the denomination, if any, to which the client belongs. The name of the denomination tells very little about the client's beliefs. Furthermore, each individual practices his or her religion differently. Many people label themselves as belonging to a certain denomination yet seldom attend services. Others are deeply involved in the theological aspects of their faith and are quite active in church endeavors.

Those who do not ascribe to a particular denomination may still have deep convictions about God or about spiritual realities. The most effective way to obtain this kind of information is by using open-ended questions and by permitting clients to tell as much or as little as they wish about their beliefs. For example, a nurse might ask if the client belongs to any denomination. The nurse could then ask the client to tell a little about what it means to be a part of that group. If the client does not belong to a particular group or does not believe in God, the nurse could expand the question: "Although some people don't believe in God or don't go to a church, they often have values that serve a spiritual purpose in their lives. I wonder if that could describe you?"

If the client seems comfortable with the initial questions, the nurse might pursue some of the other pertinent aspects of spiritual meaning. The nurse can ask the client how belief in God affects his or her personal life. If the client does not believe in God but has expressed commitment to higher ideals, the nurse can ask whether the client engages in daily prayer or meditation and how these activities enrich the client's life. The nurse can ask if the client regularly reads the Bible or some other religious book for comfort and enlightenment. Many books that are not considered religious may include content that is spiritually uplifting to certain people.

The nurse can also ask about whether the client believes that spiritual beliefs and values contribute to his or her health and well-being. Does the client rely on God or other spiritual values to enhance his or her health? Does the client turn to God or similar resources more in times of adversity than in terms of prosperity? As part of this line of discussion, the client may feel comfortable in discussing the impact of spiritual beliefs on the anticipation of death.

Identification of a Spiritual Need

Either in the initial assessment or at a later time, the nurse may become aware of a specific spiritual need. For example, a client might say, "Please pray for me." A client might express the fear that God has afflicted him or her because of a sin or might indicate a feeling of being at odds with God or with the spiritual system that has usually given him or her support. The nurse can help the client to articulate the particular concern by asking what the original comment or question meant.

In general, spiritual needs are indicated by comments or questions that touch on the meaning of life, the value of the self and others, and the significance in pain and suffering. Whenever a client raises a question or shares ideas about these issues, he or she is expressing a concern about spirituality.

PLANNING AND INTERVENING WITH SPIRITUAL NEEDS

After assessing all of a client's needs, the nurse sets priorities for intervention. Spiritual needs are often the lowest priority in nursing care, because the nurse must first minister to the physical needs of a client. When physical, safety, and security needs have been met, then it is time for the nurse to support the client's search for meaning in life.

When a client does raise questions about such deeply significant preoccupations as the meaning of his or her own life, there is usually little time for planning an intervention. Unlike questions that must be dealt with factually or with long-term emotional support, a client's difficulties with spiritual concomitants to health frequently must be met quickly. Spiritual difficulties can lead to psychological and social disruptions in a person's life. There is also a body of knowledge that demonstrates the impact of spiritual comfort or discomfort on a person's physical state.

Setting Objectives

When the nurse intervenes in a spiritual issue, he or she should have some objectives to be met within the context of a nursing intervention. For example, a nurse should not attempt to take the place of a minister or other spiritual counselor. On the other hand, assisting the client to explore the meaning of the current health care situation is quite appropriate for the nurse.

As with other areas of concern, objectives should be specific and measurable. Since spiritual values transcend material reality, the measurement will tend to be subjective. An appropriate objective for the client concerned about whether her health problem is an affliction from God would be, "Explore the meaning of the client's illness with her." A client estranged from a relationship with God might need an objective such as, "Reestablish a personal relationship with God." A client who does not believe in God but who is raising questions about meanings in his life might warrant an objective to "Identify with the client the higher values that motivate his life."

Intervening

Interventions fall into three broad categories: those the nurse does with the client; those the nurse encourages the client to do alone; and those the nurse encourages the client to do with another person or group. The interventions that the nurse engages in with the client include discussing the concern with the client and helping the client formulate a plan of action. The ability to intervene in spiritual needs is one the nurse must nurture.

The important point in talking with people about their religious and spiritual lives is to accept the client's beliefs and the nurse's limits in the situation. For example, a nurse who was an agnostic recognized that God and prayer were important to one of her clients. In addition to identifying interpersonal efforts to improve the client's relationships, the nurse asked if she had prayed about her problems. The client stated she had not but would. A few weeks later, she told the nurse that this suggestion had helped her.

It is perhaps one of the most common features of one who does not have faith or who is experiencing a crisis in faith to feel that God should not let misfortune, pain, or suffering befall those who love Him. The fact that so much misfortune, pain, and suffering befalls all of us, even those who love God, may seem to indicate that God does not exist or that He periodically ignores us

or actually causes such things to occur in order to punish us for transgressions. The interpretation that the nurse and the client make of such events is crucial to their work together on problems related to spiritual needs. If the nurse and the client have similar beliefs to begin with, it will be easier to establish a common ground for communication. If they do not have similar beliefs but the nurse is able to assess the client's belief system and work within it, the relationship will also run fairly smoothly. However, if the nurse and client have different beliefs about fundamental issues and the nurse either does not understand or does not accept the client's beliefs, additional problems may arise if these spiritual concerns become a part of the nurse–client relationship.

The following is an example of a situation in which a nurse who was strongly founded in a faith in God tried to comfort someone who did not believe in God.

The client was very depressed about family problems and self-esteem problems. The nurse listened to her recount some of the feelings she had and some of the disappointments she had been experiencing. After the client finished, the nurse said, "When I feel that way, I try to pray more and think about how much God loves me. I think about how that is much more important than any of the earthly problems we deal with. And grace lifts me up." The client looked at the nurse and said, "I know that's really important to you and you really believe it. But I don't and your telling me that doesn't help me feel any better." Both the nurse and the client ended up feeling let down.

In the above example, the nurse tried a spiritual intervention in a situation that seemed to call for it. However, given the knowledge that the client did not appreciate or value such beliefs about God, the well-meant words were impotent. The nurse felt disappointed because he had chosen an inappropriate approach, and the client felt that she was misunderstood. Fortunately, the nurse and the client had a long-standing relationship, and they were later able to redeem what could have hurt a new or less well-established working relationship.

If a nurse is willing to talk about spiritual matters, clients will perceive this. Rarely will someone pursue such issues with an unwilling listener. On the other hand, the nurse must also assess whether a client is willing to talk about spiritual aspects of a situation. The nurse can begin to assess this by asking questions and taking careful note not only of the client's verbal response but also of nonverbal cues. An example of a nurse trying to assess how much the client might be willing to discuss is given here:

In working with a depressed client, the nurse was concerned about the client's apparent isolation. During one interview, the following conversation took place.

NURSE: In talking about where you might meet new friends, you haven't mentioned church. Have you thought about church as a place to meet people?

CLIENT: I haven't gone to church in a long time. My mother thinks I still go, but I think I have to decide about that for myself.

NURSE: I think that people can have a relationship with God even if they don't go to church. What do you think about that?

CLIENT: That's true. I still feel that God is important to me even though I don't go to church.

NURSE: In what way is God important to your life?

CLIENT: (Looking at nurse) I still pray every once in a while, and I sometimes read the Bible when I feel lonely or upset.

NURSE: Have you found that to be helpful to you?

CLIENT: Yes. It usually makes me feel better. I guess I should do it more. (Looked down at hands.)

NURSE: What do you mean . . . you should do it more?

CLIENT: Well, I just feel like I don't do it enough.

NURSE: It's probably more important that you do it because you want to rather than because you feel you should. How do you feel about talking about this with me?

CLIENT: I feel okay about it. (Looking at nurse) I haven't thought about it.

NURSE: Have you ever thought about just talking to God like a friend?

CLIENT: No, I haven't. What do you mean? (Looks curious.)

NURSE: Well, I was just thinking that when you feel lonely or bad, as well as when you feel good, you could talk to God just like you would talk to a human friend.

CLIENT: No one ever said anything like that to me before.

NURSE: What do you think about it?

CLIENT: I think I'll try it. I guess I should pray more. (Looks down again.)

NURSE: I'm sort of concerned about your using the word "should." When we talk to real friends, it's not usually because we feel like we "should."

CLIENT: I don't know what you mean. (Looks back at nurse.)

NURSE: I just mean that when you talk to our Father in Heaven, I would hope that it would be because you want to, not because you think someone, even God, *expects* you to. I believe our relationship with God is just like other relationships. The best ones are usually the ones I put the time and effort into to make them good. A good relationship is mutual . . . both of us giving and receiving.

CLIENT: I just never thought about it like that. (Smiles broadly for the first time that day.) I am going to try it.

In the above example, the nurse tested the waters at various points to see whether to go on. Even though she started out by asking about meeting friends through church, she was actually trying to find out about the significance to the client of her relationship with God. The client revealed on two or three occasions that she was heavily influenced by others' expectations in regard to her relationship with God and also that she associated her relationship with God with going to church. The nurse helped her to explore another way of looking at her religious life. Early in the interaction, the nurse asked questions about the importance of God to the client and how that was expressed. After finding that the client believed that God was important in her life, the nurse was able to pursue the situation further. The nurse also gave the client an opportunity to express discomfort if she wished. The nurse introduced an idea to the client about talking to God in a certain way and let the client investigate the notion. The nurse also gently got the idea across to the client that she didn't have to live up to others' expectations about her relationship to God.

At times, it may be appropriate for the nurse to pray with a client, but only if that feels right to both the client and nurse. One nurse said:

Although I realize that I have changed a lot in what I can talk to patients about in respect to religion, there are still some things that I haven't done. For one thing, I don't feel comfortable in suggesting to a patient or client that we pray *together*. I do think that some day I will do that, but it will be when I can do it sincerely and genuinely. I wouldn't do it if I couldn't feel natural and normal about it. That is the way I felt when I began trying the other things, so I think this will come the same way.

This nurse is giving herself the same permission she would give a client. She is setting her own pace in collaboration with God, and she is not trying to fulfill anyone else's expectations. This is just as important for those who do not believe in God as for those who do: to do what seems correct spiritually according to one's own understanding of spiritual values.

All the interventions discussed thus far focus on the nurse's work with the client.

However, the nurse and the client often identify spiritual pursuits for the client to attempt by herself or himself. For example, a client may decide to try meditation in order to reach a greater sense of peace. Another client might decide to read a selection from the Bible each evening and then pray about the values contained in the passage. Another client might study various religious forms and extract the meanings from them that have significance to him. At a later point, the nurse and the client can discuss the results.

Interventions frequently call for the involvement of other people. If the client is wrestling with a specific issue of religious expression, the best resource person may be a religious leader. If the nurse feels uncomfortable with a discussion of spiritual matters, she or he should refer the client to someone who can help. However, it is important for the nurse to develop the ability to respond to some spiritual problems in order to be able to render timely assistance to clients in times of spiritual turmoil. When the nurse feels unable to help, she or he should acknowledge this and help the client to find another resource.

EVALUATION

Evaluation is used to determine whether objectives were attained and whether the interventions used were effective. If the objectives were appropriate and clearly stated, the nurse and the client should be able to identify criteria to establish whether they were accomplished. Evaluation of spiritual objectives may be subjective on the part of the client. For example, if the client's objective was to identify higher values that motivate his life, the criteria would be whether or not the client felt that he had met this expectation. If the objective was to reestablish a personal relationship with God, the client would have to determine the criteria that indicated to her that her relationship with God was intact.

The other aspect of evaluation is to consider the interventions themselves. Were they appropriate to meeting the objective? Were they timely and effective? In one of the examples given earlier, the nurse offered some spiritual wisdom he had gained that helped him to feel better in circumstances similar to the client's. Since the client did not share the nurse's beliefs, this was not an effective intervention. Once the nurse acknowledged this, he could find other ways in which he might give comfort in a spiritual context appropriate to one who did not believe in God. The nurse can assess the value of an intervention by such things as whether or not the client responded meaningfully and followed through with it. The client may state directly that a particular intervention was useful and that it helped.

FUTURE IMPLICATIONS

As nurses become more comfortable with their roles as health care coordinators as well as health care providers, they will feel more confident about intervening in spiritual matters. Society is moving toward a widespread recognition of the value of spiritual pursuits on a personal level. At present, many people are engaging in health-related pursuits that are akin to spiritual endeavors, such as the holistic health movement. The advocates of this approach are equally concerned for all aspects of the individual: the spirit as well as the mind and body.

The future will bring many more formal and informal approaches to spiritual expression. Some will be the traditional, structured forms that offer security and solace. However, as the new century approaches, there will be a greater emphasis on personal expressions of spiritual belief. There will be greater acceptance of one another's ideas and values, and this will encourage people who have avoided institutionalized religion to begin meaningful explorations of spiritual horizons. The old and the new religious forms will be revitalized and their influence on everyday life will increase.

As more and more people recognize the importance of spiritual values, we will become more comfortable with and creative in our expressions of these beliefs. Our lives will become infused with supreme values, motivated by forces of undeniable and immeasurable potency. This influence in our lives will enrich nursing practice as we endeavor to render the highest level of health care possible to our clients. Nursing care that is service-motivated will no longer seem to be a throwback to earlier times. All people will eventually perform their chosen work from a service motive.

SUMMARY

Nursing has a rich history of spiritually motivated service. Although this was undervalued in an industrial society, it will be more valued in the future. A nurse can comfortably and meaningfully approach the spiritual needs of clients, whether or not the nurse or the client believes in God. Spirituality includes and goes beyond religious form. Because the spirit is a coequal component of each person, it is an appropriate focus for nursing assessment and intervention. Our society is becoming more accepting of a variety of spiritual expressions. No doubt research will demonstrate the impact and importance of spiritual striving on the client's state of health. As science provides more and more evidence to guide us, nurses will become better able to respond to spiritual issues as a part of the healthy functioning of the client.

DISCUSSION TOPICS

1. You are working with two elderly women who live together. While you are assessing their needs, one of the women, Mrs. Montefiore, asks you to arrange for her priest to come to her home to give her communion and to hear her confession. The other woman, Mrs. Tyler, asks you to pray with her for inner strength.

     a. How would you respond to Mrs. Montefiore? What would you say? What would you do? What is your rationale for your responses?

     b. How would you respond to Mrs. Tyler? What would you say? What would you do? What is your rationale for your responses?

2. Several weeks after the visit described above, Mrs. Montefiore dies peacefully in her sleep. Mrs. Tyler asks, "Why did God take her first?" How would you respond? How would you feel? Compare your response with those of some other nurses or nursing students.

3. Describe how your personal and professional lives would be different in each of the following circumstances.

     a. Our society has no religious institutions and everyone seeks for higher meanings in life in his or her own way.

     b. Our society has one religious institution that dominates life.

     c. Our government requires health institutions and health care givers to provide for spiritual care to all clients.

4. What kind of research might nurses of the future engage in to study the relationship of health and the spiritual component of individuals? What are some aspects of this area that could be studied? Propose two hypotheses which you might investigate related to spirituality and health care.

BIBLIOGRAPHY

Carson, V.C., & Huss, K.: Prayer—An effective therapeutic and teaching tool. *Journal of Psychosocial Nursing and Mental Health Services* 17(3), 34–37, 1979.

Cox, H.: Religion. In A. Villodo & L. Dychtwald, eds., *Millenium Glimpses into the 21st Century.* Los Angeles: J.P. Tarcher, 1981.

Dickinson, C.: The search for spiritual meaning. *American Journal of Nursing* 75(10) 1789–1793, 1975.

Ferguson, M.: *The Aquarian conspiracy.* Los Angeles: J.P. Tarcher, 1980.

Ferguson, M.: The Aquarian conspiracy update. Public lecture, Norman, Oklahoma, October 1982.

Fish, S., & Shelly, J.A.: *Spiritual care: The nurse's role.* Downers Grove, Ill.: Intervarsity Press, 1978.

Hatch, J.W., & Lovelace, K.A.: Involving the southern rural church and students of the health professions in health education. *Public Health Reports* 95(1), 23–25, 1980.

Huxley, E.: *Florence Nightingale.* New York: Putnam, 1975.

Johnson, C.: Nurse in a Christian community. *American Journal of Nursing* 75(12), 2180–2182, 1975.

Lair, R.E., Jr.: Two ideas due for the ragbag. *Journal of Religion and Health* 17(4), 288–289, 1978.

McGilloway, F.A., & Donnelly, L.: Religion and patient care: The functionalist approach. *Journal of Advanced Nursing* 2, 3–13, 1977.

Marwick, C.S.: Religion and medicine draw closer. *Medical World News,* December 25, 1978, pp. 26–30.

Muller, H.J.: *Uses of the future.* Bloomington, Ind.: Indiana University Press, 1974.

Naisbitt, J.: *Megatrends.* New York: Warner, 1982.

Pumphrey, Rev. J.B.: Recognizing your patients' spiritual needs. *Nursing 77* 7, 64–70, 1977.

Richards, F.: What they believe and why (Parts 1–3) *Nursing Mirror* April 14, 1977, pp. 65–66; April 21, 1977, p. 64; April 28, 1977, p. 67.

Rosen, I.M.: Some contributions of religion to mental and physical health. *Journal of Religion and Health* 13(1), 289–294, 1974.

Stoll, R.I.: Guidelines for spiritual assessment. *American Journal of Nursing* 79(9), 1574–1577, 1979.

16

Contracting with Clients

Jo Frazer

The great thing in the world is not so much where we are but
in what direction we are going.
OLIVER WENDELL HOLMES

OBJECTIVES

After reading this chapter, you should be able to:

- ☐ Define and describe the contracting process between nurse and client.
- ☐ Understand the context, both historical and current, for contracting in community health nursing.
- ☐ Describe the significance of contracting to the nursing process and to the goals of the profession.
- ☐ Project the future of contracting under changed environmental conditions for community health nurses.

INTRODUCTION

Changes in the health care system, including changing roles for nurses, spiraling costs, the clients' rights movement, and consumer education, will revolutionize the client–nurse relationship. New definitions of responsibility are being proposed. Future shock requires stress management, and the relationship of stress to illness indicates that clients must become more fully involved in their health care. Research shows many life-style–related illnesses. To prevent disease and promote longevity, clients will have to control their diets, exercise, stop smoking, and reduce drug and alcohol consumption.

It is well documented that contracting is useful in promoting shared responsibility. It has a long tradition in nursing education, mental health care, and community health nursing. The role of the community health nurse is to help clients help themselves; therefore, the community health nurse guides, teaches, and helps, rather than doing things for the client. Historically, nurses have held the major responsibility for client health care decisions, creating a situation of client dependency. The community health nurse must help clients learn more about the decision-making process. Educated clients will, in the long run, be better motivated and better able to make intelligent choices when provided with a variety of options.

The nurse in the community will be called upon increasingly to contract with clients. This is an outgrowth of the recognition that the client bears the ultimate responsibility for his or her health. Contracting provides the mechanism for allocating responsibility to the client, at the same time validating the expertise of the health practitioner as consultant and adviser. This new form of relationship between the health care provider and the client is being supported by the public, which has become better educated and more knowledgeable about health care and is becoming oriented toward autonomy in health care decision making.

The medical model of treatment has deep historical roots, but it has not been universally successful. Under the *medical model,* the practitioner assumes full responsibility for the client, who is viewed as incompetent. The model has several flaws. People are not expected to know what is relevant to report to the physician, and the physician often does not know what questions to ask because of differences in habit and lifestyle. Client compliance to medical advice depends on a relationship in which the client abdicates responsibility to the trusted family physician. Diagnoses are sometimes inaccurate. Further, clients frequently do not actually follow through on treatments and are not necessarily helped or cured. In addition, good health care practices cannot be implemented by the physician, because such practices are inevitably connected with client self-responsibility.

An alternate model has always existed in midwifery, folk medicine, and self-care in community health nursing. In recent years, a new *self-care model* has been adopted by people who advocate such health-promotion activities as reliance on health foods, Rolfing, yoga, and exercise and fitness classes. As nurses use more contracting, they will find that the people most interested in this type of relationship include a high proportion of health-and-fitness-oriented individuals who have adopted new health care practices outside the framework of medicine.

With a highly mobile American population and less continuity among church, home, and family, we can anticipate that clients will see many different kinds of health care providers over their life spans. Without providers who have intimate and lengthy relationships with an individual, compliance cannot be obtained or ascertained, as it might have been under the historically acceptable medical model. The notion of contracting within the practitioner–client relationship is in part a product of the times and a response to an autonomy-oriented, highly educated populace.

WHAT IS A CONTRACT?

A contract is a mutual agreement between client and nurse concerning their expectations of each other. . . . Contracting is based on the premise that nurse and patient are equal partners, each with different but equal responsibilities toward common goals. A contract makes expectations, goals and responsibilities explicit. (Zangari & Duffy, 1980, p. 451)

A *contract* is an agreement between two or more parties involved in a specified objective.

A contract is designed to help clients define what they want and need and to increase clients' motivation to accomplish these goals. A contract should specify the following:

1. The specific activity to be undertaken.
2. The duration of the activity.
3. The methods to be used to evaluate the activity.
4. The mutual responsibilities of the nurse and the client.

The contract's complexity and length will depend on the client's conceptual and cognitive ability, cultural framework, communication and verbal skills, and previous experience with the health care system.

A contract should specify what will occur. Establishment of a contract begins with the parties getting acquainted with each other's perspective and follows the stages in the helping process. First, rapport is established. Second, the working phase occurs. Third is the termination phase. A successful contract includes provisions for all three steps in this process.

If contracting is new to a client, it is advisable to begin with a short and simple contract so that the client can learn and practice the process. The contract may be an informal, mutually agreed upon verbal agreement or it may be an explicit, formal, written document. Nurses have been using contracts with clients all along, but usually in an informal and implicit way. For example, a typical conversation between a new postoperative client and his nurse might be, "To avoid postop complications, it is necessary for you to turn, cough, and deep breathe. I'll give you a pain medication to make moving less painful, and in 45 minutes you must turn, cough, and deep breathe." This is a form of contracting with a client. However, for the purposes of fos-

tering autonomy, client involvement, and self-care, it is necessary to define the contract more clearly as an explicit and essential part of the nursing care plan. In the above-mentioned example, the nurse and the client would formulate a postoperative care plan before surgery with the client receiving accurate information about the postoperative process. Then, the nurse and client requirements, expectations, and behaviors during the postoperative recovery period are negotiated.

The establishment of a working relationship is the first step to any successful nurse–client relationship. The nurse must be skilled in effective communication and in interpersonal relations in order to establish a working relationship in which caring, respect, acceptance, and empathetic understanding are communicated to the client. In addition, the nurse must be able to verbalize an explicit description of her or his specific skills; what she or he can and is willing to do; and, most important, what her or his limitations are. The nurse will be viewed as the expert by the client; further, the client will expect to derive some benefit from the relationship. The importance of establishing a sense of equality—not equality of experience and professional skill, but equality of worth and dignity with mutual respect—cannot be overemphasized. There is a great difference between "we will work on it together" and "I have the answers."

Another important aspect of the nurse's responsibility and contribution to a successful contracting process is actual belief in the client's ability to change, that change is possible, and that the client has the right to define if, when, and how to change. Communicating this belief to the client is also critical. Self-assessment and monitoring are necessary in evaluating how successful the nurse is in communicating hope to the client. One's behavior—facial expression and body language—gives important clues about how believable one's words actually are. The nurse's behavior can demonstrate that the nurse does indeed believe that things will get better and that the client is able to help himself or herself. The nurse must be imaginative, creative, and flexible in order to provide accurate information, to foster self-awareness and personal growth, and to individualize care through the contract method.

What does contracting really mean? It is a tool for change rather than a means of manipulating or controlling the client. The nurse is not in a position to force values on the client, and if the nurse attempts this, the client will resist. Contracting can be complicated by the underlying dynamics of the client–practitioner relationship. For example, a client may overuse options or fail to meet deadlines, even if the contract has been carefully formulated and modified. Further, fixing of responsibility is difficult if one is rendering an old service in a new and not fully defined way. Contracting may also differ in varying circumstances: in different institutional settings; for more or less serious health problems; for emotional or physical problems; or based on the client's sex, age, ethnic group, or past experience in the health care system.

To summarize, contracting between nurses and clients requires mutual agreement and careful assessment of the nurse's and the client's strengths and abilities. The ability of the nurse to teach the client to meet his or her own health care needs is crucial to success.

NURSING PROCESS AND CONTRACTING

For the nurse to contract with a client, four stages must be carefully considered: (1) assessing the client and his or her situation, (2) planning the contract, (3) implementing and reinforcing the contract, and (4) evaluating the outcomes.

Assessment

Assessment involves collecting all significant data. The nurse must feel comfortable about asking for information, and the client must identify problems from his or her perspective, recognize the need for assistance, and develop a willingness to follow through. The client will act upon only what he or she sees as needs. Part of the nurse's assessment will be to identify the client's view of needed treatments.

It is important for the community health nurse to assess more than the medical diagnosis assigned to a client. For example: A 70-year-old male client is discharged from the hospital with the diagnosis of postoperative abdominal aortic aneurism. When the nurse visits the home, she discovers that the client has chronic obstructive pulmonary disease, is severely depressed, and refuses to get out of bed. He also needs postoperative rehabilitation. Furthermore, the client's wife is elderly and unable to cope with his physical and emotional problems. The nurse must assess the environment, the family, and the client, not just the incision and postoperative recovery. Based on the data collected, it is obvious that the whole family is in distress. It may be necessary to establish a contract with both the client and the wife. The contract will be more comprehensive and more effective if the nurse uses the holistic approach in data collection.

Assessment requires that the nurse be knowledgeable about both physical and emotional problems in order to formulate accurate nursing diagnoses. It is difficult but necessary for the nurse to create an environment in which the client can reveal all relevant information and where the nurse can communicate what is important to discuss. Assessment is a comprehensive process that forms the basis for implementation.

Planning and Negotiating

Planning care is done with the client and includes establishing mutual goals, treatment methods, a time frame, and the responsibilities of both nurse and client. Part of planning is clarifying expectations for implementation, including difficulties that can be anticipated and how they will be met. The contract incorporates the entire care plan. A suggested contract format appears in Figure 16.1. It requires that the nurse identify what she or he can and cannot offer the client in the particular situation. The nurse must recognize that time and the willingness to listen are important, as important as hands-on care. The nurse's presence and interest are real services, and the time spent in negotiating a contract yields later results in more reliable client follow through.

Establishing a contract involves making decisions about whether the contract is to be an informal verbal agreement or an explicit, formal, written document. The expectations of both the nurse and the client must be clarified. Former passive-dependent experience in the health care system

```
Client: _____

Goal #_____    Date Set _____
GOAL:


PLAN                          COMPLETION DATE
Client will:




Nurse will:




EVALUATION
```

Figure 16.1　The client–nurse contract.

may make it difficult for the client to appreciate the idea of a contract and may affect the client's willingness to agree to a contract. Some clients expect and prefer the nurse to make decisions for them. The client often must accept a redefinition of the roles of both client and nurse and must internalize the change in order to be willing to take a share of the responsibility for maintaining his or her health. The contract should be clear-cut to foster the desired behavior: client independence and full and complete agreement. The contract must be framed in language that is meaningful to the client and must specify behavior the client understands and can perform.

Client motivation for follow through must be thoroughly explored. The client must have the material resources and the knowledge base to follow through with contract expectations. For example, a young mother may wish to prepare more nutritionally complete meals. She needs information about what constitutes such meals, but she also needs choices of foods she can afford. Figure 16.2 shows how this might be a part of a contract.

Life-style assets and liabilities must be taken into account in developing a comprehensive contract plan. For example, Mrs. Washington wants to quit smoking. She has an asset in that she does believe that she will feel better if she gives up cigarettes. However, her husband smokes and does not wish to quit. Mrs. Washington has been hampered in the past because of the ready availability of cigarettes in her home. Both her desire to refrain and the temptation of ever-present smoking materials will be incorporated into the contract. Part of the contract appears in Figure 16.3.

The most difficult part of planning is probably reinforcement. Clients may want to feel better but may not want to change their behavior. Finding the right reinforc-

ers may be especially difficult, as each client has unique response patterns. Clear descriptions of the consequences of modified behavior may help. Written contracts may have more impact on some clients. Breaking the new behavior down into sequential steps can facilitate client agreement. Although this may sound time consuming, a recent study shows that it takes an average of 11 minutes for a nurse and client to negotiate a contract (Steckel, 1980). The nurse must examine the client's internal motivation, as a contract will work only if the client believes that compliance will produce specific consequences in relation to the current health care problem. It is essential for the client to realize that the first step is not feeling better; it is behaving differently.

Implementation

Implementing the contract involves translating expectations into behavior that results in improved health. If the plan is specific, the nurse and client will avoid misunderstandings in their relationship, particularly during the initial stage of implementation. Checkpoints for progress allow the nurse and the client to monitor the success of the contract and agree upon modifications. Since the client's needs will change, prior agreement and actual behavior may not always be consistent. It may become necessary to ask what kind of choice or contract the client is capable of making at a specific time. Exploration of a full range of alternatives is useful if the client does not follow through. In an earlier example, Mrs. Washington chose to quit smoking. Part of her agreement was that she would ask her husband to do certain things. She thought it would help if he smoked only in one room of the house, because she could avoid being with him when

---

Client: Mrs. Markes

Goal #1   Date Set March 7

GOAL: To provide better balanced meals for the family within budget restrictions

PLAN	COMPLETION DATE
Client will:	
1. Keep a food diary for one week.	3/14
2. Read material provided by nurse.	3/21
3. Make daily menus for one week.	3/28
4. Make a shopping list for one week to go with menus.	3/28
5. Keep food diaries for two weeks for evaluation.	4/18 & 5/2
Nurse will:	
1. Provide pamphlets about balanced diets and about preparation of menus and shopping lists.	3/14
2. Discuss food diary, food preferences, and budget for food.	3/21
3. Discuss reading matter with Mrs. M.	3/28
4. Go over menus and shopping list with Mrs. M.	3/28
5. Identify variety foods for menus within family budget	3/28
6. Evaluate food diaries.	4/18 & 5/2

EVALUATION
Mrs. Markes will prepare food diaries twice for nurse to evaluate for nutritional balance and cost.

Figure 16.2   A sample contract.

he smoked if she felt she might be likely to join him. He was not willing to limit smoking to the family room, but he did consent to smoke only downstairs. So Mrs. Washington asked him to move an easy chair and writing desk into the extra bedroom so that she would have a place to go when he was smoking and she felt the urge to do so too. The nurse praised her resourcefulness and ability to stay within her contract expectations.

Implementation involves teaching the client more about his or her health problems than is typical under the medical

```
┌─────────────────────────────────────────────────────────────┐
│                                                             │
│   Client: Mrs. Washington                                   │
│                                                             │
│   Goal #1              Date Set September 13                │
│                                                             │
│   GOAL: To quit smoking                                     │
│                                                             │
│   PLAN                            COMPLETION DATE           │
│                                                             │
│   Client will:                                              │
│                                                             │
│   1. Discard all of her own cigarettes.        9/13         │
│   2. Give away cigarette case and lighter.     9/13         │
│   3. Ask husband to do the following:          9/13         │
│       a. Keep his extra cigarettes in his car.              │
│       b. Remove all unused cigarettes from                  │
│       the house.                                            │
│       c. Smoke only in the family room.                     │
│   4. Leave the room when husband is smoking                 │
│   and she feels like doing the same.                        │
│   5. Tell friends she no longer smokes.        9/13         │
│   6. Keep a list of times when she feels like               │
│   smoking.                                     9/20         │
│   7. Identify other options for times she feels             │
│   like smoking (e.g., eat raw vegetables; do                │
│   craft work).                                 9/20         │
│   8. Tell the nurse if she slips and has a ciga-            │
│   rette.                                                    │
│                                                             │
│   Nurse will:                                               │
│                                                             │
│   1. Talk with Mr. W. if necessary to encour-               │
│   age his help.                                             │
│   2. Go over list of times Mrs. W. feels like               │
│   smoking and identify patterns.               9/20         │
│   3. Help Mrs. W. match alternative behaviors               │
│   with times she is most likely to smoke.      9/20         │
│   4. Identify support systems to help people                │
│   giving up smoking.                           9/20         │
│   5. If Mrs. W. slips and has a cigarette, nurse            │
│   will be nonjudgmental and will help to fig-               │
│   ure out how to deal with the problem.                     │
│                                                             │
│   EVALUATION                                                │
│   Client will quit smoking cigarettes.                      │
│                                                             │
└─────────────────────────────────────────────────────────────┘
```

Figure 16.3 A sample contract.

model. This requires skill, patience, persistence, and resourcefulness. Verbal and written communication and follow through are necessary to provide the client with adequate information to achieve his or her contractual agreements. This teaching process yields substantial returns when the client can manage his or her health in the long run without nursing assistance.

Evaluation

Evaluation of outcomes consists of determining how well goals and objectives have been met. Reasonable and renegotiable goals are necessary. Flexibility is crucial and must be demonstrated both during implementation and evaluation. The larger purpose of the contract is client participation and improved adherance and compliance, which can be evaluated by both parties. Evaluation allows for scrutiny of a mutually responsible relationship in terms of client autonomy and practitioner participation.

WORKING WITH A CLIENT–NURSE CONTRACT

As a community mental health nurse, contracting has been a valuable tool for the author in helping clients reach a position of self-help and responsibility. The following case illustrates how the contract method was used with a young male client who was having difficulty "getting his life together":

John Martin was a 23-year-old single man at the time of our first interview. His chief complaint was that he felt adrift and was unable to get his life organized. At first, he was rather vague about the specific problems. However, with some direct questioning and encouragement, he revealed that he had lost his last three jobs, was in financial difficulty, and was unclear about his career goals. The fact that John had made his own appointment and sought help was a positive indicator that he was ready to make changes in his life.

I told John that I believed that I could help him help himself. He seemed to like that idea. The next step was to ask John what he saw as most confusing and upsetting at the moment. He indicated that he was again working but could not seem to get his bills paid or make his money last between paydays. We agreed that that problem was a priority in our work together. The next step involved negotiating a specific contract about frequency of visits, fee, and what we might do about finances to make his situation better. I suggested that if he would agree to keep a log of every expenditure for one week, I would go over the log with him. We would look at the log together and I would help him organize his finances. We agreed upon one-hour weekly visits and a fee. The contract we initially agreed upon is shown in Figure 16.4.

On the second visit, John had a complete list of expenditures for the week and seemed rather pleased with himself. In fact, he reported that being aware of how he spent his money had helped him avoid making some unnecessary expenditures that week (which is what I had expected to happen). We listed his expenditures and I asked him to identify areas of overspending and of low priority. He spent considerable time justifying some areas of obvious low priority. After some inquiring as to what he might do differently to make his situation better, John suggested that there were expenditures he could omit for awhile, and we began to formulate a budget.

After beginning to get his financial life in order, John began to talk about a conflict he was having with his boss and his fear of again losing his job. Because of his previous work record, it seemed worthwhile to pursue John's perception of authority figures and to discuss what he might do to make the situation better. We set another goal and added this to the contract. I asked John to make a list of the people in authority with whom he had trouble. I agreed to discuss the list with him in hopes of finding some commonalities and of reaching some understanding about what precipitated these conflicts. I again placed responsibility on John for examining his own behavior. I also agreed to help him make some sense of the data so that he could find ways to make the situation better.

Client: <u>John Martin</u>

Goal # <u>1</u>   Date Set <u>April 10</u>

GOAL: Successful management of finances, demonstrated by paying bills and having money left over each payday.

PLAN

Client will:

1. Spend one hour per week with nurse.
2. Pay a set fee in advance each week.
3. Keep a log of expenditures each week.

Nurse will:

1. Be available to client one hour per week.
2. Collect fee in advance each week.
3. Review weekly expenditures with client.
4. Assist client in establishing spending priorities.
5. Assist client in formulating a budget.

EVALUATION

1. Client will keep weekly appointment with nurse.
2. Client will pay weekly fee in advance.
3. Client will bring a log of all expenditures for the next week.
4. Nurse and client will establish spending priorities and begin to formulate a budget.

Figure 16.4 A sample contract.

I saw John for six months. Many symptoms emerged, all pointing to low self-esteem, conflict with authority figures, and lack of understanding of self-responsibility.

By the time John and I ended our work, he had talked a lot about what he had learned about taking care of himself. He had changed some of his perceptions of people in authority and he had reenrolled in college with the goal of job promotion. John and I renewed and renegotiated our contract almost weekly as new material emerged. Some weeks I encouraged John to make a contract with himself about specific tasks he wished to accomplish, including organizing his time and continuing to update his budget on a monthly basis. By means of the contracting process, John developed some useful tools for getting his life together.

FUTURE IMPLICATIONS

Contracting has clearly come of age. In the future, nurses will move into the larger community as a consequence of the rise of health care costs. Community health nurses will be serving the middle and upper middle classes, with encouragement from third-party payment sources. Nurses may split their days between hospitals and home care, following individual clients throughout a health and illness cycle. This suggests that the arrangements between nurses, hospitals, and physicians will alter. Changes in the beliefs of the American public (for example, acceptance of the client rather than the patient role) will enlarge the scope of community health nursing. The need to provide cost-effective health care will be another impetus to change. With greater diversity of clients and settings, the community health nurse of the future will have to customize the contracting process. More clients will expect creative, mutual problem solving and will challenge latent authoritarianism by nurses. In order for contracting to work, community health nurses will have to be as comfortable with upper-middle-class as with lower-middle-class clients. Without the authority of superior education and income, nurses will be more frequently and critically questioned by clients who are accustomed to being in charge.

In brief, the expansion of community health nursing in the future will be tied to the adoption of contracting, a method for establishing egalitarian relationships to further the client's health care status. If nurses really believe that people are thinking beings capable of full responsibility for themselves, then contracting should become a regular mechanism for transmitting this value to clients. Health care delivery trends support the use of contracting by community health nurses as a vehicle for collaboration with clients. Table 16.1 suggests that contracting will expand because of its affinity to social and economic conditions.

In the future, clients may contract with an agency or service consortium for services to improve diet, exercise, and health habits. A variety of professionals will comprise the staff of such an agency. The clients' needs will determine the services they receive (health vs. sickness), the premiums they pay, and the type of health care provider. Some clients will be the primary responsibility of community health nurses; others will be treated primarily by other practitioners and secondarily by nurses. All of the relationships will be more explicit. Expectation levels will be adjusted, and insurance premiums may perhaps be related to incentives for enhanced health status. In brief, the contract will replace the informal community expectations of the past as a means of arranging mutual expectations with clarity and precision.

TABLE 16.1
Health Care Delivery and the Nurse in the Community

Trends in American Health Care Delivery	Impact on Role of the Community Health Nurse
Increased cost of health care	Reduced health care cost.
Intervention of private enterprise.	Community health nurses engaged in private enterprise.
Consumers more discriminating in selection of health care deliverers.	Consumers become clients of community health nurses.
Third-party payment sources available for health promotion activities.	Third-party payment sources fund expansion of community health nurse role.
Increase in personal responsibility for health.	Contracting for health care delivery.

SUMMARY

Contracting can be a valuable tool for nurses in a variety of settings. It has many implications for future trends in health care delivery and in the role of the community health nurse. Contracting fosters equality in nurse–client relations and places primary responsibility on the client for his or her health status.

Contracting requires special qualifications of both nurse and client. The nurse must be effective in communications and interpersonal relations, skilled in verbalizing her or his specific role, and able to define what she or he can do for the client. The client must be oriented to the contract approach to care and must choose to operate from within that framework for the outcome to be successful.

Contracting fosters autonomy of both provider and client and fits closely with the rising self-care movement in the United States. For the community health nurse, shared responsibility provides access to clients in all socioeconomic groups. A contract is an effective method of change.

DISCUSSION TOPICS

1. What are some of the advantages and obstacles to contracting?

2. How does contracting fit with current social trends?

3. Why is contracting important to the future of community health nursing?

4. How is the nursing process affected by nurse–client contracting?

5. How does contracting fit with historical trends in nursing care delivery?

6. Under what circumstances would you negotiate a verbal versus a written contract with a client?

7. Why would you modify a contract?

BIBLIOGRAPHY

Steckel, S.B.: Contracting with patient-selected reinforcers. *American Journal of Nursing* 80(9), 1596–1599, 1980.

Zangari, M.E., & Duffy, P.: Contracting with patients in day-to-day practice. *American Journal of Nursing*, 80(3), 451–455, 1980.

17

Teaching and Learning Principles

Victoria Schoolcraft

Man is the only one that knows nothing, that can learn nothing without being taught.
        PLINY THE ELDER

OBJECTIVES

After reading this chapter, you should be able to:

- [ ] Apply principles of teaching and learning in a variety of situations.
- [ ] Develop teaching plans.
- [ ] Select and use appropriate teaching strategies.
- [ ] Evaluate teaching and learning.

INTRODUCTION

Teaching is an often-used nursing intervention. It is a professional skill, and is one of the independent functions of nursing. The proper application of teaching principles elevates the process of mere telling to real teaching. A carefully devised and implemented effort to teach can have many worthwhile results. Effective teaching can foster healthy functioning and high-level wellness.

Professional nurses are the leaders of health care teams in many settings. They are in a position to have an indirect effect on the welfare of clients by teaching colleagues as well as those paraprofessionals they supervise. Nurses who function in the clinical setting, whether acute or ambulatory care, hospital or community, have useful experiences to share with colleagues and with students. If nurses have teaching skills, they will be able to enrich the nursing practice of others through meaningful presentations in workshops, symposia, classroom presentations, and journal articles.

LEARNING

Learning is a lifelong process of change. Bigge (1964, p. 1) stated that change might take place in "insights, behavior, perception, or motivation, or a combination of these." The dictionary defines *learning* as gaining knowledge, understanding, or skill through study, instruction, or investigation.

Although we tend to link learning with teaching, a great deal of learning occurs through experiences that are not necessarily designed to teach. For example, 4-year-old Lani may learn that the face plate of an iron is hot by reaching out and touching it. After this experience, Lani may at first be afraid to touch any part of the iron. Through additional experiences, she will learn that usually it is only the face plate that gets too hot to touch, and that even that is not always hot. She will learn ways of testing for the heat of objects by trying out methods of her own or by observing what others do, such as moistening a finger and quickly touching the heated iron. If Lani is a reasonably intelligent youngster, she will be able to transfer her learning to similar situations with other hot surfaces.

Theories of learning have evolved over many years to account for how human beings actually learn. The trend has been to acknowledge the natural propensity that people have to learn. Current learning theories and future-oriented suggestions related to promoting learning emphasize not getting in the way of people who are trying to learn. In the past, and to some extent in the present, the educational system itself has been responsible for discouraging learners from seeking and enjoying learning. Einstein once said that it was a miracle that any curiosity survived formal education (Ferguson, 1982). The educational system is on the brink of change. The nurses who are being educated today will likely work with future generations of clients who are unencumbered by many of the educationally wrought learning problems of the past. As a result, nurses of the future will work with more active and creative learners who will require progressive styles of teaching.

TEACHING

Teaching may be thought of as an activity intended to induce learning (Smith, 1960). Some theorists, however, define teaching as a process that succeeds in enabling students to learn (Dewey, 1933; Eisner, 1964; Gowin, 1961). At first, this might not seem to be a significant difference, but it is important. Consider the nursing process: a nurse sets an objective to reduce complications of immobility following a total hip replacement in a client. An intervention selected on the first postoperative day was to get the client up in a chair. However, such decisions about postoperative activity are the surgeon's, not the nurse's. Also, such activity is generally not ordered until the second or third day after surgery (Luckman & Sorensen, 1980). Such an intervention, involving a great deal of independent movement on the part of the client, could endanger the ultimate outcome of the surgical procedure. Even though the intent of the nurse, as stated in the objective, was appropriate, the result would likely be the opposite of the goal. This is an extreme example, because nurses also do many appropriate interventions that do not work in certain situations, and after these are evaluated, nurses go on to develop better approaches.

If the nurse's goals are realistic for the particular situation, eventually the nurse can succeed. If the nurse does not succeed, then she or he must examine the goals and determine whether or not they were appropriate. That brings us back to the intent. The intent might have been fine, but it might not have fit the client or the situation.

If a nurse consistently approaches client situations in which learning needs are manifested with the intent to induce learning, but is rarely or seldom successful, the interventions cannot be considered worthwhile. The nurse must be adept at identifying the learning needs, at assessing the client's capacities, and at planning and implementing a teaching project. Haphazard, poorly timed, or badly implemented efforts at teaching waste not only the client's time but also the nurse's.

In Chapter 10, Effective and Creative Thinking, a situation was described in which a student initially made an error in identifying the learning need of a client who stated that she wanted to avoid further pregnancies. With an inadequate data base, the student assumed that the woman needed information about contraceptive methods. The student gave the client too much information on methods. Although the student intended for the woman to understand enough about the various approaches to choose one, the woman did not need this information, since she already had an intrauterine device in place, a fact the student discovered later. The woman had misunderstood the purpose of the IUD; she actually needed to learn about that. The student further compounded her error by providing information at such an advanced level that the woman was more confused than enlightened. Could we call what the student did "teaching"?

In *The Aquarian Conspiracy* (1980, p. 287),

Marilyn Ferguson speaks of "transpersonal education." In this new experience, the learner is encouraged to be "awake and autonomous, to question, to explore . . . , to seek meaning, to test outer limits, to check out frontiers and depths of the self." The transforming teacher is one who senses the learner's readiness to change and responds to this by facilitating the process of learning. As people come to understand this new paradigm of the relationship between teaching and learning, they will be willing to take more risks in learning about new things. It is difficult to be a teacher now, whether that is one's primary work or a component of one's work. The difficulty is in responding to the kinds of learners most people have learned to be, while gradually trying to help them to awaken into a new way of seeing, learning, and being. We find it easy to resort to teaching as we were taught, because we too have learned to be afraid of change and its inherent risks.

The purpose of this chapter is to give the student a framework from within which to operate. As you become a nurse and increase your expertise in nursing and teaching, you will be able to change and rearrange the material presented in this chapter. As nurses evolve, and as nursing evolves, nurses will become different teachers, and nurses will become different learners, as well. The best teacher always keeps learning: from students, from friends, from every life experience.

TEACHING AND LEARNING PRINCIPLES

An understanding of principles relevant to learning is crucial to effective teaching. These are areas the nurse must consider in regard to any learner when assessing the learner and planning teaching strategies.

Readiness

Learner *readiness* refers to the learner's ability to achieve the outcomes the teacher deems appropriate. The nurse must consider factors in the physical, psychological, intellectual, cultural or social, and value realms, since all these realms impinge on the learner's ability to learn. Physical factors include mobility, coordination, general level of health, muscular strength, sensory acuity, preexisting medical conditions, stamina, stage of physical development, comfort, and level of consciousness. Psychological readiness includes factors such as attitude, self-esteem, self-concept, perception, trust, psychosocial stage of development, feelings about learning, anxiety, fear, hope, and coping abilities.

Intellectual factors relating to readiness include intelligence, education, problem-solving ability, intellectual stage of development, and verbal skills. Cultural and social factors include ethnic origin, mores, customs, family relationships, economic and social status, occupation, regional idiosyncracies, and leisure activities. Finally, value factors include religious and spiritual orientations, moral and ethical beliefs, and personal goals.

This list is not all inclusive, but it gives an idea of the many elements that can affect a person's readiness to learn. Some learner characteristics are related to more than one factor. For example, sex may have physical, psychological, and social implications. A woman may lack the neccessary physical strength to do certain things. On the other hand, she may be unwilling to learn some things because she feels they are not proper for women to do. Age can be a factor in several categories. Children are physically incapable of learning certain things at certain ages, such as sphinctor control or walking. Elderly people may have difficulty in learning some tasks because of real physical limitations brought on by age or because of negative feelings about themselves.

Motivation

The *motivation* of the learner is the actual desire to learn. An individual who values learning and who feels confident in his or her own ability to learn will be motivated to engage in the process. If the material to be learned is seen as worthwhile and useful to the learner, motivation will be enhanced. Although there is a relationship between readiness and motivation, they are different qualities. Consider a small child trying to learn to walk. The child wishes to be able to stand up and move across the room. This is motivation. However, until the bones, muscles, and neurological pathways are ready, the child will not be able to ambulate. Consider a young man who wishes to be a football player. He is determined and clear in his desire to achieve this, but until his strength, stamina, and coordination are sufficiently developed, he will not make the team. To look at it from another angle, a nursing student may have all the psychomotor ability necessary to master nursing skills; he may have all the intellectual ability necessary to learn and use the theoretical information necessary to practice nursing. If he is not really desirous of practicing as a nurse, however, his intellectual and psychomotor abilities may not even be evidenced.

The cultural, social, and value realms are clearly related to motivation, as well as to readiness. If you do not value learning, this will certainly limit your ability to learn.

Regardless of the learner's ability or the quality of the nurse's efforts to teach, if the learner is not sufficiently motivated to accomplish the goals, learning will be inadequate. Motivation is a necessary ingredient in any teaching–learning activity.

Participation

Research has shown that learning is enhanced as learner participation in the teaching–learning process increases. *Participation* is the active involvement of the learner in the process. Either learner or the teacher may first identify a learning need. Once it is identified, the two must agree that it is of significance and that they will work together to meet this need. The two collaborate in identifying the goals and objectives that will enable them to meet the need. The teacher selects strategies, which include the learner's participation. Together, the client and the nurse evaluate the client's success in reaching the goals and objectives as well as the nurse's contribution to the process. Encouraging participation will be discussed later in this chapter.

Satisfaction

A learner's satisfaction during or after a learning experience will enhance learning. *Satisfaction* is the feeling that a need has been fulfilled. As people's needs are met, they become more comfortable and their confidence is increased. If a nurse attempts to teach something a client does not see as meeting a need or that is too difficult to learn, the client may develop a sense of dissatisfaction. This may create difficulties for future efforts to work with the client. Teaching a client something he or she really wants to know, whether or not the nurse thinks it is particularly important, may enhance the relationship between the nurse and client and make the client more interested in future learning situations. The nursing student in the following situation discovered the importance of this principle:

June Wong identified a need for Ms. Washington, a client, to learn more about planning a balanced diet for the Washington family. The student thought this would help to improve the general quality of the family's health and would prevent many of the health problems they experienced. Ms. Washington was not particularly interested in learning about nutrition. However, she stated that she would like to learn to take her baby's temperature. Ms. Wong taught her how to use and read a thermometer and gave her some guidelines for deciding what to do at different temperature elevations. Ms. Washington then asked Ms. Wong to teach her something about first aid for cuts. Ms. Wong complied with this request. Finally, when the student again offered to teach the client about nutrition, the client was interested enough to ask for specific assistance in healthy nutrition.

Conducive Environment

An environment that is *conducive* to learning is one that is supportive of learning. The first concern is that the location for teaching must be physically adequate for the process. The space should be large enough for the number of people involved, but not a great deal larger than necessary for the size of the group. Another factor is the acoustic properties of the setting. Sound must carry well enough so that the teacher and the learners can communicate effectively. Considerations should also be given to the privacy needs of the learners; the interaction should not be audible by others.

Distractions, either from within the setting or from outside, must be limited. Other distractions include interruptions from visitors or indirectly from telephones. Either type of interruption is best dealt with ahead of time. This will be discussed further later in the chapter. Adequate furnishings are necessary: comfortable, flexible seating, desks or tables for writing, adequate space for exercise, if necessary.

The emotional atmosphere is also important in promoting a conducive environment. A sense that people are genuinely liked and that they can trust the teacher will help them be more open and willing to take risks. Offering positive reinforcement and encouraging exploration will promote a feeling of interest and involvement in learning.

Transfer of Learning

Transfer of learning occurs when a person uses knowledge gained in one situation to affect behavior in a new situation (Bigge, 1964). This has several implications for teaching done as part of nursing care. All clients have some knowledge that is transferable to situations in which the nurse is teaching. For example, a postcoronary client may better understand the value of an exercise program if he can relate it to past experience with exercise. Another example of transfer occurs in the teaching of problem solving. By teaching a client skills in solving a problem, such as alternative means of getting in and out of a wheelchair, the nurse gives the client some ideas about solving other problems of being confined to a wheelchair.

The nurse can aid the client in making the transfer of learning by helping the client associate a new situation with familiar situations. A good teacher is one who not only introduces new information but also helps the learner develop new ideas by putting together new information and old and synthesizing a unique understanding that is personally useful.

Individualization

In working with any learner, the nurse must take into account the individuality of that person. *Individualization* means structuring a learning activity to meet the unique needs and perceptions of the learner. Different people learn at different rates. They have unique perceptions. The nurse must assess not only what is unique about each person but also what approaches will be most useful with that particular person. Certainly, there are many qualities that most learners have in common, but readiness factors vary for each learner. The nurse's task is to make a comprehensive enough assessment to teach a client in the most effective manner possible.

A nurse may have two clients with the same apparent need, but the approach to each will be different, as shown in this example:

Bradley Johnson has two clients who both need to learn about appropriate discipline for a 4-year-old child. Ms. Kominsky is a high school graduate who enjoys reading and has willingly sought assistance for other child-rearing concerns. Mr. Johnson provided her with reading material about child development and discipline, followed with a discussion to help relate the written examples to specific problems Ms. Kominsky has encountered in disciplining her child.
The other client is Ms. Papper. She has an eighth-grade education, hates to read, and has three older children whom she has never learned to discipline appropriately. Mr. Johnson discussed with her specific issues about discipline and how they relate to all her children. He used terminology appropriate to her education and broke the teaching up into small segments with frequent opportunities for Ms. Papper to describe recent disciplinary problems.

In this example, Mr. Johnson took each client's strengths and problems into consideration before deciding on a response. Although the content he taught was the same, the manner in which he approached it was adapted to each client.

Evaluation

In order to make the teaching process a meaningful component in nursing service, evaluation must be possible and it must be carried out. *Evaluation* is the "systematic process of judging the worth, desirability, effectiveness, or adequacy of something according to definite criteria and purposes" (Harris, 1968, p. 95). The evaluation of learning is directly related to the goals and objectives that have been set. If the learner is able to achieve the established objectives, the nurse can conclude that learning has occurred. The evaluation of teaching is based on two criteria: the effectiveness of the teaching in helping the client reach the set objectives, and the nurse's ability to take into account such factors as the client's readiness, motivation, individuality, satisfaction, transfer, and participation, as well as to maintain a conducive learning environment. Furthermore, the nurse's effectiveness as a teacher may also be evaluated in terms of efficiency, timeliness, appropriateness, and skillfulness. Evaluation will be discussed at length later in this chapter.

THE TEACHING PLAN

Once a learning need is identified as part of the assessment of a client, a teaching plan is developed. This is an extension of the nursing process and is based on the data already gathered about the client. The steps in the teaching process are:

1. Assessing the client
2. Setting objectives
3. Selecting content
4. Selecting a teaching strategy
5. Implementing the strategy
6. Evaluating outcomes

Assessing the client

A learning need may become apparent through overt (direct) means, such as a client directly stating that she wishes to learn something. The nurse may directly perceive a learning need by observing the client's behavior, such as when a client demonstrates how he gives himself an insulin injection. The nurse may become aware of a need for learning in a covert (indirect) manner. For example, an adolescent girl may request information on conception control. In talking with her, the nurse may discover the girl's underlying need to learn how to handle relationships so that she does not feel compelled to become sexually active before she is emotionally ready.

Once the need has been identified, the nurse assesses the client to develop a baseline of information that will help to make decisions about the remainder of the process. Many of the elements of the data base were included in the section on teaching and learning principles. The elements would include the following information about the learner as applicable:

1. Age
2. Sex
3. Readiness
   a. Physical
   b. Psychological
   c. Intellectual
   d. Cultural and social
   e. Value

4. Motivation

5. Transferable learning

Some of these factors may seem inapplicable to a given situation, but they often create difficulties if they are not taken into account. For example, a person's feelings about being a learner and about past learning experiences may seem incidental. In practice, these feelings and memories may have a significant impact on what the client is able to learn. If a given client feels that he should be passive in a learning situation, he may not ask questions or reveal misunderstandings. He may fear the nurse will ridicule him or put him on the spot if he indicates a lack of knowledge. This can certainly lead to problems when the client later tries to apply what the nurse has attempted to teach.

After assessing the factors listed, the nurse further examines the relationships among the factors to determine possible affects on the client's learning. For example, there might be a connection between the client's relationships with significant others and the client's abilities. A woman might be intellectually capable of solving a household problem, yet she might feel that she should defer to her husband's judgment. A young man might express a desire to learn how to lose weight but might seem unable to implement a nutritional and exercise plan that he is physically and intellectually able to manage. A further assessment might reveal a lack of motivation caused by pressure from friends and family to remain overweight.

Setting Objectives

Once the nurse and client have completed the assessment phase, they are ready to set learning objectives. The objectives may be intended to meet learning needs in one or more of the domains of learning.

Domains of Learning

The *cognitive* domain is the acquisition and application of knowledge. The *affective* domain includes development of attitudes, values, appreciations, personal adjustment, and personal interests. The *psychomotor* domain involves the development of specific motor abilities. It is important to set objectives in all the domains that are applicable to a particular learning need. For example, a person who has recently been hospitalized as a result of cardiovascular disease, and who must change her daily activities, will have needs in all three domains. The client will need to understand her new physical limitations (cognitive domain), make attitudinal changes (affective domain), and change her activity patterns (psychomotor domain).

Goals and Objectives

A *goal* is the end toward which effort is directed. It may be global and somewhat abstract. For example, a goal might be that the client will not have another heart attack. Another global goal would be that the client will function optimally within the limits of her cardiovascular disease. *Objectives* are explicit expressions of behaviors or attitudes that contribute to reaching goals. Learning objectives describe what the learner will be like after completing the learning experience. They specify the behavior the learner will be able to demonstrate and the content relative to that behavior. For example, following are three objectives, each in a different domain, that are applicable to the client with cardiovascular disease. The behavior in each one is in *italics* and the content is in **boldface** type.

Cognitive domain: The client will *select and eat* **foods low in cholesterol.**

Affective domain: The client will be *willing to comply* with **exercise and diet limitations.**

Psychomotor domain: The client will *demonstrate* **exercises that promote cardiac function.**

Evaluation

In addition to clearly specifying behavior and content, the objectives must be *measurable.* This means that the presence of the behavior can be directly demonstrated. For example, the first objective above could be measured by asking the client to keep a food diary that the nurse could assess. The affective objective could be measured by the client's continued adherence to the dietary and exercise regimens. The psychomotor objective could be evaluated by the client's demonstrating the particular exercises prescribed.

In writing objectives that relate to the cognitive and psychomotor domains in particular, the nurse and the client will have a clearer idea of what is to be accomplished if the behavior is stated as explicitly as possible. For example, instead of using terms such as "know," "understand," or "recall," use words such as "list," "state," "select," or "perform." Be clear about what the nurse must see in order to determine whether the client has met the objective.

In measuring objectives in the affective domain, the nurse must rely on less direct indicators. For example, for the affective-domain objective listed above, the indicators of willing compliance would have to be indirect. Although the client might state

that she was willing to comply, the nurse must determine whether the client actually does comply voluntarily. Another affective objective might be that the client would accept the changes brought on by her cardiovascular condition. In this case, acceptance would be measured by the client's adherence to the life-style dictated by her condition and doing so with a positive attitude. Affective objectives take longer to achieve because they require attitudinal changes that affect beliefs and self-concept. A client might make an intellectual choice to change and might change his or her behavior before he or she is able to accept or appreciate the need for change.

Selecting Content

The selection of content grows from the objectives. The *content* is the material or information necessary to promote the client's meeting the objectives. If the objectives are clear, they will include a statement of the nature of the content to be used. If the cardiac client is to select and eat foods low in cholesterol, the nurse obviously must provide information about foods to choose and foods to avoid. The nurse would show the client how to obtain information from labels or other sources as to cholesterol levels of commercially prepared foods.

Determining content involves making decisions about the level of information to provide, as well as about the ways in which content can best be communicated. Some clients with limited education or with low motivation need specific guidelines to follow and a great deal of assistance. With such a client, who might become easily confused or who might make inappropriate choices when in doubt, the nurse might prepare a list of acceptable options and give a warning: "If in doubt, don't." Better-educated or highly motivated clients can obtain worthwhile information from appropriate resources besides the nurse. The nurse can give them references suitable for their educational levels and rely on them to ask questions when they have doubts.

One of the most difficult aspects of determining content is selecting the appropriate amount of information. The nurse must provide sufficient material on an acceptable level, without overloading the client and without insulting the client's intelligence. One extreme might be giving a college graduate a simplistic pamphlet meant for children or for poor readers. The other extreme would be to give a pregnant woman a college textbook on obstetrical problems. Most people do not need to understand oxygen exchange at the cellular level in order to appreciate the need for adequate ventilation. However, there is a temptation for those who teach content to teach as much as they know, whether the learner needs to know that much or not.

The nurse should have a complete, written outline of the topics to be covered and the information to be included under each topic. Having this in writing ensures that everything will be discussed. The outline will help the nurse decide how much time to allow and will give some clues about teaching methods the nurse might select.

Selecting a Teaching Strategy

Managing the Learning Environment

Managing the learning environment includes timing, pacing and providing an environment conducive to learning. The nurse who endeavors to teach clients effectively will have many opportunities for creativity in managing the learning situation. The following is an example of a nurse's response to a situation that might have adversely affected the learning environment.

A nurse planned to teach a group of other nurses about creativity in nursing practice. The room assignment had been made on the basis of the size of the class. When the nurse arrived, she found a small, windowless room with a sign on the door that read "The Dungeon." She thought that this was not the mental picture she had hoped to conjure up about creativity, so she tried to think of a more suitable designation for a small, dark, though fertile place—a place where ideas might be generated. Before the group arrived, she taped a new sign over the old one: "The Incubator."

It is always a good idea for the nurse who plans to teach a group to evaluate the surroundings in advance and to arrange for alternatives, if possible.

Although some people feel more comfortable and therefore participate more in an informal learning atmosphere, many people are made uncomfortable by such an atmosphere. The nurse may find it to be more effective to introduce physical arrangements that promote closeness gradually as the group members become familiar with one another. The nurse must assess each group and respond to that particular collection of people rather than assume that a given strategy will be useful.

It is best to prevent distractions in advance. In assessing the environment, the nurse should identify possible sources of distraction and make arrangements to circumvent them. For example, if the teaching is to occur in the client's home, the nurse can encourage the client to have radios and televisions turned off. Children may be given activities in other parts of the house to keep them occupied.

If distractions or noises become a problem during a teaching session, the nurse will have to use tact and directness to minimize or end the interruption. If the teaching is being conducted in the client's home, the nurse should ask directly that the television be turned off so that the nurse and client can better communicate. However, if the client declines to comply with the nurse's request, the nurse will have to make the best of the situation. If the noise is beyond the client's control, the nurse may be able to control it. For example, a nurse was teaching a group of clients in a community center. The session was pervaded by the loud music coming from a staff member's radio. The nurse left the room and asked the staff member to turn down the radio during the session. The nurse was assertive and explicit about the problem. The staff member quickly complied.

Occasionally, the subject matter involved in teaching may make ordinarily non-problematic environments unconducive to learning, as in the following situation.

Mary Lowe, a nursing student, had been asked by Janice Ingall to teach her about methods of conception control that do not involve devices or drugs. Ms. Lowe realized that this would entail the use of explicit terminology about sexual behavior, and she was concerned about the effect of such a discussion, since Ms. Ingall's 5-year-old daughter was always present during her visits. Ms. Ingall agreed that she would rather not have her daughter around during the conversation. The mother arranged to have the child play at a neighbor's house when Ms. Lowe returned.

Timing is an important aspect of managing the learning environment. The nurse must determine the right time for teaching to take place. If the learner is an individual client, the teaching may be done during a regular visit. If several people are to be involved, the nurse will work with them to find a time convenient to all. The nurse must consider the readiness and motivation of learners in deciding on time. Occasionally, a plan will have to be preempted because a client has a new need that takes priority over the teaching plan. On the other hand, nurses sometimes experience "teachable moments" while working

with clients. Malcolm Knowles (1970, pp. 46–47) used this phrase to describe those instances when a person is particularly open and ready to learn something. A nurse who is well prepared with general nursing knowledge and who has developed effective teaching skills will be able to take advantage of such moments.

The pacing of instruction is affected by the client's abilities, especially the rate at which the client grasps the content. It is relatively easy for the nurse to assess a single client's rate of learning. However, pacing becomes a challenge when the nurse begins teaching groups. Pacing is easier if the group members are fairly homogeneous in education, language abilities, knowledge of the topic, and motivation.

When planning to teach, the nurse should have some ideas about when to assess the appropriateness of the pace. The nurse can ask the learners for questions periodically or ask them to verify that they are following the discussion. The nurse should have alternative examples or descriptions available if clients need more explanation. The nurse should be able to perceive when sufficient examples have been given and should give only as much information as is needed. The nurse must determine in advance what material is essential and what might be deleted or summarized if time grows short or clients begin to lose interest.

Teaching Methods

The nurse must select a teaching method appropriate to the learners, the learning objectives, and the content. There are many methods, and four of the most commonly used will be discussed here.

LECTURE. At its worst, a lecture is a way of getting the information in the teacher's notes into the student's notes without having it pass through the minds of either of them. At its best, a lecture is an oral presentation of facts or ideas not readily available through other means. A lecture might present relationships among data that the learner has obtained from a variety of sources but has not been able to synthesize. A lecture might be used to emphasize important information from a vast amount available. A teacher might choose to lecture on a topic when the learners cannot read well enough to grasp material in that way.

A lecture is most suitable for groups, although the nurse may use this approach to relate specific information to an individual or family. It can be used effectively with people of any age group but must be varied in length and depth with people of various ages. Very young children can only attend for a few minutes, and even adults begin to lose interest after 20 minutes unless the subject matter or the lecturer is quite compelling. An effective lecture is concise, emphasizes no more than four or five points, and is presented in language suited to the learners.

When planning to lecture, begin by determining the main points relevant to the learning objectives. For example, a nursing student set an objective for an elderly client to be able to list three ways to avoid constipation. The student listed four kinds of foods (fresh vegetables, fresh fruits, whole grain cereals, and whole grain breads), an increase in fluid intake, and a daily walk as ways to avoid constipation. Identifying these specific things helped her to structure her lecture.

DISCUSSION. A discussion is an opportunity for an exchange of information between teacher and learner. Discussion permits the learner to ask questions and the teacher to know how much the learner understands. It is suitable for individuals or for groups. With groups, discussion may lose its effectiveness if the group is large and only a few

people actually interact with the teacher. The teacher will not be able to evaluate the learning of the nonparticipants, and they may lose interest. Even though a discussion is more informal than a lecture, the nurse should have specific objectives and content in mind. Frequently, a teacher will mingle lecture with discussion or will reserve a period of time after a lecture for discussion.

To conduct a discussion that promotes learning, the nurse must use communication techniques that encourage participation. For example, the nurse should ask open-ended questions that encourage the clients to elaborate and show whether they understand. The nursing student who taught the elderly client how to avoid constipation first told the client what kinds of foods were suitable and then asked the client what foods she thought fit into each group. The student then encouraged the client to name foods in each group she preferred and describe how she could prepare them more frequently.

Many people are shy about answering questions, because they have had unpleasant experiences in the past when they felt put on the spot by teachers. The nurse therefore should not assume that the client does not understand just because he or she is slow to respond. When the client does respond, the nurse must acknowledge and praise the contribution. If what the client says is incorrect, the nurse should point this out gently and help the client figure out the correct answer. If part of the answer is correct, the nurse should acknowledge this and build on it.

DEMONSTRATION. A demonstration is a display of behavior. Demonstration is particularly appropriate for teaching psychomotor skills. When demonstrating a skill, the teacher must demonstrate it correctly and completely. Mastering psychomotor skills includes not only learning the mo-tions involved but also the reasons behind them. For example, when a nurse changes a dressing she or he not only must be efficient in removing the soiled dressing and applying the new dressing but also must complete the task in an aseptic manner. Competence in performing the skill is determined by more than mere manual skill.

One way of teaching a skill is to begin by demonstrating the whole process, describing it as you go along. Then the teacher goes through the process again, breaking it down into its parts. After these two demonstrations, the nurse can give the learner an opportunity to attempt the parts of the process. At each appropriate point, the nurse must emphasize the other considerations besides the manual activity. As the client grasps the parts of the activity, the nurse can begin to raise questions about problems the client might encounter and suggest ways of coping with them. The demonstration sequence is completed by a final return demonstration by the client with the client explaining the process and its important aspects. If possible, the nurse should observe the client performing the skill in the actual setting. It will help to leave printed instructions or pictures of the skill being performed.

The nurse may share with the client devices he or she may use to help remember the correct sequence of steps in a technique. The client may also have had other experiences that will be useful in promoting the learning and retention of a skill. Psychomotor skills tend to be retained best if they are used frequently. However, if a nurse or client understands the principles behind a skill, it can be relearned more quickly.

ROLE PLAYING.   The simulation of a role is called *role playing*. Role playing may involve the assumption of a role usually performed by someone other than the role player, or it may involve the practicing of a new role that the role player wishes to develop. This approach is a particularly effective method to help people learn about situations involving interpersonal interactions. For example, Paul Harris, a head nurse, wanted to help Rosemary Dumas become more assertive in her interactions with other members of the health team. To accomplish this, Paul took the role of Rosemary and Rosemary took the role of one of the other nurses who intimidated her. Rosemary behaved the way that the other nurse did, a way that caused her to feel incompetent and to become tongue-tied. Paul responded in assertive ways to demonstrate alternative ways of reacting. After several practice interactions in those roles, they reversed roles, with Paul playing the troublesome nurse and Rosemary playing herself as an assertive person. Afterwards they discussed the strategies Rosemary felt most comfortable with.

It is often particularly helpful to play the role of the person you see as troublesome. This gives you an insight into that person's perspective. This alone can often improve interactions between you. Role playing also gives a learner the opportunity to try out new behaviors in a nonthreatening situation. Role playing may help the learner see that the real situation is not as threatening as it seems.

Many people feel self-conscious about role playing, even with only one other person present. This should be acknowledged if it seems to be a problem. Some people have difficulty because they cannot think of things to say or do. The nurse can assist by giving them some ideas to try. As the client begins to get involved, the nurse must stay in his or her role and reinforce the client's participation by responding in that role. After the initial attempt, the nurse might say something like, "I think you're getting the hang of this," and then suggest another interaction. If the role playing takes place in front of a group or involves several people, it is often helpful to give the observers a responsibility to look for particular things and to encourage them to remain passive. If roles have been given to several people, the nurse may give the group some time to collaborate on the general things they plan to do.

The nurse who participates in a role play should gauge her or his behavior to meet the abilities of the learner. In early attempts at role playing, the nurse may give the learner simple problems to tackle. As the learner grows more expert, the nurse can offer nuances that will make the role play more realistic. After completing the role play, the nurse and the learner, and the observers, if there are any, should discuss what was learned in terms of the objectives they were trying to achieve.

Instructional Aids

The use of instructional aids frequently enhances learning directly by providing information as well as indirectly by offering variety that maintains the learner's interest. An instructional aid is anything that contributes to the effectiveness of the teaching process. Some of the most familiar are visual aids, reading material, and mechanical devices. Equipment and models also are useful aids. An instructional aid should be appropriate to the content and should enhance the teaching process.

VISUAL AIDS. The most common visual aids are posters, photographs, drawings, slides, transparencies, and films. A visual aid should be simple, specific, and direct. A nurse who was talking to a group about car safety seats might use a slide projected in a large enough size so that all members of the group could view and discuss it at the same time. If the nurse were trying to em-

phasize the seat itself, she might show it isolated at first, and then later show a picture of it properly placed in an automobile. In general, posters and pictures should be uncluttered and should attract the viewer's attention.

READING MATERIAL. Reading material includes pamphlets, brochures, and handouts. Such material should be printed in type that is easy to read. The information should be concise and understandable. Often, pictures or graphics will help attract attention and interest a person in reading what is contained in a pamphlet.

The reading level of the material must be appropriate to the learner. In addition, uncommon or medical terms should be clearly defined. If the material is meant for people who do not read English well, the nurse should look for written materials in the language usually used by the clients.

MECHANICAL DEVICES. Mechanical devices used as teaching aids include audiotape recorders, videotape recorders, film and slide projectors, and overhead projectors. The user should be familiar with the equipment and with any problems that commonly arise with it. Immediately before using such equipment, the teacher should make sure it is working properly. The teacher should have an alternate plan in case the equipment breaks down.

Recorders may be used to record interactions or demonstrations for playback and discussion. Projectors are used in showing visual presentations to enhance an oral presentation. Another mechanical device that is sometimes used if the size of the group warrants it is a microphone. As with other equipment, it should be tested in advance to see that it is working. Whenever the space or the group size warrants it, the teacher should use a microphone.

EQUIPMENT AND MODELS. Nurses who teach clients psychomotor skills they will be using in their own homes need equipment similar to what the client will be using. The nurse may also go to the client's home and demonstrate the actual equipment. In addition, the nurse may provide samples of items which might be used to replace equipment.

Models are three-dimensional representations of objects. Nurses frequently use demonstration models of various parts of the human anatomy. For example, a nurse can use a model of a human pelvis to demonstrate the way a fetus lies within the mother's body. Models of breasts are used to teach clients how to do breast examinations and to demonstrate what different kinds of normal and abnormal tissue feel like within the breast.

The Teaching Strategy

The *teaching strategy* is the method the teacher uses to accomplish the learning objectives. Based on client needs, the nurse decides on a time, a place, who the learners are to be, and the various methods to use. The nurse makes all necessary arrangements: scheduling, securing the necessary location and equipment, and notifying the learners.

Evaluating Outcomes

The final step in the teaching process is evaluation. There are two major areas of evaluation in teaching: the evaluation of the learner and the evaluation of the teacher. The learner is evaluated for his or her achievement of the objectives that were set.

The skill of the nurse as a teacher is evaluated to some extent on the basis of the client's success in meeting the objectives. In addition, the nurse should also assess his or her effectiveness in each of the steps of the process. Starting with the assessment phase and going through to the implementation stage, the nurse should examine what he or she did and the value of each activity. For example, the nurse might consider the thoroughness of the data collection process. Was the learning need appropriate and significant? Were the objectives clearly stated and measurable? Were the correct methods chosen, and were they implemented effectively? Were the instructional aids useful and suitable? How did the nurse handle unexpected problems, such as interruptions or restlessness on the part of the client?

Before the plan is implemented, the nurse should have specific evaluation criteria in mind. Additional criteria may become apparent as the process goes on, but some of the preceding questions should be considered, and the nurse should plan to be able to answer them at the end of the process.

Evaluation may actually signal only the end of a phase of the nurse–client relationship. The evaluation may lead to the identification of further problems that warrant another teaching activity. Like many parts of the nursing process, the teaching process tends to become a recurrent strategy in working with clients.

Implementing Strategy

If the nurse has used good judgment and has made good decisions throughout the earlier steps in the teaching process, the implementation should go smoothly. The following abbreviated version of a student's plan illustrates the entire process.*

---

* The author acknowledges Pat Vernon, a nursing student at the University of Oklahoma, for giving permission to use this example.

ASSESSMENT

The client is an 83-year-old woman who has various dietary problems that she has identified. She does not drink milk and gets little calcium in any other way. She rarely drinks fluids. She sometimes skips meals because she does not like eating alone. Her vision is poor and she walks with a cane. She is eager and receptive about learning about better nutrition. She has a full set of dentures and prefers soft foods. She occasionally has problems with constipation that she relieves with Metamucil. *Nursing diagnosis:* Inadequate nutritional and fluid intake related to lack of knowledge about proper nutrition for her age.

OBJECTIVES

The client will:

1. List the four basic food groups, the number of servings needed each day per group, and four foods in each group.
2. List the reasons she should take in 1200 ml of fluids per day, and three ways she can do this.
3. List four ways to avoid constipation.

CONTENT

1. Four basic food groups; number of servings required; examples.
2. Rationale for fluid intake; suggestions for making fluids more palatable and available.
3. At least four ways to avoid constipation, including food and fluid intake and exercise

STRATEGY

Agreed on a time with the client. Decided to do the teaching in two sessions because she felt she could not learn it all at once. The home environment is quiet and few interruptions occur during regular visits, so this seemed to be a good environment. The methods chosen were lecture/discussion and demonstration. Visual aids were used, such as pamphlets and a poster.

IMPLEMENTATION

Shared the information with the client, allowing her many opportunities for questions. Periodically encouraged her to give examples of such things as favorite foods in a food group. Went to the kitchen and demonstrated measuring appropriate serving sizes and asked her to return the demonstration. Used brightly colored pamphlets with bold, easy-to-read lettering to show the food groups, and left the pamphlets with her.

EVALUATION OF CLIENT

Objective 1. Client was able to list the four food groups, specify serving sizes and numbers, and give examples.

Objective 2. Client was able to explain why she needed more fluids. She identified ways she could increase her fluids, and she started doing so.

Objective 3. Client was able to repeat four ways of avoiding constipation and she began to try two of them.

EVALUATION OF NURSE

Effective methods were used and were implemented correctly. Content selected was relevant and presented on an appropriate level. The client said the nurse did a good job and that she enjoyed the information.

In the clinical experience in which the nursing student implemented the teaching plan briefly described here, the student documented each step much more extensively. When learning to use the process, such extensive written records of the plan are necessary. The abbreviated version shown here is comparable to what a practicing nurse might actually record when working with a client.

WORKING WITH ADULT LEARNERS

Malcolm Knowles identified four assumptions about adult learners that are different from the assumptions made about child learners (Knowles, 1970):

1. Adult learners think of themselves as self-directing human beings.

2. They have accumulated a store of experiences that contributes to learning.

3. Their readiness to learn is directly related to their need to accomplish the developmental tasks of their social roles.

4. They want immediately applicable knowledge. Their orientation toward learning is problem centered rather than subject centered.

The implications of these assumptions are many. Since adults are self-directing, they must be involved in the entire learning process from planning to evaluation. Their experiences are important and useful in promoting learning. The things they want to learn have a direct application to their daily lives. They want to learn things that are useful and that will help them to solve problems.

Whether they are teaching clients principles that will improve their health, or teaching a group of nurses about a new approach to the nursing treatment of a communicable disease, nurses will find these assumptions useful. For example, a nurse who is teaching a group of colleagues must remember that these people are adults whose experiences may be applicable to the content being discussed. A nurse may be able to motivate adult learners by identifying a direct application of the information to the learners' own lives.

FUTURE IMPLICATIONS

In *Deschooling Society,* Ivan Illich stated that "for most men the right to learn is curtailed by the obligation to attend school" (p. iv). Illich advocated "learning webs," which would bring people together as necessary to learn what and when they wanted or needed. He recognized that people learn throughout their lives and that overly structured approaches to teaching and learning often discourage people from participating. Other writers have noted the excessive amount of evaluation that takes place in educational situations. Grades tend to become equated with the person receiving them. We call people "A students" and "C students" as if we could easily sum up everything about a person in that way.

Marilyn Ferguson (1980) pointed out that the uncomfortable feelings we have about learning have their origin in the classroom. Schools were designed in a time when little was known about the human mind and about learning. The scientific investigation of learning is still in its infancy, and the discoveries that are being made are slow to come into practice. Parents are fearful and suspicious of unfamiliar curricula. They are concerned about their children learning the "basics," whatever they are.

The reason that it is important to consider the schools when considering health teaching is that the nurses who are now being prepared have had their learning patterns determined by their early schooling. The learners of the present and the near future also have had their patterns set by their school experiences. However, we are on the brink of a transformation in the educational system as in other systems in our society. The new paradigm will be to look at "the nature of learning rather than methods of instruction" (Ferguson, 1980, p. 288).

Does that mean that you just read this whole chapter only to find out that you do not need to know this material? The answer is no—and yes. To work with learners now, it is useful to know how to teach in ways familiar to both teacher and learners. Nurses who will graduate in the latter half of the twentieth century need tools to function. However, it is conceivable that while those same nurses are still practicing they will begin to encounter new kinds of learners.

The new learners will have studied curricula that emphasize personal growth, flexibility, creativity, and autonomy. There are already schools that feature these transforming qualities, but not enough. Youngsters are learning to determine their own learning needs earlier in their schooling. They are interacting with highly sophisticated technology as early as the first grade. By the time they reach high school, their knowledge base is often equivalent to that of a high school graduate of 20 years ago. By the turn of the century, much, if not most, of the content offered at a college level today will be readily available to high school students.

The availability of computers will make it unnecessary for people to store the information in their own heads that it used to take them many years to acquire. In the near future, nurses will participate in designing learning packages for use on personal computer systems. For example, these resource materials may include exercise regimens or dietary instructions for a multitude of needs. Programs may assist the consumer in summarizing personal data that can be communicated to a physician or nurse to speed the process of diagnosis.

Cable television stations may carry programs to help consumers determine their learning needs and then provide information to meet these needs. Interactive television systems are already in use in some parts of the United States. In addition to requesting information, consumers will be able to obtain health-oriented materials prepared by nurses.

Marilyn Ferguson says that "if we are not learning and teaching we are not awake and alive. Learning is not only like health, it *is* health" (1980, p. 282). Health promotion is teaching. The more clients learn about themselves and their own well-being, the more able they will be to maintain or increase their level of wellness. Nursing in the future will be the process of facilitating the wellness of clients, just as teaching is the process of facilitating the learning of students. This also has broader implications: nurses must be as concerned about the schools and the rest of the educational system as they are about the health care system. Nurses must be aware of the current learning research and how it applies to teaching and health promotion.

SUMMARY

The purposes of this chapter were to enable the student to prepare, implement, and evaluate a teaching plan for a client, group of clients, or colleagues. Students and nurses should consider the more liberating educational system of the future that we can all help to build. In this system, education and health care will overlap at many points for the benefit and enrichment of both.

DISCUSSION TOPICS

1. Neal Sorensen, 25 years old, asks the nurse for some instruction or assistance on giving up smoking. Paul Moore, 48 years old, has been encouraged by his physician to give up smoking. Contrast the individual factors that might affect these two men's learning and the nurse's teaching.

2. Debbie Martin is trying to breast feed her infant but has been having some difficulty since she came home from the hospital. She feels a great deal of commitment to breast feeding, but she has received some discouraging comments from her husband

and her mother. Write three learning objectives that would be applicable to this situation. Identify the behavior and the content in each objective. Describe how you would measure each objective.

3. You have been hired by the city council to offer public classes on the topic "A Healthy Life-Style." Those attending will be adults, and the class size will be limited to 25 people. What are some of the factors you should consider in preparing your presentation? Discuss issues that relate to managing the learning environment and the assumptions about adult learners identified in this chapter.

4. How would you go about preparing a package of learning materials related to

health promotion that could be used in a personal computer system? How would you plan for individuality of the users?

5. What would you do if you were teaching a client who was more assertive and self-directed about learning than you were? What feelings would the situation evoke? How could you handle it if you felt threatened by such an independent learner?

6. Researchers have discovered that there is apparently no single place in the brain where learned information is stored. It seems that once something is learned, we know it with our whole brain (Ferguson, 1982). What is the most incredible thing you could imagine as a future discovery about human learning?

BIBLIOGRAPHY

Bigge, M.L.: *Learning theories for teachers.* New York: Harper & Row, 1964.

Bloom, B.S. (ed.): *Taxonomy of educational objectives. Handbook I: Cognitive domain.* New York: David McKay, 1956.

Dewey, J.: *How we think.* Boston: D.C. Heath, 1933.

Eble, K.E.: *The Craft of Teaching.* San Francisco: Jossey-Bass, 1976.

Eisner, E.W.: Instruction, teaching, and learning. *Elementary School Journal* 64, 115–119, 1964.

Ferguson, M.: *The Aquarian conspiracy.* Los Angeles: J.P. Tarcher, 1980.

Ferguson, M.: Aquarian conspiracy update: Personal and social transformations in the 1980s. Public lecture, University of Oklahoma, Norman, Oklahoma, October, 1982.

Gowin, D.B.: Teaching, learning, and thirdness. *Studies in Philosophy and Education* 1, 87–113, 1961.

Harris, W.: The nature and function of educational evaluation. *Peabody Journal of Education* 46, 95–99, 1968.

Hyman, R.T.: *Ways of teaching.* Philadelphia: Lippincott, 1970.

Illich, I.: *Deschooling society.* New York: Perennial Library, 1970.

Jones, D.A.: Health promotion through health teaching. In D.A. Jones, C. Dunbar, & M.M. Jirovec, *Medical-surgical nursing: A conceptual approach* (2nd ed.). New York: McGraw-Hill, 1982.

Knowles, M.S.: *The modern practice of adult education.* New York: Association Press, 1970.

Knowles, M.S.: *The adult learner: A neglected species* (2nd ed.). Houston: Gulf Publishing, 1978.

Krathwohl, D.R., Bloom, B.S., Masia, B.B.: *Taxonomy of educational objectives. Handbook II: Affective domain.* New York: David McKay, 1964.

Luckman, J., & Sorensen, K.C.: *Medical-surgical nursing* (2nd ed.), Philadelphia: Saunders, 1980.

Mager, R.F.: *Measuring instructional intent.* Belmont, Calif.: Lear Siegler/Fearon Publishers, 1973.

Mullins, L.: *Immature people with power! How to handle them,* Tulsa, OK: Actionizing, Inc., 1982.

Smith, B.O.: A concept of learning. *Teachers College Record* 61, 229–241, 1960.

18

Using Group Theory

Janet Sullivan Wilson

No man is an island, entire of itself, every man is a piece of the continent, a part of the main; if a clod be washed away by the sea, Europe is the less, as well as if a promontory were, as well as if a manor of thy friends or of thine own were; any man's death diminishes me, because I am involved in mankind; and therefore never send to know for whom the bell tolls; it tolls for thee.

JOHN DONNE

OBJECTIVES

After reading this chapter, you should be able to:

☐ Discuss the development of small group process theory.
☐ Describe the variety of groups available in nursing practice.
☐ Describe the phases of small groups.
☐ Define and describe small group process concepts.
☐ Apply group process concepts to nursing practice.

INTRODUCTION

We are all social beings; we gravitate to one another. In order to understand human behavior, it is necessary to study how people relate in groups.

A *group* may be defined as two or more people who interact and influence each other toward some common purpose or goal. The key part of this definition is com-monality. The people walking up and down a street are not a group, but if a number of them see a burglary in progress and go to help, they become a group that has some goal and purpose in common (Olmsted, 1967).

Small groups (about 6–20 people) have somewhat different dynamics than large groups. This chapter deals primarily with small groups, although some of the princi-

287

ples cited are common to both small and large groups.

All groups have two main functions: to satisfy the psychosocial needs of their individual members and to work on or complete the group's goals, whether they are stated or unstated. Research has shown that when these two tasks are not fulfilled, the group tends to dissolve (Olmsted, 1967).

A group can exert a powerful influence over an individual's behavior. Therefore, a nurse can use the group to foster a higher degree of health in individuals. Another value of groups is that their overall effect is more than the sum of their parts. This is the concept of synergy: a group, working together, can accomplish more than the individual members could alone. Growth toward health can at times be greatly facilitated in a group setting.

Historically, groups of individuals who have pursued common goals and lived and worked in the same time and place have influenced each other to produce some extraordinary outcomes. The story of the discovery of the double helix of DNA is just such an example: a group of scientists who influenced each other as they struggled against time to identify the DNA structure (Watson, 1968). Arieti (1976) identifies group interaction as a factor that can foster creativity.

THE STUDY OF SMALL-GROUP BEHAVIOR: A REVIEW

The 1940s

Before the 1940s there was a dearth of information about small-group processes. There was some interest in how problems are solved in groups, but not until the late 1930s did Kurt Lewin, a German psychologist living in America, and his fellow researchers begin studying how different methods of leadership affect group members' behavior. Group climate and norms, the impact of shared beliefs, intergroup conflict, styles of leadership (autocratic, democratic, and laissez faire) and the attraction among group members came under scientific investigation for the first time (Zander, 1979).

Lewin, in particular, was influenced by the events of World War II, and he was most interested in how people's attitudes could be changed in groups. Observing the negative impact of the Hitler youth groups, Lewin became interested in how groups could be used to produce positive attitude changes to support a democratic society.

Remember the social climate these early researchers were working under: World War II was being fought; democratic society was being threatened; there was a fear that dictators could manipulate the thoughts and actions of many people. The public was very interested in the new group research and hoped it would shed light on how a democratic society could derive strength from the effective functioning of its groups.

In 1947, the National Education Association organized the National Training Laboratory (NTL) for group development. This was where community leaders could go to learn about groups and more effective management techniques. Here the students talked with each other and their researchers about the interactions going on within their own groups. This added a dimension not foreseen in the original study of groups: personal feelings. Though the NTL did not originally intend to delve into feelings or psychology, this might have foreshadowed the later movement toward a focus on the individual's personal growth within the group.

The 1950s

The 1950s brought an outpouring of research in the social psychology of groups. Many group training labs were founded, some of which emphasized personal feelings and growth rather than group research. People who criticized these labs claimed that they engendered an overabundance of stress in the participants without providing support or benefit. Defenders said they were doing research about group behavior, not counseling individuals. By the end of the 1950s, it was evident that the group-research movement was becoming unwieldly, not only in the number of studies but also in the organization of the findings. (Zander, 1979).

The 1960s

During the 1960s, scientific investigations about group process decreased while interest in the individual increased. Although group dynamics courses were firmly entrenched in universities, major centers for the study of groups closed across the country.

There are several reasons for this shift of emphasis from the group to the individual. The social climate of the 1960s helped foster the emphasis on individual behavior and feelings. Also, early expectations that group research would provide answers to society's problems never materialized. In fact, during the 1960s, individuals questioned the larger group's right to decide their fate. We were involved in an unpopular war in Vietnam; the country at large lacked a sense of purpose or group cohesion. The general populace did not trust the outcome of group research, and social scientists' interest dwindled as well. The once-vital network of scientists who strove to provide a coherent theory of group process dissolved.

The 1970s

Group research in the 1970s continued to focus on such topics as sources of group cohesiveness, cooperative versus competitive groups, group structure, sources of social pressure in groups, and problem solving. Even though funding dried up and the number of agencies that supported group research decreased, there was still some group research taking place.

Self-help and "quickie" personal-growth groups continued to proliferate, much to the distress of many professionals, who saw them as big business for the leaders but little help (if not a hindrance) to the group members.

The 1980s and the Future

Current nursing literature describes the multitude of groups that exist, but there is little investigation of how groups function to care for the sick or prevent disease. This area is ripe for nursing researchers to explore. With increasing health care costs, group treatment becomes a more practical means for the client as well as the caregiver. Some questions that could be asked are:

1. Is medication compliance enhanced when a client participates in group versus individual follow-up?
2. What is the effect of postcoronary care group treatment on recovery rates?
3. How can we apply group dynamic concepts to health education in the community?

4. In parent support groups, what are the phases of adjustment to a child's disability?

MAJOR TYPES OF SMALL GROUPS

The community health nurse will be involved with a variety of groups whose purpose is to promote health and prevent disease. The roles the nurse may assume with these groups are varied. The nurse may be the leader or coleader of a therapeutic group. For example, he or she may lead a cancer support group, a group for parents of asthmatic children, a new-mothers' group, a stress-reduction group, an adolescent disability group, or a renal transplant recipient group. The community health nurse has the unique opportunity of assessing community needs and initiating group experience as necessary. For example, the nurse may determine that a number of clients with new colostomies might benefit from meeting with one another. This could be the impetus for a colostomy support group.

At other times the nurse will recommend and refer clients to particular groups. This means that the nurse must know what groups are available and be able to help clients find the group to meet their needs. This is true of group psychotherapy.

When a community does not have a group to meet an identified health need, the community health nurse can influence other professionals to fill the gap. For example, a community health nurse, when talking to a mother of a disabled adolescent, might identify the need for adolescents with physical disabilities to meet in a group for support. If such a group is not available, the community health nurse might stimulate some colleagues to begin one.

Psychotherapeutic Groups

Psychotherapeutic groups use the principles of group process to treat psychopathology, reduce emotional stress, and modify behavior. The group becomes a microcosm of original family relationships in that longstanding problems and strengths in interpersonal relationships are eventually transferred to members within the group. The therapist focuses on these interpersonal problems, identifying and exploring the historic precedents and alternatives to destructive behavior. Over time, the patients model the therapist's behavior. Examining problems in interpersonal relationships becomes one of the early group tasks. The relearning and practicing of healthier relationships within the group becomes the corrective emotional experience for the clients. This learning, theoretically, can be transferred to people outside the group.

How does group psychotherapy treat emotional illness? Though the research is scant, Yalom (1970) lists ten "curative factors" in groups:

1. Imparting of information about emotional health and illness, and about ways to alter behavior.

2. Instillation of hope of improvement.

3. Universality: people are more like one another than not (the "we're all in the same boat" philosophy).

4. Altruism: clients help one another and learn new ways of coping from each other.

5. Corrective recapitulation of the primary family group: reality testing with a new group.

6. Development of socializing techniques: basic social skills are learned through interaction.

7. Imitative behavior: clients copy the

therapist's behavior and can try out new ways of dealing with old problems.

8. Interpersonal learning: the group is a microcosm of the real world and members learn healthier interactions.

9. Group cohesiveness: acceptance of people as a group entity.

10. Catharsis: ventilation of positive and negative feelings.

Though Yalom examines these curative factors in the context of group therapy, they may apply to all groups. Research needs to be done to validate this assumption. How and why these factors tend to decrease psychopathology is not known.

Several factors affect the nature of the psychotherapeutic group. The theoretical framework (psychoanalytic, *gestalt*, interpersonal, etc.) determines the philosophy and type of interventions employed by the therapist. The technique and personality of the therapist and the goals, composition, and activity of the group all are variables affecting the outcome.

Wolf (1967) identifies five major types of psychotherapy groups:

1. *Reeducative Group Therapy.* Lectures and group discussion provide information and support for a homogeneous group.

2. *Psychodrama Group.* Uses psychoanalytic theory to interpret dramatizations and role plays of clients' conflicts.

3. *Experiential Existential Group Therapy.* Focuses on the experiencing and releasing of repressed feelings.

4. *Group Dynamic Group Therapy.* Group themes, communications, interactions, and reactions are explored rather than individual psychopathology.

5. *Psychoanalytic Group Therapy.* Principles of psychoanalysis—the unconscious, transference, resistance, dream material, childhood experiences—are employed.

Community health nurses do not become group therapists. However, they see many clients with emotional problems who might be referred for group treatment. Knowing whom to contact in the community and being able to interpret what group therapy is all about is necessary to the nurse.

Counseling Groups

Counseling groups use group psychotherapy techniques but have as their primary objectives prevention and education rather than treatment. While psychotherapy groups treat emotional stress, counseling groups deal with essentially "normal" or healthy individuals. The participants are people who are experiencing situational crises arising from illness, disease, or accidents or developmental crises arising from inadequate coping at a critical stage of growth (Marram, 1973).

Community health nurses are most likely to use their group knowledge in counseling groups. Groups made up of drug addicts, unwed mothers, delinquent youths, alcoholics, school phobic children, people with cancer living at home, hemodialysis homecare clients, or the elderly are some of those the community health nurse will see in the community. These groups may be located in homes for delinquent youths or unwed mothers, neighborhood centers, churches, youth centers, mental health clinics, or storefront clinics.

Groups such as these can provide factual information about community services and the health care system in addition to help with problem solving and dealing with daily activities. The community health nurse is a valuable resource to these groups.

Groups are also initiated within schools. Developmental crises very often take the form of school problems: drug abuse, sexual acting out, learning defects, and racial tensions (Marram, 1973). In such situations, groups function to provide role models, either through the leader or through stable group members who reinforce acceptable behaviors.

The selection of the group members depends upon the type of problem presented. Generally, clients known to be emotionally ill are not taken into this type of group, since the goal is not treatment.

Self-Help Groups

Self-help groups are different from other groups in that they are organized and run by the people they are helping. Professionals usually are not the leaders unless they are in the group to receive help themselves. Alcoholics Anonymous, Narcotics Anonymous, and Weight Watchers are a few well-known self-help groups. They function to inspire their members toward a more healthful way of living. This is done not by restructuring the personality but by concrete, day-to-day advice shared by members who have, for example, stopped drinking, stopped taking drugs, or lost weight. The group members themselves serve as the role models for new members and provide the support needed for improvement. Much socialization occurs within these groups, and friendly competition often develops. Sharing of "war stories" is a typical activity, and this serves to inspire other members to overcome obstacles. This is a repressive–inspirational technique. Insight and digging up the past are discouraged in these groups.

The basic premise of self-help groups is

that in order to help others with their problems, you must have gone down the same path yourself and found your way back. This attitude may be threatening to professionals who feel that they have the knowledge and expertise to solve the particular problems. Historically, self-help groups have done remarkably well in getting their members to stop drinking, lose weight, or adjust to a handicap.

How does the professional nurse work with self-help groups? First, the nurse can be a resource person, providing information about health or illness and about ways to maneuver through the health care delivery system. Second, the nurse can assist clients' efforts to attend meetings and support them in their efforts to help themselves. Ultimately, nurses should advocate their clients doing what is in their own best interests.

Colostomy, laryngectomy, and mastectomy clubs are examples of self-help groups that help with physical disabilities. They function in much the same way as other self-help groups, often providing clients and families with a wealth of practical information and support during the rehabilitation phase.

Training Groups

Kurt Lewin is the father of the *T-group*. During the 1940s, Lewin was asked to help the Connecticut Interracial Commission work on intergroup tensions. The idea was to train community leaders to deal more effectively with racial tensions and to help change negative racial attitudes. In 1946, Lewin organized a workshop in which three groups of 10 members each met with a group leader and analyzed interactional problems presented by the members. The group helped define and seek alternative solutions to the problems presented. A researcher observed and recorded the group's behavior and progress.

During the evenings, the researchers and group leaders met to discuss the group members' behavior. Eventually, group members were allowed to participate in these sessions, and it was discovered that the members profited greatly by being confronted with observations about their own behavior. They also learned about group dynamics, interpersonal relations, and the effect of their personalities on the group and vice versa. The effect was to teach the members behaviors that were constructive for the group's tasks. Lewin and his colleagues realized that they had found a method of changing attitudes by helping the trainees to see themselves as others saw them. The process was an educative experience in human relations that did not delve into individual psychopathology. Research and study of the group's behavior were two priorities of the T-group.

Today T-groups function in much the same manner. Self-awareness, intellectual understanding of group functioning, and awareness of others are the outcomes sought. The group has a leader and recorder; the leader focuses on the members' intellectual understanding of group functioning and dynamics (Marram, 1973). Such phenomena as group stages, group norms, and facilitating of group roles are applied to analyzing the members' behavior. The result is cognitive awareness of how a group works and heightened sensitivity to other people and how one reacts to others.

Over the years the T-group has been widely used in business to help managers become more sensitive to employees, and it has been used to teach professional nurses about group dynamics. Organizations, schools, governments, and corporations have all used T-group trainers as change agents. The T-group helps individuals relate more honestly to one another; the total enhancement of the individual is a goal.

Although therapy groups and T-groups have some similar functions, there are many differences between them. The basic difference is in their goals. The therapy group is meant for psychiatric clients who generally have experienced interpersonal conflicts and disruption; their capacity for relearning may be low. T-group members are generally motivated to learn and are not under as much emotional stress. T-group leaders emphasize education for improved group functioning in an organization, whereas group therapists emphasize self-awareness, self-disclosure, and personality change.

T-groups have been instrumental in helping health care professionals function more productively with one another. For example, some hospitals have their entire staffs rotate through group training sessions in order to learn skills of communication and working toward common goals.

Encounter or Self-Actualization Groups

Encounter groups, including marathon, personal growth, and sensory awareness groups, grew out of the T-group movement. Their purpose is self-actualization, personal growth, socialization, and support. They are designed for relatively healthy individuals who benefit from a catharsis of feelings or loosening of repressed material. People who have attended these groups report experiencing an emotional high, a different outlook on life, and some new skills in dealing with other people.

The purpose of encounter groups is not to treat psychopathology; unfortunately, however, encounter groups tend to attract people who are searching for easy answers to complex problems. Many leaders of these groups are untrained. Nurses can help clients evaluate whether to become involved in such a group by asking the following questions:

1. What are the leader's qualifications and credentials? (A leader should have taken courses in group theory and had a personal group experience.)
2. What is the purpose of the encounter group? What are some of the rules? What is the philosophy?
3. Who can qualify to be in the group? Is there preparation of the members?
4. How long will the group last?
5. Does the leader receive supervision?
6. What other groups has the leader led? Can you find out about former participants' perceptions of their group experience?
7. What is your reason for getting involved with the group?

Because of the influx of many different professional groups into group work, the standards for leaders vary greatly. Psychotic and severely neurotic individuals, borderline personalities, people seeking therapy, and people who are chemically dependent should not be admitted to these groups.

Professional nurses need to be aware of the differences among the groups and help the public become more knowledgeable about them. Nurses can inform people about the goals and functions of the groups and help them find professionally valid group experiences.

CONCEPTS OF GROUP DYNAMICS

There are many factors responsible for promoting group functioning and facilitating group movement toward a task. The leader is one of the most important elements in helping group members work together. Interaction among the members and with the leader constitutes the *group dynamics* or *processes* of the group. Over the years, a variety of processes have been identified as contributing to group effectiveness.

Cohesiveness is the phenomenon that occurs when members of a group find the group attractive enough to want to remain in it. Attractiveness is based on two factors: the nature of the group (the goals, programs, size, type of organization) and the needs of the individuals for recognition, affiliation, and security (Cartwright & Zander, 1965).

Cohesive groups have a feeling of "we're in this together." They can be highly productive in accomplishing the group tasks. The members generally communicate more effectively, are better motivated, are more satisfied, and remain in the group longer than members of noncohesive groups.

The *group tasks* are the processes the group must carry out in order to meet its goals. Initiating, information seeking, clarifying, consensual validation, and summarizing are all group tasks that facilitate meeting the group goals.

Group goals are the expected outcomes a group hopes to accomplish. Knowing what a group is supposed to accomplish helps the leader assess the level of productivity. It also gives direction to the group's activities.

Group maintenance functions are the behaviors the members perform that help keep the group together over time. Compromising, harmonizing, and gatekeeping (keeping communication lines open) are some of the maintenance functions that occur in small groups.

Norms are the standards or rules that develop within a group and are set by the leader. Norms are expectations about group members' behaviors, and they are highly valued. Deviation from the norms usually results in some type of reaction or censure from the group members. *Explicit norms* are clearly stated and known by all the members, whereas *implicit norms* are not clearly stated and may or may not be known by all the members.

Since norms can shape the behavior of members toward productive accomplishment of the group's goals, it is important for the leader to explicitly state the rudimentary expectations at the beginning of a group's work. The group members will also develop and improvise norms as they interact. Other norms are thus generated and the group's *moral density,* or adherence to standards is further enhanced. Group norms provide the anchorage or frame of reference that guides the judgments and actions of the group members (Olmsted, 1967).

A *role* is the learned and enacted behavioral pattern that characterizes an individual's place or position in relation to others in a group. Social roles, such as mother, father, and teacher, tell us what position a person has. In small groups the characteristic patterns of behavior for each of the members is related to the functioning of the group. *Functional roles* of group members, as described by Benne and Sheats (1948, pp. 42–49), are shown in Table 18.1.

All human interactions have two dimensions: content and process. The *content* of a group's interaction is what is being said: the subject matter or topics the members talk about. The *process* of the group is what is happening between and among the members: what is being done in the group. By recognizing and understanding both content and process, a leader can diagnose group problems or help members be more productive in their roles.

Group atmosphere is the climate or feeling the group generates. A friendly, open, accepting, informal atmosphere tends to enhance productivity and member satisfaction.

The *leader* is the person in the group whose behavior most frequently influences the group to move toward their shared goals. Some leaders are formally designated as such; some are informal leaders who emerge from the interaction of the group members. Some groups have both kinds of leaders. The development of a leader within a group occurs in the following way (Wilson, 1980):

1. People interact in a group over a period of time.

2. Members achieve some individual satisfaction from the group.

3. Group members overtly or covertly come to a consensus of common purposes based on internal needs and external pressures.

4. One or more individuals contribute the most toward the group purposes or goals.

5. Step 4 occurs repeatedly.

6. That individual is recognized and accepted by the group as the person who has the most influence over the group goal in comparison to others.

7. The individual accepts this role differentiation.

Table 18.2 illustrates the relationship of the small group concepts to effective group member behavior and to leader interventions that promote such behavior.

CONSIDERATIONS IN CONDUCTING GROUPS

Much thought and planning needs to be put into the organization of a group experience.

TABLE 18.1
Functional Roles of Group Members

Role	Behavior in Group
Group task roles	
Initiator-Contributor	Offers new ideas and suggests solutions.
Information seeker	Seeks clarification of suggestions.
Opinion seeker	Seeks clarification of values about an issue.
Information giver	Offers facts or generalizations which are authoritative or relate to the person's own pertinent experience.
Opinion giver	States belief or opinion relevant to the issue being discussed.
Elaborator	Gives examples, develops meanings and explanations.
Coordinator	Clarifies relationships among ideas, suggestions, and activities of the group.
Orienter	Defines position of group with respect to goals.
Evaluator-Critic	Relates the standards of group to problem.
Energizer	Motivates the group to action and decision.
Procedural technician	Performs routine tasks.
Recorder	Writes down suggestions, topics, decisions, and actions resulting from discussion.
Group-building roles	
Encourager	Praises, agrees with, and accepts other's ideas.
Harmonizer	Mediates intragroup differences and reconciles disagreements.
Compromiser	Operates from within to resolve conflict.
Gatekeeper	Encourages and facilitates participation of others.
Standard setter	Expresses standards for the group.
Group observer	Keeps records of group process and contributes these data to evaluation.
Follower	Goes along passively as an audience, accepting ideas of others.
Individual-centered roles	
Aggressor	Deflates status of another; may express disapproval of values, acts, or feelings of others; jokes aggressively.
Blocker	Is negativistic and resistive in an unreasonable and stubborn manner.
Recognition seeker	Calls attention to self; boasts about personal achievements.
Self-confessor	Uses group to express personal, non-group-oriented feelings and insights.
Playboy	Displays lack of involvement in group work; displays cynical nonchalance.
Dominator	Asserts authority; manipulates the group or individuals.
Help seeker	Tries to get sympathetic responses from others. Expresses insecurity, confusion, or depreciation of self beyond reason.
Special-interest pleader	Speaks for the underdog while masking feelings of bias and prejudice. Actions are contrary to verbalizations.

SOURCE: Benne, K., & Sheats, P.: Functional roles of group members. *Journal of Social Issues* 4(2), 42–49, 1948.

TABLE 18.2
Utilizing Small Group Process Concepts

Group Process Concept	Effective Group Member Behaviors	Leader Interventions to Promote Effective Member Behaviors
Cohesiveness	Members enjoy, like, trust one another; a "we-ness" is evident with much mutual support among the members. Attendance is high. Members talk readily, listen carefully, influence one another frequently.	Makes the group attractive by: 1. Helping members identify needs they may satisfy in the group. 2. Increasing the number and strength of these needs that can be met in the group. 3. Increasing the group's ability to meet these needs. 4. Helping members see how well their needs are being met in the group (Zander, 1982).
Group tasks	Members understand and will talk about the tasks at hand. They show evidence of working toward completion of the tasks.	Identifies and positively reinforces initiating, information-seeking, clarifying, and consensually validating behaviors (e.g., "You did a good job clarifying that issue for us, John. That'll make our task easier").
Group maintenance	Members attempt to keep communication open, are responsive to each others' needs, seek to reduce tension, and relinquish an individual position for the sake of the group when conflict arises.	Identifies and positively reinforces group-maintenance functions (gatekeeping, compromising, harmonizing) (e.g., "Compromising isn't easy but you and Susan worked it out, so now we can move on to our next task"; "You've suggested two different ways of handling this. How could we compromise?").
Norms	The members not only know the behavioral expectations but also remind each other verbally when deviations occur.	States norms in preparatory and beginning phases of group (e.g., "I'd like everyone to attend all eight sessions"; or "We're here to talk about you and how you're doing after your surgery").
Content and process	Members become aware of the two levels of interactions.	Teaches about the two levels of interaction and their effect on the group's goals.
Group atmosphere	Members are relaxed, informal,	Sets the mood by facilitating and stimulating rather than telling people what to

TABLE 18.2 (*continued*)

Group Process Concept	Effective Group Member Behaviors	Leader Interventions to Promote Effective Member Behaviors
	open, and enthusiastic about working with one another toward the group task. Much initiative is shown.	do. Encourages group interaction and involvement in the tasks. Is genuinely interested in people.
Group goals	Members know the group goals and will verbalize their progress toward the goals, sometimes redefining the goals.	Tells the group the goals before the group begins; facilitates ongoing discussion of the goals.
Roles	The members take group-facilitating roles (see Table 18.1).	Encourages members to play a variety of roles to facilitate completion of group tasks.
Leadership	The members know who the designated leader is and emergent leaders also develop to help with the task.	The designated or appointed leader contributes the most toward the group goals. Undesignated leaders are allowed to emerge to enhance group productivity.

Some factors to consider are composition and selection of group members, the leader, the format and structure of meetings, physical arrangements, group norms, and the group phases.

Composition and Selection of Members

Whether it is a psychotherapy group or a self-help weight-control group, certain questions should be asked about the prospective group members.

1. How many people should be in the group?
   The number of group members in part depends on the purpose of the group. Re-

search has shown, however, that a size of about 7 to 12 members will maximize group discussion and interaction. When there are too few people, conversations tend to be one-on-one, especially with the group leader. When the group becomes too large splinter groups develop, thus interfering with the overall group process. Whether the group is too small or too large, the result is limited interaction among members.

2. How old should the members be?
   The purpose of the group will have some impact on the members' ages. For example, if a nurse starts a group for adolescents with physical disabilities, the group members will all be teenagers except the leader.

In groups whose members could be drawn from a variety of age groups (e.g., cancer support groups), it is best to keep the age range from the youngest to the oldest member within a 30-year span. In this way, there will be a variety of people representing different generations but the generations will not be too far apart. Also, since homogeneous groups tend to become cohesive faster than heterogeneous groups, having members of similar ages tends to foster group unity.

3. Is the prospective group member suited for the purpose of the group?

   A nurse would probably not place a single elderly person within a group of young people formed to discuss marital problems. The goals of the group must be taken into consideration. For example, it is generally felt that brain-damaged and severely retarded individuals are not good for groups that discuss abstract topics. This type of client does better in a group with a concrete approach.

   The purpose of the group will help determine whether or not a person should be involved in it, as will motivation and prior experience. This is why it is important to talk with all prospective group members before they enter the group. The leader can orient each member to the group's goals, philosophy, and basic ground rules.

4. Should the group members have similar or dissimilar characteristics?

   Homogeneous groups are composed of people with similar problems or backgrounds. They may also be limited by age or gender. *Heterogeneous groups* vary as to all these characteristics. Most self-help and counseling groups are homogeneous in terms of the problem they address. There are several advantages to having people with similar problems all

in one group. Group members tend to offer support for one another, and group cohesiveness is enhanced because people form a better unit when they are alike.

However, members of homogeneous groups also tend to use similar defenses. Thus group process may be impeded when some or many of the members bond together to avoid accomplishing a constructive goal. For example, it is not uncommon for groups composed of all alcoholics to avoid deep problems. Though the members have not overtly said "Let's avoid talking about our problems," they have similar personality dynamics in which denial and avoidance predominate.

Heterogeneity can be useful in any group where a wide range of experiences and interactions provides the stimulation to move toward the group's goal. This is not to say that one type of group is better than the other. It is wise for the leader to remember the strengths and drawbacks of both homogeneous and heterogeneous groups and to try to enhance the strengths of whatever group is chosen.

The Group Format

In an *open group*, members can enter and leave at various times. A *closed group* has a fixed permanent membership. The choice of format depends in part on the purposes of the group. For example, a group for new mothers in the community would be open to each new mother who volunteered for the group and who had delivered recently. The group's membership would be continually changing. The difficulty with an open group is the disruption in group process caused by the rapid turnover in membership. Also, it is hard for a group such as this to have much cohesion and interaction. On the other hand, the advantage of an open group is that a large number of people can be helped in a short time. There is much peer support from a variety of people in the same life situation.

Closed groups tend to have more stable interactions. Cohesion develops and the members progress through the group phases together. Personal satisfaction can run high in these groups, because there is more ongoing interaction than in open groups. The disadvantage of closed groups is that with a fixed membership, there is a limited number of people. In many settings it is unrealistic to have a closed group, because there is a continual supply of prospective members who need what the group has to offer.

Structure of the Meetings

The organizer or leader of a group needs to determine how long each meeting will be, how frequently the group will meet, and how many people will be included. An hour is usually satisfactory for most groups. Groups that have as their purpose the analysis of interactions (e.g., psychotherapy groups) usually run one and a half hours, because it takes about that long for people to participate (Yalom, 1970). A group meeting that lasts two or more hours may make people bored and restless.

The frequency of the meetings often depends on the purpose of the group. Generally, meetings held once a week for one to one and a half hours will provide the members with the content and process needed, and are frequent enough so that members remember what has gone on before. The leader should evaluate the duration of and intervals between meetings by assessing how productive the members are in the chosen format. If necessary, the leader may suggest longer or more frequent or shorter or less frequent meetings.

Physical Arrangements

The leader needs to find a room for the time and duration of the group. The room should afford privacy and have little distraction. Obviously, the room should be accessible to the members and the temperature, ventilation, lighting, and furnishings should be comfortable. The chairs should be arranged in a circle or around a table. This enhances interaction by enabling members to see and hear each other.

Another decision to be made is about audiotape recording or videotaping. Taping can be useful for the leader to evaluate his or her performance or for members to listen to missed content or review portions of the meeting that were confusing. If the nurse decides to tape a group meeting and has a specific reason for doing so, then much preparation is necessary:

1. Before the meeting begins, tell the members why the tape is being made, who will listen to it, and how it will be disposed of after it is used.
2. Secure written permission for the use of the tape. Most agencies have a format for this, but a form can be improvised if need be. Include names, date, place, reason for the taping, and who will have access to the tapes. Have the group members sign and date the agreement. The person doing the taping should also sign it.
3. At the beginning of the meeting, again mention the tape, its purposes, and its benefits and let the members air their feelings about it. Later, let them play segments back so they can listen to themselves, if they wish.
4. Place the tape recorder so that everyone's voice can be picked up. If it is possible to do this and also be unobtrusive, so much the better. Turn the tape on and then forget it. The leader's attitude about the use of a tape goes a long way in helping the group

members feel comfortable with it. If the leader is uncomfortable, the group will be also.

5. If group members ask questions about the tapes, give them time to talk about it. The most often asked question is, "Is this tape going to be used against me?" The leader must make sure that group members are not exploited by the use of the tapes.

Group Norms

All group members should be told what to expect before they enter a group. The leader can meet with each member in a preparatory interview to discuss the following:

1. The material and occurrences within the group will be confidential. If this information will be shared, specify with whom.
2. Purposes, goals, and format and structure of the group.
3. Philosophy, if any, of the treatment modality.
4. Other expectations, such as participation, regular attendance, appropriate behavior, and fees, when applicable.

Preparation helps members fit in and be a part of a group. It is also a consumer's right to know what he or she is paying for.

The Leader

Leading groups takes much skill and experience. Nurses who decide to work with groups need educational background and ongoing experience to develop their expertise. Coursework in group theory and practice, supervision of the leader, and personal experience in a group are prerequisites for a beginning leader. The American Nurses' Association has recommended that nurses who lead psychotherapy groups have at least a masters degree in psychiatric nurs-

ing. However, many nurses without specialized training are able to lead counseling groups effectively.

The leader's role depends somewhat upon the purpose of the group. Some groups tend to be didactic rather than interactional, such as a group organized to teach groups of clients about health. All leaders, though, should be aware of the phases of the group and the tasks at hand and should facilitate members' participation throughout. Leaders who are personable and democratic tend to increase group productivity. Encouraging and guiding, rather than telling people what to do, also helps involve the members in the group activity and increase their satisfaction with the group experience.

Group Phases

Group work can be divided into four phases: preparatory; beginning; middle, or working; termination. How a group goes through these phases depends on its format (open vs. closed), the group's purpose, the length of time the members work together, the leader's ability to facilitate growth throughout all phases, and each group member's readiness.

In open groups, some members will be terminating their membership while others are beginning. In closed groups, people start and end group membership together. Also, there are individual differences in the way group members experience the different phases. Some people react more intensely to an ending than others; some seem not to react at all. Generally, the ending of any group work or the departure of a member will have some effect on all the members.

Preparatory Phase

During the preparatory phase, the leader plans for and considers the purpose of the group, potential group members, the format, the physical arrangements, and the group contract. This is also the time when the leader prepares the future members for the group experience.

The client should be given a brief explanation of the group's purposes, goals, philosophy, and format and the qualifications of the leader. The rules or norms should be reviewed and discussed with the prospective member. Clients should be allowed to question or discuss anything they wish about their participation in the group. If difficulties or particular outcomes are expected, the leader should tell the client this. For example, the leader of a short-term stop-smoking group should tell participants when to expect the most difficulty as well as what their chances of stopping smoking are.

Beginning Phase

The beginning phase is the orientation period, during which people get to know one another and learn why they are together. At this point there is little cohesion or unity. Members are guarded and polite to each other. The real group work has not yet begun. It is important for the leader to make clear the norms of the group and to continue to communicate this effectively. How long this stage lasts depends on the purpose and format of the group, the activity of the leader, and the homogeneity of the group. However, all new group members are anxious, tentative, and cautious. Knowing this, the leader can understand and help the members through this stage.

Group members look to the leader for help with their anxiety. The secure, experienced leader will not provide all the answers during this phase. Most groups benefit from the group interaction over time. A group leader helps facilitate and stimulate

communication among the members about the group's goals and norms but does not try to meet every need of the group members.

Working Phase

The group members, by interacting over time, become more cohesive and more open about the problems they bring to the group. Members begin to play recognizable roles to help the group accomplish its goals. There is a feeling of unity and a "we're in this together" spirit at this stage. This is also the time when new solutions to old problems are explored.

Termination Phase

This is the stage when the group comes to an end. This can occur prematurely, as when members leave before the specified end, or it can occur at a predetermined time. In either case, termination brings anxiety and the potential for feelings of anger, rejection, fear, and abandonment. It also brings the potential for growth.

MANAGING CONFLICT IN SMALL GROUPS

Conflict is described by Frost and Wilmot (1978, p. 9) as "an expressed struggle between at least two interdependent parties, who perceive incompatible goals, scarce rewards, and interference from the other party in achieving their goals. They are in a position of opposition in conjunction with cooperation."

Conflicts are inevitable whenever people interact. The leader's goal is not to suppress or avoid conflict or to blow the conflict out of proportion to the problem at hand. The ideal way of handling conflict is to lessen the perceived differences so that the outcome is fair to everyone involved. There are seven basic ways of managing conflict in groups: distancing, removing the conflict-causing condition, negotiating, bargaining and compromise, problem solving, mediation, and force. Table 18.3 describes these strategies and shows their applicability for the community health nurse.

If a fair outcome cannot be negotiated, it may be possible for the disputants to agree to disagree, thereby coming to some resolution. Unsatisfactory resolution of conflicts occurs when the parties involved cannot reach an agreement about what is fair for all. One or more of the members are left feeling that they have been dealt with unfairly. In such cases, there is a greater chance that members will either leave the group or disrupt the group process.

To help group members deal with conflict, the community health nurse can teach the following:

1. No matter how angry you are, do not stoop to name calling, depreciating, or making fun of what other people are saying. This only keeps a conflict going. Also, shouting never resolves a problem; it only serves to make the shouter feel better temporarily. Stay calm, look directly at the other person, and try to relax. Listen to what is being said and try to understand and acknowledge the incompatibility.

2. Communicate what you think, how you feel, and what you want from the other person. In the heat of anger, we very often say what we think and how we feel but leave out what we want the other person to do. Be sure about what you want and say it clearly.

3. Avoid bringing in past disagreements or arguments. Stay with the problem at hand. When we are angry, we tend to recall and magnify every past time we have been treated unfairly by the person we are angry with. Avoid the temptation: it will escalate the conflict. When you see this happening, say, "Let's stay on the problem at hand and figure out some resolution."

4. Try and see the conflict from the other person's viewpoint. There will always be something you can agree on. Find that common territory and build the agreement from that point.

5. If the conflict or fighting keeps going despite all efforts, stop focusing on the content and look at the process. Maybe the goal of the people involved is to fight for the sake of fighting. Some people are determined to fight and always have a great deal of conflict within their interpersonal relationships. Also, some people find it easier to gain attention by negative means. To them, arguing, fighting, or keeping a conflict going is a way to gain attention. When you see this happening, you can say, "We've tried all the ways I know to get this conflict resolved. Since the fight is still going on, I wonder if having the fight is more important than solving the problem."

LEADING GROUP DISCUSSIONS

Community health nurses meet to discuss their caseloads. Hospital nurses meet at the change of each shift to exchange information about clients and unit management. A home-care-center administrative group discusses the cost effectiveness of staff use of equipment. Nursing students take part in seminars about leadership styles and functions. A group of amputees meet weekly with a nurse to talk about their rehabilitation progress. Faculty members at a college of nursing plan each semester's course schedule.

TABLE 18.3
Strategies for Conflict Reduction

Strategy	Types of Situations in Which Strategy Applies	Examples in Nursing
Distancing: separating the people or groups of people so they cannot have a face-to-face confrontation. The need for one another therefore decreases and the warring parties' incompatibility lessens.	Used when resolution of a problem is not that important. The emphasis is on the group task, and the leader wants to minimize or repress conflict. Strategy does not work once members are deeply involved with one another.	Used in groups of children in which transitory conflicts take place. Tension is easily reduced by separating warring parties and placing them in other groups.
Removing conflict-causing conditions.	Conflicts are more likely to occur when the following conditions are present: 1. Unclear lines of responsibility. 2. Lack of policies and procedures. 3. Difficulty in communicating. 4. Large groups vs. small ones. 5. Exploitation: one person (or group) seeks to satisfy needs at the expense of the other. 6. Deprivation: group members feel they are receiving too few rewards, benefits, etc.	Conflicts often arise because of the difficulty in getting nurses together to meet. Nurses are not only geographically separated but also follow different schedules in a 24-hour period. Also, heterogeneity of background, education, and position also contributes to conflict.
Negotiating: talking over differences in order to understand and reduce them.	The parties involved must want to understand each others' viewpoints. Negotiation usually does not work when important issues are at stake (e.g., power, authority).	Should be one of the first steps taken to bring about conflict reduction. Talking over differences with a fellow employee or with an employer may reduce the conflict at an early stage.
Bargaining/compromising: bargaining is trading to reduce the differences; in compromising, each individual gives up something or makes an equal concession. The purpose of bargaining is not only to make a deal but also to compromise.	When resources or prized objects are the central issue of the conflict, bargaining and compromise are the best strategies to use.	The American Nurses' Association, as of 1980, is the largest collective bargaining representative of registered nurses. State nurses' organizations are the direct agents for bargaining. Previous bargaining efforts focused on improving salaries, fringe benefits, and working conditions for nurses. The thrust now is on improving the quality of care and

TABLE 18.3 (*continued*)

Strategy	Types of Situations in Which Strategy Applies	Examples in Nursing
		increasing the accessibility of that care to the general public (Kelly, 1981, pp. 539–540).
Problem solving: uses the following steps: 1. Describing the problem 2. Identifying solutions 3. Deciding which alternative solutions are best. 4. Taking action.	Used to get at the reasons or causes for the conflict. (Bargaining need not uncover the reasons that the conflict developed.)	The nursing process, though differing from problem solving in some aspects, incorporates the same elements: 1. Assessment (problems are identified). 2. Planning (deciding on solutions). 3. Implementing (taking action).
Mediation: using a third party to reduce differences. Usually the parties involved are desperate for a solution or are required by some authority to come to a resolution.	Usually used when negotiating, bargaining, and problem solving have failed. The mediator helps identify the issues involved, helps create the conditions needed to facilitate resolution, corrects misperceptions, and gets the parties to talk with respect and understanding.	In August 1982, when the Cleveland, Ohio, VNA nurses went on strike, mediators were brought in from the Federal Mediation and Conciliation Service to help resolve the differences. As of January 1983, the mediation process has been unsuccessful in resolving the dispute ("VNA Strike Continues," 1982, p. 7).
Force: the use of threats of some unfavorable consequence to control or modify behavior.	Used when all else fails or in emergencies. The use of force can be nonviolent or violent.	In 1968, a no-strike policy of 18 years' duration was rescinded by the ANA. Strikes have given nurses power they were not able to achieve by negotiation or problem solving. For example, approximately 40 VNA nurses in Cleveland, Ohio, went on strike to prevent excessive caseloads. The strike was the result of a breach in a two-year contract that had specified a formula for numbers of cases. VNA administrators reversed their position midway through the contract, and the nurses struck to protest the contract breach.

SOURCE: Adapted from Zander, A.: *Making groups effective.* San Francisco: Jossey/Bass, 1982, pp. 96–106.

In all of the above examples, people get together to communicate in a group discussion. It is "an opportunity for the talkers to study their personal situations, to derive what learning they can from their past, and to pool their thinking with that of associates" (Zander, 1983, p. 30). Participants in a group discussion can filter the ideas that come their way, keeping those that apply and eliminating those which do not.

Group discussion serves five purposes (Zander, 1982):

1. It helps members recognize what they do not know.

2. It helps members get answers to questions.

3. It lets people share ideas and develop common wisdom.

4. It enables members to get advice on matters that bother them.

5. It is a way for people to learn about the universality of their problems.

Steps in Leading a Group Discussion

There are five main steps in leading a group discussion: planning, introducing the topics, the discussion, closing the discussion, and evaluation.

Planning the Discussion

Deciding what topics should be discussed, how much time should be given to each topic, where to meet, and who will be involved in the group are some of the leader's first considerations. Some discussion leaders like to have a written plan to guide them (see Figure 18.1). In this plan, the topics, the objectives of the discussion, opening remarks, key questions to ask, and summary ideas can be mapped out. Also,

some physical arrangements should be made, such as obtaining a room, arranging the chairs so that everyone can see each other, bringing in audiovisual equipment, and seeing that the general atmosphere is conducive to discussion. The plan can include all these considerations in checklist form. Although planning does not ensure that a discussion will go well, it increases the probability that it will be productive.

Introducing the Subject

Creating interest in the subjects to be discussed can set the tone for the rest of the meeting. The topics to be discussed, the objectives, and the time allotted should be briefly outlined for the group in simple, direct terms. After that, several techniques can be used to get people interested. Asking questions is the most common. For example: "Who here has had trouble getting a job because of a disability?"

Another way to get people interested is to use a film, tape recording, anecdote, diagram, or role-playing situation that demonstrates the topic to be discussed. Sometimes people warm up to a topic when they can relate it to someone else's experiences before talking about themselves.

Guiding the Discussion

Once people in the group have become interested in the topic and the conversation has begun to flow, the leader's job is to facilitate the discussion around the objectives. This means that obstructive behaviors should be discouraged (see Table 18.4). A leader should not always intervene when a discussion gets off the topic. Sometimes seemingly extraneous material can be instructive for both the leader and the group members. A leader might not have assessed the group's needs correctly, and topics that should have been included might have been left out. A tangent can be a clue to this.

1. Group Members

Names	Addresses (optional)	Phone numbers (optional)

2. Topic and time allocated	Objectives of discussions	Key questions to ask	Audiovisual equipment needed

3. Physical facility checklist:

Room obtained and group members informed   _____

Chairs arranged   _____

Audiovisual equipment obtained and in working order   _____

Handouts obtained   _____

Proper lighting   _____

Ventilation   _____

4. Opening comments (or idea) to enhance interest:

5. Method of evaluation:

Questions to ask on evaluation form:

1.

2.

3.

4.

5.

Figure 18.1 Preplanning guide for group discussions.

On the other hand, getting off a subject can be a symptom of resistance. It may be easier for group members to talk about the weather, for example, than to discuss their recent bereavement. In this case, the nurse can intervene by saying, for example, "Is death a subject too difficult to discuss?"

Asking questions can be very valuable in helping the group cover the planned topics and objectives. An easy flow of ideas among the group members helps develop a team spirit that enhances the desire of members to participate.

Closing the Discussion

Discussions often deteriorate because of a leader's inability to end them. Keep to the

TABLE 18.4
Handling Obstructive Group Behavior during Discussions

Problem Behavior	Leader Response
The monopolizer: either through talking or through behavioral tactics, this person holds the attention of the group for most of the group's time.	Direct your question away from this member (e.g., "Let's let other people have a turn now"; "Let's get someone else's opinion. What do you think about that, John?"). Avoid direct eye contact. Pick up other members' nonverbal cues: "Are you getting tired, Margaret?"
The silent member: this person is usually shy in group situations and participates little, if any, verbally.	Ask direct questions of this member: "What do you think, Andy?" Pick up nonverbal cues: "You were nodding your head in agreement. Tell us your opinion." Involve such members in other ways: ask them to help set up the room, distribute papers, etc.
The group clown: makes a joke out of every communication.	Avoid responding with a joke. Reword his or her comments so they are more constructive to the group's task: "You've been joking about the group always starting late, Jim, but I think it's worthwhile to talk about why this has been happening."
The obsessional member: pays attention to the minute details instead of the overall picture. May ramble, beat around the bush, or stay stuck on a point the group has already dispensed with.	Ask "What is the point you're getting to?" or say "We only have a few minutes left. Very succinctly, what's the main idea you want to convey to the group?"
The expert: takes over the role of the leader and knows all the answers. This person can be a help to the leader, but the role also may help the member avoid being one of the group and relating to people on a feeling level.	Appreciate this person's contributions and let him or her assume some leadership functions when appropriate. If the person avoids feelings, ask, "But how does that make you feel? There's a difference between what you think and how you feel."
The fighter: has a chip on his or her shoulder and uses a tone of voice that provokes or invites an argument from other group members.	Don't argue. Reword the point this member is trying to make, but put it in a non-hostile tone: "So what you're saying, Nancy, is that you think the group doesn't listen to you." Focus on the anger: "You sound angry. What happened in the group to make you feel that way?"
The symbiotic pair: two group members who sit beside one another and start a conversation with each other when someone else is talking. The two may speak for one another; they distract the group with private jokes, etc.	Look at the two members and say: "We seem to be having several conversations going on at the same time. I don't want to miss what you have to say, so let's have one person talk at a time." If they are disruptive, try to sit between them at the next meeting.

specified time limit. Ten minutes before the meeting is to end, remind the members of the closing time: "We have only 10 more minutes. Let's have some concluding remarks, and then I'd like to make a few comments." At the end, summarize the main points of the discussion or the main decisions reached. If the group will meet again, briefly state the tasks of the next session.

The ending of a discussion can also stimulate further interest for future meetings. For example, some of the same techniques used to begin a group discussion can be used to end it. A short anecdote, poem, or quote that encapsulates or summarizes what has been said can be effective in concluding remarks. It can also help people remember the main ideas and stimulate attendance at future meetings.

Evaluating the Discussion

One effective way to improve your discussion groups is to ask the people who participated how satisfied they were with the proceedings. Some questions you could ask are:

1. Did most of the discussion relate to the topics and objectives stated by the leader?
2. Did you learn from the discussion?
3. Was your time well spent?
4. Did the discussion give you new ideas?

These or other questions can be asked informally or can be made up on a form for the participants to fill out at the end of the group.

FUTURE IMPLICATIONS

Two factors in particular will have an influence on the way groups will be formed in the future: change and the rising cost of health care.

Change

With increased social mobility, high job turnover, changing family roles, an increased number of women in the work force, and a wider and more complex range of social problems, the average person will experience greater transience in his or her relationships with other people than ever before. Gone are the days when people lived in the same house and kept the same neighbors and friends for life. In a highly mobile society, old friends will fade into the background with each successive move. Courtney Tall, a psychologist, says of friendships in the future:

Individuals will develop the ability to form close "buddy-type" relationships on the basis of common interests or sub-group affiliations, and to easily leave these friendships, moving either to another location and joining a similar group or to another interest group within the same location. . . . Interests will change rapidly. . . .
(Toffler, 1970, pp. 107–108)

Individuals will increasingly join groups that match their interests. In order to create an environment in which change can take place but does not overwhelm the basic social groupings of society, new strategies need to be employed to help people deal with the problems of change. Dr. Herbert Gerjuoy states that we should provide temporary organizations—"situational groups"—for people who are in similar transitional stages of life (Toffler, 1970). For example, situational groups could be started for families who have to continually relocate, for men and women about to be divorced, for families about to add a new member, for people facing retirement, for newly arrived families in the community, or for people about to change occupations. These situational groups would be formed to deal with an important life change. The emphasis of the group would be not on the past but on the future planning of practical, workable strategies for use in life situations.

Although situational groups are not an entirely new concept, future changes in our society will demand that nurses and other professionals use strategies such as this to help people through difficult periods of their lives. Nurses can maintain ongoing groups, although membership may change frequently.

Rising Health Care Costs

Health care costs in the future will not go down, and with waning interest in national health insurance programs, it is evident that consumers will still be paying the rising costs. How then can we maintain and increase the quality of care? One way may be through group care and treatment. Group treatment in psychiatry has been recognized as a viable approach since the early twentieth century. This strategy could be used for clients in hospitals and in the community. For example, a person who has just had a colostomy could receive instructions for self-care while still in the hospital. Several people could be instructed at one time. Upon returning home, each client could be referred to an ongoing group during the rehabilitation phase. Such a group approach to care is cost effective. Nurses have a tremendous opportunity to make some inroads in cutting costs for the consumers while ensuring high quality of care.

Prevention will be our best means of defraying the heavy costs of disease. Groups of the future will have to focus on how to stay healthy and reduce illness. No more can we presume that disease results from any one factor. It arises rather from a multiplicity of factors originating within the individual and the environment. Unless we confront the large-scale ecological problems of pollution, industrial waste disposal, overpopulation, and poverty, we will continue to treat people for diseases without getting to their causes. Community health nurses must use the influence of their positions and numbers to work together in groups which will identify and plan alternatives to community-wide problems that affect the health of their clients.

SUMMARY

A group consists of two or more people who interact and influence each other toward a common goal. Two main functions of groups are to satisfy the psychosocial needs of members and to complete the group's goals. Theory in group dynamics is relatively new. The original focus was on the functions of the group. Today the emphasis has changed to the study and enhancement of the individual within the group. Present-day research in group process is lacking in new direction and organization: old topics keep repeating themselves (Zander, 1979).

Nurses have the opportunity to be involved with many different groups of people. Our literature describes the type of group work we are doing in the community, but there has been little nursing research into what makes groups work or not work. This is a fertile area for a nurse researcher.

Types of small groups that the community health nurse might be involved with are counseling groups, self-help groups, training groups, and encounter groups. The community health nurse will probably most often work with the counseling groups.

Understanding group-process concepts

will enable the nurse to function effectively as a group facilitator. In addition, such knowledge will enhance the nurse's functioning as a member of work groups and professional groups.

DISCUSSION TOPICS

1. For each concern listed below, tell what type of group you could begin in your community to promote health or prevent disease:

  a. Accident prevention and injury control.

  b. Work-site health promotion.

  c. Alcohol and drug abuse.

  d. Smoking and health.

  e. Hypertension.

  f. Immunization.

  g. Nutrition.

  h. Physical fitness and exercise.

  i. Pregnancy and family expansion.

  j. Infant morbidity and mortality.

  k. Loss and grief.

2. State the purpose of one of the groups you identified in topic 1. How would you begin the group and select the members? What would be the structure of the meetings? What would be the basic rules? How would you prepare the prospective members?

3. After your hypothetical group has begun, how would you, as the leader, help make the group cohesive? How would you encourage group-facilitating roles? What topics for discussion would you include? Make a discussion plan format.

4. List five possible future changes that would affect the participation of individuals in groups. Choose one change and describe how nursing might influence healthy participation.

BIBLIOGRAPHY

Arieti, S.: Creativity: The magic synthesis. New York: Basic Books, 1976.

Armstrong, S., & Rouslin, S.: *Group psychotherapy in nursing practice.* New York: Macmillan, 1963.

Benne, K., & Sheats, P.: Functional roles of group members. *Journal of Social Issues* 4(2), 42–49, 1948.

Cartwright, D., & Zander, A.: *Group dynamics research and theory.* New York: Harper & Row, 1965.

Foulkes, S.H.: *Therapeutic group analysis.* New York: International Universities Press, 1965.

Freud, S.: *Group psychology and the analysis of the ego.* New York: Bantam Books, 1965.

Frost, J.H., & Wilmot, W.W.: *Interpersonal conflict.* Iowa: William C. Brown, 1978.

Homans, G.: *The Human group.* New York: Harcourt Brace and World, 1950.

Kelly, L.Y.: *Dimensions of professional nursing* (2nd ed.). New York: Macmillan, 1981.

Marram, G.: *The group approach in nursing practice.* St. Louis: Mosby, 1973.

Olmsted, M.: *The small group.* New York: Random House, 1967.

Toffler, A.: *Future shock.* New York: Bantam, 1970.

"VNA strike continues." *Ohio Nurses' Review,* December 1982, p. 7.

Watson, J.: *The double helix.* New York: Mentor, 1968.

Wilson, J.: Leadership: A review of the literature. *Nursing Leadership* 3(2), 32–38, 1980.

Wolberg, L.: *Short-term psychotherapy.* New York: Grune & Stratton, 1967.

Wolf, A.: Group psychotherapy. In A.M. Freedman & H.I. Kaplan, eds., *Comprehensive textbook of psychiatry*. Baltimore: Williams & Wilkins, 1967.

Yalom, I.: *The theory and practice of group psychotherapy*. New York: Basic Books, 1970.

Zander, A.: The study of group behavior during four decades. *The Journal of Applied Behavioral Sciences* 15(3), 272–281, 1979.

Zander, A.: *Making groups effective*. San Francisco: Jossey/Bass, 1982.

19

Settings

Carolyn J. Leman

Shine by the side of every path we tread
With such a luster, he that runs may read.
WILLIAM COWPER

OBJECTIVES

After reading this chapter you should be able to:

☐ Discuss the historical basis of settings for community health nursing practice.
☐ Identify settings currently available for community health nursing practice.
☐ Explain the nature of practice in various settings.
☐ Discuss implications for future practice in community health settings.

INTRODUCTION

Just as opportunities for nurses and nursing students today are diversified and allow for creativity, so are settings for community health practice. Settings in which nurses practice health care in the community are expanding both in number and in the variety of services offered. Preparation to practice community health nursing in the present and in the future includes:

1. Knowledge of the historical basis of community health settings.

2. Awareness of present community health settings and the nature of practice in these settings.

3. Openness to future expansion and change.

This chapter will address these areas.

HISTORICAL TRENDS

Health care has always been provided in many different community settings. The settings that were used in the past changed

313

with modernization and scientific advances, and each met a specific need at a specific time. For example, ceremonial dances were performed in caves by prehistoric peoples; priests attempted to frighten away evil spirits in temples; lepers were sent to isolated colonies; barbers performed surgery in their shops; babies were customarily delivered at home by midwives. Almost any shelter can be considered as a setting for community health practice. Settings have evolved over the years in response to human needs. The following sections discuss historical trends that continue to affect health care settings.

Increased Numbers of Senior Citizens

With increased longevity, and in many instances the lowering of retirement age, older people are using diverse health care settings in the community. The elderly population has increased, and most of the elderly are in fair to good health. Their needs include health maintenance and promotion. Meals on wheels, senior citizens' centers, and day care for the elderly are examples of resources in the community that have developed as a response to needs of the elderly. In these settings, a person's needs for food, safety and security, belongingness, and self-esteem can be assessed and interventions implemented to meet expressed needs.

Financial Changes

Realignment of government spending and changes in funding patterns have created needs for changes within agencies such as departments of health. Retrenchment of personnel, refocusing of services, and maximal utilization of human and material resources have been necessary. Also, responsibility for human needs such as health, food, and shelter has been assumed by volunteer groups in many instances. Thus, innovative settings for administration of services have evolved. Clinics held in churches, and discount clothing stores sponsored by service clubs, are examples of these responses. In the past, financial responsibility for health care shifted from the individual to state and then federal agencies. Recently, this process has been reversed, with the federal government taking less responsibility and private groups and each individual being expected to take more.

Social Changes

The increasing awareness of equal opportunity for minority groups and for women has offered an opportunity for health planning. Day-care centers, ethnic centers, shelters for battered individuals, and crisis-intervention hotlines have all been attempts to meet health needs in the changing community. The perceived value of each individual has increased, and health care is seen as a right of each individual.

Increased Knowledge Base

Laypersons today are becoming better educated about their own health and thus are more aware of disease prevention and health promotion. The communication media have responded to this awareness by providing a vehicle for health information; agencies have instigated telephone hotlines, and public schools are including health education in their curricula. More aspects of daily life are now considered to be important to promoting and maintaining health. With knowledge of facts about health, people are better able to understand the choices available to them.

Client Participation in Health Care

One result of the increased knowledge base of consumers is increased client participation in health care and decision making. In many instances, the client is a member of the health care team and is given responsibility for his or her own actions. This change is especially applicable to community health, where the client functions in a community setting. As a result of the increased awareness of health, more clients use community settings, and they are demanding expanding services.

Expanded Role of the Nurse

The role of the nurse has expanded in many areas of health care. Of special concern is the focus of care in community health nursing, which has expanded from the individual to include care of groups. Such groups may include children in schools, clients at a senior citizens' center, people attending a community mental health center, or specific ethnic groups. Human beings do not live in isolation, and optimal care requires consideration of their communities. Thus in caring for clients, a community health nurse may assume many roles, such as educator, consultant, direct provider of care, and coordinator of services.

Emphasis on Rehabilitation

With advances in health and illness care, more people are surviving what used to be terminal illnesses. Chronic conditions are amenable to interventions that prevent exacerbations and complications. These advances have increased the need for rehabilitation services. As use of support services, such as physical therapy, occupational therapy, and mental health counseling, has increased, rehabilitation has gained increasing attention. Many community health centers have added rehabilitation professionals to their staffs. In such a role, the nurse functions as collaborator and client advocate as well as caregiver. The nurse may provide direct rehabilitation services or coordinate the care given by others.

Cultural Differences

Cultural differences were once suppressed by the controlling majority or by ethnic groups themselves. Now these differences are valued, and there is an effort to promote widespread understanding and acceptance of them. In recent years, particular attention has been given to the influence of cultural patterns and cultural identification on health care. Many professional nursing programs include content relating to these concerns. Community health care has expanded to meet the special needs of ethnic groups. Centers have been established that either have health care as a primary focus, such as urban Indian health projects, or have health care as a related focus, such as Hispanic cultural centers.

Focus on High-Level Wellness and Holistic Health Care

Many of the preceding identified changes contribute to the current focus on high-level wellness and holistic care. Physical fitness and exercise, nutrition, psychosocial health, prevention of illness, and promotion of health are all being incorporated to a greater extent into the American lifestyle. The community health nurse has an opportunity to practice holistic care in a variety of settings.

OVERVIEW

For the purpose of this chapter, a *setting* for community health nursing practice is defined as the physical environment where health care is practiced. Settings may include homes, community health centers, offices and factories, religious institutions, schools, and many other environments.

Community health nursing is distinguished from other kinds of nursing by certain basic considerations about settings for practice.

1. Community health nursing is generally practiced in settings outside of acute care facilities. Community health care ideally considers each person as unique, is often family oriented, and carries an awareness of the health of the community at large.

2. Community health nursing settings function under varying sponsorships, including government authorities, ranging from local to international; private or voluntary agencies; and private industry.

3. Whatever the setting, a team approach is important, whether the team includes only two members (nurse and client) or several members. The nurse must work within the parameters of the setting but must still provide individualized, creative care.

4. Although settings differ from one another they share certain identifying characteristics.

IDENTIFYING CHARACTERISTICS OF SETTINGS FOR COMMUNITY HEALTH PRACTICE

Providing care in community settings means recognizing and making use of a variety of options. Diverse community health settings offer the innovative nurse an opportunity to individualize health care as well as to consider the health of the community at large. However, the nurse must be able to identify available resources and assess the appropriateness of services in various settings in relation to client needs.

Settings for community health nursing practice have certain identifying features that can be grouped systematically for the purpose of study. Grouping of features provides an organizational tool for examining settings for practice and offers a structure for determining appropriate settings for particular clients.

In this chapter, settings will be discussed in terms of features that various agencies and services have in common. The identifying features described in this chapter are:

1. Sponsorship of services:
   a. Official agencies
   b. Nonofficial or voluntary agencies
   c. Private providers of health care
2. Environments where services are provided:
   a. Homes
   b. Schools
   c. Ambulatory settings
   d. Occupational health settings
   e. Correctional facilities
   f. Camps
   g. Shelters
   h. Health fairs
   i. Hospices

3. Types of services provided:
   a. Direct or indirect
   b. Primary, secondary, or tertiary
   c. Short-term or long-term
   d. Single-focus or multiple-focus
   e. Individual provider or team approach
4. Target population for services provided:
   a. Cultural and ethnic characteristics
   b. Income levels
   c. Age-specific or non-age-specific
   d. Rural or urban populations

A given setting might be included in more than one grouping. For example, a senior citizens' center located in New York City might have the following features: ambulatory setting, direct services provided, multiple focus, age specific, and urban location. When caring for clients in the community, the nurse can use the characteristics of specific settings to determine sources for referral, collaboration, or utilization.

Use of a system for describing settings will assist the nurse in identifying and maximizing available resources. In applying the nursing process, the nurse can assess possible settings, plan interventions related to appropriate settings, implement the plan, and evaluate outcomes.

Sponsorship of Services

Traditionally, community health agencies have been divided into two categories of sponsorship and funding: official and nonofficial (or voluntary). There is also a third category, private providers.

Official Agencies

Agencies that are tax supported on a federal, state, or local level are *official agencies*. These agencies function within gov-

ernment hierarchies, are controlled by legislation, and receive funding from the applicable jurisdiction. Examples of official agencies are the United States Public Health Service, state departments of health, and city, county, and district health departments.

Nonofficial Agencies

Agencies that are private in nature and receive funding from nontax monies are considered to be *voluntary* or *nonofficial*. Sources of support include gifts, client fees, United Fund money, contracts with insurance companies, Medicare, and Medicaid. The sponsoring groups are diverse and may originate from educational, charitable, or welfare service organizations. The American Red Cross, the American Heart Association, visiting nurses' associations, and free clinics are examples of voluntary agencies.

Another type of nonofficial agency is the proprietary agency. *Proprietary agencies* are those settings designed to provide health care and earn a profit. They include many nursing homes, some hospitals, and health maintenance organizations.

Private Providers

The nurse may also practice in the community in an independent role without sponsorship by an official or voluntary agency. For example, nursing services may be contracted for by private clients, agencies, or schools. Private industry may also provide a form of community health nursing care. This will be discussed later in this chapter.

Environments Where Services Are Provided

Homes

The client's home has traditionally been a setting for nursing care. Often home visits originate through organizations, such as visiting nurses' associations or official public health agencies. Usually referral is made by nurses or physicians, another health agency, or the client.

The nurse utilizes all phases of the nursing process during the home visit, focuses on the family, and includes the clients as members of the team. Home visits are described in detail in Chapter 20.

Schools

Nursing practice in schools generally includes health assessment, health promotion and disease prevention, care of ill or injured people, and health education. Oda (1981) suggests that many school districts emphasize one particular area of nursing service. What that area is will be determined by available personnel, budget, local political climate, and acceptance of the expanded nursing role.

Settings for school nursing include preschools, elementary and secondary schools, and colleges or universities. Many schools hire nurses and consider them as part of the teaching staff. Others contract for nursing services from community health nursing agencies on a shared-time basis. There are advantages to each type of nursing service. The scope of nursing practice in a school is often determined by the agency employing the nurse.

When the nurse is a faculty member, more time may be available for assessment and health education. The nurse can become familiar with the specific school population and thus be aware of students' special needs. If nursing service is provided by a community health nurse who also cares for people in the community at large, the nurse will have a general awareness of the environment and the total community, including the school population.

The nurse in the school setting is often the only health provider in the building and thus performs autonomously. Flexibility, creativity, and the ability to establish positive interpersonal relationships enhance implementation of the nursing process in the school setting.

The phases of the nursing process as they are utilized in school nursing will be described at length.

ASSESSMENT OF INDIVIDUALS. Health assessment is practiced with varying degrees of complexity depending on the individual school settings and the ages and needs of students. For young children, the nurse may use screening tools such as the Denver Developmental Screening Test to evaluate fine-motor and gross-motor development, language development, and personal-social development. Many school systems develop their own assessment aids and use them either as a primary tool or in conjunction with other assessment tools. These tools are aimed at holistic assessment. Other forms of health assessment that might be used include screening for vision or hearing problems, for hypertension, for diabetes, for sickle cell anemia, and for tuberculosis.

Vision is usually checked in given grades each year. A base line can be established for each student and problems identified early. When a new student enters a school, a routine health assessment is often completed. Screening of both new and previously enrolled students allows for early detection of abnormalities and provides for positive contact between the student and the nurse. This contact provides the opportunity for health promotion activities.

Vision is tested using the Snellen E chart or a mechanical testing machine. Auditory testing can be accomplished using a tuning fork or sophisticated audiometric equipment. The nurse is responsible for learning about the equipment and its use as well as for understanding the rationale behind the testing procedure and the implications of the results.

Hypertension screening is accomplished by using the standard sphygmomanometer. Screening for diabetes and tuberculosis may require more elaborate and intrusive procedures. This not only calls for the permission of parents and guardians but may also require additional assistance to organize and implement screening procedures.

Frequently, screening procedures and their results may be misunderstood or misinterpreted by students, teachers, or parents. Difficulties can be averted, to some degree, by giving appropriate explanations before, during, and after any screening activity. Those involved should know what the procedures will be like and what the results will tell them. The nurse may do this individually, in small groups, or in large groups. The explanation should be presented in a manner commensurate with the age and background of those to whom it is given.

Spontaneous assessments may occur when a student comes to the nurse to seek nursing assistance or when a teacher consults with the nurse about a student with special needs. The nurse will also determine what community settings are appropriate for collaboration and referral. The nurse can develop a card file of such needs and agencies to permit quick access to the information. Some examples would be agencies that provide assistance for the following:

· Chronic or long-term health problems, such as diabetes, tumors, arthritis, and acne.
· Rehabilitation needs, including physical therapy and special equipment.
· Loss related to a divorce in the family or death of a relative.

Orthopedic problems, such as scoliosis, fractures, casts, and limited mobility.

The nurse assesses students in the event of accident or illness, using physical assessment skills as well as communication techniques to gather information. The nurse must decide whether the student can be treated in the school or must be sent or taken elsewhere. At times, ethical considerations enter into the situation. For example, a teenager may ask the nurse not to tell anyone she is pregnant. A child may appear to have been abused. A teenager may have signs of venereal disease (See Chapter 6, Ethical Practice).

Health education needs should also be assessed. They may be identified by means of analysis of data gathered during screening of students, staff members, and the environment. The nurse may also use questionnaires or interviews designed to target such needs.

Teachers and staff members may use the screening projects as well as other health services of the school nurse. The nurse often assesses the needs of teachers and staff members and plans special projects to meet those needs. For example, if stress is a problem, the nurse may present a workshop on stress management or may teach relaxation techniques in after-school sessions.

ASSESSMENT OF THE PHYSICAL ENVIRONMENT. The school nurse assesses the building, activities, and playground for safety and health needs. A checklist similar to the one displayed in Figure 19.1 will aid in assessing environmental safety.

ASSESSMENT OF THE PSYCHOSOCIAL ENVIRONMENT. Growth occurs best in an environment conducive to learning, including the psychosocial as well as the physical environment. Areas for assessment are interactions between students and teachers and interactions among students. These may be

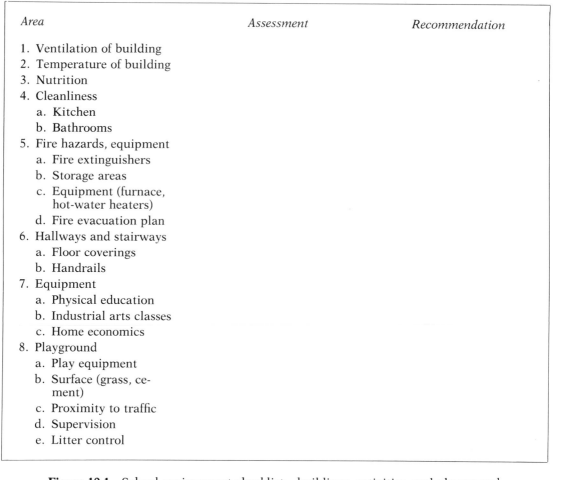

Area   *Assessment*   *Recommendation*

1. Ventilation of building
2. Temperature of building
3. Nutrition
4. Cleanliness
   a. Kitchen
   b. Bathrooms
5. Fire hazards, equipment
   a. Fire extinguishers
   b. Storage areas
   c. Equipment (furnace, hot-water heaters)
   d. Fire evacuation plan
6. Hallways and stairways
   a. Floor coverings
   b. Handrails
7. Equipment
   a. Physical education
   b. Industrial arts classes
   c. Home economics
8. Playground
   a. Play equipment
   b. Surface (grass, cement)
   c. Proximity to traffic
   d. Supervision
   e. Litter control

Figure 19.1   School environment checklist—buildings, activities, and playground.

assessed by observing classroom and playground interactions, by attending club meetings and activities available to students, and by interviewing students and teachers. This requires listening skill as well as awareness of nonverbal behavior.

PLANNING FOR SCHOOL-BASED HEALTH CARE. The planning phase is the time to prepare to respond to assessed needs. This step extends from goal setting to reserving rooms for carrying out a project to planning methods for evaluating outcomes of the activity.

The nurse establishes goals and objectives and plans for each area of responsibility:

a. Health assessment.
b. Health promotion and disease prevention.
c. Care of those with illnesses or injuries.
d. Health education.

In planning for health assessment and health promotion and disease prevention, the nurse usually has advance time to structure a project. This allows time for scheduling, education, and communication. Although each plan should be designed to meet the needs of a specific school population, a general outline for screening or teaching projects is useful. Figure 19.2 gives such an outline. Some of the components vary with the particular type of assessment used or with the age of the student.

Another responsibility of the school nurse is care of those with injuries or illnesses. Whereas screening and environmental assessments can be planned in advance, accidents and illness are unplanned. The nurse

I. Set goals
II. Preliminary preparations
    A. Review information relevant to the problem and screening procedure.
    B. Identify target group.
    C. Obtain listing of individuals in target group.
    D. Set dates and times for screening and for makeup sessions.
    E. Schedule rooms.
    F. Arrange for volunteers and for their training.
    G. Obtain equipment.
    H. Prepare educational information and presentations for students, teachers, and parents.
    I. Develop permission slips, if necessary.
    J. Prepare reporting slips (one for normal outcome, one for rescreening, one for referral).
    K. Identify referral resources.
    L. Plan for orderly screening process.
    M. Develop trouble-shooting plan (responses for things that go wrong).
III. Education
    A. Orient teachers.
    B. Talk with students.
    C. Send information and permission slips to parents.
IV. Train volunteers
V. Implement screening
    A. Set up equipment.
    B. Have students brought in prearranged fashion.
    C. Screen each student.
    D. Record results on master sheet, each student's record, and report to parents.
VI. Follow-up
    A. Rescreen students with questionable results.
    B. Screen students who missed first screening.
    C. Schedule conferences with parents as needed.
    D. Check to see that students obtained referral services.
VII. Evaluation
    A. Determine whether goals were met.
    B. Assess effectiveness of plan and its components.
    C. Evaluate volunteers.
    D. Elicit feedback from students, teachers, and volunteers.
    E. Record evaluation for future reference

Figure 19.2 Screening plan outline.

can, however, be prepared for emergencies. Preparation includes:

· Maintaining a knowledge of first aid.
· Stocking first-aid supplies including antidotes for accidental poisoning.
· Maintaining up-to-date student records, including emergency telephone numbers and records of allergies and special health needs.
· Keeping on hand a manual of communicable diseases.
· Maintaining an awareness of epidemiological principles.
· Developing and maintaining a procedures manual.
· Obtaining annual training in cardiopulmonary resuscitation.
· Having quick access to emergency telephone numbers, such as ambulance, fire, police, poison control center, and community physicians.

Health education for students and staff is a process that occurs continuously through role modeling of the nurse, planned education projects, and daily implementation of school nursing functions. Principles of teaching and learning discussed in Chapter 17 of this book are applicable to health education in the school setting.

IMPLEMENTATION OF SCHOOL NURSING SERVICES. After assessment and planning, the nurse begins to implement services. Services may be implemented as a result of a carefully designed plan or they may come as a response to general plans, such as keeping health records on students up to date. The nurse may also respond to a specific need or problem that requires rapid action. To do this, the nurse may use predeveloped plans or implement a new plan. In general, the common activities of school nurses can be placed in five categories of service:

1. Screening.
2. Treating or referring for treatment.
3. Teaching.
4. Communicating.
5. Recording.

Screening is not only an assessment tool but also an intervention. Screening is implemented when the demographic characteristics of a group indicate that it will be useful or when there are signs a problem may exist.

The second category of services are those that involve treating a student or referring that student for treatment. This would include supervision of long-term care of a student with a chronic problem, such as diabetes. The student might need daily assessment and perhaps the administration of insulin. First aid is also an example of treatment. With the assistance of physicians or other nurses, the school nurse might develop planned activities, or protocols, that she or he could put into effect for common first-aid problems. A crucial aspect of treatment is deciding when the student's difficulty requires more assistance than the nurse can render. The school nurse, in conjunction with the school administration, should have a plan for responding to such problems. This should include a system for notifying parents and a system for providing medical care if the parents were unavailable.

The school nurse is often given opportunities for teaching students, teachers, and parents, as well as other staff members and administrators. Much teaching goes on in one-to-one contacts, which may be rather informal. However, the nurse may be given time to present health education information to students, either as part of scheduled classes or on special occasions. To be most effective, the nurse must have a grasp of teaching–learning principles so that health education activities can be appropriately implemented according to the age and background of the group. A nurse would have different approaches to teaching oral hygiene to first graders than to fifth graders, for example.

Communicating with teachers and parents, as well as with the students served, is essential. In talking with students, the nurse must strive to develop a natural, easy way of communicating that is not threatening or condescending. This will promote trust and make the students likely to seek the nurse out when they have a health need or problem. The nurse must also maintain open lines of communication with teachers. They will frequently be the nurse's best resource for identifying problems and needs. The nurse must encourage interactions with faculty members and must be sure to give them feedback when their information or referrals have been useful. Communication with parents or guardians of students is often handled through notes or form letters to parents. However, it is helpful for the nurse to contact some parents directly on occasion, especially when their children have severe, chronic, or frequent problems. If possible, the nurse can also be available on parents' days or at parent–teacher association meetings. When the occasion warrants it, the nurse might make an appointment for the parents to visit the school or for the nurse to visit the home. This might be necessary if the results of a screening test are particularly alarming, if a student has frequent problems, or if the nurse feels a need to have a better understanding of the family unit in order to help a student.

Finally, recording of information is probably one of the most important activities of any nurse. It is of particular importance for a nurse who may be working with hundreds of students in one or more schools. Al-

though the nurse will usually become personally acquainted with many students and will be able to recall vital information about them, such informal methods are unsatisfactory for the vast majority. Recording helps the nurse account for her or his time and provides a basis for planning and setting work priorities. The nurse may experiment with various methods of recording until she or he finds the way that is the most time saving and useful. In addition to maintaining a record on each student who is seen for any reason, the nurse will usually maintain a daily log showing the distribution of time in relation to the nurse's goals and priorities. Whenever an extensive screening or teaching project is undertaken, the nurse may maintain a master listing of all students who are to be involved in the project in order to ensure that all will be served and that appropriate follow-up is rendered.

EVALUATION OF SCHOOL NURSING SERVICES. Evaluation, the last phase of the nursing process, assists the nurse in determining the effectiveness of nursing service, provides feedback on programs, and gives direction to future projects. A guide for the evaluation of a project plan is shown in Figure 19.3. The form shown has room to evaluate each component of the project. Some aspects can be evaluated while the project is being planned and implemented. The final evaluation should be completed as soon as possible after the project is over. The evaluation report should be kept with the other materials about the project so that it is readily available when the nurse undertakes a similar project.

Ambulatory Settings

Ambulatory settings are those the client comes to on a short-term basis. They vary in services offered, size, means of funding,

Date:

Evaluator:

Goals:

Area to be Evaluated	Subjective Data	Objective Data	Assessment	Plan for Modification
I. Preliminary preparations				
A.				
B.				
C.				
II. Education				
A.				
B.				
C.				
III. Training of volunteers				
IV. Screening				
A.				
B.				
C.				

(*continued*)

Figure 19.3 Evaluation of project.

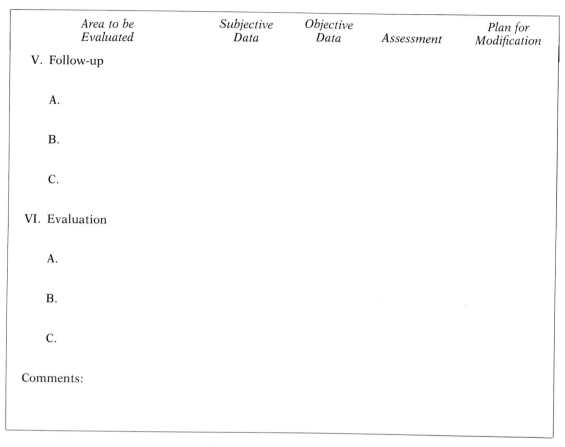

Area to be Evaluated	Subjective Data	Objective Data	Assessment	Plan for Modification
V. Follow-up				
A.				
B.				
C.				
VI. Evaluation				
A.				
B.				
C.				
Comments:				

Figure 19.3 (*continued*)

location, and target population. Engelke (1980) found that ambulatory clinics were viewed in the past as providing secondary and tertiary care but that today they are viewed as practical settings for primary prevention and treatment of chronic and episodic diseases.

Outpatient clinics, senior citizens' centers, and community health centers are examples of ambulatory settings. Ambulatory settings may be run either by official or voluntary agencies.

Comprehensive community health centers are usually located near their target population. These populations may include low-income, rural, urban, ethnic, or specific age groups. Their services include home health care; clinics providing general care, such as "medicine clinics," or specialty clinics offering well-child, immunization, or eye services; laboratory, x-ray, and pharmacy departments; and social and mental health services. Consultants, such as child development specialists, are often available on a contractual basis, as are nutritionists, physical therapists, and occupational therapists. Classes are presented to teach clients about nutrition, exercise, hypertension, and many other areas. An individual center may offer all or some of these services, and funding may come from government or voluntary agencies. Clients may be charged for services on a scale adjusted to income.

Community mental health centers provide a number of mental health services, including outpatient clinics, occupational therapy, group therapy, and day-care services. The role of these centers is described in Chapter 21.

Senior citizens' centers provide Ambulatory services during the day for senior citizens. Meals; activities, such as ceramics, knitting, and other crafts; exercises; and field trips are a few examples of services offered. Well-being clinics staffed by nurses are frequently held in senior citizens' centers; these assist in health maintenance, health promotion, and health education. The size of centers varies according to needs, facilities, and funding. Centers may be maintained by official or voluntary agencies.

As in school settings, screening for hypertension, diabetes, and hearing loss is frequently implemented. The needs of the clients must be assessed and plans made for nursing services.

A *clinic* may be one of a wide variety of settings. Outpatient clinics are usually located within a larger health facility, such as a hospital, department of health, rehabilitation center, or community health center. They may be general in nature, but they frequently focus on a specific health need, such as tuberculosis, sexually transmitted diseases, pediatrics, podiatry, well-child, and family health. Free clinics are often established by a voluntary group of health providers or interested persons to serve the needs of a low-income community. They are frequently held on weekends or evenings, and they provide a variety of services. They are generally located close to the population served. Clinics with an ethnic focus are established to meet the needs of specific cultural groups. Examples are clinics for Hispanic, Vietnamese, and native American populations.

Nursing practice in ambulatory settings is general and flexible, as the nurse must assess each situation holistically and utilize resources creatively. The nurse functions as a team member, provider of direct services, health educator, coordinator of services, epidemiologist, role model, and client advocate.

As a team member, the nurse cooperates with physicians, social workers, mental health workers, pharmacists, and laboratory personnel. The nurse may see the client at home as well as at the clinic, and the nurse shares information about the client with other team members. Team conferences provide an opportunity to communicate with other health care providers.

As a health educator, the nurse teaches the client about health behaviors, disease processes, medication, diet, and many other topics. Health education can be implemented formally, such as during planned prenatal classes at a community health center, or informally, such as during blood pressure screening at a senior citizens' center. The nurse provides direct services in clinics, such as administering medications or cleansing a wound, and coordinates services when a team of health care providers is involved. As an epidemiologist, the nurse must have a working knowledge of the community at large so that problems can be recognized early. At times, the nurse uses epidemiological principles in clinics, such as venereal disease, clinics when investigating possible contacts.

As a client advocate, the nurse facilitates health care, such as arranging for transportation to a clinic or arranging for an interpreter for a client who speaks only Spanish. Role modeling occurs in every nursing action, such as when the nurse displays caring, offers positive reinforcement, or utilizes hand-washing techniques.

Occupational Health Settings

Occupational settings vary with the nature of the industry involved. The nurse often carries out health promotion, safety, education, assessment, referral, and first aid activities as well as emergency care.

The nursing services offered are determined by each setting; however, one characteristic of all industrial settings is that the nurse focuses on a working, well population of adults. Each setting, therefore, challenges the nurse to consider problems generally associated with the working age population as well as those of the specific work environment. In the past, relates Tichy (1981), the occupational health nurse was considered a "band-aid nurse" whose role centered on first aid. Today, however, the nurse in industry is a professional functioning independently, implementing the entire nursing process with the goal of wellness for each employee. Although nursing functions must be consistent with individ-

ual company policies and procedures, the occupational health nurse generally implements the health care activities discussed in the following sections.

HEALTH SCREENING AND ASSESSMENT. The nurse assesses the total health status of employees and maintains appropriate records. On occasion, the nurse will screen employees for specific conditions, such as hypertension. Depending on the industry, the nurse will identify occupationally related diseases and institute appropriate screening measures. The nurse will also identify those with special needs, such as alcoholics, diabetics, and pregnant workers.

PROMOTION OF HEALTH BEHAVIORS. A part of the industrial nurse's role is to encourage employee participation in wellness behaviors, such as exercise and proper nutrition. A plan for identifying and responding to a wellness need is shown in Figure 19.4. The nurse will often practice or teach principles of epidemiology in order to prevent the spread of communicable diseases. A nurse

1. Assess the following:
   a. Level of wellness of employees through observations, interviews, questionnaires.
   b. Priorities of employees.
   c. Cooperation of management.
   d. Possible communication routes (posters, company newsletter, meetings).
   e. Available times for implementation of program.
2. Plan:
   a. Form committee of nurse and employees.
   b. Determine aspects of wellness to be focused upon (such as exercise).
   c. Set goals and objectives.
   d. Outline plan of action (adapt guidelines in Figure 19.2).
   e. Plan evaluation activities.
3. Implementation
   a. Communicate project to employees.
   b. Implement plan.
4. Evaluation
   a. Carry out planned evaluation of goals and objectives.
   b. Evaluate steps in plan.
   c. Establish goals for future wellness activities.

Figure 19.4 Plan for wellness promotion in an occupational setting.

in an industrial setting will find many opportunities for health education in areas such as stress management, hypertension, and cardiopulmonary resuscitation. The nurse will identify appropriate community referral sources and will assist with rehabilitation of workers who have been injured or ill.

PROMOTION OF SAFETY.   The nurse can assist in the assessment of environmental safety and can follow through by reporting the results and making suggestions to appropriate managers. The industrial nurse is responsible for being prepared for emergencies. This includes maintaining supplies for emergency treatment, such as antidotes for accidental poisoning. In addition to being ready to resuscitate a worker, the nurse should provide training so that workers can help each other when necessary. Depending on the setting, other activities might include participating in pollution control or educating employees about safety measures, such as proper handling of chemicals, equipment, or radioactive material.

Correctional Facilities

Care of those housed in correctional or other confining facilities is a part of community health nursing that is receiving increasing attention. The nurse in these facilities provides direct service; carries out health education, assessment, and screening; and collaborates with other members of the health team, such as dietitian or case manager. Correctional settings include maximum, medium, and minimum security facilities, and nurses are employed to provide care in these facilities by local, state, and federal government. Nurses may be employed directly or under contract with public health agencies.

The nurse must consider the special needs of those in correctional facilities. Fre-

quently, the pre-incarceration life-style of a prisoner has been unconducive to health. The nurse may participate in intake screening and health assessment of prisoners. The nurse will collect baseline information, such as blood pressure readings, health histories, routine medication usage, and health needs.

The nurse is concerned not only with the physical health of the inmate but also with psychosocial concerns. Prisoners have special needs because of the confinement they experience. The nurse may hold groups to address psychosocial needs. For example, the nurse may lead a group discussion about reintegration of the prisoner into family life.

Special-interest or health education groups may be held and communication established with families. The emphasis should be on holistic nursing care. For example, a nurse working with an inmate who has placed her baby in a foster home might discuss the mother's feelings and concerns with her and also might communicate with the foster family about the baby.

Prisoners often have other special problems, such as alcoholism or drug withdrawal. However, they also have the same needs as the general public for nutrition, safety, security, exercise, and rest. Thus, the nurse may monitor diet, environment, communicable disease, and exercise. Rehabilitation, including physical therapy activities, may be part of the nurse's role in this setting.

The nurse may encounter situations unique to prisoners such as hunger strikes, during which the nurse will monitor the striker's health status. Weight gain and lack of exercise may present special problems during imprisonment. In many cases, the nurse will have to decide whether to refer the inmate to a community facility for treatment unavailable in the prison. Clinics as well as hospital units may be staffed by nurses, depending on health care policy in each facility.

Attitudes of guards and other prison personnel may affect the health status of inmates, and the nurse may have an opportunity to provide inservice education about medication administration, first aid, and emergency care. The nurse may have negative feelings about the prisoners. It is necessary for the nurse to acknowledge these feelings so that they do not interfere with nursing care. Although many of the feelings will be negative, nurses may also become sympathetic to some prisoners. This is another of the many situations in which the nurse must learn to harmonize feelings, thoughts, and actions to provide the most appropriate nursing interventions.

The role of the nurse in the correctional facility varies widely, and Moritz (1982, p. 259) states that "more study is needed of nurses practicing in correctional facilities to identify their role and educational needs, define current and future practice requirements and the factors that facilitate or impede practice in these settings." She believes that a large portion of the prison population has less than adequate health care and that nursing can help resolve this problem.

Camps

The nurse functions in a role similar to that of the school nurse in camp settings. These settings include summer camps, day camps, and camps for children with special needs (such as children with diabetes or with a mental or physical handicap).

Camps are usually held during summer months and include outdoor activities that require the nurse to provide safety education. In addition, the nurse will be involved in first aid, illness screening, and counseling. The nurse may be required to set up a system to maintain needed information on the campers, or such a system may already exist. The camp may have policies about the health status of the campers. For examples, each child might have a current physical examination record on file in the infirmary. Certain immunizations may be required. There should be standard procedure for common situations if a child requires treatment. A release signed by each minor camper's parent or guardian should specify what kinds of treatment can be given without their permission. The release should also specify the way in which the nurse should contact parents or guardians if permission is needed for more extensive treatment. The name of the child's physician and how to contact that person should be included.

The camp may have an arrangement with local physicians or other health care providers to act as resources. If not, the nurse will be responsible for maintaining the information needed to locate these people if the need arises. The nurse may be responsible for supervising older campers or counselors who may assist in the care of sick children or children with special needs. This requires the nurse to be skillful at giving directions so that the campers are well cared for in the nurse's absence.

If the campers are children, the nurse should review normal growth and development for the age groups involved. The nurse should be aware of the common crises and emergencies that can occur when children are in a group living situation away from home. For example, a child may regress in an unfamiliar setting. Another child may become aggressive or behave in other antisocial ways. In a special camp, the nurse must be prepared for typical camp behavior as well as for specific problems and needs. For example, campers who are diabetic have all the usual needs of their age group but may need special attention in monitoring food intake, managing exercise, and administering medication. Part of the purpose of these camps may be to assist in the young people's adjustment to a life-long condition.

Shelters

Settings providing shelter for neglected or battered people, such as children, women, and the elderly, are another type of ambulatory setting. The nursing functions include counseling, referral, assistance with problem solving, and health assessment. Nurses may be employed as part of the staff or may be involved on a voluntary basis.

Health Fairs

In many cities, health providers participate in health fairs aimed at health assessment and education. Booths are usually set up and assessment is implemented through various screening methods for physical and psychosocial problems. Nurses interpret the results and make referrals when indicated.

Health education is accomplished in several ways. Representatives of specialty organizations may provide literature. For example, the American Lung Association may provide materials about the hazards of smoking, and a nurse may be available to help an interested person evaluate his or her own potential for developing related problems.

Hospices

Traditionally, hospices have been places where travelers, the needy, the sick, and the dying could find food, shelter, and care. The modern *hospice* provides care for the dying

client and his or her family. It includes efforts to provide emotional support as well as to control pain and symptoms of disease. The hospice concept is embodied in a variety of settings, including the client's home; hospice units in hospital buildings; freestanding, autonomous units for inpatient care; medical vans that make rounds in the community; and comprehensive programs offering inhospital service, home care, and day care for clients.

Hospice care is growing in usage and in the number of facilities and personnel available. An interdisciplinary team approach is used to implement the goal of providing holistic care to the client and family. This care does not stop when the client dies, but usually includes bereavement services for the family for a period of time.

Hospice programs are sponsored by hospitals, agencies, or volunteer groups. The goals, as delineated by Perrollaz and Mollica (1981), are applicable to a variety of hospice settings:

1. To help the client maintain physical and emotional comfort.
2. To facilitate the client's functioning at a maximal level until death.
3. To assist in meeting illness-related needs of the family and client during final stages of illness, dying, and bereavement.

Nurses function in a variety of ways as members of a hospice team. Nurses are involved in assessing clients and deciding what hospice services they need. Nurses assist in planning care and in determining who will render care. When family members or volunteers are involved in caregiving, the nurse may be the person responsible for training them. Frequently, the nurse will give direct care to hospice clients, either in their homes or in inpatient facilities. Since the hospice approach is relatively new, it is a fertile area for nursing research, and nurses may be involved as principal investigators or as collaborators with other researchers. Nurses are also involved in public education and in fund raising to increase community awareness about hospice programs and to enlist public support for their activities.

Types of Services Provided

Direct versus Indirect Services

Hands-on nursing activities are often called direct nursing care. *Direct care* includes all aspects of face-to-face service, including counseling with clients in a community mental health center, administering immunizations in a well-child clinic, and assisting with a bed bath during a home visit.

Indirect care includes coordination and collaboration activities. Some examples of indirect service include contacting various agencies to schedule transportation for elderly clients, arranging for eye exam services as follow-up to school vision screening, developing lists of referral resources, and producing health education media.

Both direct and indirect services are important to holistic, continuous care. For example, a client who has had a cerebrovascular accident and is paralyzed on one side of his body is being visited in his home by a community health nurse. The nurse gives him a bed bath, changes linens, and assists with range-of-motion exercises twice a week. These are direct services. The nurse also utilizes indirect services by teaching the client's wife to assist with personal care, by arranging for a physical therapist to make home visits, and by contacting a community service agency about lending the client a lift and wheelchair. The nurse may consult the family's clergyman about the client's spiritual needs and a psychiatric nurse about psychosocial needs.

Primary, Secondary, and Tertiary Prevention

Although the community health nurse is concerned with all three levels of prevention—primary, secondary, and tertiary—the focus for a given client may be on one particular level. *Primary prevention* focuses on health promotion and disease prevention. It includes health education, immunizations, well-child care, accident prevention, and health planning.

Secondary prevention focuses on health maintenance for people with chronic disease, early diagnosis, and intervention to limit disabilities. Some examples are follow-up activities after screening for visual or auditory deficiencies, teaching a young client to administer her own insulin, or teaching a client with cardiovascular disease to take his own pulse rate and report abnormalities.

Tertiary prevention relates to rehabilitation and restoration of functioning. The nurse who assists clients with cardiac problems by teaching them about exercise and nutrition is practicing tertiary prevention. Another example is assisting a client with range-of-motion exercises after a cerebrovascular accident to help restore function.

Short-term or Long-term Care

Whether to consider an activity short-term or long-term care may be a matter of opinion. For simplicity, *short-term care* is defined here as being limited to one contact with a client or a series of contacts over a limited period of time. This includes seeing a client once for immunizations, visiting a client three or four times after a hospitalization for an acute illness, supervising the health care of children at a summer camp, or working with a client who is dying at home. Even though these activities are time limited, the services provided may be quite comprehensive, including contacting family members, making referrals, health teaching, and so forth.

More frequently, *long-term care* is the nature of practice in community health settings. Through extended use of the nursing process, the nurse assesses, plans, implements, and evaluates care with the family and serves as a role model to them in the use of the problem-solving process. An example of long-term care is making home visits to a family that includes a member with multiple sclerosis. The client's and family's previous coping abilities, health behaviors, and health status are assessed. Resources, both material and human, are delineated. Having made an assessment, the nurse plans with the client and family for care, including activities to assist the afflicted family member to maintain his or her level of functioning. During implementation of the plan, the nurse selects the extent of care that is required as the client's or family members' needs change. At times the nurse may visit at frequent intervals and render direct care. At other times, the nurse may see the family once a month and offer health teaching or referrals as new concerns arise. Periodically, the nurse and family evaluate interventions by discussing progress and their feelings about the plan. Some long-term relationships last until a client changes residences or dies. Other long-term situations eventually terminate because the client and family become self-sufficient or no longer desire a nurse's assistance.

Focus of Care: Single versus Multiple

Many settings focus on a single health aspect of care, such as community mental health centers and hospice programs. Others have multiple foci and offer a variety of services. A comprehensive commu-

nity health center might offer mental health or hospice services plus physical therapy, occupational therapy, home health care, maternal and well-child clinics, and laboratory, x-ray, and social services.

Number of Health Providers: Individual versus Team

A public health service located in a rural setting often employs one registered nurse to serve the population of a specified geographical area. In this case, the individual nurse works as a generalist practicing many roles.

The team approach is often practiced in more heavily populated areas. Comprehensive community health centers offer a team approach through their many programs and services. Members of a team often include a nurse, physician, nutritionist, physical therapist, occupational therapist, mental health specialist, and social service workers.

Target Population Focus

Needs often relate to specific population groups, such as ethnic, income, or age groups. A discussion of settings serving specific population groups follows..

Ethnic Groups

Special settings providing care to ethnic or cultural groups are increasing in number. The native American centers and clinics and Hispanic and Vietnamese cultural centers are examples. In these settings, the nurse functions as caregiver in addition to advocate, communicator, health educator, and support person. The nurse must be knowledgeable about cultural mores and accepting of those whose beliefs may differ from her or his own. Often, the most effective nurse in such a setting is one who is of the same cultural or ethnic group, especially if the clients are outside the mainstream of U.S. culture.

Income Groups

Community health agencies are sometimes located in areas of poverty or low income. Examples are free clinics provided by volunteer groups such as the Salvation Army. Frequently, continuity of care is impossible due to mobile life-styles, so the nurse must utilize each contact opportunity for health education and care. Realistically, this education can best focus on a brief description of the illness being treated, information regarding medication or treatments, and assistance in problem solving for future health needs, such as how to seek emergency care. The nurse should assess each client's situation and adapt health teaching accordingly.

People with moderate or high incomes utilize a variety of community health resources but may need to be educated about services offered, availability of services, and sources of referral. Frequently, people in middle- or upper-income groups do not use public, tax-supported health services because of the mistaken notion that these are only for the indigent. These people need to be informed of the availability of public health resources as well as health care services available to those with large incomes.

Age-specific Groups

Many community settings provide care for persons of specific age groups only. Such settings include well-child clinics, senior citizens' centers, teenage crisis centers, and family planning clinics. Nurses can often maximize their impact by focusing on specific care to particular populations. For example, the nurse in a senior citizens' center can plan activities that relate to the aging process. If an exercise project is planned, special needs of the elderly are considered, such as limited mobility. If a program on human sexuality is planned, information pertaining to age-related changes would be appropriate.

Urban versus Rural Groups

Persons living in either urban or rural areas have some uniquely different needs. In rural areas, health needs are often related to agriculture. Farm accidents and hazards of working with chemicals such as insecticides are examples. Health care may be postponed during seasons when farmers are busy and must make maximum use of temperate weather. The nurse must be aware of the impact of an agriculturally determined life-style on health behaviors and plan interventions accordingly.

Another type of rural nursing exists for the mountain people in Kentucky, where the Frontier Nursing Service offers care. Care of native Americans living on reservations constitutes another type of rural nursing. In these settings the nurse may be the only health provider in contact with families and therefore functions as a generalist. The nurse in the rural setting often lacks face-to-face interaction with peers and must function autonomously. Nursing practice may take place in clinics or in the home.

By contrast, in urban settings multiple health resources are often available and the nurse may function in cooperation with a health team. Native Americans living in urban areas may have different needs from those in rural areas. For example, nutrition needs may become prominent when a person accustomed to gardening and growing fresh vegetables must purchase food at a city market. Urban clients often live in crowded tenements with limited recreational space. Urban dwellers may have greater control over their time than do rural people and therefore may have a different pattern of seeking health care. However, since so many resources are so readily available, city dwellers may delay meeting needs because they feel that the resources will always be at hand.

SELECTION OF SETTINGS

In community health nursing, settings are chosen for their suitability in the implementation of health care. For example, Mr. Tallchief is a native American living in a western state. He requests nursing assistance after his 10-year-old son, John-Jay, returns home from the hospital after diagnosis of and initial treatment for diabetes.

In the initial assessment of the family situation, the nurse identifies the following factors that have implications for the settings within which John-Jay and the Tallchief family can receive service:

1. The family has a limited income and no health insurance for the boy.
2. The family has minimal understanding of diabetes and its treatment.
3. Their automobile is unreliable and they try to walk to most places they need to go.
4. John-Jay is enrolled in a public school in the fifth grade.
5. John-Jay and his parents are intelligent, able, and willing to learn about diabetes. John-Jay has already expressed an interest in administering his own insulin.
6. Mr. Tallchief's sister, who is a practical nurse, has been administering John-Jay's insulin since he went home.

7. The family has a strong sense of their heritage and they socialize exclusively with other native Americans. However, Mr. and Mrs. Tallchief have worked in non-Indian situations and are comfortable but reserved with non-Indians. John-Jay has some school friends who are non-Indians and his favorite teacher is a non-Indian.

After identifying these relevant factors, the nurse begins to assess available agencies and services to find those that will make the best match with the needs of the family. Following the framework described in this chapter, the nurse could ascertain the features she or he would look for in finding resources. The sequence used to establish the necessary features to suit the needs of the Tallchiefs might proceed as follows:

1. SPONSORSHIP OF SERVICES

Because of the family's limited income and the high priority of John-Jay's newly diagnosed illness, the nurse looks for services sponsored by groups that provide free or low-cost services. Official agencies might include the local department of health; voluntary agencies would include the Visiting Nurses' Association, the American Diabetes Association, and health care centers especially for native Americans; some private providers might specialize in the care of children, diabetics, or native Americans and might put fees on a sliding scale.

2. ENVIRONMENTS WHERE SERVICES ARE PROVIDED

The family has limited geographic mobility because of unreliable transportation. John-Jay is in school. Therefore, the setting for care, including teaching, should be the home and school, with only occasional visits to a clinic or other central setting. If possible, this clinic should be relatively close to the family's home. Teachers and the school nurse should be informed of John-Jay's diabetes. The school nurse should collaborate with the nurse making home visits. The nurse making home visits should teach the mother and father how to care for their son. The nurse might need to visit the home in the evening if either or both parents work outside the home. A summer camp for diabetic children might be an option for John-Jay if a camp could be found that provides scholarships. However, this might be an unwanted service unless there were several other native American children involved.

3. TYPE OF SERVICE OFFERED

The family needs many direct services from a nurse, especially related to teaching. The nurse will provide secondary prevention services, since John-Jay already has been diagnosed with a chronic, life-long illness. The nurse will need to anticipate potential problems and help the family prevent them. Both the school nurse and the visiting nurse may have a heavier burden because of the limited time the school nurse has to work with John-Jay. Because the family lives in a metropolitan area, the nurse can avail herself or himself of many support services. Because the boy's illness is life threatening and life long, the nurse involved in giving direct service must understand the family's culture and mores. The family is accustomed to interacting with non-Indians, and they may be comfortable working with a nurse who is not a native American. However, since the nurse may have to spend time in their home, they may appreciate a native American nurse or a native American who is an assistant to the nurse, if the nurse is of a different cultural background. Direct services rendered in the home setting may be seen as more intrusive than similar activities in a hospital.

4. TARGET POPULATION

The setting may be selected on the basis of John-Jay's native American ethnicity. In addition, services particularly for school-aged children are appropriate. Services particularly for those with lower incomes would be applicable to this family. A clinic that is aware of the special concerns of urban-dwelling native Americans would be helpful to the Tallchiefs.

After the nurse has identified the important features of the setting or settings in which care could be given to the Tallchiefs, she or he would set about finding agencies that would provide these features. The nurse would help the Tallchiefs select and begin to avail themselves of the necessary services in the most appropriate settings. For this family, a nurse from the local health department might be the principal caregiver. This person would visit in the home and coordinate the use of services in other settings. How the nurse locates these resources is described in the next section.

Locating Settings for Community Health Practice

Many resources are available in community settings, and the nurse must be able to locate them and assess the value of each for meeting client needs. Locating resources often presents a challenge, since some agencies are not well publicized and others go out of business. In large metropolitan areas, a local service group may publish and update a directory of community services. In addition to this, or in place of it, the nurse can locate some services in the telephone book or through the Chamber of Commerce, the local health department, and colleagues.

If a resource book is available, the nurse will use this as a foundation for establishing a resource file. If it is not available or is incomplete, the nurse can establish a file or looseleaf notebook in which to record pertinent information about resources. Several colleagues might share a resource file. The topics that might be included about each resource are:

Resource name
Address
Telephone number
Hours of operation
Services provided
Criteria for eligibility
Costs to clients

Procedure for obtaining services

Waiting-list procedures

Referral process

Staff and roles

Strengths

Weaknesses

Other information and comments

Source of information

Date of information

The resource file can be categorized and cross-referenced based on the system outlined in this chapter for identifying features pertinent to selecting a setting for service. Some examples of settings related to the identifying features are given in Table 19.1.

Factors that Facilitate or Inhibit Use of Settings

Services provided by community settings are only beneficial if they are used. Several factors contribute to use of community health settings. One factor is trust. If a client believes that the personnel in an agency are trustworthy, he or she is more likely to use the services.

Finances contribute to whether or not a certain facility is used. The nurse may need to determine with the client how much money is available for health services. Many people who have sufficient funds to pay for health care are unwilling to spend their money unless they see direct benefits from the services provided. On the other hand, people who do not wish to pay for health-promotion activities may also be adverse to using publicly supported agencies even though they have indirectly helped to finance them.

Often health care providers as well as clients lack knowledge about services available. Therefore, the nurse must be informed about community resources and must share the information with clients and colleagues.

A service must be accessible to clients; this includes transportation to the setting, in some instances. Clients may need assistance in arranging transportation or in planning how to get to an agency. This may include interpreting bus schedules, utilizing volunteer services, or collaborating with family members. Some agencies may arrange for taxi companies to transport their clients and bill the agency. The client may not inquire about this service, or the staff of the agency may not realize the client needs it.

Many people resist change of any type; entering a community agency represents a change. The nurse must be aware of this and assist in making the change easier for the client. The nurse can act as the client's advocate by being present during initial contacts with an agency. This provides security for the client and enhances communication and trust. The nurse can help the client learn how to ask for and receive needed services.

ROLES OF THE NURSE IN COMMUNITY HEALTH SETTINGS

The nature of nursing practice in community health settings can be understood by examining roles that nurses practice in various situations. A discussion of these roles follows.

Collaborator

The nurse collaborates with members of the health team in assessing, planning, and evaluating interventions. The client may be

TABLE 19.1
Identifying Features and Examples of Settings

Identifying Feature	Setting
1. Sponsorship	
a. Official agencies	U.S. Public Health Service
	state, local, district departments of health
b. Voluntary agencies	American Cancer Society
	Arthritis Foundation, Inc.
	Leukemia Society of America
	Mental health associations
	Nursing homes for the elderly
	Health maintenance organizations
	Visiting nurses' associations
c. Private providers	Independent nurse-practitioners
2. Environments	
a. Homes	Homes
	Apartments
	Nursing home apartment
b. Schools	Elementary, secondary
	Preschools, Head Start
	Colleges, universities
	Public, private
c. Ambulatory	Outpatient clinics associated with hospitals
	Comprehensive health clinics
	Specialty clinics (maternity, well-child, family planning)
	Public health department clinics (tuberculosis, sexually transmitted diseases)
	Clinics for low-income clients
	Senior citizens' centers
d. Occupational	Industries
	Offices
e. Correctional	Maximum-, medium-, minimum-security facilities (prisons, jails, detention units)
f. Camps	Day camps
	Summer camps
	Camps for those with handicaps (mental, physical)
	Camps for those with specific diseases (diabetes)
g. Shelters	Women's resource centers
	Child-abuse hotlines and shelters
	Shelters for battered people (elderly)

TABLE 19.1 (*continued*)

Identifying Feature	Setting
h. Health fairs	At health departments, clinics, shopping centers, hospitals, and many other locations
i. Hospices	Homes
	Hospitals
	Mobile vans
	Day units
	Free-standing units
3. Type of service	
a. Direct	Comprehensive health center providing physical therapy, nutrition counseling, immunizations
	School nurse providing first aid
	Occupational nurse providing safety education
	Correctional nurse administering treatment
	Visiting nurse giving bed bath
Indirect	Comprehensive health center providing referral and consultation
	School nurse confering with administration about equipment needs
	Visiting nurse contacting senior citizens' center about transportation for a client
b. Primary	School nurse teaching a class on dental health
	Well-child clinic nurse administering immunizations
Secondary	Health fair screening for vision defects
Tertiary	Visiting nurse assisting quadraplegic client with range-of-motion exercise
c. Short-term	Community nurse following up on contacts of a child with a communicable disease
	School nurse examining children for head lice
Long-term	Nurse working with hospice clients
	Occupational health nurse implementing an ongoing safety program
	Nurse in well-child program working with abusive parents
d. Single focus	Foundations for the disabled
	Society for Crippled Children
	American Heart Association
	Society to Prevent Blindness
Multiple focus	Comprehensive health centers
	Official health departments
	World Health Organization
e. Individual provider	Community health nurse in rural area
	Independent nurse-practitioner
	Camp nurse
	Industrial health nurse

TABLE 19.1 (*continued*)

Identifying Feature	Setting
Team approach	Community mental health center
	State, local, and district health departments
	Community health centers
4. Target population served	
a. Cultural/ethnic groups	Hispanic, Vietnamese centers
	Religious-based societies
	Native-American programs
b. Income groups	Free clinics
	Religious based (Catholic Charities)
	State welfare departments
	Community health clinics using a sliding scale for payment
	Visiting nurses
c. Age specific	Senior citizens' centers
	Schools
	Youth guidance councils
	Well-child clinics
d. Rural/urban	Frontier Nursing Service
	Urban Indian Health Centers

an individual, a family, or a group of persons in the community. Collaborative activities may range from a single telephone call to arrange for physical therapy for a client to a series of meetings to prevent the recurrence of hepatitis in a community.

Consultant

As a consultant, the nurse shares nursing knowledge and expertise to help solve a problem or meet a need. For example, a community mental health nurse may be asked to present a seminar on teen-age alcoholism to a group of parents at a local school.

Coordinator

In coordinating health services, the nurse encourages use of a variety of agencies and discourages duplication of services. For instance, a nurse making home visits to a family where child abuse has been a problem will coordinate efforts of groups, such as social service, a community mental health center, and a peer-support group.

Preventer of Disease

The nurse practices disease prevention in such endeavors as conducting immunization clinics, assisting with casefinding during an epidemic, or teaching a class on dental hygiene. Prevention can be implemented in any aspect of nursing practice.

Promoter of Health

Promoting health is always a component of nursing care, whether the nurse teaches breast self-examination during a routine clinic visit or discusses nutrition with a new mother during a home visit. The role of health promoter includes consideration of the unique individual characteristics of each client as well as predictable health needs.

Provider of Direct Care

The nurse provides direct care in many ways. In clinics, such as sexually transmitted disease clinics, the nurse administers treatments according to medical orders. During home visits, nurses provide appropriate care including bed baths, range-of-motion exercises, and other treatments. In the school setting, the nurse may administer first aid.

Health Educator

Health education is another service the nurse provides in conjunction with many other roles. Education may be planned and structured, as when a nurse teaches a group of students about drug dependency, or it may be spontaneous and casual, as when a nurse teaches a child how to cleanse a scraped knee.

Manager

The nurse assumes the role of manager in a variety of situations. This calls upon many skills, including those related to communication. This may include managing a caseload of clients, managing a health clinic, or managing a staff of health providers.

Epidemiologist

A nurse uses epidemiological skills when investigating an outbreak of influenza. Like health education, epidemiology can be formal or informal, planned or spontaneous. Whatever the procedure, the nurse attempts to assess a situation and learn more about it. This process is described in more detail in Chapter 29.

Role Model

The community health nurse serves as a role model for health behaviors in many ways. Because of his or her contact with many relatively healthy people, the nurse has the opportunity to influence them by setting an example through such activities as eating properly, engaging in regular exercise, getting appropriate rest, and seeking preventive dental care.

FUTURE IMPLICATIONS

As long as there are schools, industries, correctional facilities, and so on, there will be a place for the nurse to practice. However, the nature of the settings may change, thus affecting the way nurses function within them. For example, with increased access to computers, the nurse within a school will have greater resources in making assessments. Such devices will promote more effective record keeping. A student's record could be maintained easily throughout his or her school years and would be accessible to each new school nurse. Nurses working in industrial settings often experience isolation and a lack of peer support. In the future, computer linkages may promote interchanges and sharing of knowledge among nurses working in similar settings all over the country.

Development of new industries and resources will affect health needs. Our reliance on nuclear energy has presented new health hazards, for example. Nurses will have a responsibility for promoting the well-being not only of those directly in contact with nuclear materials but also of other people who are indirectly affected. People living close to a nuclear energy plant may suffer from anxiety caused by the real or perceived dangers of the plant. Their fears may disrupt their mental health and eventually their physical health. They may also indirectly affect their children's sense of security. This chain of events might be discovered by a nurse who works with a client in a nearby workplace or community setting. Nurses should be aware of the many community factors that affect clients regardless of the setting within which the nurse comes in contact with a client.

Historically, nursing's foundations were within the community, not within acute care institutions. It is likely that nursing will be practiced more and more outside institutions. Because of the flexible nature of nursing and the many roles that nurses perform, nursing lends itself to practice within many settings. As communities change to meet the challenges of the future, nursing will accommodate new expectations. A nurse may be the health professional who collaborates most consistently with other nurses and with other caregivers to plan and coordinate the health care of many community members. This nurse would be the person to ascertain the needs of clients and to see that these needs were met within the appropriate settings. With the assistance of electronic equipment, one nurse would be able to maintain in-

formation on a large number of clients and to match clients with necessary resources.

With more public interest in and concern about health promotion and with individuals becoming willing to take on more responsibility for their own health care, health promotion centers might be established. These could be centrally located in various parts of an urban or rural area. They might be privately financed with fees for service or they might be partly or wholly subsidized by local, state, or federal government. These centers would be staffed by many health care professionals with nurses acting as specialists in planning health promotion programs for clients. Programs might be developed to suit many people of various ages and health statuses, with variations devised to meet unique needs, such as recovery from a surgical procedure.

An exciting possibility for the future is the increased involvement of nurses in the space program. Not only will they continue to function in support of people directly involved in the exploration of space, they will also become more involved in new settings. If we continue to develop space stations and space shuttles, nurses will be among those needed on such expeditions. Nutritional health, exercise, and many other types of primary prevention will be necessary. Space travel creates new health needs caused by such things as different forces of gravity, prolonged use of unconventional foods, lengthy periods of confinement, and lack of fresh air. Nurses functioning in these unfamiliar circumstances will help identify problems and develop innovative solutions. However, the nursing process and nursing skills such as being able to coordinate, teach, investigate, and render care will still provide the foundation for the nurse's activities.

SUMMARY

Settings for community health nursing practice may be grouped according to certain identifying features. The functions of nurses in individual settings vary but the nature of nursing is the same. The nurse of the present and the future must be creative in applying nursing skills and in using available resources. Regardless of the setting, the nurse's role is to respond to the needs of the client.

DISCUSSION TOPICS

1. Susan Wilson is a 16-year-old high school student who suspects she may be pregnant but does not want to get married immediately.

   a. Identify needs of Susan, her family, and her boyfriend.

   b. Use the list of identifying features to describe the settings in which these needs can be met.

2. Juan Ortega has recently moved to the United States from Mexico with his wife and two children, ages 6 and 8. The children have had no immunizations. Mr. and Mrs. Ortega speak only Spanish, and he does not have a job. The children speak minimal English. The school nurse needs to communicate with the parents about immunizations.

   a. Identify possible settings available in both rural and urban areas to assist Mexican-American families.

   b. Describe the role of the school nurse in caring for this family.

   c. Describe an ideal community setting for meeting the needs of this family.

   d. Describe local resources that would be available for health care for this family.

3. An industrial nurse employed in a factory that manufactures toxic substances has identified the need to educate workers about safety in handling these chemicals. Devise a plan for teaching the workers what they need to know.

4. Beverly Walker, age 6 months, is seen in a well-child clinic by a community health nurse at bimonthly intervals. Her mother asks the nurse about settings in the community that could help her understand stages in Beverly's growth and development. What information would be needed to determine the advantages and disadvantages of settings to which the nurse might refer Mrs. Walker?

5. Dan Littleton, RN, is employed by the health department as the only nurse in a rural county. The county jail has contracted for his nursing services on a part-time basis.

   a. Describe Mr. Littleton's role in this correctional setting.

   b. How could Mr. Littleton provide for the needs of inmates with psychosocial problems and drug and alcohol dependency?

   c. Develop an environmental checklist Mr. Littleton could use in the jail.

6. Nan Sargent, RN, has been hired by the local school board as a health educator. She has been asked to plan a wellness program for students in the junior high, age 13–15. Members of the board have told her she has complete authority over topics covered.

   a. Discuss appropriate assessments for Ms. Sargent to make in determining priority needs for wellness.

   b. Write goals and an outline of a plan for implementing a wellness project for these students.

   c. Devise a method for evaluating the long-term effects of the project.

7. Imagine you are a nurse who has helped to found Wellness Center, Inc.

a. Describe what this setting would be like using the features outlined in this chapter.

b. Describe how you as a nurse would function in the roles described in this chapter.

8. What do you think is the most innovative setting in which you might ever have to function as a nurse?

BIBLIOGRAPHY

Diamond, N.: Hospice. *Family Health* 12, 9, 28, 1980.

Engelke, M.: Nursing in ambulatory settings: A head nurse's perspective. *American Journal of Nursing* 80, 1813, 1980.

MacElveen-Hoehn, P., & McIntosh, E.: The hospice movement: Growing pains and promises. *Topics in Clinical Nursing* 3(3), 29, 1981.

Moritz, P.: Health care in correctional facilities: A nursing challenge. *Nursing Outlook* 30, 253, 1982.

Oda, D.: A viewpoint on school nursing. *American Journal of Nursing* 81, 1677, 1981.

Perrollaz, L., & Mollica, M.: Public knowledge of hospice care. *Nursing Outlook* 29, 46, 1981.

Pletsch, P.: Mary Breckinridge: A pioneer who made her mark. *American Journal of Nursing* 81, 2188, 1981.

Tichy, A.: Wellness, the worker, and the nurse. *Occupational Health Nursing* 29, 21, 1981.

Wald, F.: Terminal care and nursing education. *American Journal of Nursing* 79, 1762, 1979.

20

Visiting Clients
in the Home

Carolyn J. Leman

Health in the home can only be learnt from the home and in
the home.

FLORENCE NIGHTINGALE

OBJECTIVES

After reading this chapter, you should be able to:

☐ Understand the historical perspective of home visits.
☐ Understand the process of visiting clients in the home.
☐ Identify components of the home visit.
☐ Discuss the relationship of the nursing process to the home visit.
☐ Discuss advantages and disadvantages of the home visit.
☐ Consider the roles of the nurse during the home visit.
☐ Explore nurse–client communication during a home visit.
☐ Discuss the relationship of the home visit to other concepts and explore
implications for future nursing practice in the home setting.

INTRODUCTION

The home is a setting frequently utilized for nursing care. In this setting, where nursing practice is autonomous, all of the nurse's knowledge, skills, and experience are employed. Visiting clients in the home provides a challenge and an opportunity for both nurse and family to function as a team in the client's own environment.

This chapter discusses these opportunities, describes use of the nursing process in the home visit, and discusses the process involved in visiting clients in the home.

HISTORICAL CONSIDERATIONS

The home has been utilized as a setting for nursing care for many years. Florence Nightingale, who helped establish a training school for nurses in England, referred to graduates of that school who practiced nursing by home visiting as "health nurses" (Hanlon & Pickett, 1979).

In England, home visits began as a service to the poor in the 1850s, when William Rathbone established a visiting nursing service for the sick poor in Liverpool. In the United States, the first visiting nurses were employed in 1877 by the New York City Mission. In 1885 district nursing associations were founded in Buffalo and in 1886 in Boston and Philadelphia. Clients were the sick poor, as persons who could pay for services employed private home nursing care (Kalisch & Kalisch, 1978).

Thus professional nurses have been providing care in homes since the nineteenth century, although the focus has shifted from provision of care to the ill to emphasis on health promotion and disease prevention in addition to illness care.

OVERVIEW

In this chapter, a *home visit* is the process of providing nursing care in the client's dwelling place. This dwelling may be in a single-unit or multiple-unit structure and may be located in a rural or urban setting. The goal when visiting clients in the home is to provide appropriate nursing care leading to wellness. Wellness can mean different things to different people, just as happiness, health, and even cleanliness have various interpretations. Thus, during home visits, the goals (or level of wellness desired

by the client) are delineated by the nurse and client together.

Basic Principles

The first principle of visiting clients in the home is that the family unit is significant. Health needs of one family member, such as a newborn child with physical abnormalities, may have activated a request for nursing visits. However, each person in the family contributes to family functioning and to the level of family health. The mother, father, and other children will have added responsibilities. Each can benefit from nursing care, such as support, education, and assistance with the problem-solving process in coping with changes in their lives and family functioning. Therefore, the nurse must attempt to include each family member in all phases of the nursing process.

Second, the nurse is a guest in the client's home and makes only those nursing interventions the client agrees to. The nurse must be flexible and must respect the client's right to accept or reject care and to participate in goal setting and goal achievement.

Third, mutual nurse–client goals and interventions may require long periods of time to achieve. Patience is necessary, as the results of nursing interventions may not be immediately noted. For example, interventions for a quadraplegic teenager will include long-term physical therapy, attention to psychosocial adjustment, and career planning.

Fourth, home visits can be made by a nurse employed in a variety of ways. The nurse may be an independent practitioner, an employee of the client, or an employee of such agencies as official public health departments, visiting nurses' associations, community health centers, schools, and home health agencies.

Fifth, the nurse is autonomous in practice and often is the primary provider of health care for the family. Optimally, the family and nurse develop a positive interpersonal relationship as they work to achieve goals.

PROCESS

Visiting clients in the home gives the nurse an excellent opportunity to implement the nursing process. The home visit itself can be viewed as a process. Nursing activity begins with referral of a client for care, and, after appropriate activities, ends with termination or transfer of care.

Specific components of the process of the home visit include referral, previsit activities, entry into the home, promoting the nurse–client relationship, evaluation, concluding the visit, postvisit activities, and termination. These components may be utilized in the order described when working with a particular family, or they may be used in varying order. For example, the nurse caring for Mrs. Calhoun, age 72, who has been discharged from the hospital after a diagnosis of diabetes, would probably proceed through all the above steps. On the other hand, a neighbor present in Mrs. Calhoun's home when the nurse visits might ask the nurse to come to her house to discuss care of her elderly mother. The community health nurse would begin visits with that verbal referral and would not have time for previsit activities. The nurse can exercise his or her judgment in appropriate utilization of components described when making home visits.

Referral

The first step in the process of visiting clients in the home is *referral* of a client for

nursing care. Referral may come from a variety of sources, including other nurses, physicians, other health providers, clergymen, friends, school personnel, employees of community health agencies, and the client.

Telephone or direct referral is appropriate in many instances: when a client contacts a nurse to request a visit to explore available nursing services; when a nurse working in an agency or clinic identifies a need for home visits and refers the client to a community health nurse; when a health professional, such as a physical therapist, requests that a nurse accompany that professional on a visit. These referrals are frequently followed by written correspondence.

In other instances, written referral is necessary: when a physician's orders are required for administration of treatments or medication; when specific information and directions are needed by the nurse; when third-party payment or the employing agency requirements must be met.

Factors that determine appropriate referral sources and procedures are delineated by individual agencies, and it is the nurse's responsibility to be aware of such policies. When referral is received, the nurse begins the assessment phase of the nursing process by obtaining information such as the client's name, address, travel directions, telephone number, diagnosis, source of referral, and name and expectations of the person referring the client.

Previsit Activities

After referral, *previsit activities* begin. These activities vary depending on the individual client's and family's needs. During this stage, the assessment phase of the nursing process continues as the nurse gathers information about the client, investigates community resources, assembles supplies, and plans for the first client contact.

Information Gathering

Information gathering includes a variety of activities. First, the nurse assesses and reviews the information available on the referred client. This review includes such areas as the client's medical diagnosis. For example, when referral of Mrs. Calhoun, the diabetic client previously described, was received, the nurse assessed and reviewed these and other areas as needed:

1. The client's diagnosis.
2. Care of the aging client, including normal changes associated with the aging process.
3. Change theory, as this client is undergoing changes in many areas—diet, medication, exercise.
4. Role theory, since Mrs. Calhoun now has a new perception of herself as a person with a chronic disease. She may assume the sick role, which might be maladaptive.

After this preparation, the nurse may confer with other health providers as appropriate. The community health nurse who will be assisting Mrs. Calhoun in her home would confer with hospital personnel to learn about Mrs. Calhoun's response to medications and to her diagnosis. Consulting peers, such as a nurse who specializes in care of geriatric clients, is an option. Such consultation can enhance the nurse's knowledge and understanding of specific client situations and can assist the nurse in clarifying his or her ideas about appropriate nursing care. Feedback from peers and validation of observations and plans can enhance nursing care. A nurse who takes over care of a family from another nurse should confer with the first caregiver about needs previously assessed, interventions

implemented, and coping behaviors utilized. The nurse may confer with other professionals, such as the physician, social worker, physical therapist, mental health worker, and nutritionist.

In the case of the initial referral without prior health care contact of the family, other resources may be tapped to enhance the nurse's knowledge base and understanding of the client. For example, if the client is a member of an ethnic group different from that of the nurse, the nurse would attempt to learn about the person's culture and values. Although consideration of differences between nurse and client should be examined, Price and Braden (1978) caution community health personnel to consider common elements that both client and nurse experience. At times, both have felt happy, sad, uncertain, alone. These human emotions are a common bond.

There are instances when the nurse chooses to make an initial visit without extensive preparation or consultation with the health team. If a client has been labeled "difficult" because he refuses to comply with suggestions and the nurse feels that negative comments would predominate from team members, the nurse may choose to assess the client's behaviors during the home visit without prior consultation.

Other Activities

Other previsit activities may include investigation of community resources (see Chapter 19). In addition, the nurse may need to assemble equipment and supplies such as thermometers, catheters, bandages, and sphygmomanometers.

The nurse must decide whether to contact the client and arrange a visit time or whether to make a spontaneous visit. Each alternative is appropriate in certain circumstances. For example, if the nurse has to travel several miles, it is a good idea to make an appointment. However, if the nurse is making visits to several families to discuss vision screening results with parents, the nurse may need a flexible schedule and may visit each family on a drop-in basis.

The planning phase of the nursing process begins during previsit activities, although the largest portion of planning is usually done in collaboration with the client during the home visit.

Entry into the Home

Having completed previsit activities, the nurse is prepared to make the home visit. When a student or nurse first begins making home visits to a client, he or she may have several concerns:

· Will the family be receptive to the nursing visit?
· Will the family's goals differ from the nurse's own?
· Will friends or neighbors be present during the visit?

Being prepared by completing previsit activities will help allay the nurse's anxiety. Many agencies consider it appropriate, if numbers of staff are sufficient, to have an experienced community health nurse make an initial visit with a student.

The client and family will also have thoughts and questions about the home visit. If the visit is the first encounter between the family and the community health nurse, family members may be curious about the nurse and nursing care. If the visit was not prearranged and the family was unaware of the referral, family members may wonder why the visit is being made. Introductions and explanations of the reason for the home visit will help to prevent misunderstandings.

Feelings of both nurse and family about the home visit are important, because the initial contact is an opportunity to begin to establish trust and rapport, which are the basis of positive interpersonal relationships. These enhance nurse–client communication and must be nurtured over time. The relationship begins when the client opens the door. When first visiting Mrs. Calhoun in her home, the nurse's opening statement may be, "Good morning, Mrs. Calhoun. I'm Angela Turner, a nurse from the Visiting Nurses' Association. Your physician, Dr. Martin, asked me to visit you to follow up on your care in the hospital."

The nurse has introduced herself, she has identified herself, and she has briefly explained why she is visiting. The brief explanation at the door may be elaborated upon during the home visit. The initial introduction tells the client who you are and why you are there.

The mood for the visit will be set during entry into the home. Behaviors of the nurse that facilitate productive visits are described in the following sections.

Acceptance of the Client

Lentz and Meyer (1979) suggest that although nurses agree that personal values must not influence acceptance of clients, some values, such as cleanliness, are deeply ingrained and often nurses are unaware of how important these values are to them. When confronted with a dirty house or another environmental problem, the nurse must not correlate the level of cleanliness with the family's health in general and must be careful not to judge the family's motivation for wellness in relation to cleanliness.

Homes may have unfamiliar odors and furnishings may be in disarray. If a client does not value the same level of cleanliness as the nurse, the nurse may focus on that aspect of the environment rather than on the priority problem. For example:

A family consisting of a young mother and father and two preschool children lives in a rural two-room house with a dirt floor. Ducklings and chicks are raised in the kitchen area, and the children are unbathed. The older child has a diagnosis of developmental delay. The nurse, who highly values cleanliness, may lose sight of the primary reason for the visit, the child's developmental delay. Therefore, she must assess her personal values, identify values and priorities of the family, determine if cleanliness is a deterrent to the achievement of goals, and work within the environmental situation. In this case, cleanliness does not affect the child's development, but aspects of the environment may be utilized to enhance growth and development. For example, the child may be taught to help feed the animals, to identify feet, wings, and beaks, and to imitate sounds made by chickens and ducks.

Certain behaviors of the nurse can denote acceptance, such as a handshake, smiles, eye contact, and the nurse taking a seat in a relaxed manner. Often families will offer the nurse a cup of coffee or tea. The manner of acceptance or refusal can communicate acceptance of the family. Knowledge of cultural norms is important here, as in some cultures the sharing of food and drink is a sign of hospitality and refusal may be felt as a rejection.

Explaining the Purpose of the Visit

The primary reason for the home visit is communicated to the family at the door. In the case of Mrs. Calhoun and her recent diagnosis of diabetes, later in the visit the nurse may further explain that, during subsequent home visits, she would like to answer Mrs. Calhoun's questions about her health, review information she learned in the hospital, and assist with areas of wellness which are important to her.

Acknowledging Each Family Member

The nurse should greet and speak to each member of the family. At times this may require going to different rooms. Pets can be important to families and the nurse must be aware of their role in each family's life. For example, Mrs. Calhoun may live with a 90-year-old brother who stays in his bedroom, and she may have a pet poodle that is significant in her life. The nurse would ask to say hello and visit with the brother and would acknowledge the poodle and ask about its welfare.

Components of the home visit process discussed thus far are exemplified in the following example:

Joan Miller, RN, is a community health nurse who has received a referral to visit the King family. The family's only child, Sue, age 3, has recently been dismissed from the hospital after surgery to repair a heart defect. Mr. King has been laid off from his job at a local factory and Mrs. King earns part of the family's income by caring for four preschool children in the home. The nurse has telephoned to arrange a time for a visit, so the family is expecting her. Ms. Miller feels apprehensive, because Mrs. King asked her to visit for only a short time, explaining that Mr. King does not like outsiders in their home. Thus Ms. Miller is unsure of her reception during the home visit.

The Kings, too, are anxious, as they fear the nurse may be judgmental of their cluttered home and of the noise the preschoolers make. However, much of their anxiety is allayed the moment Ms. Miller communicates with them. As the Kings open the door, the nurse explains, "Hello, my name is Joan Miller. I'm the visiting nurse from the community health center. Ms. Williams, the nurse from the well child clinic at the center, asked me to stop and see if you had any questions about Sue's surgery and her return home."

The nurse has identified herself and has mentioned a health care provider with whom the family has had a positive experience. This provides a common bond between nurse and family. The nurse has also been careful to be nonjudgmental of the cluttered house through nonverbal communications, including smiles, eye contact, and handshakes. Since she is aware of the husband's recent job loss, she is aware of the changes he has experienced as well as the stresses associated with Sue's surgery, and she also knows of his reluctance to have her visit. Therefore, the nurse acknowledges his worth by making a positive comment about something she observes, such as Mr. King's skill in wood carving. The nurse may also verbalize her understanding of his apprehensions by saying, "I know it must be a new experience to have a stranger come to your home to talk about Sue's health."

Through her communication, the nurse has begun to establish an interpersonal relationship with the family members. As the nurse talks to the family members, she assesses their feelings about home visits and their communication patterns as well as aspects of family functioning.

The assessment phase continues as the nurse observes the home environment. Without asking questions, the nurse can obtain much information, such as the presence or absence of safety features in the home, ventilation and light, and leisure activities, such as books or television. These are examples of environmental assessment features that help the nurse understand family life-style. Figure 20.1 provides a checklist to assist the nurse in assessing the home environment. This checklist can be included in the family's chart and used by the nurse as needed.

Promoting the Nurse–Client Relationship

After entry into the home, the nurse continues to establish a relationship with the family. The developing relationship affords

Area of Assessment	Observations
Indicators of leisure activities	
Hobbies	
Crafts	
Sports equipment	
Exercise equipment	
Toys	
Books, magazines	
Television	
Other	
Indicators of work activities	
Occupational tools or gear	
Clothing (uniforms)	
Other	
Indicators of values	
Cleanliness level	
Pets	
Children	
Furnishings	
Religious items	
Cultural items	
Other	
Indicators of home safety level	
Rugs	
Plugs	
Stairways	
Ventilation	
Lighting	
Fire extinguisher	
Exits	
Electrical cords and equipment	
Other	

(continued)

Figure 20.1 Checklist for assessment of the home environment.

Sensory impressions
  Sight
  (e.g., seating
  arrangement)
  Sound (e.g., music,
  noise level)
  Smell (e.g., food, other
  odors)
  Touch (e.g., tempera-
  ture of home)

Comments:

Figure 20.1 (*continued*)

the opportunity for assessment, planning, and intervention.

Several behaviors of the nurse can aid in the establishment of the positive relationship begun during entry into the home and thus can enhance the effectiveness of the home visit. These behaviors include creativity, flexibility, follow through, and respect.

Creativity

The nurse uses creative approaches to nursing care in the home in response to unique situations that differentiate the home environment from other settings:

1. Absence of familiar institutional equipment, such as hospital beds. For example, a client's regular bed may need to be placed on blocks to raise it to a convenient height for the caregiver to give a bed bath or range-of-motion exercises.
2. Lack of institutional rules and regulations. Because the client is at home, the nurse devises plans to help the client when the nurse is not present. For example, the

nurse may develop a system, using materials available in the home, to enable a forgetful client to take medication at the appropriate times.

3. In a hospital, the welfare of other clients must be considered, but at home a client who cannot sleep at 1:00 A.M. may be able to turn on the television set without disturbing another person. A 40-year-old mother who is confined to bed but who misses her kitchen activities may participate in meal preparation from her bedroom by cleaning fresh green beans, stirring a cookie mixture, or frosting a cake, for example.

Flexibility

As previously stated, the nurse is a guest in the client's home. If the client chooses to eat meals at unusual times or to have a bed bath in the afternoon instead of the morning, he or she may arrange with the nurse or family members for a schedule change. The nurse must also respect the client's preference in such matters as timing for teaching. A friend may visit a new mother at the time the nurse had planned to teach her to bathe her baby, so the teaching plan may have to be rescheduled.

Follow Through

In order to enhance the establishment of trust, the nurse must follow through with commitments. For example, if a blizzard occurs on the day of a planned home visit, the nurse should telephone the family to explain that the visit will have to be rescheduled. Community health nurses have long recognized the importance of follow through, and on one occasion a nurse in a rural area traveled on snowy roads as far as the roads were plowed and then walked the remainder of the distance to clients' homes to keep scheduled appointments. Perhaps most of us will never have to make such extraordinary efforts, but her clients will always remember her efforts.

Respect

Respect is part of all productive relationships. Mutual nurse–client respect will help form a basis for trust. For example, the nurse should address the client with the appropriate title, such as "Mr." or "Ms." until permission is offered to do otherwise. The nurse can earn the respect of clients by being well prepared for the visit, by keeping promises, and by appearing professional in attire and behavior.

Communication

The nurse communicates with family members during all stages of the nursing process. Effective communication will assist the nurse in information gathering, teaching, contracting, and providing support. Communication is a dynamic process. The terms "helper," "helping relationship," "therapeutic communication," and "positive interpersonal relationship," are frequently used to describe productive nurse–client communication. The nursing process can be applied to assist in understanding the establishment of communication that enhances nursing care.

ASSESSING COMMUNICATION. During the assessment phase, the nurse assesses his or her own communication and that of the clients and other health team members. Honesty, value clarification, goal setting, self-awareness, sensitivity, and listening enhance communication, and assessment of these behaviors can be made. For example, the nurse must interact honestly to produce optimum communication. This implies that the nurse is honest to the self as well as others. Thus, the nurse must assess whether he or she is honest about thoughts and feelings and aware of their potential impact on working with clients.

The nurse must assess personal values and identify priorities. A nurse who values promptness in keeping appointments may be frustrated when a client is continually late for scheduled home visits. Self-awareness is closely tied to honesty and values clarification. Awareness of one's own feelings, thoughts, attitudes, and values can help the nurse eliminate those that are nonproductive and develop those that are productive.

The client and nurse work together to establish mutual goals as well as methods for implementation and evaluation of goals. When the client is a partner in health care, wellness can be enhanced. Often, we receive clues about the thoughts, feelings, attitudes, and values of others. As with awareness of self, sensitivity to others allows the nurse to intervene appropriately. For example, a nurse had planned to teach a client about his arthritis during their next visit. When the nurse arrived, the client explained that he had had a restless, sleepless night and was in pain. The nurse postponed the teaching plans and worked to eliminate the client's discomfort during this visit. The nurse also needs skill in listening and responding to people. Assessment of these skills will assist the nurse in identifying communication strengths and areas of needed improvement.

PLANNING COMMUNICATION BEHAVIORS. After communication behaviors and skills are assessed, the nurse can plan:

1. Ways to learn new skills, such as participating in communication workshops and seminars.
2. Ways to practice and enhance existing skills through application of techniques with clients or role play with peers.

3. Continued assessment of communication behaviors and values through reading journals and keeping diaries.

IMPLEMENTING COMMUNICATION SKILLS. As the nurse begins the implementation phase, the communication process continues. A discussion of four steps that can be used in the application of this process follows.

1. *Establish a helping relationship.* As discussed earlier, trust is the basis for a helping relationship, and effective communication and trust can be facilitated by applying communication ingredients (Rogers, 1962). Rogers has identified empathy, genuineness, and positive regard as essential ingredients in a helping relationship.

The ability to *empathize* with another means that the helper has an understanding of the client's private world. In other words, the helper tries to view the other person's world in the person's own terms, not the helper's terms. Complete empathy is difficult to achieve, but if the client realizes the helper's intent to understand, a positive step has been taken.

Genuineness implies understanding oneself and being oneself. This does not mean that the nurse can interact with every client as she or he would with a friend, but it does mean approaching the relationship without a facade. This is one of the arts of nursing: balancing one's personal self with one's professional self. When a nurse is still a student or is new in nursing, these aspects of self are more distinct. As the nurse matures and gains experience, the personal self and the professional self become more integrated. However, it is possible even for the novice to be genuine about such things as admitting when he or she does not know the answer to a question, or sometimes telling a client how he or she feels about something, and always using "I" statements when expressing a feeling or value of his or her own.

Prizing a person regardless of the behavior he or she exhibits is one manifestation of *positive regard*. This requires a willingness to accept people as they are. To be able to do this, one must be able to empathize with the person. To be able to demonstrate this, one must be willing and able to put value for the other person above whatever values one has about certain behaviors. For example, one common aspect of seeing clients in their homes is being confronted with different values about housekeeping. Some clients will be much poorer housekeepers than the nurse. They may have a much higher tolerance for disorder or uncleanliness than the nurse has. On the other hand, some clients may be much more meticulous housekeepers than the nurse, to the extent that the nurse feels threatened. If this aspect of the client's life-style is not a part of what the nurse and client are working on, the nurse must disregard it. The nurse's task is to exhibit behavior congruent with his or her expression of regard for the client.

Combs, Avila, and Purkey (1971, p. 215) list three ways in which helpers can function. The helper can be a *model* by setting an example of certain behaviors, such as openness in communicating. For example, Scott Major is a community health nurse who is an effective communicator. He always arranges seating so that he can maintain eye contact with clients and gives them his undivided attention. When he feels uncomfortable about a client's plan, he will say so and explain what he sees as problematic. If a client is habitually late for clinic appointments, Mr. Major states directly that this is a problem to him and asks the client what he or she can do get there on time. Mr. Major is able to communicate that he cares about the client while also making his own needs and priorities evident. His nonjudgmental approach to this not only helps facilitate the relationships with his clients but also shows them how to use this same approach in their lives.

The helper acts as a *reinforcer* by providing feedback, both verbally and nonverbally. Sarah Reynolds reinforces her clients' positive behaviors by nodding, smiling, and making comments such as, "That worked out well for you," "I'm glad you were able to follow through with your plan," "It was hard for you to stay away from that situation, but you did it," and "I agree, you've gotten a lot better at taking care of yourself."

The helper can also function as an *extinguisher* of behavior. This is the opposite of reinforcement. People tend to discard behaviors that are not responded to. The behavior is ignored, or limits are reiterated that exclude the unwanted behavior. For example:

Paula Prince, a nursing student, was working with a young man who had some chronic health problems that kept him from working. Ms. Prince was visiting him biweekly in his home. At every visit, the client controlled the conversation, and he would eventually ask her for a date. Her usual response had been to say something such as that she was busy on the night in question or that her boyfriend would object. He would persist in complimenting her and suggesting other times they could get together without the knowledge of her boyfriend. She finally talked with her instructor about the problem. The two of them worked out a new approach for her to try. Unintentionally, the student had been reinforcing the client's behaviors by simply turning down his invitations as if he were a potential date. To extinguish these advances, Ms. Prince began responding to his invitations with a simple statement such as, "Our relationship is for the purpose of helping you learn to deal with your health problems. It is not a relationship to meet your social needs." After stating this, Ms. Prince would then introduce a more appropriate topic for discussion. If the client persisted, she would state, "If you do not want to work with

me as a nurse, I will leave." (If he continued to ignore these limits, she was to leave.) Ms. Prince found that she did not have to terminate the relationship. Once she made it clear that she would not accept his invitations, the client began to respond more appropriately.

To assess your communication skills, ask yourself these questions:

· Do I have empathy for the client? What have I understood from the client's point of view?
· Do I display genuineness with my clients? Have I shared my own feelings when appropriate?
· Do I have positive regard for each client? When has it been difficult to have regard for someone? How have I communicated my positive regard to clients?
· Do I model effective communication? What behaviors of mine display effective communication?
· Do I reinforce client communication and behavior? What behaviors and words have I used to reinforce positive behavior?
· Do I extinguish behaviors appropriately? What behavior have I tried to extinguish? How did I go about extinguishing behavior and how effective was I?

2. Utilize listening skills. Giving the client full and undivided attention is a basic step in preparing for listening (Carkhuff, 1973). Several techniques help make optimal use of opportunities to listen. For example, the nurse should have a reason for listening. With the referral comes an initial reason to listen. As the relationship proceeds, the nurse listens in order to be able to make an assessment, or to evaluate the progress of the work.

The nurse must be nonjudgmental when listening. This means accepting of the client as a person without letting personal values interfere. Next, the nurse must attempt to resist distractions. Frequently, other people, pets, and noises interrupt home visits. If possible, the nurse can decrease distractions by asking if the sound on the television can be lowered, for example. Some distractions however, such as noises outside the house, cannot be eliminated, and the nurse must concentrate on attending to what is being said.

Another listening technique is waiting to respond. Carkhuff (1973, p. 37) suggests that the nurse practice waiting 30 seconds after a client speaks before responding. This allows the client to continue speaking if desired. It gives the nurse an opportunity to understand what has been said and to think about a response. As skill is gained in listening, this interval of silence will be shortened.

Recalling content is another effective technique. That is, restate exactly what the client has said to clarify what the nurse heard. Looking for themes will also enhance listening. Important themes will recur and identification of them will help the nurse to understand the client.

3. *Acknowledge and respond to the client's communication.* The nurse can respond to the client's communication both verbally and nonverbally. The nurse provides positive nonverbal reinforcement through posture (sitting or standing attentively yet comfortably), facial expressions (smiles, eye contact), gestures (head nodding), and silence (allowing time for thinking and reflecting). These behaviors communicate an interest in the client and encourage further dialogue. The nurse responds verbally by restating the client's words to demonstrate that the nurse has heard correctly what the client has said. Summarizing the client's thoughts and stating themes will let the client know what has been communicated.

4. *Practice self-disclosure.* Another technique consists of making "I" statements to disclose how the nurse feels without judging the client. For example, if the client refuses to lower the volume of the television, the nurse can respond, "I have difficulty hearing when the TV is playing loudly." If the client seems to be changing the subject frequently, the nurse may say, "I feel uncertain about what you are telling me today." These comments disclose to the client how the nurse is feeling and enhances the client's awareness in the interaction.

EVALUATING COMMUNICATION. The final step in the communication process is evaluation. This can be accomplished in several ways. First, the nurse and client can discuss the effectiveness of their communication, or the nurse can ask the client about it. For example, the nurse may ask the client which activities have been most meaningful or helpful.

Secondly, the nurse may role play a nurse–client situation with peers and ask for feedback about specific behaviors, such as positive reinforcement, listening, and genuineness.

Third, the client may grant permission for tape recording of a conversation. The nurse can listen to the recording and evaluate the communication. The tape recording might also be evaluated by a colleague.

Finally, the nurse can use tools such as the interpersonal process recording (Figure 20.2). This provides a written summary of elements of communication, including the client's and the nurse's verbal and nonverbal communication, the nurse's thoughts and feelings, techniques and concepts used, and a discussion of each element in the nurse–client interaction (Schoolcraft, 1982). Figure 20.2 illustrates a form that can be used in recording the interpersonal process.

Outline

I. Introduction
   A. Description of the client
      1. Physical appearance
         a. Posture
         b. Facial expression
         c. Body movement and gestures
         d. Body appearance and clothing
      2. Psychosocial description
         a. Age
         b. Developmental assessment
         c. Cultural data
            (1) Religion
            (2) Race
            (3) Education
            (4) Economic level
            (5) Family data and relationships
   B. Description of the setting
      1. Physical arrangements
      2. Time of day and date
      3. Body position of yourself and the client
   C. Description of your thoughts and feelings before the interaction
   D. Goal or objective of the interaction
      1. Student goals
      2. Client goals
   E. Brief summary of the interaction before the portion included in the process recording
II. Recording of the interaction
III. Conclusion
   A. Brief summary of the remainder of the interaction after the portion included in the process recording
   B. Nurse's thoughts and feelings after the interaction
   C. Evaluation of interviewing techniques used in the interaction
   D. Identification of future needs and nursing interventions
IV. Bibliography

Recording of Interaction

Communication	Thoughts and Feelings	Techniques and Concepts	Discussion
Verbatim transcript of interaction between student and client, including	Written description of conscious thoughts and feelings experienced by	List of interviewing techniques and definition of each. List of psychosocial	Explanation of student's rationale for techniques used. Analysis of effec-

(continued)

Figure 20.2 Adapted from the interpersonal process recording. (From Schoolcraft, V.: The interpersonal process recording. In R. K. Young, ed., *Community nursing workbook: Family as client.* Norwalk, Conn.: Appleton-Century-Crofts, 1982, pp. 214–215. Reprinted with permission.)

Communication	Thoughts and Feelings	Techniques and Concepts	Discussion
verbal and nonverbal communication. This should be approximately a 10-minute segment of an interview.	the student at the time of the interaction.	concepts and definition of each. Techniques are those used by the student. Psychosocial concepts may pertain to either student or client.	tiveness of techniques in facilitating or blocking the interaction. Discussion of the relationship of the psychosocial concepts to the interaction
The recording of the conversation as objectively as possible provides data for a meaningful analysis of the student's interviewing skills.	Recording thoughts and feelings helps the student: 1. Recognize the relationship of internal processes to the process of communication. 2. Increase self-awareness. 3. Examine when feelings and thoughts should and should not affect communication. 4. Increase acceptance of own thoughts and feelings.	Identifying techniques and concepts increases awareness of their meanings in communication.	Discussion helps to: 1. Increase conscious use of appropriate techniques. 2. Examine factors that improve or disrupt communication. 3. Evaluate the appropriateness of techniques. 4. Identify the effect of psychosocial concepts on communication. 5. Demonstrate the rational use of interviewing techniques related to the needs of the client.

Figure 20.2 (*continued*)

Additional Assessments

After the nurse has applied the nursing process to communication skills and has assessed the environment, other areas, including physical assessment, family functioning, cultural aspects, and psychosocial health, should be assessed. Communication skills and the client's environment have been discussed in this chapter.

Client Contract

Data assessed must be recorded and plans formulated. As the nurse continues to communicate and plan with the client, mutual nurse–client goals are established. The nurse–client contract discussed in Chapter 16 is appropriately utilized during the home visit as a guide for nursing interventions.

An example of utilization of the contract in the home setting is a situation in which the client is overweight and desires to diet. The client may contract to keep a food diary for one week, after which time the client is to meet with the community health nurse to discuss food habits and likes and dislikes and to devise a plan to reduce caloric intake, eat well-balanced meals, and begin an exercise program. Other client contracts may involve such things as range-of-motion exercises, utilization of community resources, and relaxation exercises.

John Simmons, a 40-year-old client, received a spinal cord injury in an automobile accident, resulting in paralysis of his legs. Ben Ashby, RN, is making an initial home visit after the client's dismissal and referral from the local rehabilitation center, where the client received care after his injury. The nurse and client establish the following goal and contract:

Goal: John Simmons will increase physical activities both in his home and in community settings.

Contract: Before or during the next home visit, in one week John Simmons will:

1. Utilize range-of-motion (ROM) exercises learned at the rehabilitation center twice a day.
2. Telephone the local YMCA about activities for handicapped people.
3. Select one community activity to attend accompanied by the nurse.

Ben Ashby will:

1. Observe Mr. Simmons doing ROM exercises to determine whether they are being done correctly.
2. Contact the local association for the disabled about available activities.
3. Accompany Mr. Simmons on his first trip outside the home.
4. Teach Mr. Simmons relaxation exercises.

Short-Term and Long-Term Goals

Planning can be short term or long term, and interventions can be implemented immediately or over a long period of time. Examples of short-term planning and interventions include dressing changes, teaching a mother about introduction of solid foods into her baby's diet, and teaching a father to provide care for a child in a body cast. Long-term planning and inter-

ventions include continuing assistance with range-of-motion exercises after a client's cardiovascular accident, teaching the spouse of that client the importance of mobility, discussing growth and development of a child with a mother during a series of visits, and assisting with bed baths and care of a client with a terminal illness.

Short-term goals are those that can be met in a few weeks' time, whereas long-term goals are accomplished over many weeks, or perhaps months or years. The goals established for John Simmons are short term; they are designed to be accomplished in one week's time. However, if the goal were to regain partial functioning of lower limbs, that goal would be long term.

Roles of the Nurse

During home visits, nurses practice a variety of roles when intervening in client care.

COLLABORATOR. The nurse collaborates with the client and members of the family during the home visit and with other health care providers during pre- and postvisit activities. For example, the nurse may collaborate with the client on a schedule for range-of-motion exercises and with a social service worker about rental of an overbed trapeze for the client's use. Nurse and client collaborate on goals, plans, and evaluation of interventions.

CONSULTANT. The nurse consults with another person to obtain or provide information. The nurse may serve as a consultant to the family in a variety of areas, such as use of community resources. For example, if the family of a substance-dependent teenager desires professional assistance, the nurse may discuss various alternatives for care, provide a list of community settings that provide care for teenagers, and assist the family with the problem-solving process. The nurse may act as a consultant regarding family therapy, family planning, nutrition, child care, and many other areas.

Besides consulting with clients, the nurse consults with other health professionals, such as physicians, nutritionists, occupational therapists, and other nurses. For example, a nurse is working with a client who is confined to bed. The client is frequently constipated and dislikes many foods that contain bran. The nurse may consult with a nutritionist about other foods which provide bulk. The nurse may also consult with an occupational therapist about homebound income-producing activities.

COORDINATOR. During home visits, the nurse coordinates client care by communicating with family and health care team members. If a client requires the services of several different professionals, the nurse assists in organizing care. For example, a quadraplegic client might receive services from a physical therapist, an occupational therapist, a mental health professional, and a vocational rehabilitation specialist. The nurse coordinates these services by communicating with all personnel involved to learn of their activities and to inform them of activities of other team members.

PREVENTER OF DISEASE AND PROMOTER OF HEALTH. Home visits provide excellent opportunities for disease prevention, including teaching families handwashing techniques, dental hygiene, and healthy nutrition. Nurses also practice health promotion during home visits by accepting the client's cultural values and caring for a client within his or her accepted norms. Promotion of health and prevention of disease can be incorporated into almost any nursing activity. For example, when teaching a mother about the growth and development of her toddler, the nurse may also discuss safety concerns such as keeping poisonous cleaning agents out of the child's reach.

PROVIDER OF DIRECT CARE. The home is frequently the setting for provision of direct services such as bed baths, blood pressure monitoring, catheter care, and exercise activities. Besides carrying out these activities, the nurse may also teach them to the family and the client. Although the care provided may be similar to that given in other settings, the nurse must be creative and flexible to give care under variable circumstances.

HEALTH EDUCATOR. Health education is a part of every nursing activity during a home visit. Education may be carried out formally through planned classes utilizing pictures, books, posters, or other audiovisual aids. Often, teaching occurs casually during another activity. For instance, when bathing a client who is immobile, the nurse will teach the importance of skin care and frequent turning and help the client plan for help in moving at appropriate intervals.

MANAGER. The nurse assists in management of care during home visits. For example, the nurse may manage care given to a client by family members and other nursing personnel, such as nursing assistants. Managerial activities include teaching how and why to administer care, planning for when care will be given and by whom, supervising care, and evaluating care.

EPIDEMIOLOGIST. When a nurse helps a family explore causes of disease and prevent recurrence, epidemiology is being practiced. For example, if several family members have a skin rash, factors common in each of their lives are explored. When a common cause is found, both prevention and treatment can be instituted.

ROLE MODEL. The nurse serves as a role model for holistic care during a home visit. The nurse can show a broad spectrum of concern for the client and the family. In being cognizant of his or her own practices, the nurse can show others healthy behaviors. Often the nurse has the opportunity to discuss his or her own behavior and explain the reasons for it. This enables the client and the family to learn new ways of functioning.

Evaluation

Evaluation may be formative or terminal. *Formative evaluation* goes on throughout a relationship. For example, the nurse and the client may evaluate a newly introduced self-care technique to determine whether the technique meets the client's needs and is convenient and economical. The nurse can evaluate his or her communication during an interview by noting whether the techniques used produce the appropriate results. Usually such evaluation is informal.

Terminal evaluation is done when a phase of the relationship is concluded or when the entire nurse–client relationship ends. The goals that were to be accomplished are reviewed, and the nurse and the client decide which goals were met and how effectively. The nurse should periodically review goals and evaluate efforts to achieve them. For example, a goal for a client who suffered a broken leg might have been to restore full mobility. When the client is fully mobile, the nurse can examine the various efforts made toward this end to determine what factors helped achieve it. This will assist the nurse in future situations with clients who have similar needs. Such information may also assist the nurse or a successor, if the same client has other health interruptions. For example, the nurse may have discovered that the client took suggestions more quickly when she was given a careful explanation of the rationale involved. Evaluation should be a part of the client's record.

Concluding the Visit

The correct length of time for a visit depends on the individual situation. The goals that have been agreed on will guide the nurse in setting an appropriate time limit. Some other factors that affect the time spent in the client's home include time required for direct service, such as bed making, bathing, and wound dressing; needs of other family members; emergencies, such as accidents or psychological crises; complexity of material to be taught; the client's tolerance for interacting with the nurse; and other demands on the nurse's time besides the given client situation.

Either before the visit or immediately after the nurse arrives, the nurse should give the client some idea of how long the visit will last. This will help both the client and the nurse get the most out of the time they have together. Many visits require an hour or less. If the nurse often makes visits that extend beyond that time, he or she should make sure that the time is being used productively. If the visits extend for long periods of time, this may be because either the client or the nurse is trying to meet social needs through the relationship.

When bringing the visit to a close, the nurse should summarize what has been talked about or accomplished, and the nurse and client should plan what they will do before and during the next visit. The date and time for the next visit should be set, or plans made about when another visit will be scheduled.

Postvisit Activities

After evaluating the visit, the nurse consults with members of the health care team as needed. The nurse may discuss observations and feelings and collaborate with colleagues, but the nurse must also consider the confidentiality of interactions with clients. Client situations should be discussed only in private. Records are kept where only authorized personnel can read them.

During this stage, the nurse makes necessary entries into the client's record. The nurse conducts follow-up activities such as contacting community resources and preparing for the next visit.

Termination

Termination of visits occurs when one or more of the following occurs: nurse–client goals are reached, health is restored and the client can function without nursing intervention, a client changes residences or leaves the home setting to go to another setting, or the nurse transfers the client's care to another health provider. Termination can evoke a variety of feelings. Sometimes termination may be difficult for the nurse and the client because an interpersonal relationship has been established. In anticipation of this possibility, planning for termination should begin with the first home visit. When a contract is made, termination is a part of it. If the nurse's assigned visits to the family are limited in number, the termination date is specified during the first visit and succeeding visits.

Kelly (1969) states that experiences of separation from someone with whom closeness and warmth have been shared are often remembered as very painful. However, nurses often neglect to acknowledge their own feelings when a nurse–client relationship is terminated. Both the client and nurse have feelings regarding termination. Kelly (1969) lists possible client reactions to termination:

1. *Denial* of the importance of the nurse–client relationship.
2. *Hostility* displayed to combat helplessness.
3. *Regression* or recurrence of symptoms to prolong the relationship.
4. *Withdrawal* to superficial levels of interaction.

The nurse can identify and assess these reactions and help the client through the termination process. If the client denies the importance of the nurse–client relationship, he or she may, for example, not stay at home for a scheduled visit. By denying that the relationship is important, clients insulate themselves from feelings of loss when termination occurs. The nurse can intervene by listening actively and by encouraging the client to state his or her feelings.

When the client reacts with hostility, the nurse must realize that this may be a manifestation of helplessness. The client may feel powerless about losing the relationship that has been productive and may react with anger. Again, the nurse can explore the client's feelings and help the client find other resources for continuing support.

Another possible reaction to termination is recurrence of the symptoms that initiated the referral. A client may believe that if he continues to be ill, the nurse will continue the visits. In this situation, the nurse must determine whether it is really necessary to continue the home visits, realizing that this reaction may become a habit. Finally, the client may withdraw by resorting to superficial levels of interaction and by refusing to share feelings and thoughts with the nurse. The nurse can acknowledge the difficulty in ending the relationship and share some of his or her own feelings.

The nurse must also understand his or

her own feelings about termination. The nurse may exhibit all of the same reactions as the client. For example, the nurse may forget appointments. When the client reacts with hostility, the nurse may respond in kind. When the client's problems seem to be recurring, the nurse may postpone the termination because of a need to prolong the relationship. The nurse may also respond to the client superficially or stereotypically, rather than using the accustomed relaxed and informal style of interaction.

Whenever the nurse terminates a long-standing relationship or a relationship that has aroused strong feelings (whether positive or negative), he or she should anticipate a reaction to the loss of the relationship. Talking to a colleague about the termination may help the nurse to identify any problems that are arising.

ADVANTAGES AND DISADVANTAGES OF HOME VISITS

The home has many advantages as well as some disadvantages as a setting for practice. In determining whether or not to visit in the home, the nurse must weigh these and decide which advantages will serve the client and which disadvantages can be overcome in the particular client's situation.

Advantages

In the assessment phase, the home and community environments can provide a wealth of information about the client's life-style, interests, attitudes, and values. This gives the nurse data additional to the client's verbal and nonverbal communication. Often there are features of the home or neighborhood, or of family interactions that the client does not think are important or so takes for granted that he or she does not report them.

Since clients may feel overwhelmed or rushed in agency settings, they may intentionally or unintentionally fail to communicate useful information to the nurse. The familiarity of the home setting usually decreases the client's anxiety and promotes effective communication. It is usually easier for all family members to be available for the nurse in their home. When the entire family is available, the nurse can provide more comprehensive service to the client. In addition, the interactions among family members may be more relaxed and natural in the home than in an office. The roles of neighbors, friends, and even pets in the lives of family members can also be observed and evaluated.

Communication may be facilitated and the establishment of trust enhanced in the informal and familiar setting. The nurse conveys a regard for the family and a willingness to understand and know them by visiting them in their home. Even though the family members may realize that the nurse is compensated for time and travel needed to make home visits, they often appreciate this special effort to see them and to help them.

Preventing and Handling Problems

Time Concerns

Certain aspects of the home visit may be viewed as disadvantages. The cost of home visiting is one factor that may make it an unattractive choice, and the time involved is what makes it so costly. Costs include the expense of the trip, such as carfare or gasoline. The time of a professional nurse, both while making the trip and attending to the home visit, is also expensive. Unforeseen problems, such as clients failing to be at home or the nurse getting lost, may consume time as well. These time issues may be minimized. First, the nurse can plan to visit several clients in the same general area on the same day. The nurse should have an accurate street map and should know how to use maps and street guides. The nurse should make arrangements in advance to visit the client and should get detailed directions at that time.

Second, the nurse should make as specific an appointment as possible. If the nurse will be visiting several clients throughout the day, each one should be told that the nurse could be delayed. If the delay is extensive, the nurse should call the client. A day or two before a visit, especially if the appointment was originally made some time before, the nurse or a clerk should call the client to confirm the visit. If the client does not have a telephone, the nurse might send a postcard that includes a number to call if the client needs to change the time. Sometimes people who do not have telephones have someone nearby who relays important messages. This information should be obtained at the time of the initial contact with the client. The nurse's efforts to be thorough in arranging appointments, reminding clients about them, and keeping them or being sure the client is informed of cancellations will help to promote trust as well as serve as a model for the client when the client must postpone or cancel an appointment. For this reason, it is imperative that the nurse do everything possible to contact clients when appointments must be postponed or cancelled.

Distractions

Another disadvantage of the home visit is the possibility of distractions. Children may be rowdy, telephones may ring, neighbors or friends may drop by for prolonged visits, televisions or stereos may be playing, or other unpredictable events may occur. Since the nurse is a guest in the client's home, his or her control over any of these interruptions may be limited. Some distractions, such as small children, must simply be taken into consideration in planning a visit. Other things, such as televisions and stereos, may be controlled by simply asking if they can be turned off or turned down during the visit. Telephone conversations or impromptu visits from friends may have to be endured, or, if they are extensive and seem more important to the client than the nurse's visit, the nurse may have to leave. As the nurse develops a relationship with a client, it becomes possible to deal with these interruptions more forcefully. However, early in the relationship, the nurse may have to tolerate a certain number of distractions. Whatever the stage of the relationship, the nurse should be patient about interruptions and should consider the possible consequences of any effort to eliminate a particular distraction.

Resistance

Some family members may resist having a nurse visit in the home. They may feel that their privacy is being invaded, or they may feel ill at ease about the nurse's values and attitudes. The resistance may be caused by cultural differences between the nurse and the family. Some people do not wish to have anyone in their homes other than friends or family members. Clients may feel that the nurse is "better" than they are and may feel ashamed about their homes. On the other hand, some clients feel that they are "better" than the nurse and do not want him or her rendering a service to them that they feel is usually meant for lower socio-economic groups.

To prevent resistance from developing or intensifying, the nurse should give an accurate and complete description of the purposes and nature of the home visit. The nurse must be careful about communicating attitudes that might give credence to any of the suspicious or negative feelings a client might have about the nurse. Some suggestions have already been discussed. However, the greatest contributor to promoting the usefulness of the home visit and forestalling resistance is for the nurse always to behave in a friendly and professional manner. The nurse must strive to convey an attitude of being a caring professional.

Role Confusion

Another factor that may hamper the effectiveness of home visits is the nurse's own sense of the role of the nurse in the home. It may be difficult for a nurse, especially a student or a new practitioner, to distinguish between the helping relationship and friendship when visiting a client in the home. Away from the hospital, clinic, or health department, the nurse may have difficulty in functioning as a professional. It is sometimes difficult to maintain the advantage of the informal atmosphere yet not become so informal as to undercut the professional purposes of the visit. This is one of the areas in which self-awareness is of greatest use to the nurse. Periodic self-evaluation and evaluation by supervisors and colleagues will help the nurse identify these problems early.

FUTURE IMPLICATIONS

The Near Future

In the near future, nurses will function more and more autonomously. Clients will be self-referred or will be referred by other nonprofessionals. Consumers are becoming more cost conscious, and they may find that care by a visiting nurse is less expensive in the long run than visits to doctors' offices or hospitalization. As people become more involved in health promotion, they will be able to identify needs for health teaching. In conjunction with friends or neighbors, they may engage nurses to come to their homes to provide health education. Many people already feel robbed of their individuality when dealing with systems and bureaucracies. A client who arranges for a health care giver to come to the home, demonstrates his or her individuality. Inviting the nurse into the home also gives the client a sense of having charge of his or her own life.

Private Practice

Nurses who see clients in their homes may function either as staff members of a health care agency or as private practitioners. They may supervise nonprofessionals who give care. Self-employed nurses will have more control over the actions of nonprofessionals than other nurses because they will be able to specify what training and responsibilities their assistants will have. The assistant will be directly accountable to the nurse and the nurse to the client who arranged for care. In such a situation, the nurse will need broad professional knowledge in order to practice independently. He or she will have to decide when to function without help and when to call in other professionals. Furthermore, the nurse will require skills in teaching and training assistants. Employing other personnel and managing a private practice will require administrative knowledge and ability.

Specialist versus Generalist

As long as the system permits it, professionals will probably continue to specialize. In many respects, this is advantageous. For example, a nurse who specializes in community nursing will be well prepared to plan and carry out care for people outside of institutions. By the same token, those who choose to specialize in inpatient care will be experienced and knowledgeable in acute care. However, if nurses are to take the responsibility for broad-based, holistic care of clients, those who work with clients in hospitals might visit them in their homes immediately after discharge and work directly with a community-based nurse to facilitate the transition to home care. Likewise, the community nurse could facilitate transitions to acute care settings by making visits in the hospital and communicating directly with the nurses and other caregivers to provide the best care for the client.

By continuing to be involved in the care clients receive in other settings, the nurse will be cognizant of the client's wants and needs in both situations. By keeping up-to-date on the nursing practice in both areas, the nurse will be more flexible and adaptive in the primary area. Understanding the home environment in theory and in actual practice will help the hospital-based nurse develop an appropriate discharge plan. The community-based nurse will be better able to adapt the home environment to the client's needs if she or he is aware of the way these needs were met in the hospital. This kind of sampling of other practice areas

and collaboration between specialists not only contributes to the well-being of the clients but also promotes understanding and support among nursing colleagues.

The Distant Future

We can only speculate about the role of the nurse in the distant future. A nurse may be able to "visit" a client electronically in order to determine if a personal visit is required. By visiting a client on a two-way visual communications system, the nurse can evaluate aspects of the client's status and environment that cannot be assessed over the telephone. If the client has a personal computer system, the nurse may be able to assist in programming the computer to augment care between visits. Such means may create new problems, however. Useful as they seem to be, such technical aids may create the distance that home visits have helped eradicate in the present and past. The nurse will be confronted with new problems: learning to use these technical tools judiciously and keeping the goal of the client's health and well-being at the forefront in planning interventions.

SUMMARY

Each nurse who practices in the community will approach home visits in a unique way, but the format used will usually be based on the nursing process. Creativity and flexibility will help the nurse decide when to make a home visit and to make this intervention useful for the client. The nurse who is practicing in the community and making home visits now or in the near future is helping to lay the groundwork for the future use of this strategy. As "home" takes on different meanings, the planning and interventions done by nurses will change. However, some things are not likely to change. Respect for individuals and a willingness to adapt nursing care to their needs will always be a principal aspect of nursing care.

DISCUSSION TOPICS

1. Mrs. Emma Wilson is an 85-year-old client who is being discharged from the hospital after care for a myocardial infarction. The community health nurse receives a referral for home visits.

    a. Discuss appropriate previsit activities.

    b. What is the nurse's responsibility for planning and intervention?

    c. Devise a contract for use by nurse and client.

    d. Identify community resources outside the home available for Mrs. Wilson.

2. Dan Blevis is a school nurse who is planning to make home visits to all parents of children who were discovered to have hearing deficits during audiometric screening. These are the first home visits he has made in his new job.

    a. What can Mr. Blevis do to increase his effectiveness?

    b. In what ways can Mr. Blevis evaluate his communication with clients?

3. Emil Warner, who has a terminal illness, has been visited by Joan Mayes, RN, three times per week for several months for supportive care. Bella Tyler, RN, will soon begin visiting Mr. Warner because Ms. Mayes is moving to another city. Mr. Warner and Ms. Mayes have developed a positive interpersonal relationship. Describe how Ms. Mayes and Ms. Tyler can facilitate an optimal termination between Mr. Warner and Ms. Mayes and a functional transition to Ms. Tyler's care.

4. Sammy Clark is an 18-month-old child who has been diagnosed as having developmental delay. The community health nurse receives a referral from the physician but cannot prearrange a visit, since the Clark family has no telephone.

    a. Discuss techniques for entry into the home.

    b. In what ways might all family members (mother, father, 5-year-old sister) be involved in plans for intervention?

    c. List advantages of making home visits with Sammy's family.

5. If a community health nurse were to visit your home today, what environmental assessments could be made utilizing the assessment of the home environment checklist described in this chapter? (Figure 20.1)

6. Julie Burns is a 19-year-old client referred to the community health nurse because she has gained 30 pounds in the first six weeks of her pregnancy.

    a. Devise a contract based on the client's goal of preventing excessive weight gain.

    b. Discuss how the nurse might employ change theory in nursing intervention.

    c. What are the roles of the nurse in caring for Ms. Burns in her home? How are these similar to or different from the roles of a nurse in a hospital?

7. As a result of reorganization of the local public health department, where you are employed as a community health nurse, a neighborhood nursing network is being established. A nurse will be assigned to every six-block area as a neighborhood health professional. You are planning a neighborhood meeting to communicate with clients about the new system of care. Apply the nursing process in assessing, planning, implementing, and evaluating needs for home care of clients in your area.

BIBLIOGRAPHY

Brofman, J.: An evening home visiting program. *Nursing Outlook* 27, 657, 1979.

Carkhuff, R.: *The art of helping.* Amherst, Mass.: Human Resource Development Press, 1973

Combs, A., Avila, D., & Purkey, W.: *Helping relationships.* Boston: Allyn & Bacon, 1971.

Hanlon, J., & Pickett, G.: *Public health administration and practice.* St. Louis: Mosby, 1979.

Kalisch, P. A., & Kalisch, B. J.: *The advance of American nursing.* Boston: Little, Brown & Co., 1978.

Keeling, B.L.: Making the most of the first home visit. *Nursing '78* 8(3), 24, 1978.

Kelly, H.: The sense of an ending. *American Journal of Nursing* 69, 2378, 1969.

Lentz, J., & Meyer, E.: The dirty house. *Nursing Outlook* 27, 590, 1979.

Mayers, M.: Home visit—Ritual or therapy? *Nursing Outlook* 21, 328, 1973.

Price, J., & Braden, C.: The reality in home visits. *American Journal of Nursing* 78, 1536, 1978.

Rogers, C.: The interpersonal relationship: The core of guidance. *Harvard Educational Review* 32, 416, 1962.

Smith, D., & Peterson, J.: Counseling and values in a time perspective. *Personnel and Guidance Journal* 55, 309, 1977.

Schoolcraft, V.: The interpersonal process recording. In R. Young, ed., *Community nursing workbook: Family as client.* Norwalk, Conn.: Appleton-Century-Crofts, 1982.

21

Community Mental Health

Judith Belliveau Krauss

Of all the tyrannies of human kind,
The worst is that which persecutes the mind.
JOHN DRYDEN

OBJECTIVES

After reading this chapter, you should be able to:

☐ Define community mental health.
☐ Define deinstitutionalization.
☐ Name four historical determinants of deinstitutionalization.
☐ Define and compare mental health, mental illness, the mental health–mental illness continuum, levels of prevention, and at-risk populations.
☐ Name and define nine common disturbances of mental health.
☐ Compare and critique the role of the community health nurse in three community-based models of care designed to address mental health needs.
☐ Discuss concepts of social control, social networking, and restrictiveness as they apply to community mental health.
☐ Discuss and critique alternative systems of community mental health care.

INTRODUCTION

Community Mental Health

In the early 1960s, community mental health was considered a revolutionary concept in the practice of hospital psychiatry. It was seen as the antidote to the recognized dehumanizing effects of long-term institutionalization of the seriously mentally ill. The community mental health legislation of the 1960s promised both promotion of mental health and provision of comprehensive, community-based treatment and rehabilitation of the severely mentally ill. The beginning of the community mental health movement is usually dated to the Mental Health Study Act of 1955, which directed the Joint Commission on Mental Illness and Health to conduct a five-year study of the needs and resources of the mentally ill in the United States and to make recommendations to Congress for the development of a national mental health program.

This movement evolved as the result of four primary historical forces:

1. The effects of drug and psychosocial treatment innovations on discharge rates, length of hospital stay, and the return to functional levels of patients previously believed manageable only in institutions.

2. Legislative pressure by fiscal conservatives to shift the budgetary burden of psychiatric care, which had been steadily rising since the emergence of state hospitals, from state to federal responsibility.

3. Social pressure by those who deplored the dehumanizing effects of large state mental hospitals and demanded the radical change of decarceration.

4. An acknowledgment on the part of reform-minded citizens and legislators that the stigma of a psychiatric diagnosis, particularly a long-term disabling one, had become more devastating than the illness itself (Krauss & Slavinsky, 1982, pp. 77–78).

The final report submitted to Congress on December 31, 1960, provided the framework for the Mental Retardation Facilities and Community Mental Health Centers Construction Act of 1963. That legislation, often referred to as the Kennedy "bold new approach," called for the construction of community-based mental health centers (CMHCs) that would be federally funded as long as they provided five essential services: inpatient care, outpatient care, emergency treatment, partial hospitalization, and community consultation.

The CMHCs were intended to serve two distinct populations. First, they were to address the mental illness prevention needs of the geographic populations, known as *catchment areas*, they served. It was believed that CMHCs would, through consultation and education programs, serve essentially healthy populations that had not been recipients of psychiatric care in the past but that could benefit from programs that would focus on early detection of illness, stress management and reduction, anticipatory guidance, and common child and adult developmental crises. Indeed, the early users of CMHCs did represent this group.

Second, CMHCs were intended to replace large public mental institutions by providing the alternatives of community-based hospitalization and outpatient treatment. It was expected that the inpatient population of state mental hospitals would be reduced by half over a 20-year period. That goal has been achieved. In 1955, 77 percent of mental health services were provided in inpatient settings and only 23 percent in outpatient settings. In 1975, the situation was reversed, with 76 percent of services provided on an outpatient basis and only 24 percent in inpatient settings. The greatest reduction occurred in inpatient services of state mental hospitals, which provided 49 percent of all services in 1955 and only 9 percent in 1975 (President's Commission, 1978).

Deinstitutionalization

This shift in the locus of care of the mentally ill, termed *deinstitutionalization*, represents a shift in mental health policy from an emphasis on long-term custodial care to short-term community-based care, with a focus on reintegration into society. In fact, the ink on the community mental health legislation was hardly dry when large numbers of previously institutionalized people were discharged to their communities. CMHCs and the communities they served were not ready for the onslaught. Nursing-home and room-and-board home occupancy tripled between 1963 and 1969, welfare hotels proliferated between 1965 and 1975, and local YMCAs found themselves to be the reluctant landlords of the chronically mentally ill (Armstrong, 1979; Becker & Schulberg, 1976; Greenblatt & Glazier, 1975; Ozarin & Sharfstein, 1978).

It was believed that deinstitutionalization would effectively reintegrate the chronically mentally ill into the community, that services would be available and coordinated, and that community-based care would be cheaper than long-term state hospital care. Many authors have documented that these assumptions turned into myths. Klerman (1977) suggests that deinstitutionalization was a shift in location and funding of care without the necessary support services. Talbott (1979), a psychiatrist known for his work with the chronically mentally ill, called deinstitutionalization a misnomer and created the term "transinstitutionalization" to describe the tragic shift in care from a single institution to several poor substitutes, including nursing homes, room-and-board homes, the streets, the CMHC programs characterized by lack of follow-up, dropout, and the so-called revolving-door syndrome. (The *revolving door syndrome* is the term applied when patients are repeatedly admitted and discharged from inpatient facilities after brief attempts at community living.)

Many others have documented that people who were deinstitutionalized now live lonely existences, the unwitting victims of crime, occasionally turning criminal, with inadequate or nonexistent services in the community (Arnhoff, 1975; Krauss &

Slavinsky, 1982; Slavinsky et al., 1976). About half of any discharged population return to their family of origin; the burden of caring for the ill family member and the stigma associated with mental illness cause reactive depression and anxiety in other family members (Creer & Wing, 1975; Doll, 1976; Rachlin, 1978). A large percentage of previously institutionalized people, however, do not return to their community of origin but instead cluster in low-income ghettoized areas, living a marginal existence and lacking in the high-level social competence skills required to survive on the streets (Reich & Seigal, 1978).

From a historical perspective we have come full circle. The locus of care for the mentally ill shifted from the community in the seventeenth and eighteenth centuries, to large public facilities far removed from the community in the nineteenth and part of the twentieth centuries, back to the community as we move toward the twenty-first century. Mental health services have now broadened to include the prevention and mental health maintenance needs of those who previously would not have availed themselves of services.

Nursing Roles

Krauss and Slavinsky (1982) provide a detailed summary of the historical events in nursing that paralleled the community mental health and desinstitutionalization era. In the late 1950s a public health nurse–researcher anticipated the consequences of psychiatric drugs and the therapeutic milieu and conducted a study of the use of public health nursing services by people formerly hospitalized for psychiatric problems (Gelber, 1959). She discovered that many of those released did not understand their illness, that over 40 percent did not take medication correctly if at all, that 42 percent had serious hygiene problems, and that many were parents who had adjustment problems with their children. She concluded that people with psychiatric problems had needs ideally suited to the skills of the public health nurse and recommended that nurses who cared for this population receive training in community work.

During the community mental health and deinstitutionalization era, a major controversy raged among nursing professionals and leaders: who should care for the mentally ill in the community? In the first issue of the journal *Perspectives in Psychiatric Care*, Dorothy Mereness (1963), a distinguished psychiatric nursing leader, took the position that nurses prepared at the baccalaureate level with advanced preparation in psychiatric nursing were the most appropriate care providers to the mentally ill in the community. She suggested that community health nurses lacked the training needed to serve the mental health needs of people in the community. Ilsa Wolff (1964), a public health nursing administrator, took issue with this position, noting that the needs in the community were greater than any one subspecialty group could handle, that psychiatric nurses were barely meeting the demands of hospital based-clients, and that community health nurses were already prepared in family and community care. She went on to suggest ways in which psychiatric and community health nurses could collaborate in meeting the community mental health needs of any population, with particular emphasis on use of the psychiatric nurse–clinical specialist as a consultant to community health nursing groups. As Krauss and Slavinsky (1982) point out, the debate was never resolved.

Two other events are worthy of mention. The first was a landmark study conducted by Pasamanick et al. (1967) and followed up by Davis et al. (1974) that demonstrated the use of medication and public health nursing services in the at-home care of acutely ill schizophrenics. The earlier study showed that at-home clients did better on measures of adjustment and symptom control than hospitalized controls. The public health nurses were the key care providers and data collectors in the study. The follow-up study, conducted after funding problems had caused a withdrawal of the public health nursing services, showed a return to lower precare levels of functioning. The follow-up underscored the value of public health nurses. The second event was the Arafeh et al. study (1968), which documented the liaison nursing model in which a psychiatric nurse served as the liaison between the state hospital and a public health nursing agency in the discharge planning and community-based treatment of psychiatric clients. This was one of the first publications documenting a collaborative model of care.

This chapter will address community mental health concepts as they apply to the promotion of mental health as well as secondary and tertiary prevention of illness among those who already have a diagnosed mental disorder. It reviews common disturbances in mental health and community mental health models of care and discusses the roles of the community health nurse in addressing the mental health needs of the community, both now and in the future.

OVERVIEW

Mental Health

Ramshorn and Pearlmutter (1982) present a review of four models of mental health: the normality model, the holistic model, the wellness model, and the adaptive model.

The Normality Model

The normality model (Offer & Sabshin, 1974) includes four conceptualizations of normality developed from an extensive review of the literature. *Normality* can be defined either as health, as a utopian state, as an average, or as a transactional system. Normality as health is the absence of illness. Normality as a utopian state is an idealized, unreachable state of well-being and harmony. Normality as an average is based on a standard or norm of health; this introduces the idea of deviance from a norm. Normality as a transactional system stresses process and an individual's growth over time and suggests that normal behavior is determined by a variety of interacting systems that can change over time.

The Holistic Model

Holism is a belief in the unity of mind and body. Rogers (1970) is credited with a well-known nursing theory utilizing the concept of holistic health. An individual is viewed as a unified biopsychosocial being in which alterations in one part will affect the whole. Rogers defines a human being as a unified whole greater than and different from the sum of its parts. Holism focuses our attention on the individual's culture, environment, and physical, spiritual, and mental health.

The Wellness Model

Dunn (1961) is credited with the concept of *high-level wellness*. His is one of the few positively oriented definitions of health. *Wellness* is viewed as a dynamic process of maximizing one's potential and moving toward a state of complete physical, mental, and social well-being. *Coping* is the mechanism by which one maximizes health or wellness. An inability to cope would be viewed as illness.

The Adaptive Model

Dubos (1965) utilizes the concept of homeostasis in defining health as the ability of the body to adapt to its environment. Health is thus seen as the state of being reasonably free from physical and mental discomfort and pain. This model also views health as a dynamic process involving change (*adaptation*) throughout the life cycle as one is confronted with both predictable and unpredictable events.

Mental Illness

Krauss and Slavinsky (1982) identified five models of mental illness: the medical-technical model, the epidemiological model, the sociological model, the illness as myth model, and the psychodynamic model.

The Medical-Technical Model

The medical-technical model concentrates on the organic sources and causes of dysfunction. The focus is on pathology and cure and the methods used for eradicating disease usually takes highly technical forms, including shock therapy, medications, or psychosurgery. This model can be credited with recent advances in neuropsychiatry and in the psychopharmacological management of certain forms of manic-depressive disorders.

The Epidemiological Model

The epidemiological model is a statistical model that focuses on the incidence and prevalence of disease. It is concerned not with intervention but with the identification of population groups that are susceptible to various forms of disease. *Incidence* refers to the number of new cases of a disease over a specified period of time (e.g., a year); *prevalence* refers to the number of established cases of a disease in a population at a specific point in time. Illness therefore is defined as increased incidence or prevalence, whereas health is reduced incidence and prevalence ultimately resulting in the absence of disease.

The Sociological Model

This model focuses on the ills of society and its institutional structures. Goffman's *Asylums* (1961) and *Methods of Madness* (1969) by Braginsky et al. are classic examples of the sociological approach to a definition of mental illness. This model characterizes mental illness as learned social behavior and advocates social-environmental changes to foster mental health.

The Illness as Myth Model

This model is also referred to as the antipsychiatry model. It is best represented in the writings of R.D. Laing (1967) and Thomas Szasz (1964). This model suggests that "illness" is a useless medical concept that demonstrates society's intolerance for relatively mild forms of deviance as well as the injustice and antihumanitarianism of many forms of treatment. Szasz (1964) suggests that mental illness is a medical metaphor that is no more nor less than a stigmatizing label applied to the behavior of all those who offend or annoy others. The model has been useful in raising humanitarian, moral, and legal issues relative to the care of the mentally ill.

The Psychodynamic Model

This model, originally called the intrapsychic model, can best be described as the focus on both intrapersonal and interpersonal disequilibrium. *Intra*personal disequilibrium refers to those experiences internal to individuals that negatively alter their self-concept and their view of reality. *Inter*personal disequilibrium includes those experiences occurring between an individual and other individuals or groups that impede ability to adjust to environmental demands. This model, in contrast to the medical-technical model, takes a functional view of illness and locates it in the process of interaction with others or within the abstract structures of the mind or psyche.

The Mental Health–Mental Illness Continuum

A review of the mental health and mental illness models leads to one conclusion: that one's relative state of mental health or illness exists on a continuum and is in a dynamic state of flux in interaction with the environment, both internal and external. One's relative state of health depends on one's stage in the life cycle, available resources, coping mechanisms, and the presence of organic or functional disequalibria relative to society's standards of deviance. Concepts of mental health and illness vary from culture to culture and within subgroups of the same culture. Individuals' placement on the continuum will determine the level of intervention necessary to meet their mental health needs.

Prevention

Levels of prevention in psychiatry have been borrowed directly from the fields of public health and epidemiology. Caplan

(1974) defines *primary prevention* in mental health as those interventions that seek to reduce the incidence of new cases of mental disorder by reducing harmful environmental forces and strengthening people's ability to cope. *Secondary prevention* is aimed at shortening the duration of cases of mental disorder that occur despite primary prevention efforts, thus decreasing the prevalence of mental disorder in a given population or community. *Tertiary prevention* is aimed at reducing the amount of defect that results secondarily from mental illness and thus ensuring as full a return as possible to life in the community.

Primary prevention would be utilized for those populations whose members had not been previously diagnosed with a mental disorder or who had not previously made use of a mental health facility. This is the "essentially normal" population that CMHCs were intended to serve through community education and consultation services.

Secondary prevention would be utilized for those who already carried a psychiatric diagnosis or who had been identified as having a mental disorder but whose illness trajectory could be interrupted before further deterioration took place. Individuals who are hospitalized or diagnosed for the first time fall into this category.

Tertiary prevention would be utilized for those who had a long-term downward illness trajectory and who required maintenance and rehabilitation programs to prevent the negative effects of institutionalization, the side effects of psychiatric medications and other treatments, or the family burden and drain of community resources.

At-Risk Populations

Certain categories of people are at greater risk than others for mental illness or psy-chiatric relapse. Relapse is usually defined as rehospitalization, although Krauss and Slavinsky (1982) have broadened the concept to include a transfer to a more restrictive setting or a significant increase in medication levels. The concept of an "at-risk population" allows the nurse to target certain individuals within the primary, secondary, or tertiary levels of prevention as most in need of care. A review of all of the possible at-risk populations within a community mental health framework could be the topic of a whole book. Regular review of the research and knowledge of the community assist the nurse in identifying at-risk populations. Such populations change with changes in the prevalence and incidence of mental illness and with the introduction of community education programs aimed at stress management, assertiveness, self-care, and parent-child problems, to name a few.

Common Disturbances of Mental Health

There are a variety of circumstances and conditions that challenge an individual's ability to cope. The degree to which a person is able to function effectively within living, learning, and work environments can be used as a measure of adjustment, or social competence. *Social competence* is the ability of an individual to interact with the environment through interpersonal relationships and participation in work, home, and social activities. A *social disability* results when participation in such activities and relationships is sufficiently impaired that the result is disrupted social or occupational role performance.

Psychiatric disability can be defined as physical, intellectual, and emotional skill deficits, resulting directly from a psychiatric illness, that impair functioning in the living, learning, and working environments

(Anthony, 1979; Vance, 1973). A psychiatric disability can include anything from an acute, temporary dysfunction to a severe, permanent impairment. The degree and duration of the impairment, combined with the likelihood of recovery or adaptation on the part of the individual or modification of the environment, determines the severity of the disability. Anthony (1979) has suggested that *skill behaviors* can be categorized as physical, emotional or intellectual. Physical skills are those that require ordinary physical behavior, such as driving a car, doing housework, or grooming. Emotional skills include those that are involved in interaction with others, such as controlling one's temper, explaining problems, or going to parties. Intellectual skills are those involved in problem solving, such as choosing a job, balancing the budget, or cooking. Anthony (1979) has suggested that we should not confuse skills with the environments in which they are performed. A deficit is a disability only if it disrupts an individual's functioning within the environment.

Two categories of circumstances can contribute to skill deficits and dysfunctional environmental functioning: stressful events and clinical syndromes. The following paragraphs do not constitute an exhaustive review of the common disturbances of mental health, but they serve as a brief review of those circumstances most likely to be encountered in the normal course of a community health nurse's functions. The interested student is encouraged to pursue these topics further in a basic psychiatric nursing text.

Stress Events

Stress is a well-documented precipitant of mental and physical illness. The two major sources of stress are developmental crises and life events. *Developmental crises* occur within the individual, while life events occur within the environment. Erikson's classic work, *Childhood and Society* (1963), suggests that a human life is a series of observable stages, each marked by a crisis or turning point at which time the individual is simultaneously highly vulnerable to failure and highly open to achievement and heightened potential. While Erikson's stages cover the entire life cycle, he emphasized the childhood developmental stages.

Sheehey (1976) coined the term "passages" to describe stages of adult development, while Levinson (1978) used the term "seasons." Both theorists have documented that there are predictable times in adults' life cycles when they face crises of decision that determine the future course of events in their lives. Levinson (1978), for example, suggests that somewhere between the ages of 36 and 46 a man completes a midlife transition. This is marked by evaluation of his occupational role and redefinition of his marriage.

Krauss and Slavinsky (1982) have suggested that there are four primary tasks of adult development: (1) separating from the family of origin, (2) establishing a family of orientation, (3) establishing an occupational role, and (4) facing the realities of aging. Regardless of how one labels them, it is clear that there are developmental junctures in our lives that increase the internal stress involved in making life decisions. At these times people are vulnerable to mental illness and can suffer temporary or permanent developmental lags.

Life Events

The second major source of stress in our lives is life events. There has been extensive work implicating life events as precipitants of relapse in psychiatric disorders as well as of onset and exacerbation of medical disorders (Brown et al., 1973; Goldberg et al.,

1977; Paykel et al., 1969, 1971; Rahe, 1969; Rahe et al., 1972). *Life events* are changes in relationships, interactions, living conditions, employment roles, health, economic circumstances, or life-style that are independent of the individual's control and that contribute either to a positive or negative stress valence. Individuals who have experienced one or more stressful life changes within the previous year are at increased risk for onset or relapse of mental illness.

Clinical Syndromes

DEPRESSION. In psychiatry, *depression* is a clinical syndrome characterized by an alteration of *affect* (mood). The mood alteration is dominated by feelings of sadness and apparent or expressed loss of interest in most or all daily activities. Depression is a phenomenon that is experienced by everyone at some point, and its classification as a mental dysfunction depends on the degree and duration of the depressed feelings.

Swanson (1982) has usefully categorized depression as first-level, middle-level, or severe-level dysfunction. *First-level depression* is a transitory, essentially normal condition usually accompanied by sadness, dejection, or downheartedness associated with identifiable realities such as a disappointment, letdown after an exciting activity, or loss of a meaningful object.

Middle-level depression includes a clear disturbance in affect over time, and may involve some thought disturbance as well as motor retardation, somatic complaints, and alterations in verbal interactions and social participation. People who have middle-level depression seem to have lost their lust for life, may be gloomy or pessimistic, and may weep more frequently than usual. Thinking processes are often slowed down, and there is little ability to plan for the future in goal-directed ways. Often people complain of repetitive thoughts or rumination. Motor behavior is slowed down. People complain of feeling as if they are carrying the weight of the world. Some people eat to excess, while others lose their appetite entirely. Sleep disturbances, including difficulty in falling asleep, early morning awakening, and interrupted sleep may be reported, as well as lack of interest or decreased participation in sexual activity. Verbal interaction may be characterized by negativism and an almost exclusive preoccupation with the self. Such preoccupation generally leads to social withdrawal and isolation, which is maintained and perpetuated by the depressed person until the depression lifts.

Severe-level depression is characterized either by the apparent absence of any affect or by despondency and despair. Some individuals who are severely depressed complain of having no feelings or of feeling empty. Serious alterations in thought can accompany severe depression, including delusions that confirm the individual's feelings of low self-worth and of powerlessness and emptiness. Individuals may demonstrate either extreme of motor activity: agitated, purposeless movements or practically no movement at all. Social participation and verbal communication may be nonexistent.

ANXIETY. It is somewhat misleading to categorize anxiety as a clinical syndrome, since it is a constant component of our daily lives. However, anxiety can also be identified as a primary component of almost every emotional dysfunction. It is both essential for survival and an ever-present danger.

Although anxiety was first identified as a physiological phenomenon, Harry Stack Sullivan (1948) defined it as a component of the mother–infant relationship and contributed to our understanding of it as a threat to self-esteem, prestige, and dignity. Hildegard Peplau (1952) called anxiety a potent force in interpersonal relationships and further defined it as a response to unknown danger. *Anxiety* is often described as a feeling of tension, uneasiness, jitteriness, or apprehensiveness. It is usually a feeling state that seems out of proportion to the situation at hand and it is brought on by a vague threat.

Anxiety results from a threat to either biological integrity or to self-concept (Peplau, 1963). Anxiety results from a threat to biological integrity when there is interference with satisfaction of hunger, warmth, thirst, or sexual expression. It results from a threat to self-concept when there is real or anticipated disapproval from significant others, unfulfilled expectations, or unmet needs for respect or self-esteem.

Anxiety is considered essential for survival since it can motivate change and growth. It is anxiety that triggers the response to react and change. Anxiety contributes to dysfunctional behavior when it is so overwhelming that the individual attempts to avoid or distance from the perceived precipitants. The major characteristics of anxiety are the unknown or unclear threat and the disproportionate reaction. *Fear*, on the other hand, is an identifiable response to a real threat with reactions in direct proportion to the threat.

Jimerson (1982) has identified four stages of anxiety: (1) panic, (2) acute anxiety, (3) chronic anxiety, and (4) normal anxiety. *Panic*, the most extreme form of anxiety, is characterized by personality disorganization, severe dysfunction, and immobilization or flight. *Acute anxiety* is typified by sudden onset, is of short duration, and is triggered by sudden change or loss with accompanying threat to integrity (e.g., the sudden death of a loved one). *Chronic anxiety* is consistent and persistent in nature, is

of long duration, and is characterized by vague feelings of unease and jitteriness. It is considered a part of the personality structure. *Normal anxiety* is that degree of anxiety necessary for survival that motivates us to get on with tasks.

The clinically anxious individual is the person who experiences levels of anxiety that interfere with effective everyday functioning. People who have experienced recent life events, who are in lower socioeconomic strata, who are lonely and isolated, who have experienced trauma (e.g., Vietnam veterans, victims of the eruption of Mount St. Helens) or those who have been recently hospitalized, are all at risk for high levels of anxiety. Jimerson (1982) has categorized the feelings and behaviors associated with anxiety as physiological, emotional, or cognitive. Some examples of such behaviors include diarrhea, headaches, frequent urination, sweaty palms, palpitations, fatigue, muscle tension (physiological); irritability, frequent crying, feelings of insecurity, dread or terror, preoccupation (emotional); and distractability, inattentiveness, poor reality testing, and unspecified worries and ruminating (cognitive).

SUICIDAL OR SELF-DESTRUCTIVE BEHAVIOR. Suicide is a national health problem whose proportions are far greater than reported statistics indicate. In 1978 there were 27,500 reported deaths by suicide. It has been estimated that this figure represents 12.2 percent of known attempters (Public Health Service, 1979). Shneidman (1980) suggests that suicide statistics represent an incomplete reporting of suicidal behavior and points out that high-risk behavior, including that associated with alcohol and accidents, is a clear indicator of self-destructive tendencies.

The self-destructive individual is characterized by several commonly identified behaviors: ambivalence, guilt, helplessness and hopelessness, and aggression. Ambivalence is a central phenomenon in suicidality. Suicidal individuals are known to struggle between self-destruction and self-preservation (Wekstein, 1979). In fact, the ambivalence is one of the features of the suicidal individual that allows clinicians the opportunity to intervene; for example, a suicidal individual may take an overdose of a slow-acting medication and call a suicide hotline in time to be rescued. Self-destructive individuals may carry a large burden of guilt and may express feelings of responsibility and remorse for their own and others' misfortunes. Such feelings, combined with feelings of low self-esteem and self-worth, can lead to the *helpless—hopeless syndrome*, defined by Farberow and Shneidman (1961) as the vicious cycle of feeling that problems are insurmountable and unlikely to change and that the individual is helpless to alter the course of events. Finally, there is a link between suicidality and self-destructive behavior and aggression. Suicide is often described as aggression turned inward, but there is much about suicidal acts that can be characterized as aggression turned outward. There are the obvious homicide-suicides and the more subtle acts of self-destruction motivated by revenge and anger toward others, as in the case of a successful suicide accompanied by a suicide note that implicates others in the suicide. Often the method of suicide can be evaluated as more or less aggressive or violent.

McClean (1982) has identified several groups that are at high risk for suicide and self-destructive behavior:

1. Alcoholics
2. Police officers
3. Physicians
4. Previous attempters
5. Adolescents
6. Terminally ill people
7. Accident repeaters
8. Elderly people
9. People who reject treatment
10. Attempters whose suicidalness is ignored by medical establishment

The list is long and varied; thus the community health nurse must be aware of the possibility of risk and alert to the behaviors associated with suicidality. In addition, the nurse must evaluate the degree of suicide risk or the lethality level. *Suicide risk* is determined by the presence of a plan, the availability of means, the risk of death posed by the plan, and the presence of other risk factors such as stress, psychiatric symptoms, or being a member of a high risk group. For example, a young man (adolescent risk group) who has a suicide plan with a high risk of death (a gun) and the means to carry out the plan (his father is a hunter and has guns in the home) would carry a high lethality risk of suicide. McClean (1982) suggests a four-step process in working with the suicidal or self-destructive client: (1) assess the risk of suicide, presence of stressors, and symptoms; (2) identify the problems; (3) formulate a therapeutic plan based on the risk of suicide; and (4) follow up. (Suicide intervention is discussed further in Chapter 22.)

SUBSTANCE ABUSE. Substance abuse is a psychological and/or physiological dependence on alcohol or nonalcoholic chemicals to the point that it is harmful to self and others. Alcoholism alone is said to be the third major health problem in the United States. Current estimates are that upwards of 9 to 10 million adults and over 3 million adolescents (12–17 years old) are troubled by alcoholism or problem drinking (Zamora, 1982). It is impossible to estimate the statistics on nonalcoholic drug abuse, since drug use carries greater legal and moral sanctions than alcohol use and is therefore less likely to be reported.

There is no one profile of the alcohol or drug abuser. Substance abuse cuts across socioeconomic lines and age categories. However, some common risk factors are likely to predispose someone to problem drinking or drug behavior or a combination of the two. Davidson (1979) identifies the following risk factors for alcoholism: (1) family history of either total abstinence combined with rigid moral atmosphere or alcoholism, (2) history of marital discord, (3) absent or rejecting father, (4) recurrent, cross-generation depression among the females in a family, and (5) belonging to a cultural group with higher levels of alcoholism than the population at large. The risk factors for drug abuse are the same and are often associated with heavy drug or alcohol use among adult family members and with high family anxiety levels.

Alcohol and drug abuse are often signals of family discord and may serve to draw attention away from family disharmony, marital distress, and other troubles. Substance abusers are often described as excessively dependent or passive. One can usually document a history of deprived dependency needs and lack of gratification as a child. Regardless of the etiology, substance abuse that goes undetected or untreated can result in permanent organic impairment and, in some cases, death (from drug overdose, alcohol withdrawal syndrome, delirium tremens). Like most common disturbances of mental health, substance abuse affects not only the individual client but also family members and significant others.

PSYCHOTIC BEHAVIOR. Individuals can be said to be *psychotic* when their behavior suggests that they are out of touch with re- ality. An individual who is troubled by psychotic behavior is generally sensitive to overstimulating and understimulating environments. The psychotic behavior may be seen as a means, albeit unhealthy, of coping with anxiety. Psychotic behavior causes disturbances in communication and interaction with others. Psychotic behavior is most often expressed through disordered thought, delusions, compulsions or obsessions, hallucinations, and mistaken ideas of reference. These behaviors may or may not be accompanied by altered motor activity or affect or unusual behavior. Individuals who believe that others can read their minds, or who fancy themselves to be royalty, or who describe sores on their bodies that do not exist, or who repeat certain activities, such as handwashing, to excess are exhibiting psychotic behavior. Psychotic behavior can be most troublesome to family members who must cope with the disruptions in their normal routine and who must control the behavior of their psychotic relative so as not to disturb the neighborhood or call undue stigmatizing attention to the family.

Psychotropic medications can be effective deterrents to psychotic behaviors and are still the single most effective deterrent to rehospitalization of the chronically mentally ill. Medication, administered either alone or in conjunction with other forms of treatment, can increase the number of days a chronically mentally ill individual remains in the community. Unfortunately, drug therapy is not without side effects. People who are maintained for long periods of time on antipsychotic drugs are subject to parkinsonian symptoms of motor retardation and akinesia (lack of spontaneity). *Tardive dyskinesia*, a syndrome characterized by involuntary muscular activity of the mouth, shuffling of the feet, and a variety of other abnormal posturings, is associated with prolonged phenothiazine use and can appear during use or several months after discontinuance of certain medications.

The vigilant community health nurse will be alert to such symptoms when visiting clients who are on phenothiazines. Some researchers claim that the syndrome is of no clinical significance since the symptoms disappear with time after discontinuance of drug therapy, whereas others claim that there can be irreversible organic damage (Crane, 1973). Regardless, the person who suffers from the side effects of antipsychotic medication may prefer the psychotic symptoms to the drug effects and may discontinue medication and experience a drastic increase in symptoms. The side effects can often be eliminated or reduced with antiparkinsonian drugs or with a downward titration of the antipsychotic medications, thus decreasing the client's discomfort and eliminating the attention-getting gesturing, posturing, and tremors that serve only to further stigmatize the client and family.

ABUSIVE BEHAVIOR.   The primary victims of abuse are the institutionalized, the elderly, children (especially those of preschool age), and women. Abuse takes many forms, including emotional abuse or neglect, physical abuse or neglect, and sexual abuse or exploitation. Sideleau (1982) provides an overview of the problems of abuse and neglect as well as comprehensive recommendations for nursing interventions. She defines the various forms of abuse and neglect as follows:

Physical abuse involves willful, non-accidental injury delivered with an attitude of physical harmfulness. . . .
Physical neglect is a deliberate failure to provide the necessities of life; medical care; and basic physical, physiological, and safety needs. . . .

Emotional abuse involves the use of words and actions to threaten or terrorize, or to depreciate the victim's self-worth. . . .
Emotional neglect is a failure to provide a positive emotional climate that would foster the satisfaction of love and belonging, and the need for recognition and enhanced self-esteem. . . .
Sexual abuse includes both assaultive and violent traumatic sexual contact and sexual exploitation of a non-violent type. Incest, which includes any sexual activity or intimate physical contact that is sexually arousing between non-married members of a family, is a form of sexual abuse. . . . (pp. 975–976)

The community health nurse is often able to watch for signs of abuse or neglect. The community health nurse should be observant of signs of injuries that do not match the description of the accident; injuries in the shape of handprint or thumb or fingerprints on the face or neck; burns at various stages of healing (particularly cigarette burns); bruises about the head, back, or rib cage; or poor hygiene or evidence of poor nutrition. Additionally one might notice a child who fails to seek out parents for comfort or who is wary of adults, depressed, unusually preoccupied with sexual matters, provocative, or troubled by nightmares or disturbed sleep patterns (Sideleau, 1982).

COMMUNITY-BASED MODELS OF CARE

A range of models of ways to meet the mental health needs of the community at primary, secondary, and tertiary levels of intervention currently exist. No one model meets all of the identified needs, but when taken together they represent a still developing, comprehensive, decentralized system of care. This section provides brief descriptions of the major models of community-based mental health services and details the role of the community health nurse within each model.

Community Mental Health Centers Model

Community mental health centers (CMHCs) provide five essential services to a geographically defined community: (1) inpatient treatment, (2) outpatient treatment, (3) emergency and crisis services, (4) partial hospitalization, and (5) consultation and education. Combined, the full range of services can address community mental health needs at all three levels of intervention. An example of a primary intervention service offered by a CMHC would be the provision of an educational series to a local parent–teacher organization on discipline of the school-age child or on sexuality in the latency-age child. School health nurses can be active in such programs and may initiate requests to CMHCs for timely presentations to parents and teachers. The school nurse is in a vital position to follow up such presentations with case finding, support and advice to targeted families, and reinforcement of essential principles in the school environment.

Examples of the secondary level of intervention offered by a CMHC include short-term hospitalization of a suicidal adolescent or outpatient treatment for a depressed, recently widowed man. These interventions attempt to halt or impede further deterioration in identified or diagnosed cases of mental illness as well as to restore the affected individual to a preillness level of functioning. The community health nurse can be an active case finder by identifying the common disturbances of mental health in clients and making appropriate referrals.

An example of a tertiary level intervention offered by a CMHC is a medication-maintenance program or an aftercare service aimed at treatment of the chronically mentally ill. Such services attempt to forestall further deterioration caused by the illness, monitor side effects of treatment that can contribute to social disability, and provide corrective experiences that foster community adjustment. Community health nurses are involved in these programs by providing medication supervision in the home and making periodic home visits to evaluate community adjustment. The community health nurse becomes the eyes and ears of the mental health treatment team and is a source of data which cannot be gathered effectively in CMHC settings.

Rehabilitation Models

Rehabilitation models are best classified according to the living, learning, and work environments schema (Anthony, 1979). Rehabilitation is distinguished from treatment in that its focus is social disability, not the illness itself. The intended outcome of a rehabilitation intervention is improved social competence or a changed environment.

Living Models

Social clubs, companion programs, alternative residence programs, and community drop-in centers are all aimed at improving emotional, intellectual, and physical skills that are adaptive in living environments. Such programs are generally considered to be tertiary prevention in that they attempt to interrupt or correct the deterioration caused by a known, treated illness. CMHC staff might serve as consultants to these programs, but they are often found objectionable by rehabilitation staff on the grounds that mental health professionals are too illness oriented. Although community health nurses have not had an important role in such programs, the potential for role development exists. Community health nurses might be more acceptable consultants to these programs than mental health professionals, given their orientation toward health teaching and promotion. A social club, for example, might invite a community health nurse to present an educational program on general hygiene, nutritional concerns, or community health resources. A foster placement family that is providing a home for a mentally ill adult might be more open to home visiting by the community health nurse than by a member of the mental health team. The focus of the nurses might be more acceptable consultants to these programs than mental health advice, and refer when necessary. There is no stigma attached to a visit by the local community health nursing agency, whereas a visit by the local CMHC could be highly stigmatizing.

Learning Models

Learning models rely on cognitive (educational) techniques to develop skills necessary for problem solving. Mental health learning programs may involve secondary prevention, as in the case of a long-term inpatient psychiatric service for adolescents that runs its own school; or tertiary prevention, such as special adult education courses offered at a local high school and designed to serve the learning needs of a chronic psychiatric population. This model has been used successfully with the chronically mentally ill to teach personal growth techniques and foster interpersonal skill (Lamb, 1976). Direct involvement of a community health nursing agency in such programs would be inappropriate, since the

programs are designed to address learning needs and create an atmosphere of normalcy. However, the community health nurse might be a guest lecturer in class or be available to the instructor for consultation as needed.

Work Models

Vocational rehabilitation is the cornerstone upon which psychiatric work rehabilitation programs are built. Work programs range from sheltered workshop opportunities to specialized counseling that facilitates job placement. Vocational rehabilitation can be either a secondary or a tertiary intervention, depending on when in the illness trajectory it is initiated. The occupational health nurse is likely to encounter the psychiatrically disabled person in the workplace. Many industrial organizations have special programs for alcohol and substance abusers. Sheltered workshops may employ community health nurses to provide necessary on-site health coverage. The psychiatrically disabled worker will present special problems for the community health nurse in the work setting. The illness may cause impaired movement, slowed thinking, and, worst of all, serious social disabilities that may interfere with normal employee relationships. If an employee is taking certain phenothiazines, work with dangerous machinery is prohibited. The occupational health nurse in the work setting may serve as an employee advocate or an informal counselor and may mean the difference between a successful and an aborted work attempt for the distressed psychiatric client.

Family Models

The family has been the major unit of care of the community health nurse for decades. Families of mentally ill individuals are perhaps more in need of community health nursing services than any other population, yet they are the least understood and the most underserved. Families of the mentally ill (particularly the chronically mentally ill) suffer from the stigma associated with the illness and from the etiologic theories that implicate family pathology as a major cause of mental illness.

Recent research has shown that family members are at greater risk for reactive depression and anxiety when they care for a mentally ill relative at home (Creer & Wing, 1975; Doll, 1976). In addition, such families suffer economic burdens and social rejection.

Research has also clarified the role family members have in exacerbating the psychiatric illness of a relative. Mentally ill people who live with families known to be high in expressed emotion (EE) are at greater risk for psychiatric relapse than those who live with families low in expressed emotion. *Expressed emotion* is defined as spontaneous negativity toward the ill relative and pervasive intrusiveness on the part of the high-EE family members (Brown et al., 1978). It has been found that psychiatric medications and decreased face-to-face contact with the negative relatives can reduce the risk of relapse. It has been estimated that 65 percent of discharged psychiatric clients return to their families (Goldman, 1982). Recent innovative family treatment models have been designed to reduce the risk of relapse to the mentally ill relative, reduce the incidence of reactive depression and anxiety in family members, and enable the family to remain intact in the community.

Family Surveillance

Family surveillance is a public health, not a mental health, concept defined as a "sys-tematic, continuing watch for illness, for health threatening or diminishing conditions affecting individuals, families, or population groups" (Freeman & Heinrich, 1981, p. 101). Family surveillance involves: (1) early discovery, contributing to early treatment of disease; (2) the identification and correction of health-threatening behavior; (3) supporting the family in health tasks; and (4) broadening and enriching the data base. This intervention is designed to be employed at all three levels of prevention and can be readily applied by the community health nurse to any population, including a mentally ill population. Some families of the mentally ill may require monthly or less frequent visits for the sole purpose of surveillance to make sure that the family is coping adequately with the problems associated with the illness.

Support Groups

A variety of models have been developed recently to address the needs of families living with chronically mentally ill relatives (Beels et al., 1982; Goldman, 1982; McLean et al., 1982). Parents' groups, relatives' groups, and family workshops are all examples of the new support models that combine social support with education about the illness, expression of emotion, and management of troublesome behavior. Some groups are designed just for the relatives, while others include the person identified as having a problem. All of them employ means of social support by holding their meetings in family members' homes or in community meeting places and by including families that have coped with illness in the past. Families learn that they are not alone or unique in their difficulties and benefit from helping others solve problems. Individuals high in expressed emotion can be positively influenced by those low in expressed emotion and can use the support groups to discharge negative feelings. Health professionals provide consultation to the groups and conduct educational sessions on such topics as medication, management of troublesome symptoms, expressed emotion, and community resources.

The potential role for a community health nurse in such support groups is great. The nurse is already familiar with the community and has home visiting skills. Health teaching is a normal role for the community health nurse, whereas mental health professionals need to be trained in health education techniques. A community health nurse might initiate such support activities in collaboration with a mental health nurse from the local CMHC and could employ mental health professionals to teach about technical subjects, such as medications. The community health nurse, being little inclined to interpret or manipulate group phenomena, might facilitate the self-care aspects of support groups. As more and more clients are discharged to the community after only brief inpatient psychiatric hospitalizations, family support models will become central to the community management of the mentally ill.

FUTURE IMPLICATIONS

Three major concepts guide the delivery of mental health services in community settings: (1) least restrictiveness, (2) social control, and (3) social networking. These concepts, which have grown up in the deinstitutionalization era, are directed to the needs of the individual as well as the community. They are likely to guide community mental health innovations for the next several decades.

Least Restrictiveness

The concept of restrictiveness was a direct result of the work of Goffman (1961), who, in his book *Asylums*, identified large public mental health institutions as "total institutions" that provided little in the way of real treatment. One of the results of deinstitutionalization was acknowledgment of clients' rights to receive treatment in the least restrictive environment possible. The degree of restrictiveness of an environment is the extent to which the resident is free to function independently. The more restricted a setting, the more likely it is that others will attend to a client's needs and that civil rights will be protected. The less restrictive the setting, the more it is assumed that the individual is capable of attending to such matters unassisted. Thus the psychiatrically disabled individual living at home is at greater risk of violation of civil rights than the one living in a total institution and is more in need of community health and mental health services designed to minimize disability and maximize social competence. Krauss and Slavinsky (1982) suggest that there are seven categories of restrictiveness:

1. Total institutions (inpatient settings).
2. Nearly total institutions (nursing homes).
3. Institutions where residents are partially independent (halfway houses, foster placement programs).
4. Institutions where residents are independent but isolated (room-and-board facilities, YMCAs, single-room occupancy hotels).
5. Family of origin (parents and siblings).
6. Friends or more distant relatives.
7. Family of orientation (client, spouse, and/or children).

Current and developing treatment innovations concentrate on the least restrictive settings as the best location for most mentally ill people. The further removed treatment is from traditional mental health institutions, the more likely it is that community health disciplines will need to be involved in delivery of services.

Social Control

Social control is a sociological concept defined as the influencing of human behavior to maintain social order. Sociologists debate the sources of influence used to control behavior, but in general social control is exercised through tradition, social norms, moral rules, laws, role expectations, sanctions, ceremonies, and belief structures (Wilson, 1982).

People with certain psychiatric disorders can upset the social order around them by behaving in socially unacceptable or deviant ways. The total institution was one way of exercising social control over a population viewed as disruptive of social order. In inpatient facilities (and some less restrictive institutions), social control is achieved through the distinction between staff and client roles, therapeutic community rules, the gradual earning of status and responsibility, use of medication, locked and unlocked wards, restraint and seclusion, and a specific schedule of activities.

One of the outcomes of deinstitutionalization was to decrease the use of total institutions for the purpose of social control. As increasing numbers of the chronically mentally ill people remain in or reenter the community, social control will become a pressing concern of the community members.

Wilson (1982) has suggested that a new form of social control may emerge in noninstitutional, less restrictive settings that serve the needs of the seriously mentally ill. The presence of known and trusted others, fair and equal distribution of work, and limiting the intrusion of strangers are three ways that less restrictive, noninstitutional settings exercise social control. Community-based care of the chronically mentally ill requires the exercise of social control within less restrictive environments and therefore demands a wider range of interventions that will assist individual clients in the control of their own behavior, protect them from the unnecessary intrusion of others into their lives, and protect families and the community from potentially harmful consequences of out-of-control behavior.

Social Networking

Social networking is the process of identifying both professional and natural helping resources in the community that can be coordinated to deliver comprehensive and continuous care to the chronically mentally ill. Sarason and Lorentz (1979) suggest that networking involves an open exchange of resources (not just money) that results in increased availability of resources to everyone. Organizations can engage in networking by pooling staff or sharing services. The liaison nurse who facilitates referrals between a state hospital and a public health nursing agency is an example of organizational networking.

Social networking is one way of managing the problems of social control that can result when the seriously mentally ill are treated in community settings. Pooling and coordination of resources ensures that clients and services will not fall through the cracks left by deinstitutionalization. If essential services are provided in a coordinated and comprehensive fashion, it is less likely that the behavior of individual clients will get out of control. Similarly, social networking ensures that clients will receive essential care in the least restrictive setting by providing a framework through which services can be coordinated and delivered in a decentralized system.

Alternative Systems of Care

Diers (1981) suggests that care is not delivered in a vacuum but rather reflects the attitudes and values of the institution within which the care takes place, as well as the overall culture in all its power relationships and constraints. Community health nursing takes place in a unique institution—the community. Although it is influenced by political-legal systems particular to community settings, it is free from medically dominated systems. Thus community health nursing may be more open to treatment innovations designed to focus on issues of social control and social networking in low-restriction settings.

It is possible that traditional mental health service settings (large public mental health hospitals, CMHCs, clinics) and traditional community health settings (public health and visiting nurses' agencies, departments of public health) may combine resources in the next decade and engage in organizational networking in order to better serve the needs of a growing population of mentally ill people. *Organizational networking* involves coordination of activities and exchange of information in order to maximize resources. This kind of networking involves a restructuring of traditional systems of care and arises out of a perceived scarcity of available resources (Krauss & Slavinsky, 1982).

One such network, described by Freeman et al. (1980), involved 29 separate treatment and rehabilitation agencies. These agencies formed an umbrella agency, Community Resources Consultants, whose purpose was to improve aftercare services for the mentally ill by coordinating existing resources and recommending the creation of new services to fill in existing gaps in care. This networking experiment reduced the amount of time individual caregivers spent gathering treatment resource data and making referrals and improved their working knowledge of all the treatment resources in the community. An important feature of this innovative approach to coordination of care was its relatively low cost. Existing systems of care simply pooled resources. With the money saved by resource pooling, they funded a low-cost system for coordination and evaluation of care.

Some communities employ the liaison nurse to coordinate mental health and community health care. The liaison nurse communicates discharge plans to the proper treatment agencies in the community in order to facilitate the client's transition to a less restricted environment. Although this role is not a new one, it is still not widely accepted in all parts of the country. It could be augmented if funding resources for the position were shared by each of the agencies that benefited and if the role were expanded to include identification of service gaps and coordination of efforts to create new resources. The liaison nurse could have either a public health or a mental health background, since the predominant skills necessary for the role involve interagency communication and community assessment.

In the 1980s it is clear that the problems of deinstitutionalization and the challenges of community mental health are legion and will require the talents of nurses prepared in mental health and community health. Undeniably, community health nurses were central to many innovative nursing projects that began in the 1960s and spanned a decade or more. Linda Aiken (1981) has suggested that the 1980s offer the promise of exciting contributions by nurses to the nation's health and health care system. She also points out that at the same time that nursing is coming of age, innovations in health care are becoming increasingly constrained by economic factors. Health innovations of any kind will have to either demonstrate greater cost effectiveness than existing systems or meet health needs serious enough to warrant additional expenditure.

Most nursing innovations are now taking place in community settings. Hospital innovations involve discharge planning and meeting the transitional clients' needs. Wherever we turn, we find a role for the community health nurse in the delivery of community mental health services. It would be a waste of resources to train clinical specialists in mental health to enter the community and manage at-home care of the mentally ill and their families when we already have a group of professionals prepared to do just that. It may be fortuitous that fiscal constraints will force nurses to turn to each other and begin to develop a nursing network that will extend from the most to the least restrictive treatment settings. The community health nurse is located on the boundary between traditional health care institutions and the community. It is at that boundary that new systems of care will be created. As a specialist in community care and a generalist in health care, the community health nurse is uniquely equipped to meet the mental health challenges of the eighties.

SUMMARY

This chapter provided a historical review of the events leading to the community men-

tal health movement and deinstitutionalization. Concepts of mental health, mental illness, levels of prevention, and at-risk populations were defined and discussed, as were common disturbances of mental health. Current and future community-based models of mental health care were presented within the framework of social control, social networking, and restrictiveness of care; and the current and potential role of the community health nurse in each of the models was examined.

DISCUSSION TOPICS

1. Monty Rosen is a 16-year-old with a history of attempting suicide. The last time he tried to slash his wrists, the family physician refused to see him in the emergency room and said, "Monty's just trying to get attention." You have been asked to visit Monty because he has diabetes. The disease is frequently out of control because of his own failure to manage it properly.

a. What factors in Monty's history would contribute to your assessment of his suicide risk?

b. How would you respond to Monty in the most therapeutic way in order to decrease the possibility of a successful suicide attempt?

c. How are Monty's suicide attempts and his lack of control over his diabetes related?

d. How might you use support groups to help Monty?

2. Describe a network of professionals in the community where you live and work that could promote mental health in people who are not already having problems with their mental health.

3. In what ways might both professional and natural helping networks be developed

and utilized in the community to benefit the chronically mentally ill?

4. How might total institutions be used in the next century?

5. How might the common disturbances of mental health be different in the first part of the next century?

BIBLIOGRAPHY

Aiken, L.H., ed.: *Health policy and nursing practice.* New York: McGraw-Hill, 1981.

Anthony, W.: *The principles of psychiatric rehabilitation.* Amherst, Mass.: Human Resource Development Press, 1979.

Arafeh, M., et al.: Linking hospital and community care for psychiatric patients. *American Journal of Nursing* 68, 1050, 1968.

Armstrong, B.: St. Elizabeth's Hospital: Case study of a court order. *Hospital and Community Psychiatry* 30, 42, 1979.

Arnhoff, F.: Social consequences of policy toward mental illness. *Science* 188, 1277, 1975.

Becker, A., & Schulberg, H.: Phasing out state hospitals—A psychiatric dilemma. *New England Journal of Medicine* 294, 255, 1976.

Beels, C., et al.: Family treatments of schizophrenia: Background and state of the art. *Hospital and Community Psychiatry* 33, 541, 1982.

Braginsky, B., et al.: *Methods of madness: The mental hospital as a last resort.* New York: Holt, Rinehart and Winston, 1969.

Brown, G., et al.: Life events and psychiatric disorders. Part I: Some methodological issues; Part II: Nature of the causal link. *Psychological Medicine* 3, 74; 3, 159, 1973.

Brown, G., et al.: Influence of family life on the course of schizophrenic disorders: A replication. *British Journal of Psychiatry* 121, 241, 1978.

Caplan, G.: *Support systems and community mental health.* New York: Human Sciences Press, 1974.

Crane, G.: Clinical psychopharmacology in its 20th year. *Science* 181, 124, 1973.

Creer, C., & Wing, J.: Living with a schizophrenic patient. *British Journal of Hospital Medicine* 16, 73, 1975.

Davidson, S.V.: The assessment of alcoholism. *Family and Community Health,* 2, 1, 1979.

Davis, A., et al.: *Schizophrenics in the new custodial community.* Columbus, Ohio: Ohio State University Press, 1974.

Diers, D.K.: Nurse-midwifery as a system of care: Provider process and patient outcome. In L.H. Aiken, ed., *Health policy and nursing practice.* New York: McGraw-Hill, 1981.

Doll, W.: Family coping with the mentally ill: An unanticipated problem of deinstitutionalization. *Hospital and Community Psychiatry* 27, 183, 1976.

Dubos, R.: *Man adapting.* New Haven: Yale University Press, 1965.

Dunn, H.L.: *High level wellness.* Arlington, Va.: Beatty, 1961.

Erikson, E.: *Childhood and society* (2nd ed.). New York: Norton, 1963.

Farberow, N., & Shneidman, E.: *The cry for help.* New York: McGraw-Hill, 1961.

Freeman, R., & Heinrich, J.: *Community health nursing practice* (2nd ed.). Philadelphia: Saunders, 1981.

Freeman, S., et al.: An agency model for developing and coordinating psychiatric aftercare. *Hospital and Community Psychiatry* 31, 768, 1980.

Gelber, I.: *Released mental patients on tranquilizing drugs and the public health nurse.* New York: New York University Press, 1959.

Goffman, E.: *Asylums.* New York: Doubleday, 1961.

Goldberg, S., et al.: Prediction of relapse in schizophrenic outpatients treated by drug and sociotherapy. *Archives of General Psychiatry* 34, 171, 1977.

Goldman, H.H.: Mental illness and family burden: A public health perspective. *Hospital and Community Psychiatry* 33, 557, 1982.

Greenblatt, M., & Glazier, E.: The phasing out of

mental hospitals in the United States. *American Journal of Psychiatry* 132, 1135, 1975.

Jimerson, S.S.: Anxiety. In J. Haber, et al. eds., *Comprehensive psychiatric nursing.* New York: McGraw-Hill, 1982.

Klerman, G.: Better but not well: Social and ethical issues in the deinstitutionalization of the mentally ill. *Schizophrenia Bulletin* 3, 617, 1977.

Krauss, J.B., & Slavinsky, A.T.: *The chronically ill psychiatric patient and the community.* Boston: Blackwell, 1982.

Laing, R.: *The politics of experience.* New York: Pantheon, 1967.

Lamb, H.: *Community survival for longterm patients.* San Francisco: Jossey/Bass, 1976.

Levinson, D.: *The seasons of a man's life.* New York: Knopf, 1978.

McClean, L.J.: Guilt and fear of self-destruction. In J. Haber, et al. eds., *Comprehensive psychiatric nursing.* New York: McGraw-Hill, 1982.

McLean, C.S., et al.: Group treatment for parents of the adult mentally ill. *Hospital and Community Psychiatry* 33, 564, 1982.

Mereness, D.: The potential significant role of the nurse in community mental health services. *Perspectives in Psychiatric Care* 1, 34, 1963.

Offer, D., & Sabshin, M.: *Normality.* New York: Basic Books, 1974.

Ozarin, L., & Sharfstein, S.: The aftermaths of deinstitutionalization: Problems and solutions. *Psychiatric Quarterly* 50, 128, 1978.

Pasamansick, B., et al.: *Schizophrenics in the community: An experimental study in the prevention of hospitalization.* New York: Appleton-Century-Crofts, 1967.

Paykel, E., et al.: Life events and depression: A controlled study. *Archives of General Psychiatry* 21, 753, 1969.

Paykel, E., et al.: Dimensions of social adjustment in depressed women. *Journal of Nervous and Mental Diseases* 152, 158, 1971.

Peplau, H.E.: *Interpersonal relations in nursing.* New York: Putnam, 1952.

Peplau, H.E.: A working definition of anxiety. In S.F. Burd & M.A. Marshall, eds., *Some clinical approaches to psychiatric nursing.* New York: Macmillan, 1963.

President's Commission on Mental Health. *Task panel reports (Vol. II).* Washington, D.C.: U.S. Government Printing Office, 1978.

Public Health Service, *Monthly vital statistics report, provisional statistics, annual summary for the United States, 1978.* Office of Health Research, Statistics, and Technology, National Center for Health Statistics, U.S. Department of Health, Education and Welfare, August 13, 1979.

Rachlin, S.: When schizophrenia comes marching home. *Psychiatric Quarterly* 50, 202, 1978.

Rahe, R.: Life crisis and health change. In R. May & J. Witterborn, eds., *Psychotropic drug response: Advance in prediction.* Springfield, Ill.: Thomas, 1969.

Rahe, R., et al.: Illness prediction studies. *Archives of Environmental Health* 25, 192, 1972.

Ramshorn, M.T., & Pearlmutter, D.R.: Social, cultural, and historical aspects of mental health. In J. Haber, et al. eds., *Comprehensive psychiatric nursing.* New York: McGraw-Hill, 1982.

Reich, R., & Seigal, L.: The emergence of the Bowery as a psychiatric dumping ground. *Psychiatric Quarterly* 50(3), 191–201, 1978.

Rogers, M.: *An Introduction to the theoretical basis of nursing.* Philadelphia: F.A. Davis, 1970.

Sarason, S., & Lorentz, E.: *The challenge of the resource network.* San Francisco: Jossey/Bass, 1979.

Sheehey, G.: *Passages.* New York: Dutton, 1976.

Shneidman, E.: *Voices of death.* New York: Harper & Row, 1980.

Sideleau, B.F.: Abusive families. In J. Haber et al. eds., *Comprehensive Psychiatric Nursing.* New York: McGraw-Hill, 1982.

Slavinsky, A., et al.: Back to the community: A dubious blessing. *Nursing Outlook* 24, 370, 1976.

Sullivan, H.S.: The meaning of anxiety in psychiatry and life. *Psychiatry* 11, 1, 1948.

Swanson, A.R.: Depression. In J. Haber et al. eds., *Comprehensive psychiatric nursing.* New York: McGraw-Hill, 1982.

Szasz, T.: *The myth of mental illness.* New York: Hoeber-Harper, 1964.

Talbott, J.A.: Deinstitutionalization: Avoiding the disasters of the past. *Hospital and Community Psychiatry* 30, 621, 1979.

Vance, E.: Social disability. *American Psychology* 28, 498–511, 1973.

Wekstein, L.: *Handbook of suicidology: Principles, problems and practice.* New York: Brunner/Mazel, 1979.

Wilson, H.S.: *Deinstitutionalized residential care for the mentally disordered.* New York: Grune & Stratton, 1982.

Wolff, I.: The psychiatric nurse in community mental health—a rebuttal. *Perspectives in Psychiatric Care* 2, 11, 1964.

Zamora, L.C.: Anger. in J. Haber et al. eds., *Comprehensive psychiatric nursing.* New York: McGraw-Hill, 1982.

22

Crisis: Danger and Opportunity

Victoria Schoolcraft

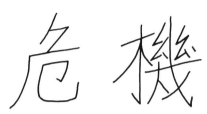

OBJECTIVES

After reading this chapter, you should be able to:

- [ ] Define crisis and stress.
- [ ] Discuss the relationship between stress and crisis.
- [ ] Describe the six classes of crises and give an example of each.
- [ ] Describe the process of crisis development and resolution.
- [ ] Discuss the relationship between loss and crisis.
- [ ] Discuss the meaning of vulnerability in crisis.
- [ ] Describe strategies for crisis prevention.
- [ ] Describe the steps in crisis intervention.
- [ ] Describe the assessment of suicide potential.
- [ ] Describe strategies for intervening in each class of crisis.
- [ ] Discuss the implications of future societal trends for prevention of and intervention in crisis.

The Chinese word at the beginning of the chapter represents "crisis" and is a combination of the characters for "danger" and "opportunity." It was drawn by Keen Ming Ling, RN, BSN.

INTRODUCTION

The two theorists responsible for describing the phenomenon of crisis are Erich Lin-

391

demann and Gerald Caplan. Lindemann's first significant contribution came in 1944, when he presented his findings on the symptomatology and management of acute grief (Lindemann, 1944). He became aware of the frequent need for intervention with essentially normal people who were experiencing significant loss. Gerald Caplan elaborated these concepts and developed a model for crisis intervention that serves as the basis for this important aspect of preventive mental health (Caplan, 1951, 1961, 1964).

In the late 1950s and early 1960s, numerous programs were started to provide community mental health services. At first, each tended to be single focus, such as day hospitals for part-time psychiatric care. Gradually, the services provided became more comprehensive and included a number of services for people without diagnosed psychiatric illnesses.

By the late 1960s, some of the principal services for mental health promotion were crisis hotlines and walk-in crisis centers which were provided especially for young people. This was the era of the hippie counterculture, when many young people left their families to live in communes, on the streets, or to roam about the country. Many experimented with drugs, especially hallucinogenics. Most of these adolescents felt alienated and had no sense of meaning in their lives. These problems were magnified by the usual disruptions of adolescence. Their needs were best served by nonauthoritarian, no-hassle resources such as free clinics and crash pads (places where youths could stay and sleep for a short time).

Out of many of the resources originally established for youth grew ongoing crisis hotlines and walk-in clinics for anyone who felt the need for them, regardless of age. Although there are still some specialized crisis resources for such people as rape vic-

tims or victims of abuse, the generalized crisis hotline, available 24 hours a day, 365 days a year, has remained.

Even though techniques of crisis intervention were developed by professionals in psychiatry and mental health, the model for intervention can be taught to nonprofessionals. In fact, many crisis lines can be kept open only through the efforts of volunteers trained and supervised by professionals. Even though there have been some problems with using volunteers, the majority of programs have successfully assisted many people in crisis. These volunteers have prevented suicide, promoted comfort, assisted in problem solving, and referred people for professional counseling.

Another trend in crisis care has been teaching people who are not in psychiatry or mental health to recognize and intervene in crises. Crisis theory is now a common component of programs for physicians, nurses, teachers, clergy, police officers, firefighters, and other people who frequently come into contact with those who are under stress or are in crisis. These people are often in the position to prevent or mitigate a crisis.

Future shock occurs when an individual feels stressed and disoriented when experiencing too much change in too short a time (Toffler, 1971, p. 2). With personal and societal change occurring so rapidly, future shock is becoming a common phenomenon. This reaction is becoming a frequently identified stressor that leads to crisis development. The burgeoning number of best-selling future-oriented books attests to the fact that people are interested in and concerned about the future. They are attempting to foresee and prepare for changes so as not to become overwhelmed. However, there are still a majority of people who do not perceive the value of planning and prevention.

Nurses are in a position to foster the advent of community-wide efforts at preventing all kinds of crises, including those brought on by future shock. A basic knowledge of crisis theory will greatly help nurses in the community make a worthwhile contribution to their fellow citizens.

DEFINITION AND CLASSIFICATION

Definition

The word "crisis" has its root in the Greek word *krinein,* which means "to decide." Crisis is indeed related to making decisions and to solving problems. Caplan (1964, p. 39) defines *crisis* as a situation in which a person is unable to cope with an interruption in the meeting of "interpersonal needs" in his or her usual manner. Crisis is characterized by feelings of tension and helplessness.

Stress and crisis are significantly related but they are not the same thing. *Stress* is "the nonspecific physiological response of an organism to any demand made upon it" (Selye, 1955, p. vii). Stress is the response of the individual to *stressors,* which are the causative agents. Stressors may be physical, psychological, or social. Stress may persist for a period of time, taking a toll on the individual, but without necessarily causing a crisis. On the other hand, some stressors result in crisis for a given individual because they are perceived as hazardous. Therefore, stress does not always result in a crisis, nor does any given stressor necessarily cause crisis to occur.

Generally, stress is considered to be an undesirable occurrence that has short-term or long-term negative consequences for the individual. Crisis is not necessarily a negative experience, because it may lead to a higher level of functioning.

The Chinese character at the beginning of the chapter represents the word "crisis" and is a combination of the characters for "danger" and "opportunity." The potential danger in a crisis is that the individual may choose destructive mechanisms to cope with or relieve anxiety. The individual may become so disorganized that severe psychiatric problems occur or may resolve the crisis by functioning at a lower level than before the crisis. For example, a young person attending college may experience a crisis as a result of the stress of living away from home for the first time. He may cope with the stress by dropping out of college and by avoiding further attempts to attend. In addition, he might incorporate a perception of himself as being a failure because of the incident and thus make future decisions based on this negative view of himself.

A person in crisis may also resolve the situation in a way that is clearly growth producing and positive. A person often learns new skills by working through a crisis, and these skills increase that person's repertoire of skills for dealing with future stresses. For example, the first child of a couple dies unexpectedly in infancy. The man and woman may learn through their grief to deal constructively with their feelings of anger, guilt, and helplessness. As a result, they may be willing to risk having other children, either biologically or by adoption. In addition, they can provide support to other people who experience the same tragedy. This is an example of an opportunity presented by a crisis.

Classification of Crises

Baldwin has provided a classification system to help in identifying the relative seriousness of crises (Baldwin, 1981c). This is a significant contribution to crisis theory because it helps determine the kind of intervention that is appropriate. Table 22.1 pro-

TABLE 22.1

TABLE 22.1
Classification of Crises and Nature of Interventions

Crises	Precipitant Events	Nature of Intervention
Class 1 Dispositional crises	Situation problematic to the individual (e.g., child rearing, environmental disruption, transient impotence, alcoholic family member).	Provide information or education; make referrals to specific agencies or professionals; apply administrative leverage to situation.
Class 2 Crises of anticipated life transitions	Normal life situations over which client has inadequate control (e.g., change in role status, including leaving home, marriage, divorce, parenthood, maternal–child separation, infertility, school or college entry or completion, return to work force, career change, retirement; change in body image, including chronic illness, disfigurement, weight change).	Help client to develop understanding of the changes and their impact; discuss the emotional impact on client; provide anticipatory guidance to plan adaptive responses to problems.
Class 3 Crises resulting from sudden traumatic stress	Strong, externally imposed stresses or traumatic situations that cause sudden, unexpected disruption (e.g., death of significant other, job loss, diagnosis of terminal illness, disaster, war or combat, rape, assault, murder).	Provide or mobilize support initially; help client acknowledge need for assistance; help client recognize and express negative emotions about the situation; provide anticipatory guidance.
Class 4 Maturational/ developmental crises	Inability to resolve attempts to attain emotional maturity (e.g., dependency, value conflicts, sexual identity, emotional intimacy, power issues, self-discipline).	Help client identify and understand the underlying and unresolved developmental issue; help client respond more adaptively; help client cope with the underlying problem.
Class 5 Crises resulting from psychopathology	Unresolved problems rather than stressor per se (e.g., borderline personality disorder, severe neurosis, characterologi-	Respond primarily to present problem; emphasize problem-solving skills and environmental manipulation; avoid producing or reinforcing client dependency or regression; acknowl-

TABLE 22.1 (continued)		
Crises	*Precipitant Events*	*Nature of Intervention*
	cal problem, psychosis, multiproblem family).	edge deeper problems but do not attempt to resolve them; stabilize client functioning; after crisis is resolved, refer client for therapy.
Class 6 Psychiatric emergencies	Acute disorganization or impairment of functioning, sometimes with physiological as well as psychological disruptions (e.g., drug or alcohol intoxication; impulse-control problems, including suicidal or homicidal impulses; acute psychosis).	Assess client's psychological and physical condition quickly and accurately; clarify precipitating situation; mobilize all resources necessary to help client; arrange for follow-up or coordination of services.

SOURCE: Baldwin, B.A.: Crisis intervention: An overview of theory and practice. In A.W. Burgess & B.A. Baldwin, eds., *Crisis intervention: Theory and practice*. Englewood Cliffs, N.J.: Prentice-Hall, 1981, pp. 35–40.

vides examples of precipitating events and describes interventions for each class. The crises increase in severity from Class 1 to Class 6.

Dispositional crises (Class 1) result from problematic situations that are distressing to the individual but are sharply defined and cause minimal disruption. They are responsive to educational, informational, and administrative intervention. Examples of dispositional crises are a person disturbed by noisy neighbors, an adolescent who is fearful about physical changes, or a parent with child-discipline problems.

Class 2 is constituted of crises of anticipated life transitions. These crises are caused by anticipated but normal life transitions and may occur before, during, or after the transition. These transitions usually include a change in role status or body image or both. Some examples are leaving home, parenthood, and retirement.

Class 3 is comprised of crises resulting from sudden traumatic stress. Strong, unexpected, externally imposed stresses or events cause these crises. Examples are rape, sudden death of a significant other, or a disaster such as a fire or flood.

Maturational or developmental crises (Class 4) result from attempts to deal with interpersonal situations that are determined by deep, unresolved developmental issues related to the attainment of emotional maturity. Examples include dependency, sexual identity, and emotional intimacy.

Class 5 includes crises resulting from psychopathology. These crises are precipitated or intensified by preexisting psychopathology. The apparent stressor is less important to the development of the crisis than are the client's unresolved problems. For example, the event that preceded the crisis might be typical of another crisis class, such as a life transition. However, the degree of disorganization or dysfunction is greater because of the client's severe neurosis or character disorder.

Finally, Class 6 is psychiatric emergencies. People in these crises are severely impaired in their functioning and are incapable of assuming responsibility for themselves. These crises may be related to intended or unintended intoxication by drugs or alcohol. They frequently involve problems with impulse control, such as suicidal or homicidal attempts. Like Class 5 crises, Class 6 crises may be a severe reaction to an event similar to one of those named earlier. For example, an unexpected pregnancy, or the loss of a loved one, might result in a reaction typical of Class 2 or Class 3, respectively. However, some people might become extremely disorganized and out of control, as in Class 6.

CRISIS DEVELOPMENT AND RESOLUTION

Crises are self-limiting and last from one to six weeks (Caplan, 1964). This is the period during which the individual experiences emotional disruption and is psychologically vulnerable. Since the feelings of tension and anxiety are so uncomfortable, the individual seeks to resolve the crisis. The resolution will diminish the tension, but as a result, the individual may be at a functional level equivalent to, lower than, or greater than the precrisis state.

Regardless of the level at which the crisis itself is resolved, the events or issues that precipitated it may require long-term attention. For example, a rape victim may resolve the crisis caused by the trauma within a few weeks but may continue to feel guilt or loss for months. By the same token, when a person experiences the death of a loved one, which results in a crisis, the crisis period ends in about six weeks, but the mourning period may last for a year or more.

Loss in Crisis

An important component of crisis theory is the recognition that an actual or anticipated loss is part of any crisis and that the individual must become reconciled to this loss as part of resolving the crisis (Baldwin, 1981c). The significance of the loss to the individual is a factor in his or her perception of the danger of an event. Understanding the loss the client has experienced can facilitate the nurse's assessment and intervention in a crisis and may even assist in crisis prevention.

Strickler and LaSor (1970) have identified three types of loss common to crisis situations. Loss of self-esteem occurs when an individual feels unable to maintain a sense of self-worth in social roles and relationships. Loss of sex-role mastery occurs when an individual experiences a change in a role or relationship that results in the need to perform at a new, unacceptable level (higher or lower). An individual sustains a loss of nurturing when he or she experiences a change that diminishes the amount of nurturing the individual gives or receives. It is important to note that the nurturing lost might have been given by the person in crisis. For example, a grandmother who was responsible for caring for her grandchildren while their mother worked becomes disoriented and depressed shortly after the mother quits her job and stops bringing the children to the grandmother's home on a regular basis.

Ipema (1979) identified loss of choice and loss of consent as the crucial issues in the rape experience. The victim is not only deprived of the right to select between options but also has a traumatic event forced upon her or him. (It is important to realize that men as well as women may be victims of rape.)

The loss a person feels results in a disruption in life-style and relationships. A person who experiences a loss feels vulnerable, distrustful of others, and unable to make decisions. Morris (quoted in Ipema, 1979) characterized this combination of effects as a loss of meaning. Other losses result in the individual's difficulty in finding meaning in experiences and in relationships.

The loss of control inherent in losses of choice and consent is part of the experience of a person whose crisis results from a sudden traumatic stress. For example, assaults, automobile accidents, combat experiences, and natural disasters are beyond the control of victims, who feel that the direction of their lives has been changed by the event and its aftermath.

Recognizing the significance of loss as a part of any crisis experience helps promote understanding of why particular events cause crises in some people but not in others. An event that is a real or symbolic loss to one person may not be perceived as such to another. On the other hand, some experiences are almost universally associated with loss, such as the death of a significant other. Since these events can be predicted to precipitate crises, prevention of crisis or early intervention in crisis is more likely to occur.

Those who intervene must be sensitive to the pain caused by the client's loss. The resolution and outcome phases must incorporate a certain amount of grief work, during which the individual acknowledges the loss, deals with the significance of the loss, and begins to reestablish connections with his or her social world to meet the needs that have gone unmet since the loss. Finally, whenever a person experiences a loss of any kind, it can reactivate unresolved feelings from previous losses. This factor can intensify a loss and precipitate a crisis that may seem to be an inordinant response to the stressor. The following example illustrates this:

A woman client became extremely distraught when a box of books was lost during a move. The books had no particular intrinsic value. In the course of trying to ascertain why this loss caused an extreme response, the nurse learned that several of the books had belonged to the woman's father, who had died a few years earlier. The woman had repressed and denied many of her feelings about her father. The books were the only things of his she had, and they represented her last symbolic tie to him.

Vulnerability in Crisis

Lindemann (1944), Caplan (1964), and Erikson (1963) have all noted the vulnerability of the person in crisis. *Vulnerability* refers to the individual's capacity to be both harmed and enriched by the experience (Erikson, 1963). Because of this vulnerability and because the intense discomfort of the crisis, the individual has a greater capacity for cognitive and affective learning (Baldwin, 1981b). The learning that occurs during a crisis state persists; therefore, the individual does increase his or her skills for dealing with future stressful events.

The vulnerability of people in crisis is what makes them need to trust and depend on someone else. Since such people need help so badly, they may get it either in constructive or destructive ways. Well-intentioned friends may compound the problem with inappropriate or unhealthy solutions. Other people may try to exploit those in crisis. For example, Ms. Politz's aunt demanded that Ms. Politz buy a very expensive dress for her mother to be buried in, even though there were many dresses in the mother's wardrobe that would have been suitable. On the other hand, an unscrupulous real estate dealer pressured her to sell her mother's home at a loss. He assured Ms. Politz that this would help her to deal with the grief by "getting rid of this painful reminder." Fortunately, the person in crisis is equally amenable to appropriate interventions. One can help an individual in crisis by being somewhat directive and helping the individual make appropriate decisions or put off decisions that can be delayed. The importance of this will be discussed further in the section on crisis intervention.

Because the person in crisis is so amenable to outside influence, a very small amount of activity can result in a remarkable degree of response: "A little help, rationally directed and purposefully focused at a strategic time is more effective than more extensive help given at a period of less emotional accessibility" (Rapoport, 1965, p. 30). This principle accounts for some of the opportunity a crisis presents: the individual has the chance to grow and change much more rapidly than at other times. Even though the experience as a whole may be painful, the eventual outcome can be beneficial.

Phases of Crisis

Every theorist has observed that crises proceed in an identifiable sequence of phases (Aguilera & Messick, 1982; Baldwin, 1981c; Caplan, 1964). Figure 22.1 illustrates the process.

Precipitation Phase

The first phase is the *precipitation phase*. In this phase, the individual experiences an event that is perceived as hazardous. It is important to note the role of perception in this process. Some events may seem hazardous to one person and not to another. It is also possible for a given event to be seen as hazardous to a person at one time but not at another time. In addition, some stresses, such as sudden trauma, are perceived as hazardous by almost anyone. When an individual perceives an event as hazardous, he or she attempts to respond. If the person's ability to respond is hampered by inadequate internal resources, problem-solving and coping skills, and external resources, perceptions of the event and particularly of its meaning become even more distorted.

Crisis Phase

The *crisis phase* is the period within which the individual experiences tension, disorientation, and helplessness. The severity of this part of the process depends on the classification of the crisis (Class 1 crises are the least severe, and Class 6 crises are the most severe). This phase lasts from a few days to a few weeks—until the individual becomes uncomfortable enough to attempt resolution.

Resolution Phase

When the tension and other discomforts become intolerable, the individual begins the *resolution phase*, during which the individual makes efforts to resolve the crisis, whether healthy or unhealthy. Healthy attempts include seeking help, clarifying and changing perceptions of the hazardous event, identifying the problem, learning new skills for solving problems and coping, and mobilizing previously untapped internal and external resources. These efforts lead to a considerable decrease in discomfort.

Unhealthy attempts at resolution include not seeking help or getting inadequate help, further distorting the hazardous event, fail-

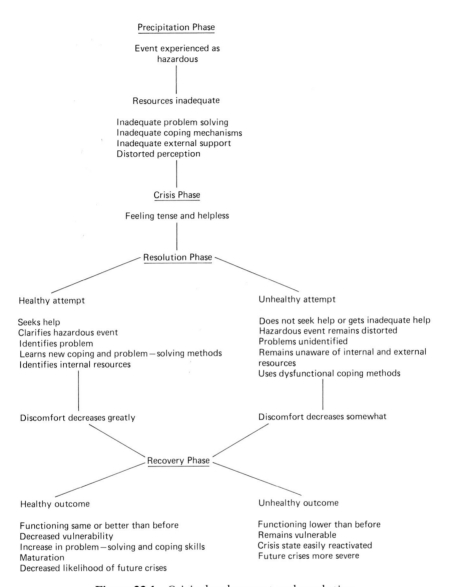

Precipitation Phase

Event experienced as
hazardous

Resources inadequate

Inadequate problem solving
Inadequate coping mechanisms
Inadequate external support
Distorted perception

Crisis Phase

Feeling tense and helpless

Resolution Phase

Healthy attempt

Seeks help
Clarifies hazardous event
Identifies problem
Learns new coping and problem—solving methods
Identifies internal resources

Discomfort decreases greatly

Unhealthy attempt

Does not seek help or gets inadequate help
Hazardous event remains distorted
Problems unidentified
Remains unaware of internal and external resources
Uses dysfunctional coping methods

Discomfort decreases somewhat

Recovery Phase

Healthy outcome

Functioning same or better than before
Decreased vulnerability
Increase in problem—solving and coping skills
Maturation
Decreased likelihood of future crises

Unhealthy outcome

Functioning lower than before
Remains vulnerable
Crisis state easily reactivated
Future crises more severe

Figure 22.1 Crisis development and resolution.

ing to identify the problem, remaining unaware of internal and external resources, using dysfunctional problem-solving or coping methods (e.g., denial, avoidance, projection, repression). Even unhealthy efforts lead to resolution, but the decrease in discomfort is not as great. The individual may continue to feel somewhat anxious or depressed.

Recovery Phase

The *recovery phase* is the postcrisis period. Whether or not this part of the process has a healthy or unhealthy outcome is determined by the nature of the resolution: a healthy resolution leads to a healthy outcome; an unhealthy resolution leads to an unhealthy outcome.

A healthy outcome is characterized by the individual's functioning at the same or a higher level than before the crisis. In addition, the individual is less vulnerable, has learned new skills in problem solving and coping, has matured, and has a decreased likelihood of future crises.

The person who experiences an unhealthy outcome functions at a lower level than before the crisis. This person is also still vulnerable to emotional distress. A crisis state for this person can be reactivated more easily than before the crisis, and future crises are likely to be as severe or more severe than the recent crisis.

CRISIS PREVENTION

Even though crises have desirable outcomes in many instances, it is often desirable to prevent a crisis from occurring. For example, if the individual has little opportunity to get assistance, is responsible for the welfare of others, or is already attempting to cope with a crisis, it is preferable to avoid the burden of further upheaval.

Assessment of Crisis Potential

The first step in prevention is to identify life events that are stressful and that individuals might perceive as hazardous. The general categories of precipitant events are problematic situations, changes in role status or body image, sudden traumatic stress, deficits in attaining emotional maturity, preexisting personal problems aggravated by another stressor, and acute disorganiza-

tion and impairment. A number of specific examples of each are given in Table 22.1.

Another way to identify potential crisis precipitants is to determine what events might activate feelings of loss. The major kinds of loss that lead to crisis are loss of self-esteem, of sexual role mastery, of nurturing, of choice, of consent, of control, and of meaning. Contributory losses include the loss of one or more of the following: a love relationship, a job, money, health, a body part, an ability, youth, a friendship, faith, a dream, ambition, respect, a belief, sexual drive, energy, support, a hope, a goal, an ideal, physical capacity, a home, spirit, and virginity (Downey, 1983).

A final component of crisis precipitation is change. Lippitt (1973, p. 37) defines *change* as "any planned or unplanned alteration in the status quo in an organism, situation, or process." Change is a part of each of the events and losses listed above. However, change in itself may precipitate crisis: there are life events that are overtly positive and may be highly desirable and energetically sought but that nevertheless include an element of loss. For example, even though a couple is enthusiastic about their new marriage, they may still feel loss of freedom. Other changes hold a threat of loss. For example, a person who has just been promoted may fear that he or she will not live up to the requirements of the new position and thus may suffer a loss of self-esteem.

Holmes and Rahe (1967) identified several life events that necessitate readjustment and that are potentially stressful whether a given change is seen as a benefit or a loss. Many of these have already been included in the discussion, but some of the others are marital reconciliation, business readjustment, outstanding personal achievement, revision of personal habits, vacation, holidays, and changes in the following: health of one's self or of a family member, one's occupation, number of arguments with spouse or lover, living conditions, work hours or conditions, residence, school, recreation habits, religious activities, social activities, sleeping or eating habits, and number of family get togethers (Holmes & Rahe, 1967). These occurrences are not all equally important in predisposing people to stress or precipitating a crisis. Holmes and Rahe have found that such events have a cumulative effect and that many of the changes are significant only in conjunction with more disturbing events. This helps to explain why a seemingly minor occurrence may be the most immediate event before a crisis: the straw that broke the camel's back.

Continual assessment of the presence or absence of the precipitant events, losses, or changes helps to provide an ongoing indication of the susceptibility to crisis of an individual, family, group, or community. Early identification or recognition of the actual or potential event enables the nurse to promote healthy functioning.

Crisis Avoidance Interventions

Some nursing activities may be implemented with individuals or families, while others have implications for promoting healthy functioning and crisis avoidance in populations.

Interventions for Individuals and Families

EGO SUPPORT. *Ego support* includes activities aimed at reinforcing and strengthening already existing capacities in essentially healthy individuals (Cyr & Wattenberg, 1965). For example, a senior nursing student is fearful of taking his first professional position. Ego-supporting activities might include helping the student assess his nursing abilities and knowledge, emphasizing other successful work experiences, and encouraging review of nursing school content specific to the area in which he will work.

CLARIFICATION. *Clarification* is the process of bringing meaning to a confused or poorly understood situation. This includes giving an appropriate amount of accurate and timely information. For example, as young people mature, they have changing degrees of curiosity about sexual behavior. Information given in proper increments at various times helps allay fears and misunderstandings that can lead to crises.

EDUCATION. *Education* is the process of facilitating learning. This includes imparting information, but usually with the goal of fostering a certain behavior. It may include helping the individual identify and utilize community resources. For example, classes for expectant parents help them to predict normal feelings and behaviors in themselves and their children. It is usually easier to handle an unavoidable experience if a person can anticipate it, recognize what things do and do not help deal with it, and realize that it will eventually be resolved.

EMOTIONAL EXPRESSION. In many normal life situations, the emotions aroused are suppressed or repressed. The nurse can facilitate *emotional expression* by helping the individual identify his or her feelings and talk about them. The loss of a loved one is much more likely to develop into a crisis if the mourner feels that her feelings are abnormal or if she does not want to "bother" anyone with them. Similarly, a new parent may be reluctant to acknowledge his or her fears or resentments about the child.

ANTICIPATORY GUIDANCE. *Anticipatory guidance* means identifying possible future events and preparing the individual to cope with them in a healthy manner. This strategy may include ego support, clarification, emotional expression, and education. It also includes planning and organizing activities. For example, the nurse may assist a family in preparing for the arrival of an adopted child by helping them realize not only what material resources are necessary but also the emotions and situations which are predictable on a short-term as well as a long-term basis. The adoptive family must eventually decide what they will tell the child about the adoption and about the biological parents. The nurse can help them learn about issues common to parenting as well as issues specific to adoption so that they can plan how to meet these situations before they become problems.

MODIFICATION OF THE ENVIRONMENT. *Modification of the environment* refers to changing the living or working environment in such a way as to make it more facilitative of physical and emotional health (Cyr & Wattenberg, 1965). For example, a client worked for a company as a lobby attendant in the evening hours. During most of the hours she worked, no one else was on the same floor, and the entry door was unlocked. She was aware of becoming increasingly fearful of being alone in the area when virtually anyone could walk in off the street. The nurse who served as an occasional consultant to the company suggested that an electronic lock be installed and that the attendant be given a beeper activator to enable her to signal the security guard if she was in danger. The company initiated both recommendations.

FUTURE AWARENESS. *Future awareness,* which incorporates education, clarification, and anticipatory guidance, is helping individuals, families, and groups to arrive at broader views of the future. This involves helping them to learn about societal changes and trends that can affect their lives and to put their own experiences into the larger context of the community. For example, a young woman may express an interest in getting training as a card-punch operator. Although this sounds like a promising area since it is related to computers, the woman needs help in evaluating whether this field will continue to be a viable employment area throughout her working life.

Interventions for Populations

Crises can be prevented by determining what groups of people have a high risk of being affected by a stressor. Once at-risk groups are targeted, nurses can plan and implement activities to help these people bolster their strengths and mitigate their weaknesses.

CONSULTATION. *Consultation* is "a collaborative effort on the part of the consultant and the consultee which utilizes the problem-solving process for the purpose of creating change" (Torres, 1974; see Chapter 8 of this book). Nurses can indirectly prevent crises in populations by providing consultation to such groups as school systems, city councils, disaster-planning groups, industries, or virtually any group responsible for providing services to or meeting needs of large numbers of individuals. Not only may the consumers of the services potentially be at risk, the staff may be in need of preventive strategies to forestall crisis development as well.

PROGRAM PLANNING. Nurses are frequently involved in planning programs of educational, informational or supportive services. For example, a nurse might plan an educational program in a modular format for the use of public school teachers in teaching human sexuality. Other nurses have helped to establish telephone services for a variety of purposes, from helping elderly people find out about community services to providing sympathetic listeners for people with problems. Nurses serve as members of boards for mental health centers and help to plan preventive programs.

AIDING VOLUNTARY RESOURCE GROUPS. Voluntary resource groups are comprised of people who, because of a similar need or interest, organize themselves to meet their needs collectively. Although they are usually established by non-health professionals, the groups may include varied social and economic mixes of members, including health professionals who are interested in the principle focus either personally or professionally. For example, groups such as Parents Without Partners, Mothers of Twins, and ostomates' clubs provide support and information to help members cope with predictable and unpredictable situations common to their respective foci. Nurses may help plan overall programs, present educational programs, or assist in other ways to help such groups fulfill their goals. In addition, nurses do well to be aware of these resources for their clients.

FUTURE AWARENESS. Nurses can promote future awareness when working with population groups as well as with individuals. By being aware of trends in economics, society, and other areas, nurses can help service organizations prepare for changing mental health needs. The nurse can recommend and participate in developing future scenarios to be presented in educational programs for lay groups as well as for professional organizations. Being prepared for the future will enable people to cope in healthier ways with the stressors they may encounter. Some of these are discussed in the "Future Implications" section of this chapter.

CRISIS INTERVENTION

Nurses frequently encounter people who are in crisis. A nurse may make a home visit to a usually well-adjusted client and find him distressed and disoriented. A client may come to a clinic for a seemingly routine request and exhibit great distress when she starts talking with the nurse. An employee may see the nurse in an occupational setting for a small cut and in the course of the visit begin talking about his impending layoff from his job. A friend may confide in the nurse about an unwanted pregnancy. The nurse may be the most accessible helping person in the individual's environment, and the nurse must be able to respond appropriately.

The steps in crisis intervention are the same as in the nursing process. Because crisis intervention is limited by time, the steps seem to blend into each other when put into practice.

Baldwin's Assessment Model

Baldwin (1981a, p. 74) has proposed a model for assessment of crisis that integrates many previous approaches to assessment. The model includes the following components:

ASSESSMENT OF THE PRECIPITATING EVENT

1. Time and place of precipitating event.
2. Interpersonal aspects of the problem (involvement of significant others; loss component).
3. Affective response to precipitating event.
4. Client's request of the nurse.

ASSESSMENT OF PSYCHODYNAMIC ISSUES IN THE CRISIS

1. Event is directly analogous to an unresolved conflict or trauma.

2. Event activates fear of reexperiencing past conflict or trauma.

1. Examine what the client has accomplished through the use of unhealthy coping skills.
2. Define alternative, healthy coping skills.
3. Analyze risks involved in attempting healthy coping skills.

1. Usual coping behaviors.
2. Emotional style and communication skills.
3. Existing social support system.
4. Personal vulnerabilities.
5. Self-description of personality.

1. Suicide assessment.
2. Drug use.
3. Recent medical history (at least six months).
4. Recent psychiatric history.
5. Mental status (ability to function and make decisions).

Sometimes the process of assessment is therapeutic enough to begin to relieve the client significantly. For example, just by introducing the formal structure of the assessment process, the nurse indicates that help is coming. Beginning with assessment, and throughout the entire intervention process, the nurse must be direct and in charge. The client needs this approach in order to feel secure and confident that he or she is going to be helped.

The nurse must verify that the client has a problem and that he or she can solve the problem with some help. The nurse offers herself or himself as a helping person and assures the client that the nurse will either help directly or get help for the client. If the nurse has had limited experience in crisis intervention, he or she may be reluctant or unable to intervene. If this is the case, it is the nurse's responsibility to get the client appropriate service. However, the nurse who has opportunities to apply the principles of crisis intervention will find himself or herself to be competent in this area.

The nurse should establish a contract with the client specifying how long they will work together on the crisis. If this intervention takes place within the context of an ongoing relationship, the contract may be an addition to an already established agreement. For example, it may include adding some interim visits instead of seeing the client only once a month. Many interventions take only one or two contacts with the client, and the last one may be a follow-up.

Clients may be frightened about feeling so helpless and dependent. It is appropriate to reassure them that when the crisis is resolved they will no longer be in the dependent position.

Suicide Assessment

In assessing a person for suicidal potential, the nurse must ask direct and specific questions. Some clients make statements: "I'm going to shoot myself." Others are indirect: "My family would be better off if I were out of the way." Other people give coded cues, "I won't be here the next time you come." When the client in crisis has not said anything about suicide, the nurse should raise the subject. Clients in Class 1 crises seldom have a severe enough disruption to cause them to consider suicide. Before the intervention is concluded, the nurse can tell without inquiring that the person is safe. In other classes of crises, when the client is more distressed, the nurse can make a statement to the following effect: "Sometimes when people are in this much distress, they feel desperate enough to kill themselves. Have you had any feelings like that?"

When the nurse finds that a client has thought about suicide, the potential for it must be ascertained. There are three factors to assess first of all:

1. *Method.* The more *lethal* the method, the more at risk the client. For example, someone whose method is a gun, jumping from a tall building, or setting himself or herself on fire is at high risk. A person whose method is to take pills, slash the wrists, or starve is not at as great a risk because there is time for someone to intervene even after an attempt is made. Another aspect of the method is its potential for *disfigurement or disability* if the person attempts it and does not die. The more lethal examples given above also have more potential for disfiguring or disabling than the less lethal examples.

2. *Means.* If the means to carry out the method are immediately available, the person is at greater risk than someone who does not have ready access to the chosen method.

3. *Plan.* The person who has worked out a specific plan for committing suicide is more at risk than someone who has only a vague notion about how he or she would actually do it. Elements of a specific plan include time, place, means, writing notes, saying goodbye, and getting affairs in order.

Planning

Planning is part of both assessment and intervention. The nurse and client work together to resolve the crisis in a healthy manner. The nurse assists the client in identifying an appropriate and attainable outcome. Together they plan how to make use of untapped or newly developed internal and external resources to achieve the desired outcome.

During the intervention stage, the client and nurse may redefine the problem. For example, even though the most immediate stressor apparently caused the crisis, further investigation may reveal other problems. The goal of crisis intervention is to help the client resolve the immediate crisis before attempting to cope with other issues. Long-term problems or inadequate coping patterns may require attention from a professional with expertise in psychiatric nursing.

Intervention

The nature of the intervention is determined by the class of the crisis (see Table 22.1). The following sections give an example of each class of crisis and discuss the method of intervention.

Dispositional Crisis

Virginia Columbo, RN, visited a client, Joan Slater, the mother of a 5-year-old daughter, Lisa. Ms. Slater was moderately distressed because Lisa had developed a habit of throwing temper tantrums when she did not get her way. This had gone on for about a month. The tantrums were not frequent, but Ms. Slater was afraid they might become so, since she did not know how to respond. Ms. Slater had tried spanking Lisa, but this seemed to lengthen the tantrum.

Ms. Columbo determined this was a Class 1 crisis that mostly required information. She suggested a technique she had read about in a journal (Melichar, 1980). She recommended that Ms. and Mr. Slater impose a "time out" period during which Lisa would sit for two to five minutes without talking or being spoken to when she started to throw a tantrum. The parents explained to Lisa that this would be done if she failed to calm down after one warning.

Ms. Slater was relieved to have a plan for dealing with Lisa. Ms. Columbo followed up a few days later and found that the plan was effective.

In the above example, the nurse assessed the nature of the crisis, found out what methods had been attempted, and suggested a new coping skill. Since the client was experiencing minimal distress and the problem did not appear to be complicated by preexisting difficulties, the crisis quickly abated.

Crisis of Anticipated Life Transition

Shirley Adams, age 34, was seen in the women's clinic of the city health department for a routine vaginal examination. After the examination, she started to cry uncontrollably for no apparent reason. The nurse, Minita Feather, encouraged her to talk about what was upsetting her. Ms. Adams said she felt confused and sad. She had been feeling this way increasingly for about a month. The precipitating event was having sexual intercourse for the first time.

Ms. Adams stated she usually coped with problems by talking about them, but she did not have a friend to whom she had felt she could confide this. She had enjoyed the experience but felt somewhat guilty about it. In describing herself, she said, "I worry a lot about what other people will think of me. Usually I can handle my own problems, and I don't like being dependent on anyone." She had few close friends, and the man with whom she had had the sexual liaison had moved to another town.

Ms. Feather encouraged Ms. Adams to talk more about her feelings about becoming sexually active. Ms. Adams revealed she was afraid she would start "hopping in bed with anyone in pants." This brought on more tears. Ms. Feather helped her to acknowledge that she was able to decide whether or not to become sexually involved with anyone else. She had been able in the past to decide not to have sexual relationships and she still could control that aspect of her life. Ms. Feather also encouraged her to examine whether or not she wanted to find another sexual partner. Ms. Adams was able to

say that she did want to have that within the context of a more complete relationship.

Ms. Feather suggested that Ms. Adams come back to talk with her in a week to look at ways to increase her social contacts with both women and men.

In this example, the client needed assistance in integrating new role expectations and a body image change: becoming sexually active and no longer being a virgin. Since she had been impulsive, she feared that she might make future decisions about sexual activity in the same way. The nurse helped her to begin to understand her experience and to look for meaningful relationships.

Crisis from Sudden Traumatic Stress

Kim Fraser called Bobbie Walker, RN, who was working as a volunteer for a rape crisis center. She had been abducted while walking home from a college class. She was taken by the rapist to a deserted area and raped by him and another man who was waiting there. They hit her several times, leaving her unconscious. When she recovered consciousness, she had made her way to a road. She followed it to a service station where she called a friend to come and get her. Her friend took her to an emergency room where she was treated and questioned by a police officer. This happened two days before she called the center.

Kim told Bobbie that she was afraid that somehow the rapists would find her and attack her again. Bobbie encouraged her to talk about her feelings and told her that most women were very angry about being raped. At first, Kim would merely say she felt sorry for them. She felt she should be coping better with the experience and felt guilty for causing "so much trouble." Bobbie continued to urge her to talk about it. Kim gave Bobbie her telephone number and Bobbie said she would check with her the following day.

The next day, when Bobbie called, Kim told her she had thought a lot about what Bobbie said about being angry, and she finally realized she was. She began crying but also talked about how furious she was that those two "animals" could disrupt her life. Bobbie encouraged her to ventilate these feelings.

Bobbie explained to Kim that it took time to recover from an experience like hers and that she would probably find it helpful to talk with someone periodically. She also helped Kim to identify future events that might be more distressing because of this experience, such as seeing movies with rape scenes, and they discussed how Kim could deal with these instances.

Because she recognized the role that loss and anger play in crises caused by sudden traumatic stress, the nurse was able to help the client work through her feelings. She gave the client time to think about the experience and kept communication open. She provided anticipatory guidance so that the client would be less susceptible to possible stressors in the future.

Maturational/Developmental Crisis

Mark Eaton, RN, was on his way to a class when he saw a young man sitting on a bench with a dazed expression. Although it was below freezing and there was snow on the ground, the young man was in his shirtsleeves. Mark sat down beside him and introduced himself. The other man told Mark that his name was David Lewis. Mark told him he looked as if something was wrong. David said, "I just can't handle this place anymore." Mark proceeded to draw him out until he learned that this was David's third try at going to college and living away from home.

Mark encouraged David to talk about his experience and what seemed to have precipitated his feeling of not being able to "take it anymore." David said he had run out of money and did not have enough to buy meals for the remainder of the month (four days). He did not see how he could solve his problem and was afraid to call his parents.

Mark helped David figure out some possible solutions for getting some money for food for the rest of the month. He then suggested they go to the counseling center and make arrangements for him to see someone on a regular basis to work on developing skills so that he could live away from home and finish college. David told Mark he was the first person who had ever made him feel he could solve his problem.

In the above example, the nurse helped most by fostering the quality the client felt he lacked—the ability to function independently. The nurse helped the client recognize that with some of the right kind of support, he could eventually function independently. By helping him to find some solutions to the most immediate problem—finding money for food—the nurse helped the client feel more able to confront the developmental issue behind it.

Crisis from Psychopathology

Pete Norris was an airman stationed on an air force base far from his home. He was at a local shopping mall where several community agencies had screening booths, many of which were staffed by nurses. Pete approached John Feldman, RN, who was checking blood pressure readings. After his blood pressure was taken, Pete asked John if he could talk to him for a while. John agreed and the two went for coffee. Pete told John that he felt he had a problem but that he did not want to go to the mental health clinic on the base because he did not want them to think he was "nuts."

The precipitating event he identified was a warning that if he continued to get into trouble (such as fighting with other men in the barracks), he would be discharged. Pete's usual way of coping with things was to "punch people out." He denied feeling guilty about this and felt it was really beyond his control. He use stereotypical language to describe himself and his behavior, such as "I'm a man's man," "I hit first and ask questions later," and "I'm not gonna take anything off some wimpy lieutenant."

Pete said he wanted to stay in the service, that it was his "whole life." Finally he mentioned, almost offhandedly, that his father had been a career military man. John asked if his dad was still in the service and Pete said, "Oh, no, he blew his brains out two months after he got retired."

John helped Pete formulate a plan for dealing with situations in which he tended to get mad enough to punch someone. For example, Pete could take a shower instead, or go for a walk. John also gave Pete the number of a crisis telephone service and encouraged him to call and talk to someone when he felt himself getting out of control. John said, "You really are in control of yourself. One of the myths of our society is that 'real' men work things out with their fists. It takes a lot more courage to talk it out or walk away. If you want to stay in the air force, you've got to show you're strong enough and smart enough to learn some new things."

Pete agreed to try what John suggested and also agreed to go to the mental health clinic on base for additional help. John gave him his work number and said he would like to hear from him.

In the above example, the nurse recognized that severe problems were at the root of the client's crisis. He also realized that circumstances limited what he could do to help. He talked directly to the client and used terms and concepts that had meaning to the client. He emphasized that the client had not only the ability to control his own behavior but also the responsibility.

Psychiatric Emergencies

Helen Johnson, RN, had been visiting Jack Fife in his home since he had an accident that confined him to a wheelchair. At first he had seemed optimistic about coping with his disability, but lately he had been more depressed about his life. At the end of one visit, Jack said, "You'd better call before you come next time. I might not be here."

Helen asked if he was planning to go somewhere. Jack said, "You can never tell." Since he was usually not vague and evasive, Helen was concerned. The following conversation occurred:

H: Jack, what are you thinking about doing?

J: (laughed) I just might get out. . . .

H: What do you mean, "get out"?

J: You know, my brother's a pharmacist. If things get too bad. . . .

H: Are you telling me you're thinking about killing yourself?

J: You nurses, you always take things too seriously.

H: Well, Jack, I care about what happens to you. Sometimes people who are thinking

about killing themselves say things like you did.

J: Why should I kill myself? I've got so much to live for.

H: That isn't what you were talking about earlier. Have you gotten some pills from your brother or someone else?

J: No.

H: Things are really tough for you right now. What have you thought about doing?

J: I have thought about committing suicide.

H: Tell me about it.

J: I really did think I could get some pills from my brother, but I haven't asked him.

H: Can you talk to your brother about this, and ask him to help you stay alive?

J: I've already been such a bother.

H: Let's talk about how you can get some more support.

Helen then assisted Jack in identifying some more resources in his environment. Finally she closed with this:

H: Jack, we've made contracts before that have helped and I want you to make a contract with me now. I want you to make the following statement: "No matter what happens, I will not kill myself, accidentally or on purpose, at any time."

J: OK, I won't.

H: No, I want you to repeat it just the way I said it.

J: OK, I promise that no matter what happens, I won't kill myself on purpose or by accident at any time.

In this example, the nurse first of all determined that the client might be giving a clue that he was planning to kill himself. Next she assessed his suicide risk. Since he did not have the means or a plan, and since the proposed method had the possibility for reversal, she felt his immediate risk was low. She made it clear that she took him and his problems seriously and helped him to find other people to add to his support system. Finally, using a no-suicide contract, she was able to ascertain that he would be able to control his impulses (Twiname, 1981).

Evaluation and Follow-up

While intervention is being implemented, the nurse evaluates the effectiveness of the technique. This includes making sure that you are direct and specific when requesting particular information. If you do not get appropriate information, perhaps your questions are too vague or open ended or are not couched in terms that are familiar to the client. When the nurse tries to encourage the client to ventilate and describe feelings but receives short responses, the questions may be too specific and not open ended.

The most crucial factor in evaluating outcome is verifying that the client returned to at least the precrisis level of functioning. If the nurse and client have made plans that must be carried out outside their meetings, the nurse must check in for a progress report. This is often done with a telephone call. For example, if they identified a need for the client to seek long-term counseling, the nurse should support this by expressing a continuing interest in the client.

FUTURE IMPLICATIONS

Because of the continuing rapid rates of change in culture, demography, and technology, people will continue to be prone to future shock. People are often unable to change as rapidly as the things around them. Young people in our society are already experiencing the discomforting problem of reaching their goals only to find they are no longer applicable because the world changed faster than they expected (Lesse, 1981). This is likely to continue to be a problem for the adolescents and young adults in the next generation.

Lesse (1981) has identified several aspects of our changing societal values that will cause stress in the future. Some problems may arise because of rigid adherence to old values, efforts to adapt to new values, or resistance to new values. It is difficult for most of us to tell for sure if newly emerging values are good, malevolent, or merely ahead of their time. The age gap between groups with different values has grown smaller. For example, seniors in college may be unable to understand the values of seniors in high school.

The young people of today have grown up in a period of affluence and unbounded expectations. They have acquired values that emphasize individualism and work as a means of gaining status. Many feel that they should not have to tolerate physical or emotional discomfort, and they expect immediate relief. These values have not prepared them well for a more group-oriented society with shrinking resources for increasing numbers of people.

Some of the other potential stressors and their implications, as identified by Lesse (1981) are:

- *Crowding*
  - Lack of privacy
  - Lack of space
  - Oversatiation with human contacts
  - Limited mobility
  - More restrictions on behavior

- *Incapacity to choose*
  - Restricted choices due to decreased goods
  - Limitation on possessions
  - Sparseness of resources may produce feelings of deprivation
  - Individualism may be defined as an "illness" by society

· *Overinformation*
  · Need to know what *not* to read
  · Increased information-handling capacities
  · No controls over quality or reliability of information
· *Mass media*
  · Control of thought patterns by those who control media
  · Need to teach journalists to function ethically and responsibly
· *Threatened family*
  · Depreciation of family as primary unit of society
  · Group methods of rearing children
· *Male–female relations*
  · Changing relative statuses
  · Evolving interpsychic and intrapsychic similarity
  · Role confusion
  · Greater freedom of sexual expression
  · Increase in recreational sex; decrease in romantic sex
· *Automation and cybernation*
  · Increased leisure
  · Increase in number of nonlaboring people
  · Need for educational system to prepare people for increased leisure

All of these potential patterns entail change and loss. These trends may affect large numbers of people at a time, thus creating massive upheaval and disruption. However, nurses can have a substantial role in preparing people to anticipate and cope with such changes. People will need help to cope with their sense of loss in ways which do not prove unhealthy to themselves or to their community. Prevention of crisis will become more important than ever.

As our society moves from a product-oriented to a service-oriented economic system, nurses can help identify and provide essential and meaningful services to individuals, groups, and populations. Many of these services will be health producing and health promoting, with an ever-increasing focus on mental health.

SUMMARY

This chapter has discussed introductory crisis theory. Emphasis was placed on the prevention of crisis. A classification system was introduced to aid in identifying the appropriate style of intervention in a crisis. A number of potential future stressors were described in order to provide some direction for crisis prevention in the future.

DISCUSSION TOPICS

1. Jill Michaels has found out that she is pregnant. She is not married and does not want to have the child. She is distressed and confused when you see her in the clinic.

   a. What are the roles of stress and crisis in this example?

   b. In which classification does this crisis belong?

   c. At what stage is Ms. Michaels in the development of the crisis?

   d. What loss or losses might Ms. Michaels be experiencing? Give your rationale for your conclusion.

   e. With a partner playing the role of Ms. Michaels, go through the assessment, planning, intervention, and evaluation steps. Discuss your skills in applying theory to this situation.

2. Lennie Ginnco is 5 years old and about to enter kindergarten. He says he will not

go. His mother, Ms. Ginnco, asks you what to do. She is anxious and says her husband has told her he does not want to hear about the situation anymore.

    a. How can you prevent this stressful situation from becoming a crisis? List at least two strategies you would use. Describe what each one would entail.

    b. What kind of follow-up is indicated?

3. Marty Hogan is the college-age son of Dottie Hogan, a client you have been visiting for several months. You arrive at the home one morning to find Ms. Hogan extremely agitated. Marty has locked himself in his bedroom and says he has a gun. When you go to the bedroom door, Marty tells you that he has a loaded gun and plans to shoot himself.

    a. How do the assessment factors apply in determining the risk of Marty's shooting himself?

    b. Describe how you would intervene.

4. In 1982, a well-known pharmaceutical manufacturer had to take a popular analgesic off the market because cyanide was found in some capsules. The scare lasted for weeks, with daily publicity about deaths from adulterated capsules. Following this, there were instances of "copy cat" crimes with similar tampering. This incident stimulated a great deal of anxiety and fear in the American public.

    a. Discuss the relationship of at least one of the potential stressors listed in the "Future Implications" section to this incident.

    b. Describe how this threat fits the model of crisis development and resolution in the population as a whole.

    c. What are some of the outcomes of the resolution of this crisis?

5. How can you use the information of possible future stressors in your professional nursing practice

    a. With clients?

    b. With colleagues?

    c. With yourself?

6. What could you do with your nursing education if nursing ceased to exist as a profession?

BIBLIOGRAPHY

Aguilera, D.C., ed.: *Coping with life stressors: A life-cycle approach. Family and Community Health* 2(4), 1980.

Aguilera, D.C., & Messick, J.M.: *Crisis intervention* (4th ed.). St. Louis: Mosby, 1982.

Baldwin, B.A.: The assessment of emotional crises. In A.W. Burgess & B.A. Baldwin, eds., *Crisis intervention: Theory and practice.* Englewood Cliffs, N.J.: Prentice-Hall, 1981a.

Baldwin, B.A.: Creating structure for the crisis intervention and resolution process. In A.W. Burgess & B.A. Baldwin, eds., *Crisis intervention: Theory and practice.* Englewood Cliffs, N.J.: Prentice-Hall, 1981b.

Baldwin, B.A.: Crisis intervention: An overview of theory and practice. In A.W. Burgess & B.A. Baldwin, eds., *Crisis intervention: Theory and practice.* Englewood Cliffs, N.J.: Prentice-Hall, 1981c.

Barrell, L.M.: Crisis intervention: Partnership in problem-solving. *Nursing Clinics of North America* 9(1), 5–16, 1974.

Burgess, A.W.: Family reaction to homicide. *American Journal of Orthopsychiatry* 45(3), 391–398, 1975.

Burgess, A.W., & Baldwin, B.A.: *Crisis intervention: Theory and practice.* Englewood Cliffs, N.J.: Prentice-Hall, 1981.

Burgess, A.W., & Brodsky, S.L.: Applying flight

education principles to rape prevention. *Family and Community Health* 4, 45–51, 1981.

Burgess, A.W., & Holmstrom, L.L.: Rape trauma syndrome. *American Journal of Psychiatry* 131, 981–986, 1974.

Burgess, A.W., & Holmstrom, L.L.: *Rape: Victims of crisis.* Bowie, Md: Brady, 1974.

Caplan, G.: A public health approach to child psychiatry. *Mental Health* 35, 235, 1951.

Caplan, G.: *An approach to community mental health.* New York: Grune & Stratton, 1961.

Caplan, G.: Emotional crises. In A. Deutsch & H. Fishbein, eds., *The encyclopedia of mental health* (Vol. 2). New York: Franklin Watts, 1963.

Caplan G.: *Principles of preventive psychiatry.* New York: Basic Books, 1964.

Cronin-Stubbs, D., & Velsor-Friedrich, B.: Professional and personal stress: A survey. *Nursing Leadership* 4(1), 19–25, 1981.

Cyr, F.E., & Wattenberg, S.H.: Social work in a preventive program of maternal and child health. In H.J. Parad, ed., *Crisis intervention: Selected readings.* New York: Family Service Association of America, 1965.

Downey, A.M.: Living, loving, and losing: Implications for health and well-being. *Health Values: Achieving High Level Wellness* 7(1), 7–14, 1983.

Edelhart, M., et al.: The business sector. In R. Weil, ed., *The omni future almanac.* New York: Harmony Books, 1982.

Ellis, E.M., et al.: An assessment of long-term reaction to rape. *Journal of Abnormal Psychology* 90, 263–266, 1981.

Erikson, E.H.: *Childhood and society* (2nd ed.). New York: Norton, 1963.

Ewalt, J.R., & Crawford, D.: Post-traumatic stress syndrome. *Current Psychiatric Therapies* 20, 145–153, 1981.

Gaston, S.K.: Death and midlife crisis. *Journal of Psychosocial Nursing and Mental Health Services* 18(1), 31–35, 1980.

Haber, J.: Crisis theory and application. In J. Haber, et al.: *Comprehensive psychiatric nursing* (2nd ed.). New York: McGraw-Hill, 1982.

Hall, J.E., & Weaver, B.R.: *Nursing of families in crisis.* Philadelphia: Lippincott, 1974.

Hefferin, E.A.: Life-cycle stressors: An overview of research. *Family and Community Health* 2(4), 71–101, 1980.

Holmes, T.H., & Rahe, R.H.: The social readjustment rating scale. *Journal of Psychosomatic Research* 11, 213–218, 1967.

Holmstrom, L.L., & Burgess, A.W.: Assessing trauma in the rape victim. *American Journal of Nursing* 75, 1288–1291, 1975.

Ipema, D.K.: Rape: The process of recovery. *Nursing Research* 28, 272–275, 1979.

Johnston, M.: *The health of families in a culture of crisis.* Kansas City, Mo.: American Nurses' Foundation, 1981.

Josephson, J.W.: The male rape victim: Evaluation and treatment. *Journal of American Council of Emergency Physicians* 8, 13–15, 1979.

Krauss, J.B., & Slavinsky, A.T.: *The chronically ill psychiatric patient and the community.* Boston: Blackwell Scientific Publications, 1982.

Lesse, S.: *The future of the health sciences.* New York: Irvington, 1981.

Lindemann, E.: Symptomatology and management of acute grief. *American Journal of Psychiatry* 101, 141–148, 1944.

Lippitt, G.: *Visualizing change: Model building and the change process.* Fairfax, Va.: NTL Learning Resources Corp., 1973.

Maloney, E.M.: The subjective and objective definition of crisis. *Perspectives in Psychiatric Care* 9(6), 257–268, 1971.

Melichar, M.M.: Using crisis theory to help parents cope with a child's temper tantrums. *American Journal of Maternal Child Nursing* 5(3), 181–185, 1980.

Murray, R., & Luetje, V.: Crisis intervention to promote psychological adaptation. In R.B. Murray & M.M.W. Huelskoetter, *Psychiatric/mental health nursing.* Englewood Cliffs, N.J.: Prentice-Hall, 1983.

Norris, J., & Feldman-Summers, S.: Factors related to the psychological impact of rape on the victim. *Journal of Abnormal Psychology* 90, 562–567, 1981.

Pisarcik, G.K.: Psychiatric emergencies and crisis intervention. *Nursing Clinics of North America* 16(1), 85–94, 1981.

Rape in another gender. *Emergency Medicine* July 15, 1980, pp. 106–107.

Rapoport, L.: The state of crisis: Some theoretical considerations. In H.J. Parad, ed., *Crisis intervention: Selected readings.* New York: Family Service Association of America, 1965.

Sarrel, P.M., & Masters, W.H.: Sexual molestation of men by women. *Archives of Sexual Behavior* 11(2), 117–131, 1982.

Selye, H.: *The stress of life.* New York: McGraw-Hill, 1955.

Sneidman, E.S.: Preventing suicide. *American Journal of Nursing* 65(5), 111–117, 1965.

Strickler, M., & LaSor, B.: The concept of loss in crisis intervention. *Mental Hygiene* 54(2), 301–305, 1970.

Toffler, A.: *Future shock.* New York: Bantam, 1971.

Torres, G.: *The consultation process in higher education.* Memo to members, Council of Bacca-laureate and Higher Degree Programs, National League for Nursing, New York, 1974.

Twiname, B.G.: No-suicide contract for nurses. *Journal of Psychosocial Nursing and Mental Health Services* 19(7), 11–12, 1981.

Vinokur, A., & Selzer, M.L.: Desirable versus undesirable life events: Their relationship to stress and mental distress. *Journal of Personality and Social Psychology* 32(2), 329–337, 1975.

Williams, F.: Intervention in maturational crises. *Perspectives in Psychiatric Care* 9(6), 240–246, 1971.

Zilberg, N.J., et al: Impact of event scale: A cross-validation study and some empirical evidence supporting a conceptual model of stress response syndromes. *Journal of Consulting and Clinical Psychology* 50, 407–414, 1982.

23

Health Promotion

Victoria Schoolcraft

> To ward off disease or recover health, men as a rule find it
> easier to depend on the healers than to attempt the more
> difficult task of living wisely.
>
> RENÉ DUBOS

OBJECTIVES

After reading this chapter, you should be able to:

☐ Define health and high-level wellness.
☐ Define disease.
☐ Define and describe holistic health.
☐ Identify and discuss the factors that influence health.
☐ Define health promotion and the determinants of willingness to promote one's own health.
☐ Describe the changing perspective on the role of the professional in promoting health.
☐ Define and describe levels of disease prevention.
☐ Describe goals related to health promotion.
☐ Carry out a health assessment with clients.
☐ Describe ways of promoting health.
☐ Discuss the nurse's role in health education.
☐ Identify research needs in regard to health promotion.
☐ Identify difficulties in promoting health.
☐ Discuss the future evolution of health promotion in relation to the growth and change in nursing.

INTRODUCTION

Once Western, scientific medicine began to find causes of disease, its approach became heavily weighted toward the cure and prevention of diseases by means of medical interventions. This method of looking at a particular aspect of a person—such as a disease—is sometimes called "reductionism." This term refers to the reducing of the field of study to a single focus, such as an organ or body system. Because this viewpoint has prevailed, an enormous amount of study has been devoted to agents of disease, such as microorganisms, while the determinants of health and disease within the person and the environment have been neglected.

There have always been holistic health practitioners who have focused on health promotion, self-responsibility, holism, and alternate approaches to health and healing. The movement toward a new paradigm of personal health has been gathering momentum, particularly over the last 20 years. The velocity of growth has been affected by groups who have felt neglected, mistreated, or exploited by the health care system and who have instituted new approaches to health supervision and health promotion. For example, the women's health movement has flourished as women have reclaimed control over their own bodies. In the early 1970s, women independently established health collectives in which they learned about themselves and met their own health needs (Mulligan, 1983). Such groups organized significant assaults on the male-dominated health care system. They did a great deal to make people aware that what is good for women's health is also good for children's health and men's health. There is little published evidence of nursing involvement in this consumer-originated movement, but the values within it are akin to common public health nursing concepts: "mutual decision making and responsibility for one's own health state" (Mulligan, 1983, p. 3).

Other groups have sprung up as part of the holistic health movement that are providing options to people who want to take more responsibility for their own health. Although they are often started by consumers without formal medical or nursing credentials, many of these health centers use the teachings and resources of nurses, physicians, psychologists, and public health professionals. They offer a wide array of practices, from Western scientific models to native American, Eastern, and metaphysical approaches. One such center is in California: the Berkeley Holistic Health Center, which has published two resource books which are compilations of a wealth of health information (Bauman et al., 1978; 1981).

Physicians have also established health-oriented practices. One of the best known is John W. Travis, founder of the Wellness Resource Center in Mill Valley, California. Travis focuses only on wellness and does not use drugs or treat disease. Clients who require illness care are referred to other physicians (Ardell, 1978). Another physician who has made a significant impact is Bill Hettler of the University of Wisconsin-Stevens Point. He has been the director of a highly successful wellness-promotion program on the university campus and has spearheaded the development of a Wellness Commission in the community of Stevens Point (Hettler, 1980; Rentmeester & Hall, 1982).

Where are the nurses in this burgeoning field of health promotion? To begin with, few nurses work in community-oriented settings. In 1980, only about 25 percent of employed nurses worked outside of inpatient settings (hospitals and nursing homes). Of these nurses, less than 7 percent worked in public or community health (Levine & Moses, 1982). Although many of the nurses in community and public health promote health, they tend to do so in ways that have limited impact on their communities and that do not attract much attention.

The time has come for nurses to acknowledge a commitment to health for all. This means that nurses must become concerned with the health of all people in the community. Not only nurses in community health practices have this responsibility, but also nurses in hospitals, nursing homes, physicians' offices, and mental health centers. It is time for nurses to cease being preoccupied with illness and instead to become occupied with health.

This chapter defines the basic concepts of health, introduces some of the tools used in assessment and promotion of health, and describes some of the prospects for the future of health promotion. Health planning at the community level is covered more extensively in Chapter 30 of this book. Approaches described here are oriented to individuals, families, and groups with some recommendations for community involvement. Other sources are listed at the end of this chapter.

HEALTH

Dwore and Krueter (1980) state that it is important to understand that the nature of health is complex and often cannot be reduced to a simple definition. They believe that the components that must be considered in defining health are:

· The ability to adapt to changing situations
· The capacity to perform valued tasks

· Multidimensional causality of health
· A relative state of being

Two of the definitions of health cited by Dwore and Krueter, if combined, seem to meet their criteria. *Health* is:

a relative state that represents the degree to which an individual can operate effectively within the circumstances of his heredity and his physical and cultural environment. (McDermott, 1977, p. 136)

the expression of the extent to which the individual . . . maintain[s] in readiness the resources required to meet the exigencies of the future. (Dubos, 1962, p. 111)

Although the words "health" and "wellness" are frequently used interchangeably, these concepts have been differentiated by some important theorists. Halbert L. Dunn defines *high-level wellness* in this way:

High-level wellness for the individual is defined as an integrated method of functioning which is oriented toward maximizing the potential of which the individual is capable, within the environment where he is functioning. (1977, p. 9)

Dunn differentiated wellness from health in that he saw the former as dynamic and the latter as a relatively passive state in which the individual was free from illness and at peace with the environment. Many of the programs that emphasize comprehensive approaches and self-responsibility include this distinction. In this chapter, the term "health" will be used inclusively and the term "wellness" will be used to quote or restate the words of a writer who preferred that term.

Since health promotion is frequently linked with disease prevention, it is appropriate to define disease. *Disease* means a "specific physical or emotional malady linked to selected causal factors" (Dwore &

Kreuter, 1980, p. 105). This definition of disease implies that even though someone has a disease, it may have a limited effect on that person's health, which is related to many different factors. For example, a person might have diabetes yet still be healthy. By the same token, many people do not suffer from any disease yet experience poor health.

Illness is not always a completely negative experience. Much of the literature on holism and new paradigms of health treats disease as a life experience. Therefore, it can provide useful learning about a life-style problem or increase our sensitivity to others who suffer. It can be growth producing and have beneficial outcomes.

Holistic Health

One of the most significant trends in the medical and health care systems has been the recognition and integration of the holistic view of people. The *holistic* concept is the consideration that within each person is a dynamic, continual interaction of the biological, emotional, intellectual, and spiritual dimensions of identity. Furthermore, holism includes the recognition of the influence of the psychosocial and physical environments on the individual.

The factors that affect an individual's health are usually grouped in four classes:

· Life-style factors
· Biological/genetic factors
· Physical environment factors
· Medical care system factors

Of these, the medical care system has the least impact. Generally, that system is utilized only when a person has some interruption in health.

Perhaps the most important class of factors is the cluster of behaviors related to life-style. *Life-style* "consists of the aggregation of decisions by individuals which affect their health and over which they more or less have control" (LaLonde, 1980, p. 446). Hancock (1982, p. 6) adds that it is not "merely personal behavior" but "personal behavior modified and influenced by a lifelong process of socialization." Thus the individual's apparently independent choices of behavior have been greatly influenced by family and social determinants. Life-style includes patterns of diet, physical activity, sleep, and personal safety; work; use of tobacco, alcohol, or drugs; interpersonal relationships and social activity; spiritual and religious expression; emotional expression; attitudes about health and use of medical care system; response to stress; recreation; and residence.

HEALTH PROMOTION

Health promotion includes the active and purposeful bringing about of necessary changes, marshalling required resources, and carrying out whatever activities are necessary to develop, sustain, and increase healthy functioning. It also includes activities that support the health-producing activities of others.

Dwore and Kreuter (1980, p. 106) define health promotion essentially as "advocating health in order to enhance the probability that personal, private, and public support of positive health practices will become a societal norm." Since such a large proportion of preventable health problems are influenced by societal norms, as manifested in personal life-styles, one must look for ways to influence aggregate populations as well as individuals and families.

Health Promotion and Health Professionals

Silverman (1980) has articulated six presuppositions that affect the field of health care and that he challenges. First, he points out that health professionals are not taught much self-care as part of their professional education. It is as if they were immune to health problems, when in fact they have a significantly high incidence of disease, especially stress-related diseases. The second presupposition is that health care professionals are responsible for their clients' health. This view fosters reliance on the medical care system and deprives people of self-responsibility. It casts doubt on any other source of health information or assistance.

The third assumption is that the medical care system heals people. Silverman points out that this is merely a way of viewing things. An equally satisfactory way of looking at the same process would be to view health professionals as "creators of a field in which healing may occur" (p. 97). This acknowledges the limits of the health professional and the importance of the uniqueness of each individual in participating in his or her own healing.

The last three assumptions have to do with viewing disease as a threat. The first involves the primacy that has been given to fighting disease as the role of the health professional. This "oppositional" point of view does not encourage understanding of the human beings within which disease may occur. It is more beneficial to strengthen the person to resist disease and to be able to manage some imbalances without outside intervention.

The next presupposition is that the end justifies the means if it saves lives. Silverman points out that a disease-oriented system results in health professionals' thinking that to help people with diseases, they have "to *do* something to them," "to take responsibility for *changing* them." The result has been that many people end up the same or even worse than they were before they sought help. For example, since health professionals feel that they must do something to change the person, they become angry and resentful toward clients who do not follow instructions. Indeed, sometimes the cure is worse than the disease.

Finally, to health professionals, death is the enemy, particularly if the victim is not elderly. This is the final criterion of success or failure for the health professional. It has justified untold suffering and many ethical entanglements because of the belief that health professionals should prolong the quantity of material life by any means. This neglects the consideration of quality of life.

In order to promote health, presuppositions such as these must be examined, challenged, and replaced with new assumptions. An alternate set might be:

1. Health professionals are responsible for their self-care, and this should be an integral part of their professional education.
2. Clients are responsible for their own health; health care professionals may help them promote it.
3. The healing process takes place within the client, cofacilitated by the client and the health professional.
4. Promoting health is the key function of health professionals.
5. Health professionals care for clients and do things with clients only with the clients' support.
6. We must accept and understand death as a part of life, find meaning in death, and help clients find meaning in death.

The integration of these kinds of assumptions must take place within the context of a profession that largely subscribes to the first set. For this reason, this chapter also presents precepts about health promotion that incorporate the concepts of disease prevention. Even though the reader has one foot in tomorrow, he or she still has to take note of the conditions of today.

Self Health Promotion

The willingness of an individual to select and to participate in health promotion is influenced by a number of intrapersonal, interpersonal, and situational factors (Pender, 1975).

Intrapersonal Determinants

1. *Importance of health.* Health tends not to have an intrinsic value; instead, it is important in enabling a person to accomplish things that are valued.

2. *Perceived vulnerability.* An individual is more motivated if the probability of developing a particular health problem seems high.

3. *Perceived value of early detection.* People are more likely to participate in screening if they feel that early detection improves their chances of recovery.

4. *Perceived seriousness.* An individual is more likely to engage in prevention if the health problem is threatening, can cause visible changes, can alter family or occupational roles, or is communicable.

5. *Perceived efficacy of action.* Given the options of which he or she is aware, the person will choose the one that is most effective and that has the least risk and inconvenience.

6. *Perceived level of internal versus external control.* Internally controlled people be-

lieve in their power to influence health; externally controlled people feel powerless.

Interpersonal Determinants

1. *Concern of significant others.* Either loving concern or irritating persistence from family members is motivating.

2. *Family patterns of utilization.* Parents, and particularly mothers, have a high degree of influence on health patterns.

3. *Expectations of friends.* Peer pressure and friends' values influence health decisions.

4. *Information from professionals.* The greater the credibility of the source, the more likely the person is to follow recommendations. People tend to act negatively toward a health behavior advocated by someone who lacks credibility.

Situational Determinants

1. *Cultural acceptance of health behaviors.* U.S. culture has tended to discourage concern about oneself until pronounced symptoms develop.

2. *Societal group norms and pressures.* Approval or disapproval by society is a strong influence on behavior.

3. *Information from nonpersonal sources.* Information gained through media may make people feel more vulnerable to certain health problems as well as more confident in the efficacy of preventive measures.

4. *Availability of resources and options.* Regardless of motivation and willingness to engage in promotion activities, if resources are limited or if people are not aware of their options, they will not change their behavior.

As this list indicates, the determination of a person's, family's, or community's motivation to engage in health promotion is quite complex. The variety of these factors as well as their number makes plain why the role of the health professional in encouraging health promotion can be so challenging.

Disease Prevention

Although much of health promotion is positively oriented toward enhancing health states, a portion of it is still related to the prevention of disease and premature death. Some criteria for the success of health promotion are couched in terms of disease prevention. These criteria will be discussed later in this chapter.

Levels of Prevention

The concept of levels of prevention is a familiar one in the literature of public and community health. *Disease prevention* is the action involved in stopping disease from occurring or progressing. Three levels of prevention are usually identified: primary, secondary, and tertiary. What varies among these levels are the goals, the target and nature of preventive activities, and the population involved. Table 23.1 summarizes these factors.

Primary prevention is the prevention of disease or dysfunction. It includes health promotion activities instituted by the individual, family, or group, by health professionals, or by the community. The popula-

TABLE 23.1
Levels of Prevention

Level	Goal of Prevention	Activities	Population	Examples
Primary	Decrease vulnerability; reduce risk factors. *Prevent* disease and dysfunction.	Health promotion; reduction of risk factors.	Healthy people.	Health education, exercise, stopping smoking, immunizations, stress management, understanding emotions.
Secondary	Halt pathological process, shorten duration and severity of disease, limit or delay disability. *Prevent* progression of existing disease.	Screening for early diagnosis and prompt treatment.	People with undetected disease or disability.	Self breast examinations, blood pressure checks, PKU tests, sickle cell anemia screening, crisis intervention.
Tertiary	Restore person to highest level of functioning within limits of disease. *Prevent* further deterioration from a fixed or irreversible disease.	Rehabilitation.	People with fixed or irreversible disease.	Environmental modifications for those with cardiovascular disease, amputation, multiple sclerosis, chronic psychiatric illness.

tion involved consists of healthy people. *Secondary prevention* halts the pathological process and limits the duration and severity of the disease. The methods used are aimed at early detection through screening and prompt treatment. The population involved consists of those who have few or no symptoms of a disease and require some diagnostic procedure. *Tertiary prevention* is rehabilitation, the restoration of the client to the highest level of functioning possible. The target population includes those who have a disability that is fixed or irreversible and who require assistance in attaining their optimum level of functioning.

The levels of prevention fall along a continuum (Shamansky & Clausen, 1980). This means that some activities may overlap between two levels, especially the secondary and tertiary levels. For example, foot care may be seen as secondary prevention in the long-term care of a diabetic client, because deterioration due to circulatory problems common in advanced stages of diabetes may occur. The client already has diabetes and the nurse attempts to limit disability from the disease. This intervention is also an attempt to prevent further deterioration, which is tertiary prevention.

With another client, efforts may be aimed at two or three levels at once. For example, a young woman delivers twins prematurely. Within 24 hours, one baby dies. The other survives. The nurse who works with the client would have some goals that involved primary prevention, such as teaching the mother about the normal growth and development of a premature infant. In addition, the nurse would help the client deal with the crisis of a premature delivery and the death of one infant, which are secondary prevention activities.

Shamansky and Clausen (1980) have questioned the value of the continued use of this classification concept in nursing. They think it has complicated rather than clarified the description of preventive activities. This seems to be especially true with the secondary and tertiary levels. Use of this sometimes "fuzzy" terminology has affected the focus of nursing activities. For example, many prevention programs focus on preventing disease at the secondary level when they could be influencing prevention much earlier, at the primary level.

Goals of Health Promotion

The overriding goal of health promotion is to have healthy individuals and ultimately a healthy society. Some criteria are necessary to evaluate the attainment of that goal. Dwore and Kreuter (1980) cite Blum's eight aspects of health that characterize a healthy society:

1. Low rates of premature death.
2. Low rates of disease or deviation from physiological or functional norms appropriate to age and sex.
3. Low rates of discomfort or illness.
4. Low rates of disability or incapacity.
5. High rates of internal satisfaction (joy of living, self-realization).
6. High rates of external satisfaction (satisfaction with the environment).
7. High rates of positive health (resistance to ill health and creation of reserve capacity).
8. High rates of participation in personal and community health activities (Blum, 1974).

These criteria can be extended to the assessment of individual health.

National goals that relate to health promotion and disease prevention have been set forth in *Healthy People: The Surgeon General's Report on Health Promotion and*

Disease Prevention (1979) and are listed in Table 23.2. These goals relate to some of the general concerns that recur in the literature and contain a mix of promotion and prevention.

As with other nursing activities, the goals appropriate to a given client, family, or community are determined by an assessment. However, it is important for nurses to balance concern and activity related to individuals or communities with concern for and activity to promote the health of the population at large.

HEALTH ASSESSMENT

Health assessment means gathering and analyzing data about the health status of an individual, a family, a group, or a community. Although assessment tools vary depending on the situation, those applicable to individuals and families generally take into account information in the following categories:

1. Biological
    a. Medical and dental history

TABLE 23.2
National Health Goals

  I. To continue to improve infant health, and, by 1990, to reduce infant mortality by at least 35 percent, to fewer than 9 deaths per 1,000 live births.
     Subgoal: Reducing the number of low birth weight infants.
     Subgoal: Reducing the number of birth defects.

  II. To improve child health, foster optimal childhood development, and, by 1990, reduce deaths among children ages one to 14 years by at least 20 percent, to fewer than 34 per 100,000.
     Subgoal: Enhancing childhood growth and development.
     Subgoal: Reducing childhood accidents and injuries.

  III. To improve the health and health habits of adolescents and young adults, and, by 1990, to reduce deaths among people ages 15 to 24 by at least 20 percent, to fewer than 93 per 100,000.
     Subgoal: Reducing fatal motor vehicle accidents.
     Subgoal: Reducing alcohol and drug misuse.

  IV. To improve the health of adults, and, by 1990, to reduce deaths among people ages 25 to 64 by at least 25 percent, to fewer than 400 per 100,000.
     Subgoal: Reducing heart attacks and strokes.
     Subgoal: Reducing death from cancer.

  V. To improve the health and quality of life for older adults and, by 1990, to reduce the average annual number of days of restricted activity due to acute and chronic conditions by 20 percent, to fewer than 30 days per year for people aged 65 and older.
     Subgoal: Increasing the number of older adults who can function independently.
     Subgoal: Reducing premature death from influenza and pneumonia.

SOURCE: *Healthy People: The Surgeon General's Report on Health Promotion and Disease Prevention,* 1979, pp. 21–78.

b. Physical assessment

c. Family history

d. Immunization status

e. Use of medications and drugs

f. Personal health practices

g. Use of conventional care systems (medical, dental, ophthalmological, chiropractic, osteopathic, etc.)

h. Use of alternate care systems (homeopaths, folk healers, reflexologists, herbalists, etc.)

2. Psychosocial

a. Marital status and family relationships

b. Parenting status and patterns

c. Significant others (extended family, lovers, friends)

d. Emotional status

e. Sexual history

f. Self-esteem

g. Education

h. Developmental tasks

3. Life-style

a. Dietary patterns and weight

b. Sleep patterns

c. Physical fitness and exercise patterns

d. Safety awareness

e. Work history, both in and out of the home

f. Motor vehicle use

g. Patterns and history of tobacco use

h. Patterns and history of alcohol or mood-altering drug use

i. Recreational activities

j. Amount and quality of social activity

k. Residence (kind and suitability)

l. Travel (amount and frequency)

m. Stress and stress management

n. Spiritual and religious involvement

4. Environmental

a. Exposure to pollution (air, water, radiation)

b. Quality of environment (living and working)

5. Other

a. Community interest and involvement

b. Economic security and resources

c. Specific cultural, personal, or regional health influences

Specific questions that can be used to elicit information can be found in a variety of resources or developed by the nurse. The questions should be straightforward and unambiguous. Although the nurse may ask the client the questions, it is often satisfactory to ask the client to respond to a written questionnaire. This gives the client more time to formulate responses, and the client may feel more comfortable in writing some answers than in expressing them orally. Another benefit of the client's responding in writing is increased involvement in the process. This benefit may be further enhanced by using an instrument that provides a health rating or identifies risk factors.

A number of instruments have been developed to permit health assessment both independently and interdependently. One example is the Lifestyle Assessment Questionnaire from the University of Wisconsin-Stevens Point. This inventory has four sections that assess components of life-style, interest in personal growth, risk appraisal, and medical, behavioral, and emotional problems (Hettler, 1980). Another widely used assessment tool is the Health Hazard Appraisal, which helps a person identify his or her own health risks, analyzes the person's life expectancy, and gives individualized recommendations for reducing risks and prolonging life expectancy (Snyder, 1982; Wagner et al., 1982). Information about these and other instruments follows the Bibliography at the end of this chapter.

An assessment of the individual's or family's openness to health promotion in general or to specific kinds of health promotion can be made by identifying the applicable intrapersonal, interpersonal, and situational determinants of health promotion. These were listed earlier in the section on self health promotion. Some of these may become apparent from responses to the health assessment questions or through observations and information obtained while working with clients. The nurse may have to ask direct questions to establish the significance of some of the determinants.

Assessment of the aggregate population of a community can be carried out in a variety of ways. One way is to assume that the quality of health of the community is similar to the national picture of the health of Americans. Statistical reports on particular aspects of national health status can be obtained from a variety of federal agencies, such as those listed at the end of this chapter.

Other groups such as the American Cancer Society, the American Heart Association, and the National Safety Council also have useful statistical information. This type of data may provide a point of comparison for a nurse's community. By being aware of typical health needs, the nurse can target certain concerns for investigation. For example, knowing that cigarette smoking is a common activity that may compromise health status, a nurse might undertake a study of the prevalence of that activity in his or her community.

Another approach would be to do a broad-based community assessment to identify the presence or absence of indicators of health or disease. Priorities for the community can then be set on the basis of the data obtained. Community-specific factors include the existence of certain kinds of industry that may contribute to environmental pollution or safety hazards. Indirect indicators of the health of a community include age (the very young and the very old are most susceptible to disease), income (lower-income people are generally in poorer health than affluent people), and race (the life expectancy of nonwhites is considerably lower than that of whites) (Cordes, 1978).

ACTIONS FOR HEALTH

Part of the Surgeon General's report on health promotion (*Healthy People*, 1979) included priority activities to meet the national health goals. These are listed in Table 23.3. They give a sense of the focus in health promotion, as determined by the assessed needs of an individual, family, or community.

In a landmark study of 11,000 adults over a long period of time, Breslow identified seven rules for healthy living that became apparent in comparing healthy people and those with health problems (Belloc & Breslow, 1972). In addition to two other rules, these simple measures are effective in prolonging and maintaining the quality of life:

1. Eat three meals a day at regular times; do not eat snacks.

2. Eat breakfast every day.

3. Get seven to eight hours of sleep once out of every 24 hours.

4. Engage in exercise two to three times per week.

5. Do not smoke.

TABLE 23.3
Actions for Health: Priority Activities to Meet National Health Goals

Health promotion
  Smoking cessation
  Reducing misuse of alcohol and drugs
  Improved nutrition
  Exercise and fitness
  Stress control
Health protection
  Toxic agent control
  Occupational safety and health
  Accidental injury control
  Fluoridation of community water supplies
  Infectious agent control
Preventive health services
  Family planning
  Pregnancy and infant care
  Immunizations
  Sexual transmissible disease services
  High blood pressure control

SOURCE: *Healthy People: The Surgeon General's Report on Health Promotion and Disease Prevention*, 1979.

tend to persist in doing what they have learned to do and what they have incorporated into their life-styles. The processes involved in influencing both the development of and change in life-style components are not entirely logical or rational: many of the underlying factors in life-style decisions are emotional. That is why a very intelligent, well-educated physician or nurse may be an overweight smoker who fails to learn relaxation techniques.

In order to be successful at promoting health, a nurse must have realistic expectations. Furthermore, the nurse must balance a sense of professional responsibility for promoting health in individuals and populations with a realization that people are responsible for changing themselves. However, health professionals have brought about change by instituting measures that did not require the active participation of the population. For example, fluoride has been shown to be an effective agent in reducing tooth decay. Adequate fluoride application through regular mouth rinses, dietary administration, or use of fluoride toothpaste can provide protection. However, the fluoridation of public water supplies requires no additional daily expense in money, time, or effort and is much more effective than most personal fluoride applications.

6. Maintain weight within 10 percent of optimal range.

7. Consume alcohol in moderation or not at all.

8. Practice some kind of stress management technique, such as daily meditation (Pelletier, 1980).

9. Drive safely and wear seat belts whenever riding in an automobile.

The rules listed above seem simple to identify and to follow. However, people

Methods of Health Promotion

The principal method of promoting health is education. This ranges from information campaigns to make the public more aware of healthy behavior and health risks to classes in schools, youth organizations, religious institutions, and community centers. Increasing awareness and providing information do influence many people to change their behavior. The use of some of the assessment instruments, in conjunction with individual and group activities, has helped people to lead healthier lives (Ferguson, 1980; Hettler, 1980; Travis, 1980).

Nurses working in the community—visiting clients in their homes, seeing clients in ambulatory settings, working in occupational health—have many opportunities for assessing needs for health promotion and intervening with educational strategies. The nurse may share appropriate health information or help the client to evaluate other resources, such as reading material, health collectives, or wellness workshops. Nurses who work in agencies or other settings can advocate the use of an assessment process and the development of complementary educational activities. In addition to their teaching skills, nurses can use a variety of other concepts, such as change theory, group process, political activity, and assertiveness.

Even though the emphasis of health promotion is to help people remain independent of the medical care system, people will continue to have contact with physicians and will on occasion require hospitalization. Therefore, one crucial locale for health education is within the medical care system. It is estimated that 75 percent of the population sees a physician at least once a year (Nelson & Simmons, 1983). With the high rate of contact and the esteem in which people hold their personal physicians, this is an excellent place for health education.

Schools and other places where young people gather are crucial sites for health education. Increasing general public consciousness of the importance of early determination of health habits will promote the inclusion of a well-organized, appropriately paced health curriculum. Nurses can develop contacts with parents' groups, teachers' groups, and school officials to generate and maintain an interest in health education.

Many private industries have already responded to the rationality and value of health education. Knobel (1983) cites several examples of large corporations that have instituted programs to teach employees about the benefits of proper nutrition, exercise, and of not smoking. They have followed through by supporting health-related behaviors on the part of employees.

Industry's response leads into the consideration of another technique of promoting health—*subsidization*. This involves rewarding people for engaging in healthy activities. For example, employees might earn bonuses for participating in company-sponsored exercise classes. Although this is generally unavailable at present, third-party payers could reimburse health education expenses. Most insurance companies have special rates for people who are low health risks. Eventually, government subsidies, in the form of reduced taxes, may be available for health promotion as it already is for certain kinds of medical treatment.

Taxation is a way of punishing people for engaging in unhealthy activities. An example is taxation of tobacco and alcohol. Another example is the proposal to decrease or eliminate tax deductions for more than two or three children or to increase the tax for people who have more than a certain number of children.

Regulation is accomplished through legislation that compels people to engage in healthy activities or restrains them from unhealthy activities. Such regulations are often accompanied by provisions for heavy fines for noncompliance. Examples include the requirements for the use of certain kinds of automobile fuel and pollution-control devices. There are also regulations about environmental quality that are aimed at industry. Laws about child abuse and neglect are meant to control unhealthy personal behavior.

Research Directions

The three areas in which research about health promotion is most needed are: (1) studies to demonstrate the efficacy of health-promoting activities; (2) studies to determine the factors that contribute to health habits; and (3) studies to identify ways of motivating people to adopt healthy life-styles.

Many of the activities people engage in to promote their own health or the health of others lack a scientific basis. Therefore, studying these activities will enrich the knowledge base from which nurses function. There is also a need to sharpen educational approaches and to develop effective educational programs for a variety of clients and population groups.

As more studies are conducted to determine the factors that facilitate health promotion, the information obtained will enable nurses and others to be more effective at identifying points of intervention. For example, one approach to this kind of research question has been to examine the relationship of locus of control to health life-style (Hallal, 1982; Pill & Stott, 1981; Wallston, 1978). *Locus of control* refers to whether a person is motivated by internal or external factors. A person with internal locus of control feels capable of having an effect on his or her own life and feels competent to cope with difficult situations. One who has an external locus of control tends to feel powerless and at the mercy of others. Such aspects of self-concept have great significance in health decisions and perceptions of disease.

Finally, motivation is an issue in many interpersonal enterprises. This is related to what influences people to adopt healthy or unhealthy life-styles. As professionals gain a deeper understanding of such factors, this will indicate what efforts might be successful in influencing health behavior. For ex-ample, there is already a body of knowledge that shows the powerful influence of family, friends, and societal determinants on health behavior. Further research is needed to develop precision in measuring these influences.

Constraints on Health Promotion

Questions have been raised about the ethical implications of trying to control personal behavior, even for individuals' "own good." The United States has a long history of personal freedom. Many issues surrounding health, particularly environmental health, have shown us that there is no such thing as total freedom. Eventually there comes a point at which one's efforts to express one's freedom conflict with the rights of another person. Inappropriate health decisions affect not only the individual but also potentially those in the immediate and distant communities. For example, people who neglect their own self-care not only deprive themselves of some of the quality of their lives, they also diminish the quality of life for their families, friends, employers, and others, both directly and indirectly. Given the possible effects on individuals and the community, does the community, through its government or through some other mechanism, have the right or responsibility to take some action for health promotion? Who will determine the priorities and the extent of such intervention?

Another difficulty in promoting health is inconsistencies or confusion over existing government policies. A commonly cited example is the continuing contradiction between the longstanding war on smoking from the Surgeon General's office and the continuation of government subsidies to tobacco growers.

The greatest difficulty arises from the American norm of seeking short-term, uncomplicated solutions and permitting potentially destructive behavior, such as reckless driving, alcohol abuse, and freedom without responsibility. It is certainly valuable to teach a class of second graders oral hygiene or to teach young parents about growth and development. However, health promotion must also be of community-wide and nation-wide proportions to make the necessary impact on the quality of life of the American people.

A HEALTH-PROMOTING NURSING PRACTICE

This section describes the nursing practice of Dana Gray, RN, and Robert Radtke, RN, two graduates of the University of Oklahoma College of Nursing whose partnership is in Hyampom, California. It is an independent practice that emphasizes health promotion for individual clients and for the community. The practice incorporates many traditional and nontraditional nursing interventions, but what they do is based on principles of nursing that were a part of their baccalaureate education. Their practice is in a rural community in which the only industry is lumber. Many people are out of work, and they rely on their own ability to produce what they need or barter. What follows is mostly in Gray and Radtke's own words.

As for education, we have done various activities: teaching classes at the grade school; teaching foot reflexology at the local fair; setting up CPR classes, first aid, and assembling emergency information for the town. We also give (and receive) information about diet and nutrition to people as they ask for it—without trying to advocate any particular type of diet. Herbs are in common use around here, so we are learning more about them than we are teaching.

The clients who come to us are generally of two types: those who know what kind of service they want and those who come with some sort of "problem." If they have a particular problem, we take a history of it and decide whether we should treat it or not. We frequently make referrals to different practitioners, such as physicians, chiropractors, homeopaths.

We explain what we have to offer and let the client decide whether it will help. All the methods we use are aimed at stress reduction and relaxation. We use three different types of massage—full (or part) body muscle, foot reflexology, and polarity. During massage, we teach deep breathing, and it enables us to do an excellent physical assessment. These massages last a long time (1–2 hours for muscle, 30–45 minutes for foot reflexology), and it has turned out to be a good time for talking with the client. We do a lot of listening.

As their description shows, these nurses have incorporated the perception of the client or community as partners who work with the nurse to determine what they need. The nurses emphasize health education and the adoption of a healthy life-style. They encourage their clients to focus on promotion and prevention, although most clients seek the nurses' assistance when they have already identified a problem.

Mrs. B. came to us complaining of numbness and weakness in the right arm intermittently for several weeks. She requested foot reflexology. We also gave her hand reflexology. She reported a great deal of improvement and relief from reflexology and later muscle massage. She confessed during treatment that her marriage was rocky, she saw no future in it, felt dominated, and wanted to gain the strength to split up. We stayed away from giving marital advice. Recently, we found out that she divorced her husband and that she is doing "just great."

As far as payment, we tell people that in the city the rate of pay is anywhere from $20–60 per session for therapeutic massage. We realize that most people don't have jobs, so we are willing to accept other things besides money. Corn, grape juice, help with fence building, and rare seeds are some of the things we've bartered for. We try to be open and versatile about payments, but we're still not sure about the rabbit one man wants to give us! Best of all, massage is no longer just for the rich and elite!

Gray and Radtke are discovering the interrelationship of the physical with the emotional and spiritual. They chose to go to this community and are finding out how they can meet the health needs there in harmony with the people's own life-style, rather than trying to superimpose their own values. They have adopted a life-style characterized as voluntary simplicity and have incorporated their nursing practice into this mode of living. When they talk about their own feelings about the community, their clients, and their nursing practice, it is obvious that their holistic, health-oriented practice is conducive to promoting their own health.

FUTURE IMPLICATIONS

There are already hopeful signs that Americans are becoming more involved in and committed to healthy life-styles. Many are trying weight-reduction and weight-control methods that incorporate greater concern for nutritional value and long-term benefits, for example. Spas and health clubs are not opening or expanding rapidly enough to meet the demands of people interested in exercise and athletic activity. This kind of interest and willingness to make financial investments in health-oriented activity foreshadows a community initiative to provide more public as well as private facilities. Nurses are becoming more aware of the value of physical fitness and are encouraging it for their clients. The present generation of young adults is on the crest of this important trend.

In the future, nurses and other health professionals will have to acknowledge and test new health-oriented models for their practice. The nursing curricula of the near future will incorporate methodology on health promotion and self-care for the nurse. This is already occurring gradually. Some curricula may become completely health oriented and will require the reexamination of the definition and practice of nursing. At present, most nurses who want eclectic practices incorporating techniques such as reflexology, homeopathy, or polarity must study these approaches outside of nursing. The future nursing curricula will incorporate interdisciplinary or elective opportunities to include these alternate methods. As nurses increase their range of knowledge in health-oriented fields, they will be more imaginative and creative in fostering health.

As general developments in society increase the length of life, it will be even more important for people to learn ways of increasing the quality of life. Social change is a reflection of the cumulative behavioral changes made by individuals. As more and more individuals become concerned about their own health and the health of others, they will support methods to sustain the trend toward a healthy population.

The example given in the preceding section above demonstrates a new life-style—voluntary simplicity. The rules for living a healthy life include acquiring and consuming only what you need. This requires questioning previous notions that have linked health with wealth. Until now, the affluent have had the resources to be healthier than others. Now there are people who look at affluence as unhealthy and are willing to find a new kind of communality.

SUMMARY

This chapter has defined health and disease and discussed the multiple determinants of both. Approaches to assessing and promoting health have been introduced and examples given. Promoting health is as complex as the factors that determine health. The health of each member of the population is important; efforts to promote health for the whole population will result in benefits for each person.

One of the most important tasks for nursing is to incorporate a health orientation into nursing practice. Nurses and other health professionals must act as role models by promoting their own health. In order to have credibility as health promoters, nurses must successfully advertise their own product in their own life-styles.

DISCUSSION TOPICS

1. Compare and contrast health and high-level wellness. Give examples of each.

2. Choose a client you have worked with and describe how the concept of holistic health applies or does not apply to your work with that person.

3. Describe your own life-style in regard to the components listed in the chapter. How do these patterns affect your health?

4. Select a client in your community experience and assess that person's openness to promoting his or her own health, based on the determinants from Pender (1975).

5. What are the differences between promotion and prevention? What are the similarities?

6. Select one of the subtopics under "life-style" in the health-assessment categories. (If a group is working together, each person should select a different one.) Make up 10 questions that the nurse could use to obtain useful information. (For example, "Tell me about a typical work day.")

7. Discuss the nurse's role in health education. Give two examples of health teaching you have done or are planning to do.

8. State a case for or against the use of regulation in promoting health. State a case for or against taxation in promoting health. Take the opposite position on each method.

9. Identify a constraint on health promotion and discuss some future changes that might affect it.

10. Describe the "healthy society" of the year 2000. What will your personal life-style be like? How will your nursing practice relate to the rest of the society? What changes will have to occur for the healthy society to come about?

BIBLIOGRAPHY

Allanson, J.F.: The dubious values of community health fairs: A position paper. *Health Values: Achieving High Level Wellness* 6(4), 17–19, 1982.

Ansari, R., et al.: Ethnic group response to preventive health education. *Urban Health* 11(6), 33–48, 1982.

Ardell, D.B., ed.: *High level wellness.* Emmanus, Pa.: Rodale Press, 1977.

Ardell, D.B.: John Travis: Doctor of wellness. In E. Bauman, et al., eds.: *The holistic health handbook.* Berkeley, Calif.: And/Or Press, 1978.

Bauman, E., et al., eds.: *The holistic health handbook.* Berkeley, Calif.: And/Or Press, 1978.

Bauman, E., et al., ed.: *The holistic health lifebook.* Berkeley, Calif.: And/Or Press, 1981.

Belloc, N.C., & Breslow, L.: The relation of physical health status and health practices. *Preventive Medicine* 1, 409–421, 1972.

Bezold, C.: Health care in the U.S.: Four alternative futures. *The Futurist* 16(4), 14–18, 1982.

Blum, H.L.: *Planning for Health.* New York: Human Sciences Press, 1974.

Boots, S., & Hogan, C.: Creative movement and health. *Topics in Clinical Nursing* 3(2), 23–31, 1981.

Carlaw, R.W., & DiAngelis, N.M.: Promoting health and preventing disease—Some thoughts for HMO's. *Health Education Quarterly* 9(1), 81–93, 1982.

Carlson, R.J.: Holistic health: Will the promise be realized? In E. Bauman, et al., eds., *The holistic health lifebook.* Berkeley, Calif.: And/Or Press, 1981.

Cordes, S.M.: Assessing health care needs: Elements and processes. *Family and Community Health* 1(2), 1–16, 1978.

Diekelmann, N.: *Primary health care of the well adult.* New York: McGraw-Hill, 1977.

Dilloway, D., & Kenny, P.A.: National health service: A new concept in health-care delivery. In E. Bauman, et al., eds., *The holistic health lifebook.* Berkeley, Calif.: And/Or Press, 1981.

Downey, A.M.: Living, loving and losing: Implications for health and well-being. *Health Values: Achieving High Level Wellness* 7(1), 7–14, 1983.

Dubos, R.: *The mirage of health.* New York: Doubleday, 1959.

Dubos, R.: *Torch of life.* New York: Trident Press, 1962.

Dubos, R.: *Man adapting.* New Haven, Conn.: Yale University Press, 1965.

Dunn, H.L.: What high-level wellness means. *Health Values: Achieving High-Level Wellness* 1(1), 9–16, 1977.

Dunton, S.: Evaluating a risk reduction program: Well aware about health, a controlled clinical trial of health assessment and behavior modification. In M.M. Faber & A.M. Reinhardt, eds., *Promoting health through risk reduction.* New York: Macmillan, 1982.

Dwore, R.B., & Kreuter, M.W.: Reinforcing the case for health promotion. *Family and Community Health* 2(4), 103–119, 1980.

Faber, M.M.: Sharing responsibility: The new health care partnership. In M.M. Faber & A.M. Reinhardt, eds., *Promoting health through risk reduction.* New York: Macmillan, 1982.

Faber, M.M., & Reinhardt, A.M., eds.: *Promoting health through risk reduction.* New York: Macmillan, 1982.

Ferguson, T.: Medical self care: Self responsibility for health. In P.A.R. Flynn, ed., *The healing continuum.* Bowie, Md.: Brady, 1980.

Fink, D.: Holistic health: The evolution of western medicine. In P.A.R. Flynn, ed., *The healing continuum.* Bowie, Md.: Brady, 1980.

Flynn, P.A.R.: *Holistic health.* Bowie, Md.: Brady, 1980.

Ford, L.C.: Influencing health values. *Health Values: Achieving High-Level Wellness* 1(1), 17–22, 1977.

Halfman, M.A., & Hoynacki, L.H.: Exercise and the maintenance of health. *Topics in Clinical Nursing* 3(2), 1–10, 1981.

Hallal, J.C.: The relationship of health beliefs, health locus of control, and self concept to the practice of breast self-examination in adult women. *Nursing Research* 31(3), 137–142, 1982.

Hancock, T.: Beyond health care: Creating a healthy future. *The Futurist* 16(4), 4–13, 1982.

Healthy people: The Surgeon General's report on health promotion and disease prevention. Washington, D.C.: U.S. Government Printing Office, 1979.

Hettler, B.: Wellness promotion on a university campus. *Family and Community Health* 3(1), 77–95, 1980.

Hilario, M., & James, S.M.: The children of Blythe Street. *Nursing Outlook* 30(3), 175–177, 1982.

Holmes, T.H., & Rahe, R.H.: The social readjustment rating scale. *Journal of Psychosomatic Research* 11, 213–218, 1967.

Hojnacki, L.H.: Fitness evaluation. *Topics in Clinical Nursing* 3(2), 11–22, 1981.

Israel, B.A.: Social networks and health status: Linking theory, research, and practice. *Patient Counselling and Health Education* 4(2), 65–79, 1982.

Jaffe, R.M.: Health in the 80's: Toward optimum human existence. In F. Feather, ed., *Through the 80's: Thinking globally, acting locally.* Washington, D.C.: World Future Society, 1980.

Knobel, R.J.: Health promotion and disease prevention: Improving health while conserving resources. *Family and Community Health* 5(4), 16–27, 1983.

Kreuter, M.W., et al.: Moral sensitivity in health promotion. *Health Education* 13(6), 11–13, 1982.

LaLonde, M.: The traditional view of the health field. In P.A.R. Flynn, ed., *The healing continuum*. Bowie, Md.: Brady, 1980.

Lancaster, J., ed.: *Change and health promoting activities for the 1980's. Family and Community Health* 5(4), 1983.

Leppink, H.: Health risk estimation. In M.M. Faber & A.M. Reinhardt, eds., *Promoting health through risk reduction*. New York: Macmillan, 1982.

Levine, E., & Moses, E.B.: Registered nurses today: A statistical profile. In L.H. Aiken, ed., *Nursing in the 1980's*. Philadelphia: Lippincott, 1982.

McDermott, W.: Evaluating the physician and his technology. *Daedalus* 106(1), 136, 1977.

Milio, N.: A framework for prevention: Changing health-damaging to health-generating life patterns. *American Journal of Public Health* 66(5), 435–439, 1976.

Miller, P., et al: Development of a health attitude scale. *Nursing Research* 31(3), 132–136, 1982.

Mulligan, J.E.: Contributions of the women's health movement. *Topics in Clinical Nursing* 4(4), 1–9, 1983.

Murphy, M.M.: Why won't they shape up? Resistance to the promotion of health. *Canadian Journal of Public Health* 73(6), 427–430, 1982.

Naisbitt, J.: *Megatrends*. New York: Warner, 1982.

Nelson, E.C., & Simmons, J.J.: Health promotion—The second public health revolution: Promise or threat? *Family and Community Health* 5(4), 1–15, 1983.

Pelletier, K.: Toward a holistic medicine. In P.A.R. Flynn, ed., *The healing continuum*. Bowie, Md.: Brady, 1980.

Pender, N.J.: A conceptual model for preventive health behavior. *Nursing Outlook* 23(6), 385–390, 1975.

Pender, N.J.: *Health promotion in nursing practice*. Norwalk, Conn.: Appleton-Century-Crofts, 1982.

Pill, R., & Stott, N.C.H.: Relationship between health locus of control and belief in the relevance of lifestyle to health. *Patient Counselling and Health Education* 3(3), 95–99, 1981.

Popkess-Vawter, S.A.: Holistic weight control. *Nurse Practitioner* 7(4), 26–29, 1982.

Rentmeester, K.L., & Hall, J.B.: Organizing a community for health promotion. In M.M. Faber & A.M. Reinhardt, eds., *Promoting health through risk reduction*. New York: Macmillan, 1982.

Sedgwick, R., & Hildebrand, S.: Family health assessment. *Nurse Practitioner* 6(2), 37–54, 1981.

Shamansky, S.L., & Clausen, C.L.: Levels of prevention: Examination of the concept. *Nursing Outlook* 28(2), 104–108, 1980.

Shephard, R.J., et al.: Health hazard appraisal—The influence of an employee fitness program. *Canadian Journal of Public Health* 73(3), 183–187, 1982.

Silverman, J.: On the meta-physical aspect of health care: Attitudes, values, and other thoughts we use to think. *Family and Community Health* 3(2), 93–103, 1980.

Snyder, R.D.: Health hazard appraisal. *The Futurist* 16(4), 25–29, 1982.

Tausig, M.: Measuring life events. *Journal of Health and Social Behavior* 23(1), 52–64, 1982.

Travis, J.W.: Wellness education: A new model for health. In P.A.R. Flynn, ed., *The healing continuum*. Bowie, Md.: Brady, 1980.

Wagner, E.H., et al.: An assessment of health hazard/health risk appraisal. *American Journal of Public Health* 72(4), 347–352, 1982.

Wallston, K.A., et al.: Development of the multidimensional health locus of control (MHLC) scales. *Health Education Monographs* 6, 160–170, 1978.

Young, R.: *Community nursing workbook: Family as client*. Norwalk, Conn.: Appleton-Century-Crofts, 1982.

ASSESSMENT TOOLS

This list is provided for information only and does not constitute endorsement or recommendation of any of the tools.

John Travis, M.D.
Wellness Resource Center
42 Miller Avenue
Mill Valley, CA 94941
(*Wellness Workbook* and Wellness Inventory)

Institute for Lifestyle Improvement
University of Wisconsin-Stevens Point Foundation
2100 Main Street
Stevens Point, WI 54481
(Lifestyle Assessment Questionnaire)

Medical Datamation
Southwest and Harrison
Bellevue, OH 44811
(Health Hazard Appraisal and computer evaluation)

Pacific Research Systems
P.O. Box 64218
Los Angeles, CA 90064
(Nutrition, Health and Activity Profile; Computer evaluation and information.)

Prospective Medicine, Inc.
3901 N. Meridian
Indianapolis, IN 46208
(*Prospective Medicine* includes Health Hazard Appraisal for self-scoring)

In addition, the following Bibliography entries include health assessment guides:

Ardell, D.B. (1977): Wellness–Worseness Continuum
Bauman, E., et al. (1981): Lifestyle Survey
Diekelman, N. (1977): Health History
Flynn, P.A.R. (1980)
Hettler, B. (1980): Lifestyle Assessment Questionnaire
Holmes, T.H., & Rahe, R.H. (1967): Social Readjustment Rating Scale
Sedgwick, R., & Hildebrand, S. (1981): Family Profile
Young, R. (1982): Several specialized assessment guides in addition to assessment tools for each developmental level

RESOURCES FOR HEALTH STATISTICS

Center for Disease Control
Atlanta, GA 30333

Clearinghouse for Occupational Safety and Health
4676 Columbia Parkway
Cincinnati, OH 45226

Consumer Information Center
Pueblo, CO 81009

National Clearinghouse for Mental Health Information
5600 Fishers Lane
Rockville, MD 20857

National Clearinghouse on Alcohol Information
P.O. Box 2345
Rockville, MD 20852

National Clearinghouse on Drug Abuse Information
5600 Fishers Lane
Rockville, MD 20857

National Institutes of Health
Bethesda, MD 20205

Office of Health Information and Health Promotion
200 Independence Ave. S.W.
Washington, D.C. 20201

Technical Information Center for Smoking and Health
5600 Fishers Lane
Rockville, MD 20857

U.S. Bureau of Labor Statistics

U.S. Census Bureau

24

Network Analysis

Ruth Kramer Young

The family only represents one aspect, however important an aspect, of a human being's functions and activities . . . . A life is beautiful and ideal or the reverse, only when we have taken into our consideration the social as well as the family relationship.

HAVELOCK ELLIS

OBJECTIVES

After reading this chapter, you should be able to:

☐ Identify and discuss environmental factors that influence a client's health and illness.

☐ Describe the network analysis model.

☐ Discuss application of the network analysis model by the community health nurse when the client is an individual, a family, or a larger entity, such as a neighborhood, city, state, or country.

☐ Compare and contrast present and future implications for use of the network analysis model.

INTRODUCTION

Community health nursing practice involves viewing an individual as part of a social system that is influenced by the physical and social environments. The practice of community health nursing involves knowledge of the individual client's total systems, including health and illness fac-tors. In nursing, we now recognize that a problem in any area of a client's life, whether biological or social, can cause problems in other areas. In community health nursing, this principle is demonstrated whether the nurse works with an individual, a family, a neighborhood, or larger entity such as city, state, or country. Isolated data must be interpreted in terms of other related data, whether on the individual level, such as a hemoglobin report, or on a national level, such as an epidemic of influenza. The community health nurse classifies each bit of data as either particularistic or general. To facilitate this, the nurse uses a conceptual model to describe the essential features of a health care situation. The use of a model makes it easier to know what is significant in each situation.

Historically, nurses have defined the nursing role in terms of the environmental factors that have affected the health needs of an individual, family, or larger entity. As early as the 1870s, nurses in New York City recognized that many of their clients' illnesses were caused by economic and social problems, such as inadequate housing and food, poor sanitation, and unfair labor conditions. In 1893, New York immigrants made up 42 percent of the total population and 63 percent of the inhabitants of slum districts. Nearly 30 million immigrants entered the United States between 1910 and 1920. Of all the large cities, New York was perhaps the most concerned with problems experienced by these immigrants (Dolan, 1978; Kalisch & Kalisch, 1978).

Nurses responded to these environmental problems. For example, Lillian Wald (1867–1940) made a profound contribution to the development of community health nursing through her work in New York City. In 1893, she was instrumental in establishing a visiting nurse service as a part of the Henry Street Settlement in New York City. In 1902 she persuaded the city council to adopt a full-time school nursing program for a community health nurse. She also persuaded the Metropolitan Life Insurance Company in 1909 to begin what became a highly successful program of home nursing service for its policyholders. Finally, in 1912 she became the first president of the National Organization for Public Health

Nursing, which became part of the National League for Nursing in 1952 (Dolan, 1978; Kalisch and Kalisch, 1978).

As scientific discoveries and technological development occurred, the role of nursing changed. Community health nurses have adapted new knowledge about understanding, treating, and preventing health problems, into their nursing practice.

ENVIRONMENTAL DETERMINANTS AND COMMUNITY HEALTH NURSING

People interact continually with their physical and social environments, and these environments play an important role both in health and illness. A comprehensive model for the community health nurse to use in gathering data is shown in Figure 24.1.

The *physical environment* includes information about the location: urban versus rural, climate and geography, resources, and industrial attributes. Industrial pollution or rural dust storms may affect clients' health. A dry climate may be more healthful for an individual with allergies than a humid one.

Technology and resources are specific to the historical period as it affects the community in which the client resides. For example, community health nursing practice in places such as Appalachia, Indian reservations, or remote villages in Alaska are affected by the limits of transportation, which results in the need to airlift clients and nurses on occasion to tertiary care centers. Whether the most current methods for caring for the sick and maintaining individual health are available within the client's environment will affect the nurse's approach to health and illness care. Technology and resources include methods of

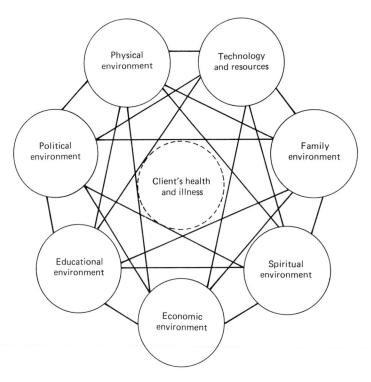

Figure 24.1   Interacting environmental determinants.

transportation and communication; availability of electricity and safe water system; and access to airports, television, and mechanical devices commonly used in and near major medical centers, such as dialysis machines, infusion pumps, and nuclear-powered hearts.

The *political environment* includes leadership, legislation, and public policies that affect health care services. Further, whether there is war or peace is an important factor in the health of a community.

The *educational environment* concerns society's systems for educating its members. Education determines health care knowledge as well as awareness of health needs and utilization of health care. Informal and formal education are the major channels for dissemination of new health care knowl-

edge. For the nurse to be effective, he or she must be a credible part of a community's informal and formal systems of health care education. Clients' reception of health teaching is affected by their cultural beliefs regarding who should teach and who is expected to learn. Finally, the level of educational sophistication that individuals have regarding health and illness influences their motivation and readiness to learn.

The *economic environment* sets the outer limits of a community's participation in the mainstream of American life, where wealth is a critical determinant of health and of availability of needed health services within reasonable geographical limits. The economic environment affects the community's life-style, which enhances or detracts from physical well-being. Who has adequate resources and who does not? How many people do not have adequate resources? Is there a system for helping those who have no means of obtaining food, shelter, and health care?

The *family environment* constitutes the parameters for family norms: roles, behaviors, responsibilities, and so on. These parameters shape the expectations family members have about their own families. These expectations include health and illness behavior, whether it is permissible to be sick, to go to a physician or nurse, to take medication, to be hospitalized, and to receive innoculations. Different family units attach varying meanings to food, clothing, shelter, and economic well-being. Diverse family values and economic levels complicate the nurse's role.

The *spiritual environment* refers to the religious, philosophical, and ethnic beliefs that heavily influence health and illness care decisions. How individuals view significant events such as birth and death in part reveals their spiritual beliefs and practices as they are related to health care maintenance and treatment of illness. The spiritual environment provides one way for the individual to interpret significant events and especially influences decisions about whether to maintain an active or passive stance in responding to life's vicissitudes.

Consideration of all environmental determinants, as shown in Figure 24.1, assists the nurse in making a more accurate assessment and therefore facilitates a more productive implementation of the nursing process. The cycle of assessment, planning, implementation, and evaluation requires information about all dimensions of the environment. These environmental factors set the background for the individual client's own personal network interaction.

INTEGRATION OF NETWORK ANALYSIS

In using the network analysis approach, the nurse attempts to determine the client's existing network of relationship interactions and the existing or potential resources for help present within the network that are available when needed by the client. The client for the community health nurse can be an individual, a family, a neighborhood, or a larger entity.

The Individual Client

The community health nurse most typically initiates interaction with an individual client rather than with a whole family unit. In using network analysis, the logical progression is to move from basic information about the individual to information about the individual's network of significant relationships. *Network analysis* is a method of determining what the client's significant relationships are and of describing these fully in order to provide optimal care for the client. Personal groups in which the individual client has significant relationships are identified. This network of groups, which includes all of the individual's meaningful community ties, typically includes the family, the kinship group, the work group, the neighborhood group, and the social group. Figure 24.2 shows the individual in relation to his or her personal and institutional resources. The client's perceived closeness to personal and institutional resources is a function of five factors: identification, affiliation, duration, intensity, and extensiveness of the relationship. Personal and institutional resources can operate singularly or collaboratively, and each can assist with time, money, facilities, knowledge, availability, and geographic proximity. The community health nurse of-

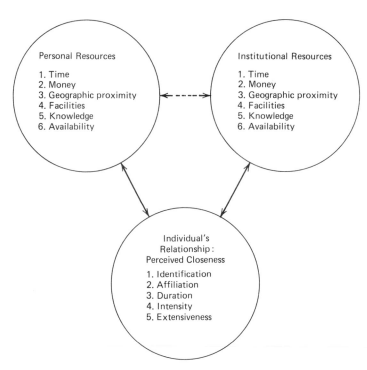

Figure 24.2   Network analysis: individual relationship to personal and institutional resources.

ten promotes articulation between the client and his or her potential personal and institutional resources.

The nurse of the future will need to orchestrate networks to aid clients even more than now, because of the breakdown of family and community ties and the increasing indifference of institutional structures, especially during difficult economic times. The interacting environmental determinants (shown in Figure 24.1) are the broad sociological determinants of the institutional and personal resources (Figure 24.2). Figure 24.1 shows the large-scale (macro) perspective; Figure 24.2 shows the small-scale (micro) perspective for the network analysis model. The connection between the client and the client's personal and institutional resources is largely dependent on the client's willingness to tap the available resources. This willingness is a result of past experiences that show the client that reassurance, nurturance, and assistance will probably follow the request for help. In a broader way, the environmental determinants influence the personal interaction of all individuals within the environment, including that of the client.

Network analysis is basically a perspective that focuses on structured relationships between individuals or collectivities. An individual is connected with others by different kinds of relationships. These connections to others constitute the individual's social network (MacElveen, 1978). Within an individual's network, a variety of relationships typically exists to meet different needs. Network analysis provides a systematic way for the community health nurse to gather data about the client and to organize this information. It is especially valid in periods of social change.

A *community* may be defined as a social system whose members experience significant relationships with each other (Parsons, 1960). Each individual has a unique network of communities. A community's boundaries may be determined by kinship, geographical, ethnic, religious, economic, or political groupings. Nisbet (1966) defines "community" as a fusion of feeling and thought, of tradition and commitment, of membership and volition. He states further that the archetype of a community, both historically and symbolically, is the family. Individuals are members of more than one community at a time. The nurse first identifies the communities to which an individual client belongs and then formulates a data base that includes information about the beliefs, norms, and overall support systems of that individual. The network of communities for an individual could include kinship group, church group, friendship group, work group, or some other type of group in which the individual finds significant relationships. In these groups, the individual runs into trouble, gains support and encouragement, experiences health and illness, develops his or her identity, and has an opportunity to realize his or her potential.

The Family as Client

The family unit is often the community health nurse's client. When a family is the client, the family is viewed as a functioning system. The nursing process is applied in a way that considers each individual and the interaction patterns among family members. Using network analysis with a family as client involves assessing the social network of each family member and of the family as a unit. The resulting constellation of networks of individual family members comprises the family network system. As general systems theory indicates, an individual family member's relationships and interactions within any given group included in his or her social network affects other members of the family.

With the family as client, the nurse's initial referral might have regarded a problem such as diabetes or child abuse. In either of these examples, the original contact would be with individual family members, and then the nurse would move toward finding out about and helping the whole family, since an individual's illness or problem affects the whole family system.

Figures 24.1 and 24.2 also apply when working with a family as client. Assessing the interacting environmental determinants gives the community health nurse a macroperspective of the family's environmental influences and resources. Assessment of all family members' relationship networks regarding perceived closeness to personal and institutional resources provides a microperspective of the family situation.

Larger Entity as Client

When the client is a larger entity such as a neighborhood, city, state, or country, the nurse can apply network analysis in order to obtain the desired outcome, whether it is resolution or control of an identified problem or prevention of potential problems. The initial reason for the nurse's involvement may vary from an outbreak of infectious hepatitis to natural disasters such as floods, tornadoes, or hurricanes.

The social network of a neighborhood, city, state, or country is more complex and larger in scope than that of an individual or family. This social network is made up of individuals and groups who have responsibilities to maintain the activities of the five social institutions: government, economics, education, religion, and family. The environmental factors of place (physical environment) and time in history (technology and resources) are the environmental determinants that the nurse should define first, since they have a profound influence on the interaction patterns of the five social institutions within the environment. In general, leaders, followers, and participants take part in the interaction patterns within these social institutions that comprise the total social network of neighborhood, city, state, or country. In gathering data about the network of the entity considered as a client, the nurse needs to determine the role of each social institution and the individuals and groups that have the most influence on other members. A large entity requires a macroperspective in assessment.

Types of Communities and Network Analysis

Countries, states, cities, and neighborhoods are all communities that influence each other and differ in size, scope and complexity. They may have some of the same health problems. The community health nurse may be responsible for health care problems in any of these communities. As one moves from the individual and family to the nationwide level, the nurse's role involves statistical, public relations, legal, and policy making activities.

For the community health nurse of the present and future, integrating different community types with opposing special interests remains a difficult challenge. Figure 24.3 shows the change in characteristics of clients as the nurse moves from individual and family to larger entities. These charac-

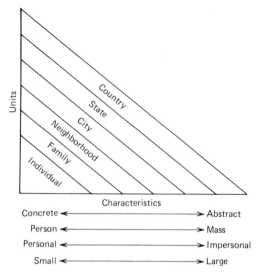

Figure 24.3 Network analysis: units for application and their contrasting characteristics.

teristics may be viewed on a continuum. For example, the nurse's role becomes more abstract and less concrete as one moves toward the national level. Further, one goes from the concerns and needs of a particular person to those of a mass of people, society at large. There is a personal relationship as contrasted to an impersonal, often bureaucratic relationship as the nurse moves from working with an individual or family to working with a nationwide aggregate.

Individuals, families, neighborhoods, cities, states, and countries have many common health and illness determinants and consequences. Network analysis suggests many connections among communities of different types and ways of analyzing these connections. For example, the identified environmental determinants affect families as well as larger groups of people. Existing social networks can be identified for all types of clients when needed for maintaining health or resolving health problems.

FUTURE IMPLICATIONS

For the future-oriented nurse, analysis of community networks for clients is essential for activating the resource support needed for the health care of clients. Clients are often mobile, have multiple health needs, often have unstable personal relationships, and live in environments where institutional regulations governing assistance change rapidly. Fragmented networks are more likely to occur in the future, as economic dislocations affect clients' relationships and health statuses. Development of client coping abilities and building supportive networks may be a large part of what community health nurses will be expected to do in the future.

With clients having increasingly complex and fluid relationships, the nurse will be asked to describe and evaluate clients' networks with increased sophistication and specificity. Computerized systems for rapid network analysis based on forced-choice questions are likely to be developed. Nurses will need skill in computer data management and quantitative applications of systems analysis in order to work effectively in communities in the future. Technological education will become imperative under these circumstances.

Technology will impel the community health nurse to work with aggregate health needs of larger population groups, especially in view of the identification of national health care problems. Statistical competencies, such as analytic and computational skills, will be required if nurses are to retain their traditional domain. As more and more of the usual community health nursing clientele becomes concerned about self-care, there will be a shift in emphasis toward more teaching and providing more information to clients than ever before.

Naisbitt (1982) states that American society is moving from an industrial society to an information society in which wealth is based on the creation and distribution of information. He states further that this new information society will be highly influenced by what he terms "high tech/high touch." By this he means that new technology introduced into our society must be counterbalanced with the introduction of human response. If this new technology, or high tech, is not accompanied by humanizing aspects, or high touch, it will be rejected. The community health nurse is in a unique position to provide this high touch to balance the high tech in health and illness care. By considering individual needs and situations, the community health nurse can utilize social networks to maximize human response to technological developments.

Since nurses are facilitators of communication and of the mobilization of health care activities, they will become even more active in wedding technology and concern for aggregate care. For networks to function, facilitators are essential. Advances in technology and familiarity with technology will enable nurses to adopt macroperspectives in responding to the health needs of aggregates.

Bezold (1982, p. 14) states that "there is no one set future for the health care system in the United States. Rather, the future will be shaped by current trends in society at large and in the field of health care and by the choices we make." Nursing must develop models that will provide us with the tools we need to meet the challenges of the future. The network analysis model will help us focus on clients' existing and evolving networks. This will enable us to adapt the nursing process to the health and illness problems the future brings.

SUMMARY

Network analysis permits the community health nurse to examine a client's relationships in a dynamic rather than a static capacity. Sociological variables such as perceived closeness, potential for resources, and resource availability related to location may differ for different clients or the same client over time. The community health nurse can measure or estimate the relative importance of various relationships as they affect the ability of a client's network members to be of assistance.

Network analysis is a mechanism for ordering the potential overflow of random information about a client and his or her environment. It provides a systematic approach to assessment that can be adapted to different kinds of clients with different kinds of health problems. Such a structure simplifies the nurse's role without oversimplifying the client's situation.

Network analysis is a practical tool for community nursing practice since it can be applied with various kinds of clients including individuals, families, neighborhoods, cities, states, or countries. It can also be used for better understanding of various time periods in history. It can be used to understand client interaction patterns and nursing practice in the past, to apply the nursing process with the present client, or as part of a futuristic approach when we are trying to prepare models that will prepare us for the application of the nursing process in the future.

DISCUSSION TOPICS

1. What environmental factors influence your own health and illness?

2. How can network analysis help the community health nurse of the future in his or her work with clients?

3. Why will it be increasingly important in the future to understand a client's broader network, including factors relating to all environmental determinants?

4. Describe a hypothetical or real client situation and explain how you could use network analysis for assessment and planning care.

BIBLIOGRAPHY

Bezold, C.: Health care in the U.S.: Four alternative futures. *The Futurist* 16(4), 14–18, 1982.

Dolan, J.A.: *Nursing in society: A historical perspective.* Philadelphia: Saunders, 1978.

Ferguson, M.: *The aquarian conspiracy: Personal and social transformation in the 1980s.* Los Angeles: J.P. Tarcher, 1980.

Hancock, T.: Beyond health care. *The Futurist* 16(4), 4–13, 1982.

Hazzard, M.E.: An overview of systems theory. *Nursing Clinics of North America* 6(3), 385–393, 1971.

Kalisch, P.A., & Kalisch, B.J.: *The advance of American nursing.* Boston: Little, Brown, 1978.

MacElveen, P.M.: Social networks. In D.C. Longo & R.A. Williams, eds., *Clinical practice in phychosocial assessment and intervention.* New York: Appleton-Century-Crofts, 1978.

Naisbitt, J.: *Megatrends: Ten new directions transforming our lives.* New York: Warner, 1982.

Nisbet, R.A.: *The sociological tradition.* New York: Basic Books, 1966.

Parsons, T.: *Structure and process in modern societies.* New York: Free Press, 1960.

Wellman, B.: The community question: The ultimate networks of East Yorkers. *American Journal of Sociology* 84(5), 1201–1227, 1979.

Wellman, B., & Leighton, B.: Networks, neighborhoods and communities: Approaches to the study of the community question. *Urban Affairs Quarterly* 14(3), 363–390, 1979.

Young, R.K.: *Community nursing workbook: Family as client.* Norwalk, Conn.: Appleton-Century-Crofts, 1982.

PART III
NURSING WITH AGGREGATE POPULATIONS

Concern for the health of populations was an early focus of nursing in the community when it was known as public health nursing. The field is experiencing a resurgence of interest in health issues that have an impact on populations. Part III deals with issues that affect entire communities as well as cities, states, and the nation.

Chapters 28 and 29 cover basic tools in considering health on a wide scope: statistics and epidemiology. These chapters introduce the ways in which these tools are used in assessing and describing the health and health problems of populations.

Chapter 26 describes the influence of various levels of government on health care issues and discusses the role of nursing in governmental processes. Chapters 25, 27, and 30 discuss community assessment, environmental health, and health planning. Each chapter emphasizes the role of nurses, particularly how nurses can be involved in promoting healthy environments for large populations.

25

Community Assessment

Thomas H. Cook, Dorothy Jacobson Baker,
and Sherry L. Shamansky

Conscience is the guardian in the individual of the rules
which the community has evolved for its own preservation.
WILLIAM SOMERSET MAUGHAM

OBJECTIVES

After reading this chapter, you should be able to:

☐ Develop an operational definition of "community."
☐ Differentiate between client assessment and community assessment.
☐ Delineate the steps in the community assessment process.
☐ Recognize the parallels between inductive systematic inquiry and community assessment.
☐ Discuss situations in which community assessment strategies are applicable.
☐ Recognize the limits of community assessment in light of available time, energy, and other resources.

INTRODUCTION

This chapter on community assessment differs from others in two ways. First, it is guided by teaching–learning principles: learners must perceive the goals of the learning experience to be their goals (Knowles, 1977); learners must demonstrate a need to learn (Redman, 1976); goals must be clear and achievable (Redman, 1976); learners must participate in selecting and planning what they are learning (Postman & Weingartner, 1969); new material must be based on what the learner already knows; and differences and similarities of content are highlighted (Redman, 1976); and new material must not repeat previously developed information (Postman & Weingartner, 1969).

Second, the material presented is only

447

that which is relevant to the beginning student of community assessment. It is not always feasible for the beginner to complete an assessment, determine a plan, and develop interventions at the community level in the brief time of a community health nursing rotation; hence, information on planning and intervention are not included in this chapter. Remarks focus on how to select a community for study and emphasize the *process* of community assessment. A review of community health nursing literature reveals a multitude of definitions of community, a variety of community assessment strategies, and a blurring of the differences between the student experience and the professional experience. The literature states that community assessment is done to determine the health problems of a given community (Tinkham & Voorhies, 1977), that community assessment determines what needs exist, what goals are achievable, and what resources are available. The literature further states that community assessment is done to analyze the way existing community services meet the identified nursing needs of the community or to determine the priority of nursing needs within a designated community (Tinkham & Voorhies, 1977). However, it seems unreasonable to expect a student to do this because it often leaves the nursing student with an overwhelming feeling of confusion about where to begin and what needs to be accomplished.

THE WHAT AND WHY OF COMMUNITY ASSESSMENT

Moe (1977) has defined community in a manner which is most functional. He states that a community is "people and the relationships that emerge among them as they develop and use in common some agencies and institutions and a physical environment" (p. 128). *Community assessment*, then, is the process by which nurses estimate the magnitude of selected health problems in a selected community. Both the definition and the steps in this process will be elaborated later in this chapter. *Community diagnosis* is the summary statement or conclusion derived from the community assessment. It provides a description of the health status of the selected community.

Nurses should learn the skills of community assessment in order to fulfill their roles, as defined by Virginia Henderson:

Nursing is primarily helping people (sick or well) in the performance of those activities contributing to health, or its recovery (or to a peaceful death) that they would perform unaided if they had the necessary strength, will, or knowledge. It is likewise the unique contribution of nursing to help people to be independent of such assistance as soon as possible.

(Henderson & Nite, 1978, p. 34)

An example may serve to illustrate how community assessment is part of the nurse's role. Individuals who work in a common setting may have similar or related health problems that they cannot recognize as having a common etiology. They lack the knowledge to change their setting so that others are not similarly affected. The nurse who works in that setting would have the perspective to assess, plan, and treat the affected individuals and to begin to speculate about what was causing the problem in the first place. To gather data aimed at identifying group health needs is to do community assessment. To have the knowledge and skills needed to carry out community assessment is, therefore, basic to nursing practice.

Nurses have access to clients in the hospital, in their homes, in the workplace, in nursing homes, and in schools. This access, coupled with experience and perspective, logically positions them to identify group health issues. Because they work closely with the ill and see the many ramifications of disease and disability, nurses are motivated to think about prevention. Whatever nursing specialty one chooses, the skills of community assessment will help nurses look for trends and patterns in the health problems they see. By being knowledgeable about community assessment, nurses learn to collect thorough, pertinent data and plan relevant interventions aimed at preventing illness, detecting it earlier, and promoting health. Community assessment skills assist nurses in looking beyond the needs of any one individual to the actual or potential needs of groups or communities.

Community assessment skills enable nurses to conduct formal or informal projects with immediate implications for their own practice. By questioning how effective her practice in contraceptive counseling is, for example, a family planning nurse might devise methods to determine which clients are returning for counseling about an unwanted pregnancy. By determining how large that group is and what its demographic characteristics are, one might identify the need to reevaluate one's teaching strategies for a specific client or group of clients. Here, community assessment can serve as a formal data collection process whereby the nurse identifies the health needs of a given group and determines which variables are most important in practice. The process of community assessment leads logically from attention to the individual to a concern for larger health issues located in groups and communities.

LEARNING COMMUNITY ASSESSMENT

The first step in the process of caring for an individual is assessment. A plan is then formulated, and interventions are applied and evaluated for effectiveness. In the process of community assessment, the same course is followed. However, Kark (1981) outlines important differences, as shown in Table 25.1. Although the terms used (assessment and diagnosis) are the same, the process is much different in scale and complexity. In caring for an individual, the health care provider readily knows who the client is. In caring for a community, the client is more elusive. In order to care for hypertensive people in the community, one must first locate them.

Another difference is apparent in providing care to individuals and communities: access to health information. In caring for an individual client, a standard history and physical data base exists. No such standard data base exists for a community. The data-gathering process is far more laborious. The client is now a group rather than an individual; pulse and temperature readings are replaced by a series of statistical measurements—birth rates, death rates, incidence of particular diseases. A woman is pregnant or not pregnant; a community is always between 2 and 4 percent pregnant. A client does or does not have hypertension; a community always has hypertensive disease, although the rate varies (Tinkham & Voorhies, 1977).

Given the difference in individual and community health assessment, it is not always realistic for a beginning community health nursing student to expect to complete a community assessment, determine a community diagnosis, develop a plan of care, and implement and evaluate the effec-

TABLE 25.1
Comparison of Individual and Community Assessment

Clinical (individual)	Epidemiological (population group)
Examination of a patient.	Survey.
Interview and examination of individuals by history taking, physical and psychological examinations, laboratory, x-ray, and other special techniques.	State of health of community and families, using questionnaires, physical and psychological testing, and specific facilities for such investigations.
Diagnosis: Health and Illness	
Usually of a client. Differential diagnosis to determine main causes of client's complaints.	Usually problem-oriented. Differential distribution of a particular condition in the community and the causes of this distribution.
Appraisal of health status of a well person, such as a pregnant woman or well child, periodic health examinations of adults.[a]	Health status of the community as a whole or of defined segments of it, such as health of expectant mothers, growth and development of children, birth and death rates.

SOURCE: Kark, S.: *The practice of community-oriented primary health care.* New York: Appleton-Century-Crofts, 1981.

[a] Assessment includes an appraisal of both health and illness.

tiveness of that plan. What is possible, however, is to conduct an assessment in microcosm—to select a small group in which one is interested, to use the language and skills of community assessment on that group, and perhaps to plan appropriate interventions. The process of community assessment is different from most student nursing experiences in that no actual therapy is given; however, the community may derive some positive benefits, and many communities do become "healthier."

CARRYING OUT COMMUNITY ASSESSMENT

Systematic Collection of Data

The father of logical thought, Aristotle, identified two ways by which we learn—deduction and induction. Those who learn deductively do so by reasoning from the general to the particular. Many approaches to community assessment in the past have been based on deductive reasoning: for example, students have been asked to draw conclusions about families from studying data about neighborhoods.

Those who reason inductively do so by drawing general conclusions from particular occurrences. This seems to be the way most of us learn. Therefore, community health nursing students who have progressed from the care of individuals to the care of families might now best learn community assessment by studying small groups. For example, the community health nursing student might well be providing home care to a diabetic client. It is apparent that the student should examine the effect of this long-term illness upon the family members. A logical question, then, is "How many other diabetic individuals and families are similarly affected in the larger community?"

The profession of nursing shares with other sciences the process of systematic inquiry or problem solving. There is a set of recognized steps in the formal scientific method of inquiry. These include: (1) understanding the problem, which necessitates delimiting, defining, and describing it; (2) collecting data; (3) formulating a hypothesis; (4) evaluating the hypothesis; (5) testing the hypothesis; and (6) developing conclusions.

These steps are part of the research process, the nursing process, and other problem-solving approaches. Thus community assessment includes the same systematic approach, beginning with sorting and classifying information, comparing and analyzing relationships among the facts, and summarizing data in order to arrive at a logical conclusion about the community's disparate parts.

Little and Carnevali define the nursing assessment as

a compact information seeking and giving transaction between two or more people involving subjective and objective data, usually in predetermined categories relevant to nursing care. It is, at least on the part of the nurse, a skilled activity requiring thinking and observing as well as interpersonal activity (verbal and nonverbal) in which the direction of observation and the nature of responses are modified on an ongoing basis in accordance with the data being received. At the same time, the Nursing Assessment requires the nurse to behave toward the client in a manner which successfully initiates the relationship needed to deal effectively with the problems of health and illness.

(Little & Carnevali, 1976, p. 97)

Assessment is assessment, whether it be individual or community. However, there is no such thing as a routine assessment. In every situation, new information is organized according to the most accurate and productive set of relationships.

IDENTIFYING A POPULATION

The community assessment assignment is designed to help the nursing student develop a concern for ways of reaching everyone in a population—those who seek help and those who do not. The student will seek to answer the following questions: How can groups at risk for developing problems be identified? How can the problems common to a designated group be defined? Williams states that

there is more to community health nursing than family-oriented care delivered outside the institutional setting; it's a matter of focus on group health problems, present and projected, in contrast to individual, clinically oriented care.

(Williams, 1977, p. 250)

It follows, then, that one begins with the question "Who are included in the group?" or, "Who are included in the community?" People are the "who" at the heart of an operational definition of community. This dimension of community includes information about socioeconomic and demographic characteristics, together with ethnocultural factors, values, and ideals. The people factors go hand in hand with the spatial and temporal considerations about a community (the "where" and "when"). Any collection of people is influenced by the passage of time and space. Space is often defined by well-established boundaries, such as census tracts, neighborhoods, counties, or other familiar designations. Finally, every community has a purpose (the "why" and "how" dimensions) which usually includes such needs as support, participation, socialization, or the production, distribution, and consumption of goods (Shamansky & Pesznecker, 1981).

ASSESSING A GIVEN COMMUNITY

In carrying out the assessment, you should select a community that is accessible, a health problem of interest to you, and one for which data are obtainable.

Selecting a Community

1. Select an age group of particular interest.
2. Select a health problem of particular interest in that age group.
3. Select a community in which the given age group with the given health problem can be found.
4. Briefly describe the community you have chosen. Why are you calling it a "community"? Using the most recent data you can locate, what is the size of your community? What are the demographic characteristics of your community: the age, sex, and racial distribution? If appropriate, what can you say about birth and death rates in your community? How has your chosen community changed in the last 10 years?

Analyzing a Health Problem

Now that the community has been located and described, the next step is to analyze the health problem that affects it.

1. Through a brief literature review, examine the natural history of the selected health problem in the at-risk group (etiology, signs and symptoms, diagnosis.)

2. Determine what other populations are at risk for this problem; determine the basis for these risks. Why have you chosen the group you did? Is it at highest risk? Do demographic characteristics, such as age, sex, and race, seem to make a difference in what is known about the risks for this particular problem?
3. Determine whether environmental factors, occupational factors, or behavioral factors contribute to the risk of this problem and if so, how.
4. Determine the appropriate health indicators to apply to the group at risk: morbidity or mortality rates, disability days, indices of nutritional status, measures of population pressures such as crime statistics.
5. Use the correct epidemiologic methods to gather the necessary data.
6. Discuss pitfalls in interpreting the data.

Having determined the magnitude of the problem in the designated community, the next step is to review what is already known about treatment for this health problem.

1. What approaches to treatment have been used in the past? Were they effective? Why? Why not?
2. What primary prevention strategies (risk reduction) have been employed?
3. What secondary prevention strategies (early diagnosis and treatment) have been employed?
4. What tertiary prevention strategies (reduction of long-term disability) have been employed?
5. Conduct a brief survey of health resources available in the community for the at-risk group.

Formulating a Diagnosis

Finally, formulate a diagnosis based on your assessment of the target group. How would you describe the health status of your selected community at this point in time? What are the implications of your diagnosis?

ONE NURSE'S EXPERIENCE IN COMMUNITY ASSESSMENT

Many examples serve to illustrate the application of community assessment. A pediatric nurse-practitioner (PNP) working in a neighborhood health center screened all toddlers for lead poisoning. During one week in the late spring, she noticed an upsurge in the frequency of elevated lead levels. She began to wonder whether there were any patterns discernible in these cases. Here her community was a group of toddlers, all of whom were apparently exposed to an environmental risk factor: lead-based paint. The ages of the toddlers ranged from 11 months to 29 months; boys and girls were equally affected. The cases were divided between black and Hispanic children.

The children were not related to each other by blood. None lived in the same house. When the environmental health expert analyzed the samples of paint taken from each of the homes, none of the paint chips contained lead. The literature clearly shows that toddlers are the group at greatest risk of permanent damage; therefore, the source of this exposure had to be located. Although lead poisoning can cause death among small children, illness (specifically, neurological damage), is the more common result. This group could be described in terms of the morbidity related to

the health hazard rather than its mortality.

Now it was time for the detective work. What other common factors existed among this group? A careful record review revealed that all of the children lived within four blocks of one another. It was also noted that in all cases, the parents of those toddlers worked full-time. Listed on all of the records was a name of the babysitter. Here was the common source. All of the children shared the same babysitter, whose apartment contained many areas where paint and plaster were peeling off the walls. Analysis of these samples revealed dangerous levels of lead.

This finding paved the way for a variety of strategies for prevention at all levels, primary, secondary, and tertiary. The landlord was forced to paint the apartment, thereby reducing further risk for the children. At the same time, parents of the toddlers, along with the babysitter, were counseled about pica, or the habit of chewing nonfood substances. Safety and appropriate toys were discussed. The original screening done by the PNP is an example of secondary prevention, or early detection. None of the children required treatment, so tertiary prevention was not necessary at this time.

In this example the nurse began to think beyond the one child in her examining room. The question "How many others are there like this one?" led her to a community diagnosis: toddlers at risk for lead poisoning secondary to a commonly shared environmental hazard. A logical, systematic appraisal of each of the dimensions of who, where, when, why, and how of community assessment followed. The nurse described a problem she was interested in, collected data about it, formulated, tested, and evaluated a hypothesis, and developed a diagnosis that directed her interventions toward a significant health problem.

FUTURE IMPLICATIONS

Community assessment, regardless of any future changes in the nature of communities, must be approached in the logical and systematic manner we have set forth in this chapter. The age, sex, and racial distribution of given populations will change. Some form of national health insurance, a cure for cancer, and the threat of nuclear war, could all change the face of society. But whatever the world looks like 50 or 100 years from now, populations can still be assessed using the operational definition of community we have provided as well as the assessment steps we have outlined. That should provide some level of comfort: knowing that however the "community" appears in the future, it can still be evaluated in terms of its who, when, where, why, and how.

SUMMARY

This chapter has illustrated the differences and similarities between assessment of an individual and assessment of a group, outlined how to choose a community to study, and indicated some of the variables that should be considered when defining the magnitude of a health problem in a given community. Having discussed how community assessment is a part of nursing practice, the chapter described the process of performing an assessment. It provided an operational definition (who, why and how, where and when) and examples. The effort throughout was to emphasize the process of community assessment rather than the product. Finally, the authors suggested that whatever the future of the community, the steps of logical thinking and systematic inquiry will provide a reasonable and responsible approach to that community's assessment.

DISCUSSION TOPICS

During an informal discussion with the community health instructor, a student in community health nursing commented on the number of class members who were smoking cigarettes. The student and instructor began to wonder whether smoking was perceived as a problem among the other students and, if so, what could be done about it.

1. What data would the student need in order to decide whether smoking is a serious problem in this age group?

2. How would the student determine the magnitude of the problem?

3. What diseases are associated with smoking?

4. Given the natural history of these diseases, when might college students develop symptoms?

5. What environmental risk factors are associated with smoking in college-age students?

6. What other information should be considered in developing a list of risk factors associated with smoking?

7. What are the students' health beliefs about smoking?

8. What trends and patterns are apparent in smoking behavior in this group?

9. What are the overt and covert sanctions concerning smoking, both positive and negative?

10. How would you organize this material to describe the problem, determine its magnitude, and develop a diagnosis?

BIBLIOGRAPHY

Henderson, V., & Nite, G.: *Principles and practice of nursing* (6th ed.). New York: Macmillan, 1978.

Kark, S.: *The practice of community-oriented primary health care.* New York: Appleton-Century-Crofts, 1981.

Knowles, M.: *The modern practice of adult education.* New York: Associated Press, 1977.

Little, D., & Carnevali, D.: *Nursing care planning* (2nd ed.). Philadelphia: Lippincott, 1976.

Moe, E.O.: Nature of today's community. In A.M. Reinhardt & M.D. Quinn, eds., *Current practice in family-centered community nursing* (Vol. 1). St. Louis: Mosby, 1977.

Postman, N., & Weingartner, C.: *Teaching as a subversive activity.* New York: Dell, 1969.

Redman, B.: *The process of patient teaching in nursing* (3rd ed.). St. Louis: Mosby, 1976.

Shamansky, S., & Pesznecker, B.: A community is. . . . *Nursing Outlook* 29, 182–185, 1981.

Tinkham, C., & Voorhies, E.: *Community health nursing evolution and process* (2nd ed.). New York: Appleton-Century-Crofts, 1977.

Williams, C.: Community health nursing—What is it? *Nursing Outlook* 25, 250–254, 1977.

26

Governmental Influences

Yoshiko Shimamoto

Democracy, which shuts the past against the poet, opens the future before him.

ALEXIS DE TOCQUEVILLE

OBJECTIVES

After reading this chapter, you should be able to:

☐ Describe the role of government in influencing nursing and the health care delivery system.
☐ Describe the effect of local, state, and federal legislation on nursing.
☐ Describe the process by which a bill becomes a law.
☐ Describe the ways in which nurses can influence legislation.

INTRODUCTION

Nursing as an organized, legislated system would not exist as it does now without the influence of government. Who is the government? The government is the people whom nurses serve. It is this public that accords nursing the privilege to serve. It is important to keep this in our minds as we carry out our nursing practices. The government or the people give nursing the license to serve. The various levels of government, with their licensing mechanisms and financing of health care, all have profound influences on nursing and tend to set the parameters of the profession unless nursing can interpret to the people its nature and values.

HISTORICAL BACKGROUND

Human beings are social, interdependent beings. Living in social groupings, we have been prey to epidemic diseases. In antiquity, Greeks and the Romans were involved in personal hygiene practices and in sanitation. Religious groups also contributed

456

greatly in providing public health by their commitment to serving others.

When Henry VIII ruled England during the sixteenth century, municipalities assumed the responsibility for the ill and cared for them in infirmaries. During the seventeenth century, John Graunt introduced the concept of vital statistics. By statute, the Elizabethan Poor Law in 1601 laid the basis for care of the lame, impotent, old, and blind. During the colonial period, Massachusetts passed laws providing for the isolation of smallpox victims and the quarantine of ships and passengers.

In 1846 the first public health act was passed after Edwin Chadwick made such a recommendation in his "Report of the Sanitary Conditions of the Labouring Population and on the Means of Its Improvement" (1842). Yellow fever and cholera were the two catalysts to such social and sanitary reform. Boards of health were established in the late eighteenth and early nineteenth centuries in New York, Massachusetts, Connecticut, Virginia, Philadelphia, and other cities and states.

The Marine Hospital Service was created by Congress in 1798 and became the United States Public Health Service in 1912. The principles of public health practice, including sanitary regulation, immunizations, and health education, were recommendations taken from the "Report of the Sanitary Commission of Massachusetts" (1850) by Lemuel Shattuck.

States gathered at quarantine conventions to establish a uniform code for maritime quarantine. One of the byproducts of these conventions was the American Public Health Association, which was established in 1872 with Dr. Stephen Smith as its first president. The organization is still active today. Its Public Health Nursing Section, to which many community health nurses belong, has a large membership.

A devastating yellow fever epidemic in 1879 served as an impetus to the formation of a national board of health. It passed out of existence, perhaps because of the controversy over state versus federal authority, four years later.

With the discovery of the vaccine in the eighteenth century, the United States passed laws requiring immunization for smallpox; there were stringent quarantine laws for many diseases by 1915. In 1912 the Children's Bureau was created by the federal government to be responsible for the welfare of all children in the United States. Later the Maternity and Infancy Act of 1921 and the Social Security Act of 1935 were passed. Physical examinations were required for school children in the early 1920s, and the federal government started school lunch programs to combat malnutrition. The United States Labor Department, formed in 1913, investigated the health of workers. By 1910 most states had occupational health programs.

Financing mechanisms for health care evolved on a voluntary basis. Compulsory health insurance in the form of Medicare in 1965 provided benefits to persons age 65 or older.

GOVERNMENTAL STRUCTURE IN THE DELIVERY OF HEALTH CARE

Health care as a basic commodity essential to all people is a matter of concern to all levels of the governmental structure. The roles and responsibilities of the United States government are carried out by three branches: Congress, a bicameral legislature that makes laws; the executive branch, headed by the president and aided by a cabinet of secretaries who are responsible for carrying out the intent of the Constitution;

and the judicial branch, composed of the Supreme Court and other federal courts that interpret the Constitution. This distribution of functions is also found at the state and local levels.

States are individual units of one nation. Certain powers are delegated to the federal government and prohibited to the states. The Supreme Court decides when questions of states' rights arise. The United States government handles interstate issues and problems that are beyond the control of the states. In 1953 the United States Department of Health, Education and Welfare was created and took over the Federal Security Agency. It is now the Department of Health and Human Resources and is responsible for all health functions.

Each state has a constitution and has the responsibility to protect the health of its people. The governing body of each state health department adopts regulations that are monitored and enforced by appointed officials. Each department of health in each state has a health officer and a board of health, all appointed by the governor. The key role of the health officer is to maintain relationships with the governor and the legislature. The board serves in an advisory capacity. It represents the public and helps establish policy. The state health department supports local health units that provide services to local communities.

Local health units must meet the needs of the community by providing the leadership for comprehensive health services and delivering such services. Local health units operate on limited tax resources and look to the state unit to support them with adequate financing. The federal government also assists in financing the state health units by awarding grants.

All health departments establish policies that affect the functioning of community health nurses. These policies are set to enable staff members to carry out the objectives of the health department. They must conform to laws, statutes, and ordinances as well as meet expectations of the public, based on local traditions and mores.

With the increasing rate of change in society, a nurse may find certain policies obsolete. Because of his or her understanding of the bases of certain policies and review of local and state laws and regulations, a nurse may bring information to the health officer via appropriate channels to instigate change in policies that may hinder effective nursing practices.

MAJOR HEALTH LEGISLATION

In the twentieth century, the expansion in the volume and variety of federal health legislation has had a major impact on community health nursing practice. Over the years the federal government has increased its role in influencing the health care practices of local and state governments. The intent of all this legislation has been to integrate health programs at all levels and to strengthen the roles of the local and state units as effective instruments of health policy. A few of the laws will be discussed as examples of major legislation that has affected and continues to affect nursing practice.

On April 9, 1912, President Taft signed a bill establishing the Children's Bureau. Enactment of this law was recommended by two public health nurses, Lillian Wald and Florence Kelley; and it has had a profound influence on child care practices and maternity care. Over the years, infant mortality attributable to diarrhea, infectious diseases, premature births, and congenital defects has been greatly reduced. Next came the Sheppard-Towner Act of 1921, which authorized appropriations for state programs in maternity and infant care and for child care centers. This initiated federal–state–local relationships to provide maternal and infant protection. Today, public health nurses work in well-child clinics subsidized under this arrangement that provide preventive health care to mothers and children.

The Social Security Act of 1935 provided for welfare insurance and welfare assistance programs. Its categorical welfare assistance programs include Aid to the Blind (AB), Old Age Assistance (OAA), Aid to Families of Dependent Children (AFDC), Aid to the Permanently and Totally Disabled (APTD), and Old Age and Survivors Insurance (OASI). Title V of the Social Security Act was enacted into law on August 19, 1935. It provided federal aid to states for programs in maternal and child health, medical care for crippled children, and child welfare services (Goerke & Stebbins, 1968).

The Public Health Service Act of 1944, as amended, coordinates national public health legislation. It provides financing for the building of health care facilities, traineeships for health care professionals such as nurse training acts, and traineeships for graduate students in public health, grants-in-aid to schools of public health, national comprehensive health planning and resource development, and the development of health maintenance organizations. It also provides for health services for migratory workers, family planning services, communicable disease control, emergency medical services, and research facilities for the prevention and control of conditions such as heart disease, cancer, stroke, kidney disease, sudden infant death syndrome, arthritis, Cooley's anemia, sickle cell anemia, and diabetes mellitus (Goerke & Stebbins, 1968).

The Economic Opportunity Act of 1964 was known as the law to fight poverty. As an antipoverty program, it established the Office of Economic Opportunity (OEO), authorized Volunteers in Service to America (VISTA), the Job Corps, Upward Bound, Neighborhood Youth Corps, Head Start, neighborhood health centers and community action programs (CAPs). Neighborhood health centers offer comprehensive health care easily accessible and available to residents. Operation Head Start, for preschoolers, offered health examinations, follow-up care for adverse health conditions, dental treatment, free lunches, and health education through parent participation.

In 1965 amendments to the Social Security Act provided for the establishment of Medicare (Title XVIII) and the health assistance program of Medicaid (Title XIX). Medicare consists of two parts, A and B. Under part A, anyone over 65 years of age who applies for Medicare is covered for hospital insurance prepaid through Social Security contributions. Part B is medical insurance, and the insured individual pays the required premium. Over the years the basic structure and benefits under Medicare have not changed, except for the amount in the deductibles and the amount of premiums paid for part B.

Medicaid covers medical costs for all persons who are eligible for federally aided public assistance programs—the aged, the blind, the disabled, and families receiving AFDC assistance. Some states also include medically indigent children under the age of 21 years (Hanlon, 1974).

In 1971 the Comprehensive Health Manpower Training Act and the Nurse Training Act provided assistance to increase health manpower. The aim of these acts was to increase the number of practicing physicians to 436,000 by 1978 and the number of nurses to 1.1 million by 1980. Schools were awarded special funds if they pledged to increase student enrollment. These acts also provided direct loans of up to $3,500 and $2,500 a year to medical and nursing students. There was a provision for loan forgiveness if the students agreed to work two years in an area suffering from manpower shortage (Wilner, Price, & O'Neill, 1978). The 1982 federal support for nursing education as well as research and special projects fell below $50 million, compared to $106 million in 1981.

In 1974 the passage of the National Health Planning and Resource Development Act combined aspects of the Hill-Burton Act, the Regional Medical Programs Act, and the Comprehensive Health Planning Act into a single new program of state and local planning and development featuring a national network of Health System Agencies (HSAs). Congress identified health care problems, such as lack of uniformly effective methods of health care delivery, maldistribution of health care facilities and manpower, and increased costs of health care. To correct these problems, this act covered underserved areas, coordination and consolidation of institutional health services, development of group practices, use of physician assistants and nurse clinicians, sharing of support services, promotion of preventive activities, adoption of uniform cost accounting, and effective methods of health education (Novello, 1976).

This is a representative sample of major health legislation that has greatly influenced nursing practice. To carry out legal and current nursing practices, the community health nurse must be continually aware of changes in existing laws and introduction of new laws. To be knowledgeable about current health legislation is as important as being abreast of new medical and clinical nursing practice.

THE LEGISLATIVE PROCESS

Health care laws are made by the people, through their legislators. Community health nurses who have the health of the people in mind, as they serve the community, are keenly aware of the health needs of the population they serve. Nurses can bring these needs to the attention of legislators and be instrumental in creating laws that can meet these health needs. They can participate and affect legislation by being familiar with and involved in the process.

The role of the government in influencing health care can be seen by analyzing the delivery system. The majority of community health nurses work for official agencies and hence derive their income from official bodies. Clients' health care is greatly influenced by third-party payers; reimbursement by the government is a major funding source. This demonstrates the importance of community health nurses having a working knowledge of the political and financial systems that directly influence the parameters of community health nursing practice. When change is indicated, these parameters can be altered only by an understanding of and involvement in the legislative process.

Federal Level

The real work of Congress occurs in the office buildings that flank the Capitol rather than on the floors of the House of Representatives and Senate. The House is divided into 22 standing committees; the Senate has 18 similar committees.

A bill or legislative proposal sponsored by one or more members of Congress is introduced when it is dropped into the "hopper," a large box set up on the floor in the House or Senate. The bill is referred to the appropriate committee, where it may die quietly unless it has strong backing from committee members or the president. The committee members and their staffs decide which bills deserve further consideration. These bills are studied to determine further action. Public hearings are scheduled, at which time official witnesses and private citizens are heard. At this point in the process, constituents communicate with legislators about their opinions of bills under consideration. The committee amends and refines the bill and sends it to the House or Senate floor. The bill is identified with a number prefaced by SR or HR to indicate its origin. It is accompanied by a House Report or Senate Report.

The House rules committee is the legislative traffic director. This committee reviews and approves bills before they reach the House floor and decides whether amendments can be offered on the floor, what form the bill will take, as well as how long the bill can be debated. The Senate does not have a rules committee; its bills go straight to the Senate floor. After debate, which in the Senate is not limited in time and after which amendments may have been made, the bill is approved or disapproved. When a bill is passed by the House or Senate, it is sent to the other body for consideration. Both Senate and House must pass the bill in identical form before it becomes a law. If there is disagreement about the bill, a joint conference committee appointed by House and Senate leaders try to reconcile differences. The modified bill is sent back to both chambers for a final vote. If the differences are irreconcilable, the bill dies in conference.

When the bill is approved, it is sent to the president. If the president signs it, it becomes public law and the legislative process is completed. If the president rejects (vetoes) the bill, Congress can overrule him by a two-thirds vote of both houses.

If a law requires federal spending, Congress must adopt an authorizing bill that may contain a spending limit and a time limit. After this authorization and the signing of the law, Congress introduces an appropriation bill to fund the program. This is usually done for one fiscal year, which starts on October 1. The president may delay spending by deferral or by asking Congress to rescind legislation that has been passed (Nathanson, 1975).

State Level

The states' governments are arranged in three branches of government—executive, legislative, and judicial—like the federal government. The legislative processes carried out in each state are similar to those of the federal government.

A bill is a proposal to the legislature. If and when it is approved, it becomes a law of the state. Each state has a state constitution that must be consistent with the federal Constitution.

A bill may be drafted by a private individual, an organization, a legislator, a lawyer, or a legislative reference bureau. It is introduced in the legislature by a legislator. The bill is assigned a number by the chief clerk. After the first reading, it is printed and referred to an appropriate committee to be studied. The public may testify at a public hearing sponsored by the committee. The bill must pass the second and third readings in both houses. If there are differences between the houses, a joint conference is held and compromises made. The bill is sent to the governor, who signs it or vetoes it. If the bill is signed, it becomes a law and is prepared for publication.

Local Level

The state legislature creates local units of government. The various local units vary from one section of the country to another. The primary units of local government are the city, village, township, county, and special-purpose district. Local units have no legislative powers. They have limited authority to enact certain local ordinances. Ordinances are local laws or regulations enacted by a city council or other similar body under powers delegated to it by the state.

THE IMPACT OF GOVERNMENT ON NURSING

The federal and state governments have had a direct influence on nursing practice in the areas of manpower, licensing, research, and the delivery of health care.

Manpower

A major manpower problem in the health field across the nation is the shortage of nurses. Since 1963 several national commissions have conducted major studies of health manpower and have made recommendations concerning nursing education and services. As a result, nursing, along with other health disciplines, has received federal support, such as the Nurse Training Act of 1964 and the Health Manpower Act of 1968. Currently the Institute of Medicine of the National Academy of Sciences has a committee to study the role of the federal government in nursing education. This is a mandate of the Nurse Training Act Amendment of 1979, Section 113. The recommendations of this committee will determine whether there is a need to continue specific programs to support nursing education. The results of this study will be the basis for further governmental support of nursing.

Under the Division of Nursing, Health Resources Administration, Bureau of Health Manpower, schools of nursing have received and are receiving federal assistance for special projects, graduate and practitioner programs, traineeships, and student loans and capitation grants. With the recent drastic cutback in the federal budget, nursing has suffered greatly. Students have lost traineeships for graduate education, particularly in the field of psychiatric nursing. Support for practitioner programs has also been eroded. Schools of nursing that depended heavily on capitation grants for support services now must do without this aid.

Licensing

The most direct way in which government influences the delivery of nursing care is in the licensing mechanism. All nurses must obtain a registered nurse license in the state in which they practice. One of the functions of a profession is to determine credentials for its members, its educational programs, and the organizations that utilize its professional services. The profession sets standards for licensing individuals for entry into professional practice and into specialty practice and for institutions that offer educational programs to prepare people for entry into professional practice and specialty practice (Study of Credentialing in Nursing, 1979). The nurse practice act of each state defines nursing and establishes the minimum knowledge and competency necessary to ensure the health, safety, and welfare of the consumer:

Licensure is a process by which an agency of state government grants permission to individuals accountable for the practice of a profession to engage in the practice of that profession and prohibits all others from legally doing so. It permits use of a particular title. Its purpose is to protect the public by ensuring a minimum level of professional competence.

(Study of Credentialing in Nursing, 1979, p. 266)

Before the twentieth century, anyone could legally call himself or herself a nurse without any requirement for formal education, state examination, or state license. In 1903, North Carolina became the first state to register nurses. In that same year, New York also passed a law that called for "inspectors" to ensure minimal standards for nursing education.

Each state has a board of nursing that is a department or unit of state government created by the legislature to administer the nurse practice act. The following are elements of nurse practice acts (Notter & Spalding, 1976):

Definition of nursing.

Identification of qualifications for nursing.

Procedure for approval of nursing schools.

Procedure for state examinations.

Requirements for license issuance and renewal.

Procedure and grounds for complaint and license revocation.

Stipulations about reciprocal licensure.

State laws have differing regulations for licensure. Although certification of nurses beyond the recognized minimum competencies is the function of the American Nurses' Association and should not be included in the licensure laws, 36 state acts refer to specific "categories" of nurses, such as pediatric nurse associates and practitioners. Therefore, a nurse falling within a specific category must be cognizant of such requirements and parameters of practice.

The board has considerable power in carrying out the intent of the law to safeguard the consumer. The board has the power to revoke, suspend, or renew any license or to place on probation or discipline a licensee because of violations of the act or rules and regulations of the board pertaining to nursing practice.

"Sunset laws" have been adopted by many states that require that all government agencies and programs undergo periodic review and evaluation and that those not necessary to the governmental processes be abolished or modified. The purpose of the sunset law is to guarantee meaningful and thoughtful program evaluation. This process has direct implications for the current licensure and regulatory activities of state boards of nursing. The New Hampshire State Board of Nursing was "sunsetted" in the 1981–1982 legislature. Nurses in that state pooled their efforts and were able to reinstate the act and the Board of Nursing during the following session. A last-minute Senate bill in the 1981 legislative session in Texas saved the nursing board from suffering the effect of the sunset law. All legal authorization for the board was due to end in August 1982. The bill extended the operations of the board through 1993.

Research

Nursing research received a significant push in 1955 with the Special Nurse Research Fellowship Program in the National Institute of Health, Division of Nursing (Batey, 1973). The objectives of the Division of Nursing, Bureau of Health Manpower at the Health Resources Administration, Public Health Service are improved client care and well-being through systematic study of problems in nursing education, practice, and administration. Under the Nursing Research Grants Program, three types of grants are available: (1) regular research projects, (2) research conference grants to communicate findings to the professional and scientific community, and (3) institutional research projects to strengthen institutions in the development of sound research. Since 1955, much federally supported nursing research has been done.

Results of research have improved client care. In publications distributed via the Public Health Service publication of the United States Government Printing Office research projects that are supported by the Division of Nursing are listed and described. These research projects cover organization, distribution and delivery of nursing services, recruitment, selection, education and characteristics of the nurse supply, and research development.

Besides funding, the government figures significantly in all research in the protection of the rights of human subjects. Federal funding agencies, institutions, and universities have systematic procedures to assure that the rights of human subjects are protected. Applications for federal funds are not reviewed until the project has been cleared at a local level by an institutional review committee (Diers, 1979).

National Health Insurance

The government has a long history of interest and involvement in the financing of health care. The first movement for government health insurance was launched by the American Association for Labor Legislation in 1915 in New York State. This movement received strong support from the State Federation of Labor, civic and women's organizations, and Governor Alfred E. Smith. It was opposed by merchants and the medical society. With the reaction to socialism and "Bolshevism" which permeated society at that time, it was impossible to enact any type of health insurance. Since that time, other attempts have been made to enact government health insurance, including a provision of the Social Security Act of 1935. That endeavor was shelved after opposition from the American Medical Association. The Wagner-Murray-Dingell bill for national health insurance was introduced

during World War II but was never passed. For many years, there have been great efforts to institute national health insurance without much success. Today the United States is the only major western country without a comprehensive national health insurance program (Schroeder, 1981).

Situations in which gaps occur in the delivery and financing of health care might be remedied by a comprehensive national health insurance program. With the patchwork approach to health insurance in Medicare and Medicaid, there are clients who lack sufficient coverage for high hospital expenses or long hospital stays or long-term health care such as nursing homes. Although governmental programs have impressively increased access to medical care by the poor and the elderly, recently there has been a reduction in federally sponsored programs for the poor and the elderly as government reduces federal spending and transfers the responsibility for social welfare programs to the states. Health coverage is a political issue and decisions about health insurance will be made by political means.

The concern about rising inflationary costs of health care is a real one that has generated much activity and concern for cost containment. Because of the great financial burden to the government, the question of financing national health insurance has been an obstacle. The quest for reasonably priced, comprehensive health care that can reach all segments of American society will continue.

Community health nurses who are directly involved in delivering health care and influencing their clients to seek appropriate health care are keenly interested in the direction the government will take to improve the health care system. It is imperative that nurses know the current provisions of the law and that they become directly involved in making changes. Both the American Public Health Association and American Nurses' Association have issued statements in support of national health insurance. Through these professional organizations as well as through the legislative process, we can support movements that will make comprehensive health care available and accessible to all our clients.

CHANGE AND THE ART OF LEGISLATION

If we are to participate in the development of a health care system that is oriented to maintaining health, we must apply the principles of planned change. *Planned change* is a deliberate change effort in which those variables that make a difference in the performance of the system are identified and manipulated by the change agent (Bennis, 1969).

Change is exciting, stimulating, interesting, and enlivening. It is also hard, painful, unsettling, scary, unpredictable, and disruptive. Whether one participates in it or not, change occurs continually, often with negative effects, such as painful disruption. Nurses must participate in planned change.

How do nurses promote planned change in the governmental process? To begin, we must study the situation as we find it and envision the way we would like it to be. We must identify alternative solutions, decide what change is needed, and plan a design that will guide the change. In other words, we must employ the nursing process.

To direct the change in the governmental process, nurses must develop the art of influencing legislation. This is the way in which a concerned citizen can most effectively use political power and responsibility. There are at least three distinct phases in the art of affecting legislation. These are: (1) the presession preparation period, (2) the session activity, and (3) the activity after a bill has passed both houses of the legislature.

Preparation Period

During the presession period, much preparation must be done to lay the foundation for effective action. The initial task is to define the program accurately and concisely. Does the program affect a large segment of the population, and does it have their approval? Is it easily definable and explainable? Is it practical and can it be financed through available state funds?

Other information that will be needed is:

1. What is the problem of concern?
2. What are the facts or statistics underlying the problem?
3. What are the alternative solutions to the problem?
4. What solutions have already been attempted?
5. Which alternative solution is the most feasible?
6. Why is it most feasible?
7. Why should government instead of private groups or organizations undertake the program?
8. What will be the effect of this program on other programs or groups?
9. How much will it cost?
10. Is there a need for specially trained personnel or for special facilities?
11. Are such skills and facilities available?
12. Where are the funds to come from?
13. What is the experience of other states that have attempted the same kind of solution?

It is important to anticipate the answers to questions that will be posed and to formulate responses before making the presentation. The proposal should be put in writing.

The next step is to seek a legislator who is sympathetic to the program and have that person draft the bill. Simultaneously, it is advantageous to take a political survey of friends, co-workers, colleagues, and other associates who are active in party politics. This will help to determine who is a supporter, friend, or constituent of what legislators and who might support the proposed program. Encourage these people to become involved with their district representatives, and tell them how to go about it. Legislators listen and respond to their friends, supporters, and constituents.

If there is a particular program the professional association or nursing community is supporting, it may be possible to get the program into the party platform. The political parties are most amenable to suggestions before the beginning of a political campaign when the platform is being drafted, especially if the proposal affects a large number of voters. Once the legislators convene, it is easier to promote the program if it is part of the party platform. If the program fits into an existing department in the governmental structure, the supporters should try to persuade the department head to include it in the administrative program. Passage of the program through the legislature is facilitated if it is part of an existing program. It is essential to obtain support in writing from as wide a base as possible within the community. This includes other organizations that have an interest in the program. The strength of a bill is often measured by the number of voters who support it.

Lobbying is the main tool citizens use to affect legislation. Lobbying includes activities such as engaging in personal contacts or the dissemination of information with the objective of influencing public officials and members of a legislative body. To work effectively, one must work closely with a professional organization. The organization may have a legislative committee and one must work with the committee and the assigned lobbyist. Get to know the legislators, their track records, and their legislative synopses. Know their backgrounds, interests, occupations, friends, and positions in the legislature. It also helps to know legislators' administrative assistants, since often the assistants can expedite the process, provide information, and notify you about upcoming hearings.

Contacts with legislators should begin before the legislative session begins. Once the session begins, legislators are under tremendous pressures and may be too harassed to listen and talk to constituents in a relaxed manner. Members of the organization who are friends of the legislators should be assigned to them. Other members can be assigned to specific legislators: the Republican to the Republican, the Democrat to the Democrat, and the constituent to the representative. The following points will be helpful in making the meeting with the legislator most effective:

1. Always make an appointment by phone or letter and outline issues you plan to discuss.

2. Be prompt for the appointment and identify yourself.

3. Be prepared to present the issues directly and concisely. Take no longer than 15 minutes. Offer suggestions and possible solutions to problems. These should be presented in a written statement including facts and data supporting your position.

4. Ask for the support of the legislator; commend the legislator for his or her support.

5. Offer to provide additional information or do any necessary follow-up.

6. Show appreciation for the time and attention given.

Correspondence with the legislator is important. This is an effective way to inform a legislator of your feelings on the issues and bills before the legislature. Letter writing can be an effective form of lobbying. These suggestions for letters can serve as a quick checklist:

1. Address the letter correctly. For Congress: Representative _____, U.S. House of Representatives, Washington, D.C. 20515; Senator _____, United States Senate, Washington, D.C. 20510. For state senate, delegate, or assembly members, write care of your state capital.

2. Mention your state and congressional or legislative voting district. Also give affiliations, when appropriate, such as the state nurses' association.

3. Specifically cite legislation by bill number or name. If you are unsure of this, briefly describe the issue pending legislation.

4. Explain how you perceive the bill and how it will affect the community and nursing or other groups. State clearly whether you are for or against the bill.

5. Write when the issue is current, not after a key vote has been taken.

6. Urge the legislator to take action and request a response to the letter. You are entitled to know the position of the legislator on the issue.

7. A one-page letter is usually the most effective. Address only one issue per letter.

8. Mail the letter right away.

9. Thank the legislator for support for the bill (How to Meet with Your Legislator, 1981).

During the Session

During the session, find the proper sponsorship for the bill. The best person to introduce the bill will be the speaker of the house, the president of the senate, a chairperson of a committee, or a majority legislative leader in either house. Try to get a sponsor who will wholeheartedly support the bill and will be willing to fight for it. Have the bill introduced in both houses. Maintain contact with the chairperson of the committee to which the bill is referred after its introduction. You will want to know the number of the bill and its status in its passage through both houses. Continue to indicate an interest in the bill and press for an early public hearing. Attend the hearing and present your case. The following are guidelines in preparing testimony:

1. Be prepared to discuss:
   a. What the bill is about.
   b. What the cost of the program is.
   c. How the program can be financed.
   d. What public interest can be served by the bill.
   e. Who will be affected by the bill.
   f. What other states have similar legislation.
   g. What significant groups favor or oppose the bill and why.

2. Keep the testimony brief. One page is sufficient.

3. Be prepared to submit whatever number of written copies of the testimony the committee may request.

4. If you do not know the answer to the question, offer to look it up and send in the answer. Be sure to follow through on this.

5. Represent an organization or numbers of people whenever possible.

6. Find someone who lives in the same district and is of the same political party as the chairperson of the committee to present the testimony.

7. Attach data as an appendix. Do not give many detailed statistics in the body of the testimony.

8. Type testimony triple spaced so it can be easily read.

9. Give positive views. Be polite and respectful.

10. Read your testimony first. When questioned, address the chairperson first.

11. Do not antagonize a questioner or get into an argument.

12. Get other people and organizations to testify in favor of the bill.

Follow the bill through the various committees and maintain contacts with chairpersons and committee members. Discuss the status of the bill with friendly legislators to determine the bottlenecks and legislators who are opposed to the bill so that you can contact them. The most effective method of influencing them is through personal contacts by their constituents, party members, or friends. Obtain favorable newspaper publicity for the bill. Be present in the gallery to indicate interest as well as offer moral support to the legislators who have supported the bill.

Follow-up Activity

Develop a strong relationship with the executive branch, since the governor may veto the bill. See the governor and explain the bill. Let the governor know which organizations are supporting it. After the bill becomes law, be sure to thank the governor, the legislators, and organizations and individuals who supported it. Our form of government is predicated on active and intelli-gent citizen participation. If the system is to work effectively, one must participate in the political and legislative process.

An Example

The following is an example of strategic planning in the legislative process to promote nursing aims in one state. This particular state board of nursing had difficulty in interpreting limits of function of aides and in offering legislative assurance to independent nurse-practitioners because of ambiguities in the nurse practice act. The nurses felt that major changes were needed in the act. A nurse practice act coalition was formed with representatives from the board of nursing, the professional organization, the union (which was a separate body allied to the professional organization and representing the majority of nurses in the state), and other health care organizations encompassing a broad base of nurses in the community. For two years this coalition carried on research and received information from various sources on ways to revise the act.

The act was then presented to all nurses in their various work settings, discussed at the annual nurses' convention, and shared with other professional groups to elicit their support. The legislative lobbyist from the nurses' organization approached the chairman of the consumer affairs committee in the legislature and asked him to introduce the bill. The chairman felt that he could not wholeheartedly support the bill because it called for a nurse as executive secretary to the board. Having a nurse as executive secretary was in direct contradiction to the current practice of the state's department of regulatory agencies, and that department was not in favor of having a nurse as executive secretary. The committee chairman also felt that a nurse practice act should rightfully be introduced as an administrative bill.

In testing out the political waters before introducing the bill, the coalition withdrew its action to introduce the bill in this particular session. The coalition then worked with the board to introduce the bill as an administrative bill and to compromise on the issue of the qualifications of the executive secretary to the board. This compromise allowed the coalition to accomplish some of its goals. In politics tradeoffs are part of the game.

FUTURE IMPLICATIONS

As long as governmental structures have existed, the government has affected and influenced the provision of health care services. At the beginning of this century, the government licensed nurses to ensure minimum safety in nursing practice. In programs such as Medicare and Medicaid, the government greatly influences the provision and financing of health care. If continued discussion and promotion of national health insurance by the American Nurses' Association and the American Public Health Association are successful in establishing such a program, this will have a vast impact on health care delivery in the future. Government influence in nursing practice is omnipresent. Nurses must actively participate in governmental processes as they affect nursing.

In *The Third Wave* (1981), Alvin Toffler observes that it is no longer possible for one person to represent a "majority." Our society has become too diverse for people to mass into a uniform group that allows us to predict their positions on emerging issues. Although one might assume that such diversity always leads to conflict, such fervor and interest can actually strengthen our so-

ciety. If many people have different but compatible goals, they can accomplish much more by collaborating than by struggling to extinguish each other.

Toffler hypothesizes about the use of voting in an altogether new fashion. Instead of voting yes or no on an issue, citizens would have the power to negotiate with their votes. For example, if the county were trying to expand the services of the department of health and asked for a tax increase, a voter would be able to communicate a counterproposal. The voter might specify that he or she was willing to support an increase in taxes if the health department would extend services into an underserved area of concern to the voter. Another possibility might be that the voter could agree to support the tax increase, but would specify that part be used for the health department and part be used for some other county improvement. With the increasing sophistication of computers and their availability to many more citizens, this type of polling could be done from the citizen's own home, or from a convenient location at a time of the voter's choosing. This would move us toward the participatory government that so many people have as their ideal of democracy.

Another strategy for changing our present system is Toffler's approach of "decision division." This concept recognizes that the locus of decision making is not static. Some decisions should be made at a national level; however, many decisions that should be made by state or local governments are now in the hands of Congress. By the same token, there are issues that now are within the purview of the states that might be better served by making them national issues. For example, some threats to health are controlled by state laws and by state bodies. However, because of the mobility of the American population, severe problems can occur if states have diverse methods of reporting and treating health problems that are easily transmitted. In such instances, nationally regulated investigation and reporting of such ailments may be appropriate. On the other hand, state regulation is appropriate for health problems that are apt to be confined to a specific state or region and that are not communicable.

Health-related decisions that affect large numbers of citizens regardless of their residence and that may have some implications for constitutionally guaranteed rights should be controlled by the Federal government. An obvious example of this would be whether or not the choice of abortion is the right of the woman involved. The future may bring us other dilemmas in which we must decide whether or not health care is a right, and if so, who is responsible for ensuring that everyone's rights are protected.

The government-supported health care of the future is likely to be a system that provides publicly financed community health centers that are primarily geared to maintenance of good health. These centers would be administered and staffed by nurses especially prepared in primary prevention strategies. People are already taking more responsibility for improving their life-styles. In the future, government support in the form of tax breaks and low-cost health maintenance insurance may further encourage this development. Those who experience illnesses that are highly correlated to an unhealthy life-style would have to take more personal responsibility in paying for their acute and chronic care. Their "illness insurance" would require much higher premiums than "wellness insurance."

As people become more concerned about health and illness care, they will also become more concerned about the accreditation and licensure of those who provide services in both areas. Government on all levels, but especially on local levels, will be responsible for instituting and maintaining the boards involved in accreditation and licensure on an even broader scale than presently. There will be greater consumer participation in the accreditation process, and this will be provided for by changes in the laws that determine the composition of accreditation and licensing boards. Nurses will be in the forefront of those who will educate the public about appropriate expectations for health care professionals.

The teaching skills nurses have always learned will enable them to help consumers increase their involvement in their own health care. In a system where health is public policy, many more nurses will become involved in community-based practice in endeavors such as teaching health care skills in workshops for lay persons, managing community health centers, and supervising community health aides. Community residents will not only expect their local governments to facilitate such developments, they will also be assertive in planning and implementing health programs that are government supported and are community based. There will be a greater sense of involvement, and citizens will use their governmental structures as tools rather than consider them as obstacles to be surmounted.

SUMMARY

Government influences on nursing include the licensing mechanism, the funding of health care and of nursing research, and the passage of laws that affect health and illness care. The future invites us to make the government more responsive to our changing needs and life-styles. As government evolves, the relationship between nursing and government will also evolve. Nurses can have a strategic role in determining the direction and outcome of the governmental impact on the delivery of health care and the treatment of disease.

DISCUSSION TOPICS

1. Several nurses are planning to form a partnership to establish a private for-profit agency to administer community nursing services. What state laws would affect their ability to establish such an agency? If there are restrictive laws that prohibit them, how would they go about effecting changes in the laws to make it possible for them to establish their agency?

2. In carrying out the intent of the sunset laws, the legislature in your state has decided that there is no need for a board of nursing. How would you respond to such an action? What organizations would you work with to curb such an action? What can you do as an individual? Identify legislators whom you would contact. Plan the content of a letter to legislators. What would you say to one of them in a personal interview about the issue?

3. One consideration in planning for the future is the relationship of resources to population. The decision about allocation of resources will be a negotiable issue that may have farreaching effects. A federally funded program will grant a certain amount of money to your local community for a health-related project. One group in the community wants to build an exercise center. Another group wants to establish a stress-reduction clinic. Develop a plan to present to the funding group to win support for one of these projects. How could you develop a plan to win support for both projects?

BIBLIOGRAPHY

AFL-CIO: *When you write your legislator.* Publication #116. Author (n.d.).

Aiken, L.: *Health policy and nursing practice.* New York: McGraw-Hill, 1981.

Batey, M.V.: Reflections—And the way ahead. *Communicating Nursing Research* 6, 215–221, 1973.

Bennis, W.G.: Theory and methods in applying behavioral science to planned organizational change. In W.G. Bennis, K.D. Benne, & R. Chin, eds., *The planning of change.* New York: Holt, Rinehart & Winston, 1969.

Bezold, C.: Health care in the U.S.: Four alternative futures. *The Futurist* 16(4), 14–18, 1982.

Bloch, D., Gortner, S.R., & Sturdivant, L.W.: The nursing research grants program of the division of nursing. *Journal of Nursing Administration* 8(3), 40–45, 1978.

Blum, H.L., & Leonard, A.R.: *Public administration: A public health viewpoint.* London: Collier-Macmillan, 1963.

Cowart, M.E.: Teaching and legislative process. *Nursing Outlook* 25, 777–780, 1977.

Diers, D.: *Research in nursing practice.* Philadelphia: Lippincott, 1979.

Ellison, J.: Anticipatory democracy in action. *The Futurist* 15(6), 25–28, 1981.

Goerke, L.S., & Stebbins, E.L.: *Mustard's introduction to public health* (5th ed.). New York: Macmillan, 1968.

Goodman, L.J., & Steiber, S.R.: Public support for national health insurance. *American Journal of Public Health* 71, 1105–1107, 1981.

Hancock, T.: Beyond health care: Creating a healthy future. *The Futurist* 16(4), 4–13, 1982.

Hanlon, J.J.: *Public health administration and practice* (6th ed.). St. Louis: Mosby, 1974.

Health is a community affair—Report of the National Commission on Community Health Services. Cambridge, Mass.: Harvard University Press, 1966.

How to meet with your legislator. *The Oklahoma Nurse* 26(5), 13–14, 1981.

Klay, W.E.: Nurturing foresight in government. *The Futurist* 15(6), 25–28, 1981.

McClure, W.: National health insurance and HMOs. Nursing Outlook 21(1), 44–48, 1973.

Milio, N.: *The care of health in communities—Access for outcasts.* New York: Macmillan, 1975.

Nathanson, I.: Getting a bill through Congress. *American Journal of Nursing* 75, 1179–1181, 1975.

Notter, L.E., & Spalding, E.K.: *Professional nursing foundations, perspectives and relationships* (9th ed.). Philadelphia: Lippincott, 1976.

Novello, D.J.: The National Health Planning and Development Act. *Nursing Outlook* 24, 354–358, 1976.

Schroeder, S.E.: National health insurance—Always just around the corner? *American Journal of Public Health* 71, 1101–1102, 1981.

Stevens, B.J.: *The nurse as executive* (2nd ed.). Wakefield, Mass.: Nursing Resources, 1980.

Study of credentialing in nursing: A new approach. *Nursing Outlook* 27, 263–271, 1979.

Toffler, A.: *The third wave.* New York: Bantam, 1981.

U.S. Department of Health, Education, and Welfare: *Report on licensure and related health personnel credentialing.* DHEW Publication No. HSM 72-11, Washington, D.C., U.S. Government Printing Office, 1971.

Waddle, F.I.: *Legal regulation of nursing practice.* Kansas City, Mo.: American Nurses' Association, 1981. (Unpublished report)

Wilner, D.M., Price, R., & O'Neill, E.J.: *Introduction to public health* (7th ed.). New York: Macmillan, 1978.

27

Environmental Health Hazards

Diane J. Mancino

Man–environment interactions are characterized by continuous repatterning of both man and environment.
MARTHA E. ROGERS

OBJECTIVES

After reading this chapter, you should be able to:

☐ Identify and describe the health aspects of exposure to radiation, toxic chemical waste, and air and water pollution.
☐ Identify and describe nursing interventions that focus on prevention, identification, and treatment of illnesses related to environmental pollution.
☐ Locate additional information on specific environmental health hazards.

INTRODUCTION

The practice of nursing evolves to meet the complex health needs of the society it serves. Society's needs are dependent upon many interacting variables, one set of which is environmental factors. Our modern life-style, with its dependency on technological achievements and products, exposes large populations to disease-producing pollutants in the environment. While it is easy to recognize and appreciate the many advantages of modern living, the diseases and discomforts that result from pollution and other stresses imposed by technological achievements, increasing world population, and other sociopolitical forces cannot be overlooked.

The term *environment* is defined to include all that is external to the human body. The definition of *environmental hazards* in this chapter will be limited to artificially produced contaminants that threaten the health and well-being of humans. Because of limited space, environmental health hazards covered here are those most commonly found in the United States. Most environmental pollutants, however, do not

473

have boundaries that keep them in a specific location. Many pollutants migrate around the globe, transported in the atmosphere and the oceans. DDT and other pesticides found on the polar ice caps are examples of how pollutants can travel thousands of miles away from their points of origin.

The recognition and study of the health effects of environmental pollutants is just beginning. It takes many years for illness to appear after low-dose exposure to a pollutant that occurs over a long period of time. By the time an illness does appear, the contributing factors of the disease are not easily discernible. Long-term epidemiological and laboratory studies are currently in progress that will reveal the relationships between pollutants and health in years to come.

Until the facts are known, many authorities believe that care must be taken to identify possible environmental health threats and to eliminate them or limit human and wildlife exposure. Government regulations and enforcement of standards have become a costly bureaucratic maze as officials sort out who is responsible for the economic impact of pollution, the diseases related to exposure, and the many complex sociopolitical implications.

The role of the nursing profession and particularly the community health nurse in the prevention, identification, and care of illness caused by environmental contaminants is just beginning to be defined and implemented. Development of this role will accelerate by the end of this century as more environmentally related diseases are identified and treated. Prevention and early detection of diseases related to pollution and environmental health hazards is becoming a new specialty for community health nurses.

This chapter will explore in some detail the health implications of radiation in the environment, air pollution, water pollution, and toxic wastes and will introduce ways in which nurses have responded and can respond to these health hazards.

DEFINITION OF TERMS

Biological magnification refers to the concentration of some synthetic chemicals as they move up the food chain. As a result, organisms at the top of the food chain receive large quantities of the chemicals. For example, plankton contaminated with DDT are eaten by small fish, the small fish are eaten by larger fish, and humans eat the larger fish. Since DDT is not degraded or excreted, it remains in an animal's system. A nursing mother may pass on high dosages of DDT to a nursing infant through her breast milk.

Conservation is the preservation and protection of natural resources to extend availability and prevent destruction, exploitation, and neglect so that the resources will be available over as long a period of time as possible.

The *ecosystem* is the interaction of organisms within the environment, which sustains and regulates itself and the organisms within it. The *environment* is all that is external to the human body. This does not mean that humans are separate from the environment. Humans and all living and nonliving systems are inseparable and interdependent.

Pollution is the artificially produced contaminants that threaten the health and well-being of humans. While it is recognized that pollutants also threaten all biological, organic, and inorganic systems, only human health will be considered in this chapter.

Synergism refers to the interaction between two or more contaminants when mixed together. It is important to note that little is known about the possible health implications when two or more contaminants are mixed together to produce another compound.

RADIATION

Public awareness of the health aspects of radiation has come about as a result of the increased use of radiation. *Radiation* is energy moving through space as invisible waves. The *frequency* of these waves (the number of waves per second) helps to determine the characteristics of the radiation and how it can affect people. Frequency is also a basis for classifying radiation, such as x-rays, ultraviolet light, infrared rays, or microwaves. The frequency scale from least energetic to most energetic is called the electromagnetic spectrum (Britain, 1974).

Ionizing and nonionizing radiation are the two major categories of radiation. *Ionizing radiation* (such as x-rays and radiation found in radiopharmaceuticals and fluoroscopy) has the ability to strip electrons from atoms, creating electrically charged *ions* that are capable of disrupting the life process. Radiation which is *nonionizing*, such as microwaves, cannot create ions, but may disrupt the body processes through other means (Britain, 1974).

Since the discovery of x-rays by Wilhelm Konrad Roentgen in 1895, the discovery of radioactivity by Henri Becquerel in 1896, and the early work by Pierre and Marie Curie with radium in 1898, a vast amount of literature has explored the use and effects of ionizing radiation. Today, the medical and dental use of x-radiation accounts for over 250,000 installations in the United States alone (Purdom, 1980). A few examples of beneficial application of radiation are the application of x-rays and radioisotopes in clinical diagnosis and therapy; the use of radioisotopes in industry for measuring, testing, and processing; electric power generation; microwave cooking equipment; and lasers used in science, industry and medicine (Hafen, 1972).

Effects of Radiation on Humans

Sufficiently large doses of radiation will produce death (Trieff, 1980). Many scientists believe that there is no safe level of radiation exposure and that the threshold for biological effects varies among individuals. The federal government has strict standards and regulations for exposure to ionizing radiation, and these exposure limits are adjusted as scientific research reveals evidence that shows that exposure limits require alteration. Adverse health effects on people from exposure to ionizing radiation are believed to have a direct relationship to the amount of radiation received (Britain, 1974). Ionizing radiation exposure is cumulative—one dose adds on to the preceding dose, no matter how small (*Procedures to Minimize Diagnostic X-ray Exposure*, 1981). Therefore, it is necessary to keep exposure levels as low as reasonably achievable (ALARA) (Shapiro, 1981).

Health risks associated with ionizing radiation include cancer (particularly leukemia), genetic mutations, and damage to the fetus of a pregnant woman. While these effects are recognized, it is difficult to prove that ionizing radiation was the direct cause, since there is a latency period between exposure and symptoms (Gofman, 1981). Individual sensitivity to radiation makes it even more difficult to determine what may be a safe exposure; however, children are more sensitive to radiation than adults, and the developing fetus is highly sensitive (*Procedures to Minimize Diagnostic X-ray Exposure*, 1981).

There is evidence that diagnostic x-ray examinations resulting in exposure of the fetus increases the chance of leukemia or other cancer during childhood (Shapiro, 1981). Such injuries to the unborn are known as *somatic effects* and are limited to that particular child. *Genetic effects* result from damage to genes, which affect not only immediate offspring but future generations as well (Hafen, 1972).

Data on the effects of low-level ionizing radiation on humans come from a variety of sources, including studies of survivors of the atomic bombing of Hiroshima and Nagasaki, children exposed prenatally as a result of abdominal x-ray examination of the mother during pregnancy, children treated for enlarged thymus glands by irradiation of the thymus, adults who underwent x-ray treatment to the spine for ankylosing spondylitis, adults who received radioactive iodine for treatment of thyroid conditions, individuals with radium implants, and uranium miners exposed to high levels of radioactive gases and radioactive particles (Shapiro, 1981). Currently under investigation are the health effects to soldiers exposed to high levels of radiation during atomic weapons testing in the 1950s (J. Miller, 1982) and to persons living near radioactive materials waste storage and disposal sites such as the one in West Valley, New York.

Sources of Ionizing Radiation

Natural Background Radiation

Everyone is exposed to natural background radiation from cosmic rays and natural radioactivity from materials in the earth (soil, stones, water) and building materials (*Radiation Protection*, 1976). Background radiation exposure averages 100 millirems (mrem) per year. The range of background dose accumulated per year in the United States varies from 80–250 mrem depending on location, altitude, and geological composition. For example, in Denver, the average is 180 mrem per year. Cosmic radiation at sea level is 35–50 mrem per year.

Certain aspects of background exposure can increase this natural radiation exposure. Frequent air trips can add additional millirems because of high altitudes. Living and working in stone buildings also increases exposure because of the close contact with the stone.

X-ray Radiation

Exposure to x-rays comes from either x-ray machines (cathode ray tubes) or high-energy particle accelerators (cyclotron and betatron used for deep therapy in cancer cases) (Purdom, 1980). X-rays can penetrate opaque materials and affect a photographic film. When a photographic plate is placed behind the person radiated and then is developed, the darkening is proportional to the amount of radiation intercepted and absorbed by the plate, and this produces an image related to the internal structure of the person being examined. X-ray pictures are produced because a variable fraction of the x-ray energy is absorbed by different kinds of tissue as the x-rays penetrate the body. This absorbed energy produces a *dose distribution* in the irradiated person that has the potential for producing injury coincidental with its use in promoting health (Shapiro, 1981).

Uranium Mining, Milling, and Enrichment

The first step in the nuclear cycle is the exploration and mining of uranium ore. The earliest record of human damage from ionizing radiation dates back to the year 1500, when it was observed that the pitchblend miners of Saxony and Bohemia had a very high incidence of a fatal lung disease. In 1879 Herting and Hesse performed the first postmortems on these miners and reported malignant growths in the lungs (McKee, 1974).

The main health danger posed by mining is worker exposure to radioactivity in the form of uranium byproducts known as *radon daughters*. Radon daughters are the decay products of radon-222, a radioactive gas formed from the natural decay of radium found along with uranium-238, the main type of uranium in natural ore (Gyorgy, 1979). Miners who breathe in the radon gas or radon that has attached to water droplets are exposed to the risk of lung cancer. Approximately 30 percent of premature deaths in uranium miners are caused by lung cancer. Studies show that the number of lung cancers in miners is highest when there are large concentrations of radon daughters in the mines, when miners have worked for 10 years or more, and when the miners are moderate to heavy cigarette smokers (Gyorgy, 1979). A study published in 1971 by the Public Health Service found that lung cancer rates in Colorado uranium miners were 5 to 25 times the normal rate ("Virginia delays permit," 1982). Deaths among uranium miners from nonmalignant respiratory diseases as well as an excess in skin cancers have also been documented (Gofman, 1981).

When the uranium ore is processed to remove the uranium, a sandy material called *tailings* is produced. This byproduct of milling was until recently used in landfills and construction materials. Since the tailings are radioactive, they expose people living near or downwind from the waste piles to radon byproducts. In addition, people living on landfills of tailings or in homes manufactured from construction materials that contain tailings are also in danger of exposure. While some scientists argue that the radiation exposure is small, others say that continuous exposure over a period of time could significantly increase lung cancer death rates (McKee, 1974).

Uranium mine tailings were used in the construction of 5,000 homes in Grand Junction, Colorado. The home owners were not warned that their health could be in danger. The Colorado State Department of Health calculated "that the lungs of the occupants in 10 percent of those 5,000 houses are known to have been exposed to the equivalent of more than 553 chest x-rays per year" (Metzger, 1971).

It takes approximately one ton of uranium ore to produce one pound of enriched uranium. Because of the large amount of tailings produced, there are an estimated 90 million tons of tailings at 30 mines in western states, including New Mexico, Wyoming, Colorado, Utah, Arizona, Oregon, Washington, South Dakota, and Texas. There also appears to be a danger of long-term genetic effects and cancer in future generations as a result of exposure from the slow release of radon from the tailings (Gyorgy, 1979).

After the uranium is mined and milled, it is enriched for use as reactor fuel (uranium-235). Once this is accomplished, the fuel fabrication process prepares fuel rods loaded with pellets of the enriched uranium, which is then used to produce heat through fission in nuclear power plants. During both the enrichment and fabrication processes, workers are in danger of radiation exposure and strict enforcement of safety regulations is necessary to prevent exposure to the uranium-235.

Because of the high price paid for uranium products, theft is common. As of September 1976, nuclear facilities in the United States could not account for more than 8,000 pounds of plutonium and highly enriched uranium. The danger of improper handling by thieves could expose large populations to the risks of radiation exposure.

At least two states, Virginia and New Jersey, have enacted temporary moratoria on uranium mining. These states fear that such mining could damage underground water supplies and threaten public health ("Virginia delays permit," 1982).

Nuclear Power Plants

The total number of nuclear reactors in the world in operation or planned now stands at 762. In the United States as of September 30, 1981, there were 70 nuclear power plants licensed to operate, 4 licensed for testing, and 78 construction permits issued (Solon, 1982). The development of nuclear power was the outgrowth of the Atoms for Peace program initiated in 1953 by President Eisenhower. The first nuclear reactors built for commercial use in the United States were pressurized water reactors (PWRs).

Atomic power is the energy that is released when atoms are split. The splitting of atoms is called *fission*. In a nuclear power plant, steam is produced by the heat coming out from the controlled chain reaction that takes place inside the uranium fuel rods within the reactor core (Gyorgy, 1979). The heat boils water, producing steam, which turns a generator, thus producing electricity.

HEALTH THREATS FROM NUCLEAR CYCLE. Potential health effects from radiation exposure can occur during several steps in the nuclear cycle, including mining and milling of uranium ore, enrichment for nuclear fuel fabrication, transportation of nuclear fuel, accidents at the power plant, and transportation, storage, and disposal of radioactive waste materials from spent power plant fuel. The health hazards of nuclear power can result from releases of radioactive poisons (including strontium-90, iodine-131, cesium-137, and plutonium) into the environment; accidents at the power plant that release radioactive materials into water and air; or inadequate storage systems and disposal of radioactive wastes.

Radioactive materials enter the food chain through releases into the air and water supplies. *Plutonium*, the radionuclide produced in nuclear reactors, is one of the most toxic materials known, and one millionth of a gram of plutonium (an invisible particle) can cause cancer several years after the particle is inhaled. It is estimated that one pound of plutonium, if deposited in the lungs of people throughout the world, would be enough to kill every person on earth (Gyorgy, 1979). The half-life of plutonium-235 produced in contemporary U.S. reactors is 24,000 years (Solon, 1982). During the reprocessing of spent nuclear reactor fuel, the plutonium is purified and may be used either as fuel for atomic bombs or fuel for breeder nuclear reactors.

Other radioactive byproducts produced in nuclear reactors are radioactive iodine, strontium-90 and cesium-137. Radioactive iodine is absorbed through the bowel into the blood and is deposited in the thyroid gland where it can cause thyroid cancer. In the event of accidental release of radioactive iodine into the environment from reactor malfunction, a precaution that can be taken to prevent thyroid cancer is administration of potassium iodide. Seven thousand families within a five-mile radius of the Sequoyah nuclear power plant received vials of potassium iodide and instructions for use in the event of a nuclear accident at the plant ("People near reactor get pills,"

1981). Potassium iodide would prevent uptake of the radioactive iodine released into the air from such an accident.

Strontium-90, which is absorbed by the bowel after people drink contaminated milk (milk containing strontium-90 is produced by cows that have eaten contaminated grass) is deposited in the bones, where it fools the body by resembling calcium, thus predisposing the person to osteogenic sarcoma and leukemia. Cesium-137 is deposited in the muscles, where it can cause malignancies.

Since nuclear power plants require tremendous amounts of cooling water, thermal pollution results from the discharge of heat into the environment. This has been known to kill fish when water used for cooling is discharged back into a river, ocean, or lake near the plant (Gyorgy, 1979). Water temperature may increase by as much as 20 degrees Fahrenheit.

Although nuclear power plants are equipped with sophisticated safety systems and have strict safety regulations, accidents have occurred from systems failure and human error. There were 2,300 nuclear power plant malfunctions reported by the Nuclear Regulatory Commission (NRC) in 1979 and 2,800 in 1978 (Greater N.Y. Council on Energy, 1980). Nuclear accidents, shutdowns, and leaks of radioactive water are reported routinely in daily newspapers. The Three Mile Island accident, which occurred in 1979 in Harrisburg, Pennsylvania, marked the beginning of public and national concern over the health dangers associated with nuclear power. The location of nuclear power plants in densely populated areas, such as the Indian Point plant, which is 30 miles from New York City, raises important questions about evacuation in cases of core meltdown, the worst-case reactor malfunction.

NURSES' RESPONSES TO POWER PLANT HAZ-ARDS. The professional nursing community has expressed its concern about the public health and safety impact of nuclear power plants. In three separate actions, the Delaware Nurses' Association, the Michigan Nurses' Association, and the National Student Nurses' Association took positions that highlight the public's concern about the safety of nuclear energy. They recommend a variety of actions, including asking Congress to impose a moratorium on the construction of nuclear power plants until safe disposal of spent nuclear fuel can be assured, imposing more effective safety controls, comprehensive evacuation plans for those living in the vicinity of a nuclear power plant, funding of research to determine the health effects of nuclear power plants on those living near them, and funding for the research and development of safe, renewable energy resources.

Nuclear Weapons Testing

Since the first nuclear bomb was tested on July 16, 1945, in a desert 200 miles south of Los Alamos, New Mexico, 230 atmospheric and 380 underground experimental nuclear detonations have taken place in the United States. Atmospheric blasts were halted in 1963 after the signing of the Limited Nuclear Test Ban Treaty by the United States and the USSR. Today, six countries (the United States, the USSR, Britain, France, China, and India) have built and tested nuclear devices ("Debate over nuclear testing," 1982).

An estimated 250,000 servicemen took part in the atmospheric tests from 1945 to 1963. In addition, civilian populations around test sites viewed the blasts. Civilians downwind from the test sites were exposed to radioactive fallout. The Defense Nuclear Agency denies that illnesses reported by veterans who were present during the bomb testings are a result of radiation. At this time, significant investigations are going on. The Senate Committee on Veteran's Affairs has agreed to explore claims that diseases suffered by participants in early atomic weapons tests were brought on by exposure to radiation (J. Miller, 1982). Health problems reported by veterans who witnessed the explosions include cancer, muscle and joint deterioration, internal disorders, lung problems, disabilities in offspring, miscarriages, sterility, and birth defects.

In a mammoth civil suit charging that the United States government negligently damaged westerners by failing to adequately protect them from fallout from the Nevada test site, 1,200 plaintiffs claim that cancer cases resulted from the bomb testings among residents of southern Utah, northern Arizona, and Nevada. A study done by Dr. Joseph L. Lyon, epidemiologist at the University of Utah, found extraordinarily high rates of childhood leukemia in southern Utah in the period of intense testing. He found that from 1951 to 1958, the number of childhood leukemia deaths was 2.4 times higher than in nontesting periods and that in five Utah counties closest to the Nevada border and the testing region, the rate was 3.4 times greater than it was in nontesting years ("Trial hinges on safety," 1982).

Nuclear War

In August 1945, one month after the first bomb test, the United States dropped a uranium weapon on Hiroshima, Japan. Three days later, a second uranium weapon was dropped on the Japanese city of Nagasaki. No one knows all the long-term health effects on the people who survived. The Hiroshima bomb resulted in 70,000 immediate civilian deaths and an additional 80,000 deaths within one month of the blast. The Nagasaki bomb resulted in 40,000 immediate civilian deaths and 20,000 additional deaths within one month. Within a 1-kilometer radius from ground zero, casualties were about 95 percent of the total population in both cities (*Nuclear Weapons*, 1980).

Higher-yield nuclear explosives, such as those used in modern nuclear weapons, would increase the impact and number of deaths and casualties. A single weapon today might have the power of 1,000 Hiroshima bombs. A 20-megaton bomb, for example, detonated over a major city, would vaporize, crush, incinerate, or burn to death almost every person within a radius of 5 or 6 miles of the center of the blast—perhaps 2 million people. Within a radius of 20 miles, a million more or so would either die instantly or suffer fatal wounds. If the bomb exploded on the ground, countless others who live miles away, far beyond the reach of the initial blast and searing heat wave, would be killed by radioactive fallout drifting away from ground zero (Lifton & Erikson, 1982).

Deaths and injuries would be caused by intense heat, flying debris, crushing wounds, inhalation of dense dust, hurricane-force winds, and acute radiation exposure (which would kill most people almost immediately). Third-degree burns, broken bones, contusions, open wounds, blindness, internal injuries, and acute radiation sickness would also result.

If an all-out nuclear war were waged between the United States and the Soviet Union, one can imagine the intense disruption of the present social, political, and economic system. Nuclear bombs would be detonated in several cities at one time. Radioactivity and physical destruction would leave cities uninhabitable. Hospitals, medical supplies, and wound dressings would not be available. The types of wounds and injuries resulting from nuclear war would require sustained medical and nursing attention that would not be available. In addition to physical injuries, there would be intense psychological damage in survivors. Dr. Jay Lifton describes the survivors of the Hiroshima bombing as follows:

In Hiroshima, survivors not only expected that they too would soon die, they had a sense that everyone was dying, that the world was ending. Rather than panic, the scene was one of slow motion—of people moving gradually away from the center of destruction, but dully and almost without purpose. They were, as one among them put it, "so broken and confused that they moved and behaved like automatons . . . a people who walked in the realm of dreams." Some tried to do something to help others, but most felt themselves to be so much a part of the dead that, as another remembers, they were "not really alive."

(Lifton & Erikson, 1982, p. A17).

Current public controversy has raised questions about the survivability of nuclear war, the moral, ethical and political issues surrounding nuclear war, and the medical and health consequences. A study published by the International Institute for Strategic Studies in London asserts that if a tactical nuclear war erupted in Europe, it could not be controlled (Middleton, 1981).

NURSING AND MEDICAL RESPONSE TO NUCLEAR WAR. Nurses and physicians have publicly debated the issue of responding to the complex injuries and social disruption that would occur from a nuclear invasion. Both the American Nurses' Association and the American Medical Association have addressed this issue in position statements, passed by their respective voting bodies, alerting the health care community of the need to inform the government and the public that there can be "no adequate med-

ical response to a nuclear holocaust" (Butterfield, 1981).

In addition, health professionals have begun to educate the public about the consequences of nuclear war and the importance of disarmament and prevention. Examples of organized efforts include the following: Nurses' Environmental Health Watch, Nurses' Alliance for the Prevention of Nuclear War, Health Network Against Nuclear War, and Physicians for Social Responsibility. (Refer to Appendix B for details about these organizations.)

Public demonstrations in both Europe and the United States reflect the public's wish for a nuclear arms freeze and express the fears of the general population over potential world destruction. Many nurses, scientists, physicians, and people from all walks of life believe that a nuclear war is the one issue that faces everyone and that prevention is the only solution to impending holocaust.

Radioactive Waste

The disposal of *radwaste* (radioactive waste) is a growing problem. Radioactive wastes are produced by all phases of nuclear weapons production, industry, nuclear power, and nuclear medicine. As of 1981, there were 100 million gallons of high-level wastes from 8,000 tons of spent fuel temporarily stored around the country. These amounts are expected to increase to 107 million gallons and 63,000 metric tons, respectively, by 1995 (*Report by the Comptroller General*, 1981). Some nuclear power plants are nearing the limits of their storage capacity for spent fuel and face shutdown in a few years because of lack of temporary storage space.

Thoughtless and irresponsible waste disposal practices have led to the contamination of ground water supplies, the condemnation of wells and other sources of drinking water, and tragic illness for many persons living near waste disposal sites (Shapiro, 1981). Adding to the problem of regulation of disposal of radioactive waste is illegal dumping of these materials. One example was a situation in which past and current employees of a waste removal company in Connecticut accused the company of secretly burying thousands of gallons of toxic and radioactive substances and flushing them into municipal sewers or rivers. The company, according to the employees, falsified records to hide the illegal dumping ("Cops and dumpers," 1982). Ineffective disposal of radioactive wastes has activated some states to pass moratoria on the licensing and building of power plants until safe disposal methods are available.

Contact with radwaste can occur at every stage of the nuclear cycle. In addition to mining and milling dangers, contamination of humans and the environment can occur from illegal dumping, transportation, storage, sabotage, and occupational exposure to radwaste.

Transportation has received national and international attention in the media in the past few years. Several communities have expressed concern that accidents involving trucks that carry radwaste could force evacuation of an area, long-term radioactive contamination, and exposure of humans, animals, and crops. People in densely populated areas fear that they would be unable to leave if there were an accident. Most communities do not have viable emergency escape plans. Many small and large community hospitals are not equipped to respond to the emergency needs of contaminated victims from any type of accident involving radioactive materials.

Low-Level Radwaste

Most low-level radwaste consists of ion-exchanging resins, rags, clothing, tools, paper, wood, uranium mill tailings, and biological material contaminated in facilities where radiation is used. A limited quantity of low-level radwaste may be disposed of by release into the atmosphere, inland or tidal waters, sewage disposal, or burial. *Radionuclides*, which have a short half-life, are often stored and allowed to decay until they can be disposed of as nonradioactive wastes (Shapiro, 1981). Currently three low-level repositories are operating in the United States: Barnwell, South Carolina, Beatty, Nevada, and Hanford, Washington.

The Nuclear Regulatory Commission recently approved the first federal regulations for burying low-level radwaste. The new rules divide low-level radwaste into three categories based on the radiation they emit and set up criteria for the disposal of each. The regulations require that the sources of wastes, such as laboratories, hospitals, and nuclear power plants, classify the wastes and ship them separately. The rules serve as guidelines for state officials in setting up their own rules, since most states have agreements with the NRC to regulate low-level radwaste disposal facilities on their own ("U.S. adopts first disposal rule," 1982).

High-Level Radwaste

High-level radwaste includes both liquid residue from reprocessing reactor fuel and irradiated or spent fuel rods periodically removed from reactors (Salzman, 1978). These wastes remain hazardous for an extremely long time and permanent isolation from the biosphere is required to prevent contamination of water and air.

There are currently no repositories available for high-level radwaste. It is stored temporarily on the site of power plants in metal containers placed in pools of water. These containers were originally planned for storage for a few months. Military radwaste is held at government storage sites. Several methods for disposing of high-level wastes and spent fuel have been considered, including disposal in geological repositories, the ocean floor, polar ice regions, and outer space (*Report by the Comptroller General*, 1981). At this time authorities believe that geological repositories, such as salt domes, are the best sites for high-level radwaste.

Under investigation in the United States and other countries are methods to solidify certain liquid radwastes into either glass or ceramic containers. After solidification, the material would be placed in corrosion-resistant containers that must be able to last 250 to 1,000 years (Garmon & Peterson, 1982). These containers would then be buried in geological repositories.

Suitable potential repositories of salt, basalt, granite, and tuff (a volcanic rock) have been found in the states of Washington, Louisiana, Mississippi, Texas, and Utah. Government scientists believe that these sites have the subterranean geology and hydrology required to provide a safe million-year containment for the accumulation of nuclear waste (Franklin, 1982). As of this time, Congress has not decided on the locations of the repositories. It is estimated that the first repository will not be ready until 1993.

Nursing Intervention: Education

Nurses in the community have a responsibility to educate themselves, their clients, their peers, and other community members about the health aspects of radiation. The following teaching points will be helpful in designing an education program in the community.

X-rays

1. Learn how to protect yourself from excessive x-radiation. Resources are provided at the end of this chapter.

2. Encourage people to question the need for x-rays when they are ordered and to keep an ongoing personal record of date and x-ray received and why it was taken. When people change physicians, they should request that their x-rays be transferred to the new physician.

3. Discourage people from insisting that x-rays be taken. Many people think that an exam is not complete without an x-ray.

4. Advise people to request a tuberculin skin test instead of chest x-ray screening.

5. Recommend that people insist on proper shielding and protection of areas not being x-rayed if x-ray procedures must be performed. Lead aprons and thyroid shields should be provided routinely for radiographic procedures. Nurses working in hospitals should insist that clients, children as well as adults, are shielded and that x-rays are not overused.

6. Encourage the avoidance of mammography examinations for women under age 50 who neither exhibit symptoms nor have a personal or strong family history of breast cancer (Shapiro, 1981).

7. Prevent women who are pregnant from being x-rayed unless it is an emergency. The developing fetus is highly susceptible to cell damage from x-rays. This rule applies to women who are not certain if they are pregnant (for example, before the first

missed period or while awaiting pregnancy test results).

Transportation of Radioactive Materials

1. Advocate that radioactive materials not be transported through densely populated areas since accidents in these areas would expose large numbers of people to radioactive contamination.
2. Learn decontamination procedures and the health effects of contamination from radioactive materials.
3. Get involved in disaster planning in the event of an accident involving radioactive materials.

Nuclear Power Plants

1. Be aware of disaster plans in the event of an accident at the plant.
2. Define nurses' roles and involvement in disaster and evacuation plans.
3. Know the emergency treatment for people who are contaminated with radioactive materials from a power plant accident.
4. Participate in disaster planning along with other community members and plant representatives so that the role played by nurses is determined by nurses.
5. Be familiar with the somatic and genetic effects of radiation and be aware of these when assessing the health of people who live around nuclear power plants. In addition, be aware of the psychological reactions of people who live near nuclear power plants where an accident has already taken place (such as Three Mile Island) or where there is potential for accidents.
6. Take a leadership role in informing the public about the actual and potential health hazards that result from the production of power using radioactive materials.

AIR POLLUTION

History

Several pre–industrial revolution industries, such as metallurgy, ceramics, and animal product preservation, were associated with air pollution (Stern, 1973). The burning of coal in England was frequently prohibited in the early tenth century; as early as 1300, a royal decree was issued in London prohibiting the use of low-grade coal for heating because it created excessive smoke and soot. In 1600 sulfur dioxide (from coal burning) was the first chemical specifically recognized as an air pollutant (Hesketh, 1973).

The steam engine, fired principally by coal, emitted smoke and ash and tainted the air of homes and workplaces. Beginning in 1848 public health acts in Great Britain imposed restrictions intended to abate smoke and ash production. In the United States, the first municipal ordinances and regulations limiting the emission of black smoke and ash appeared in the 1880s and were directed toward industrial, locomotive, and marine rather than domestic sources (Stern, 1973).

As technology advanced, steam-powered engines were replaced by electricity generated from central plants. Oil replaced coal, and smoke and ash emissions significantly declined. As chemical technology advanced, the number of byproducts polluting the air increased. Pollution sources continue to increase. They include the return to the use of wood burning stoves for heat, contamination of the stratosphere with carbon dioxide from jet contrails, radioactive byproducts from nuclear power generators, automobile emissions, and the return to coal burning in some power plants.

Most air pollution control activities began with the Clean Air Act of 1963 (Hesketh, 1973). The act was amended in 1965, 1966, 1967, 1970 and is currently slated for revision. The Environmental Protection Agency, established in 1970, oversees the Clean Air Act and is responsible for enforcing standards.

Statistics show that air quality has significantly improved since the passage of the Clean Air Act. The available national index of air quality indicates that progress in controlling air pollution has been significant, at least on the basis of the number of days in which pollution levels are very high in a number of major metropolitan areas (*State of the Environment*, 1982).

Composition

Air pollution is the discharge into the atmosphere of airborne substances that are actually or potentially hazardous to humans, animals, plants, and inanimate objects. Polluting substances may be naturally occurring, but most of those that concern us are produced by people. Sources of natural air pollution include forest fires, decaying vegetable matter, volcanic eruptions, and pollens. The major cause of air pollution is from human sources, such as emissions from motor vehicles, energy production, industry, and heat generation.

Growing populations that are more and more dependent on technology to satisfy life-style needs will cause air pollution to continue to be a serious health hazard unless strict standards are mandated and enforced. While technological advances (such as emission control devices on automobiles) can reduce pollution, economic, social, and political circumstances often make pollution control a low priority. U.S. society generally focuses on short-term needs, such as sanitation, economics, transportation, crime, communicable disease control, and

housing, and ignores the long-term goal of ensuring safe resources. Without clean air and adequate food and water resources, communities cannot survive.

Air pollution exists on several levels: the personal and home environments, the industrial and workplace environments, the community or neighborhood environments, and the global environment. Weather conditions, such as precipitation, temperature inversions, and wind patterns, as well as geography determine the effects air pollutants have on human health. Very little is known about the effects of pollutants combining and acting synergistically.

The substances that pollute the air can be broken down to two major categories: particulate matter and gaseous matter.

Particulate Matter

A *particle* is a small, discrete mass of solid or liquid matter that may consist of dust, aerosol droplets, fly ash, fog, fumes, mist, smoke, soot, or sprays (Parker, 1977).

Inhalation of particles irritates the respiratory tract and can predispose an individual to chronic respiratory diseases. About two-thirds of the nation's manmade particulate emissions are from stationary industrial sources, about 18 percent are from vehicles, and about 5 percent are from solid waste disposal (*State of the Environment*, 1982).

Gaseous Matter

This category of pollutants includes sulfur dioxide, nitrogen oxide, carbon monoxide, carbon dioxide, fluorides, hydrocarbons, hydrogen cyanide, and tobacco smoke. See Table 27.1 for a more complete description of the health hazards from some common gaseous air pollutants.

The prevalence of tobacco smoke in both the personal and occupational environment

TABLE 27.1
Health Hazards from Five Common Air Pollution Sources

Pollutant[a]	Primary Source	Health Effects	Comments
Sulfur dioxide	Burning coal and high-sulfur oil.	Thought to produce increased death rates, particularly among those with heart and lung diseases. Associated with increases in acute and chronic respiratory diseases.	Contained in acid rain; is one of the air pollution vapors of greatest concern because of damaging effects.
Carbon monoxide	Emissions from motor-vehicle exhaust.	Interferes with the absorption of oxygen by red blood cells and alters judgment, slows reflexes, and causes drowsiness. Inhalation of high levels causes death.	Emission controls have helped lower ambient levels.
Ozone	Product of photochemical reactions, nitrogen oxides and volatile organic compounds produced by industrial processes, and motor vehicles.	Severely irritates mucous membranes of nose and throat and impairs breathing.	In 1977, over 140 million people lived in areas exceeding the primary air quality standard for ozone.
Nitrogen oxide	Motor vehicles and power plants.	Lung irritant contributing to lower resistance to respiratory infections and breathing impairment.	Levels have increased in recent years.
Suspended particulates	Motor vehicles, coal burning, industry, and solid waste disposal.	Irritation to respiratory system leads to acute respiratory illness. Prolonged inhalation can increase likelihood and severity of chronic respiratory diseases.	Conversions from coal to cleaner-burning fuels and mandated emission reductions have decreased ambient levels of particles.

SOURCE: *State of the Environment: A Report from The Conservation Foundation*, 1982.

[a] The five pollutants outlined in this table are the five "criteria pollutants" that are routinely evaluated to determine the pollution standards index (PSI). The PSI is a national index used to determine pollution levels in metropolitan areas.

makes it one of the most common pollutants people are exposed to. Tobacco smoke contains carbon monoxide, nitrogen dioxide, fly ash, nicotine, formaldehyde, and organic tars (Hesketh, 1973). People who do not smoke but who are exposed to exhaled smoke and the smoke from burning cigarettes, cigars, and pipes involuntarily absorb the same toxic materials in tobacco smoke that the smoker inhales directly. The health consequences of tobacco smoke have been widely researched and documented. They include cancers of the lung, larynx, pharynx, oral cavity, esophagus, pancreas, and urinary bladder; cardiovascular disease, chronic bronchitis and emphysema; complications of pregnancy, retardation of fetal growth, spontaneous abortion, premature delivery, fetal death, and perinatal death; other ailments ranging from minor respiratory infections to stomach ulcers. Recent reports have recognized smoking as the chief preventable cause of death in the United States (*Smoking*, 1982).

Of growing concern to environmentalists and scientists is the problem of *acid rain*. While the cause of acid rain has not been confirmed, acidic sulfur and nitrogen compounds reacting with moisture to form weak nitric and sulfuric acids are believed to be factors in the chemical process. A recent increase in the burning of high-sulfur coal in electric generating plants is expected to add to the problem. Acid rain killed aquatic life in at least 10 percent of New England's 226 largest freshwater lakes ("Storm over a deadly downpour," 1982). Loss of fish and contamination of drinking water by acid rain are public health threats in northeastern United States and Canada.

Health Effects of Air Pollution

Air pollution has been directly and indirectly associated with the following diseases: premature aging, asthma, berylliosis, emphysema, mesothelioma, bronchitis, and cancer of the respiratory and gastrointestinal tracts (Stern, 1973). While a variety of predisposing factors interact to produce disease, air pollution is a contributing factor in many human illnesses and in the destruction and loss of wildlife and vegetation.

In addition to the direct effects to the respiratory system, the skin and eyes are also susceptible to damage from pollutants in the air. The body has protective mechanisms, such as tearing, which washes irritants from the eyes, and ciliary action in the upper respiratory tract, which filters particles from the air. The mucous lining of the respiratory tract helps remove gaseous pollutants and particles from the air entering the lungs. If polluted air is inhaled continually, the body's natural defenses slow down and become less effective.

Temperature inversions and accidental releases of toxic air pollutants have caused human deaths. Any time dispersement of pollutants is minimized because of weather or topographic entrapments, the incidence of illness from pollutants increases.

Recognizing that air pollution is implicated in human disease, especially conditions involving the respiratory tract, nurses need to include this as a consideration in initial and ongoing client assessment. Assessing a client's personal and home environment as well as the workplace and community environments may give clues to factors that affect respiratory and other conditions associated with air pollution.

WATER POLLUTION

Potable water for drinking and clean water for personal, industrial, and recreational use is essential to life and health. Contamination from a variety of sources, including industrial, biological, natural, and agricultural, plus overuse by an increasing population, threatens both ground and surface water supplies.

It was not until the nineteenth century cholera epidemics took over 260,000 lives in Great Britain that contaminated water was recognized as a transmitter of disease-producing organisms. Today, pathogens are removed from drinking water by filtration or chlorination. Routine water testing and treatment for disease-producing organisms have reduced the occurrence of disease outbreaks associated with contaminated water. Recreational water use, however, may occasionally be prohibited because of high bacteria counts.

Modern technology and industrialization have created a serious health threat to our water supply. Toxic substances originate from a variety of sources, including industrial and household wastes, dissolved soil minerals, sludge, atmospheric emissions, metals dissolved from pipes and other pumping equipment, nuclear wastes, radioactive fallout, mining effluents, pesticides, and natural sources (Lehr, Gass, Pettyjohn, & Demarre, 1980).

Experts estimate that industrial and domestic waste water introduces up to a million different pollutants into natural waters (Forstner & Wittmann, 1979). While many of these pollutants may not adversely affect health, they may impair the color, odor, and taste of drinking water. Common sources of water pollution are listed in Appendix A.

Surface Water Supply

Lakes, rivers, and the ocean are actual and potential sources of surface water supply. River water is a source of drinking water for many communities. Pollution from in-

dustry, sewage, and recreational uses threaten the potability of river water. River water must be constantly monitored and must be treated before it is used for drinking. Strict enforcement of environmental protection laws and regulations will help protect river water from contamination.

Lakes are another source of drinking water; in most instances lake water must be treated before use for drinking. Pollutants can enter lake water from industry, sewage, and contaminated stream runoff. Treatment varies depending on the location of the lake and the substances in the water. Algae blooms (overgrowth of algae), associated with nitrates and phosphates resulting from sewage effluents and commercial fertilizers, are a common problem of lake water supplies (Purdom, 1980). The presence of certain kinds of algae alters the color, taste, odor, and toxicity of lake water and can affect fish, animals, and humans.

As the world population increases, the use of sea water for drinking becomes more likely. Treatment to convert sea water to fresh water is much costlier than conventional treatment of fresh water. Methods of conversion include evaporation, freezing, ion exchange, electrodialysis, reverse osmosis, and distillation (Purdom, 1980).

Ground Water Supply

Approximately 25 percent of the U.S. population obtains its drinking water from ground water resources, and this percentage is growing. Ground water is desirable for drinking because it is usually consistent in temperature and chemical content and is generally less affected by drought and other weather conditions than surface water. Ground water supplies that come from deep wells are generally biologically pure (Purdom, 1980).

Although pollution of ground water is

less common than pollution of surface water, it would require years or decades for polluted ground water to return to its natural state. Any change in taste, color, or odor of ground water should be reported immediately to the local health department and the water should be analyzed. Possible pollution sources of ground water include land fills, irrigation, waste disposal, road salting, oil well drilling, excavations, explosions, and fires. Shallow wells are commonly contaminated by effluents originating at cesspools and privies (Lehr, 1980).

Radioactivity is another source of pollution of both ground and surface water supplies. Mining of uranium releases radon gas, which is readily absorbed in water. Radon gas is released and inhaled when the water leaves the pipes. Radioactive tailings from uranium milling contain 85 percent of the original radioactivity; this can also enter water supplies. Radium-226, another byproduct of uranium-238, is soluble in water and accumulates in bones once it enters the body.

Water Standards

The Safe Drinking Water Act and the Clean Water Act contain provisions that enforce standards for water purity and protection of drinking water resources from pollution. Water standards have been developed by the U.S. Public Health Service and are mandated in most states. Under the current rules of the Clean Water Act, states must ensure that specific bodies of water meet federal requirements to protect clean water from being degraded and to improve waters that are already polluted.

With the number of hazardous waste sites being created and abandoned sites discovered, protection of ground water from contamination is a growing problem. Public control over the quantity and quality of ground water is exercised principally at the state level, and most states have a minimum regulatory program designed to address ground water contamination problems (*State of the Environment*, 1982).

While standards and laws exist to ensure safe water resources, illegal dumping of chemicals into streams, rivers, lakes, and the ocean are difficult to police. In some cases, fines are not high enough to prevent the dumping, and enforcement officers are unable to patrol adequately. Examples of illegal dumping appear almost daily in newspapers across the country.

Water Supplies and Conservation

Vast differences in climate and geology account for variances in regional water supplies. In areas with adequate precipitation, water shortages are uncommon, although shifting populations, industrial development, and water pollution have altered regional water usage. Water use throughout the United States increased 35 percent between 1965 and 1975. The fastest growing uses have been for public water supplies (covering most residential and commercial uses) and for generating electricity (*State of the Environment*, 1982).

During the 1970s, severe droughts occurred in California and New York, forcing officials to take steps to conserve water. Many environmentalists advocate conservation of water as an ongoing program rather than as an emergency measure. Conservation of water includes the practices listed in Table 27.2 (Powledge, 1982).

As technology advances and people become more dependent on products produced by technology, accumulations of toxic wastes will continue to grow and enter the ground water and surface water resources. Nurses, acting as public health advocates, must be aware of diseases related

TABLE 27.2 Methods to Conserve Water
Place a dime-shaped disk with a hole in it in a bathroom shower head to reduce the volume of water passing through the shower.
Use devices available for reducing the amount of water stored in a toilet tank.
Do not flush a toilet that has been used only for urination.
Place a bucket in the shower to collect shower runoff and use for flushing toilets, watering house plants, and filling humidifiers.
Use low-cost water-treatment to improve both the quality and taste of drinking water.
Fill basin when washing dishes rather than allowing water to run continuously.
Turn water off when brushing teeth.
Repair leaking faucets.
Teach children water-conservation habits.

to water pollution and monitor community disposal practices for chemical and radioactive wastes. The availability of potable water should be part of the home assessment made by community health nurses. Nurses working in the community should familiarize themselves with the local department of health's activities concerning water supplies and work closely with health department officials to be certain that standards are enforced. Community health nurses can serve as environmental conservation teachers in the community and promote water conservation at the local level.

CHEMICAL WASTES

About 30,000 chemicals are now in commercial production and 1,000 new chemicals are introduced each year (G. T. Miller, 1982). In 1980, about 63 million tons of hazardous industrial wastes were produced in the United States by approximately 750,000 different producers. These included lead, mercury, cadmium, radioactive materials, acids, cyanides, and pesticides (G. T. Miller, 1982). The Environmental Protection Agency (EPA) estimates that only 10 percent of the toxic wastes produced are disposed of properly. The remaining wastes are dumped illegally into rivers, streams, sewers, and oceans, along roadsides, and in landfills and vacant lots.

Love Canal, located in Niagara Falls, New York, was used for dumping over 22,000 tons of chemical wastes. Part of the 15-acre site was then donated to the local school board for an elementary school to be built. Houses were built on much of the remaining land in the vicinity of the canal. Following a period of high rainfall, which raised the water table, the chemicals surfaced in the school playground and in the basements of homes built near the canal. Evacuation of families, whose lives and health became endangered from the chemicals, called the entire nation's attention to what was soon identified as a major problem all over the United States: chemical waste dumping.

The discovery of abandoned waste dump sites from the nineteenth century industries reveals that dumping is not a new problem. Arsenic, lead, and mercury compounds used in many products made a century ago remain in the environment and continue to threaten health. Disposal of wastes was unregulated, and manufacturers freely poured waste products into running water and into dumps on vacant land. Years of uncontrolled waste dumping is currently a source of water and soil contamination.

Illegal dumping is another major source of uncontrolled waste disposal that has contaminated an unknown number of land fills and vacant lots as well as water sources. In addition, inadequate disposal practices, leading to ruptured drums and subsequent leakage of toxic substances into the ground, complicate the already complex problem of controlling environmental contamination from billions of tons of hazardous substances. By 1980, the EPA had estimated that there were 32,000 to 50,000 sites in the United States that contain hazardous wastes, with an estimated 1,000 to 2,000 of these sites believed to pose significant risks to human health and the environment (G. T. Miller, 1982).

Methods of treating and reducing hazardous chemical wastes include neutralization, precipitation, solidification or fixation, oxidation-reduction, and ion exchange. In addition, incineration, deep well injection, solvent recovery, and distillation hydrotreating processes can also be utilized to treat and reduce wastes.

Polychlorinated Biphenyls (PCBs)

PCBs are highly toxic and persistent chemicals primarily used as insulating fluids in heavy-duty electrical equipment in power plants, industry, and large buildings across the country (Winter, 1979). PCBs have been widely used in a variety of products, such as fluorescent lights, television sets, carbonless duplicating paper, printing inks, plastics, adhesives, paints, insulating tape, caulking compounds, air conditioners, microwave ovens, hydraulic and heat-transfer fluids, and radio sets.

Although manufacture of PCBs was halted in 1979, it is estimated that 1.25 billion pounds of PCBs were purchased by industries since their introduction in 1929 and that 750 million pounds are still in use (Winter, 1979). Three hundred million pounds of PCBs have been placed in landfills and dumps. One hundred fifty million pounds are unaccounted for and presumed to be contaminating the environment (Kiefer, 1981). Since they do not break down easily, PCBs contaminate the food and water supplies and accumulate in the food chain.

Although the tolerance level for PCBs is currently 2 to 5 parts per million (ppm), several U.S. locations have concentrations ranging from 20,000 ppm in some landfills (which lead into water sources) to 50 ppm in some parts of the Hudson River in New York State.

PCBs are particularly hazardous to human health because they accumulate in larger amounts as they move up the food chain. PCB's are stored in fat and have been found in the milk of nursing mothers. Harmful health effects of PCB's include liver lesions and tumors, birth defects, neurotoxicity, immunological defects, enzyme disturbances, rashes and depigmentation of the skin, eye discharge and swelling of the upper eyelids, acne-type skin eruptions, swelling, jaundice, numbness of limbs, hearing and vision disturbances, gastrointestinal disturbances, reproductive disorders, and cancer.

There has been widespread contamination from PCBs over the last 40 years. The greatest problem from PCBs results from long-term, low-level exposures. Since PCBs do not mix with water, they tend to settle at the bottom of rivers and lakes and migrate when sediment is disturbed by rainfall, dredging, or water currents. They are swallowed by fish feeding on the bottom and thus enter the human food chain. Wind currents also pick up the highly volatile PCBs and deposit them far from the original source. PCBs have been found in all the Great Lakes, especially Lake Michigan, as well as in air samples taken 2,000 miles off the Atlantic Coast and in ice samples extracted from the Antarctic ice sheet (Winter, 1979).

Cleanup of PCBs is an expensive and slow process. For example, in 1980 the General Electric Company agreed to fund remedial actions at seven PCB-contaminated land disposal sites in the upper Hudson valley, New York. It is estimated that the program will take three to five years to complete and that it will cost $27.6 million to clean up the estimated 350,000 pounds of PCBs contained in the Hudson River sediment. The PCBs will be placed in encapsulation sites where they will be stored until some future time when an effective and practical method for ultimate disposal is available (*PCB's in the Land*, 1980).

Dioxins

Dioxins are byproducts of manufacturing processes such as the manufacture of herbicides, pesticides, and some disinfectants. Dioxins are created, for example, as unwanted byproducts in the production of the antiseptic hexachlorophene. Dioxins were also contained in the herbicides (e.g., Agent Orange) used to defoliate trees and kill crops in South Vietnam.

In the United States, dioxins contaminate the environment as a toxic waste found in land fills and toxic waste dump sites. They have been illegally mixed with and unknowingly added to oil mixtures used to keep down dust on roads and in arenas. Dioxins were identified at Love Canal in Niagara Falls, New York, at levels as high as 17.2 parts per million (Cionne, 1982) and in areas in Missouri at levels of more than 100 parts per billion (Reinhold,

1982). Although the danger level of dioxins is presently unknown, amounts of one part per billion are said by the Center for Disease Control in Atlanta to pose a health risk (Biddle, 1982).

Exposure to dioxins can occur by means of inhalation of herbicides or pesticides containing them; ingestion of contaminated food (dioxin biomagnifies in the food chain and is believed to be stored in fatty tissue); and possibly by absorption through the skin (*CIP Bulletin*, 1980). Horses and other farm animals died when oil containing dioxin was used as a spray for dust control.

Environmental Protection Agency officials call dioxins "the most acutely toxic compound made by man." The effects of dioxins are not fully understood at this time, but animal studies have associated them with mutations, nervous disorders, birth defects, spontaneous abortions, cancer, skin disorders, and kidney and liver failure. In humans, dioxin is directly linked to chloracne, a skin condition similar to adolescent acne but much more severe (Reinhold, 1983). Recent studies also show an unusually high incidence of soft tissue sarcomas among workers exposed to dioxins at two chemical plants in Michigan and West Virginia (Biddle, 1983).

Veterans exposed to Agent Orange during the Vietnam war have reported health problems including cancer, deformed children, miscarriages, still births, liver and kidney disorders, fatigue, tingling and numbness in the hands and feet, nerve damage, abdominal pain, depression, loss of sexual drive, sterility, skin rashes, headaches, and dizziness (Boffey, 1982). Several studies are now underway to determine the health effects of Agent Orange and dioxins on Vietnam veterans, but results are not expected for several years. The latency period between exposure and development of disease makes it difficult to pinpoint the health effects of toxic chemical exposure.

Regulation of Chemical Wastes

Through tighter regulation and law enforcement, chemical waste producers will be forced to take responsibility for the cost of waste treatments and disposal. The Resource Conservation and Recovery Act and the Comprehensive Environmental Response, Liability and Assistance Act of 1980 are recent examples of the government's efforts to clean up existing dump sites and to prevent illegal dumping.

Resource Conservation and Recovery Act

On October 21, 1976, President Ford signed into law the Resource Conservation and Recovery Act (RCRA). This act gives the Environmental Protection Agency the authority to regulate the generation, transport, and disposal of hazardous wastes and requires that hazardous wastes be controlled from the time of production to the time of final disposal. The law mandates the design of a system to eliminate open dumping, inventory waste sites, regulate how landfills are constructed and monitored, require private funding for long-term care of the dumpsites, send grants to rural communities to improve solid waste management, and institute a system to track wastes from production to disposal (Brown, 1980).

The EPA has been criticized for inadequate implementation of the RCRA. Of concern are the criteria for listing hazardous wastes that are affected by the law. In addition, because enforcement of regulations is costly and the EPA budget has been significantly cut in recent years, there is doubt that adequate protection will be implemented.

Superfund Legislation

In 1980 Congress passed the Comprehensive Environmental Response, Liability and Assistance Act (known as the Superfund), which created a federal program for waste-site cleanups (Shabecoff, 1983). The fund, authorized for five years, provides that federal money spent on cleanups be recovered from responsible parties or from the $1.6 billion Superfund collected from industry through an excise tax on chemicals.

There are an estimated 1,400 toxic waste dumpsites throughout the country. The EPA has listed 418 of them as the most hazardous waste dumps and has earmarked Superfund monies to clean them up. These sites are considered to require immediate cleanup since they pose threats to human health.

NURSING IMPLICATIONS

Community Assessment

Using the nursing process, the community can be assessed for environmental health hazards. In addition to assessment guidelines provided in other chapters, consider the following:

1. What are the population size and growth rate of the community?
2. What are the morbidity and mortality rates?
3. What are the disease incidence and prevalence rates?
4. *Water Resources*
   a. What is the source of the community's drinking water?
   b. Is the supply adequate?
   c. Is there a history of drinking water contamination in the community?

d. Are there rivers, streams, lakes, or oceans available for recreational use, and is this water safe?

e. Does commercial or recreational fishing occur, and is it known if the fish are free from toxins? Are there warnings not to eat fish from certain bodies of water?

5. *Air Quality*

a. What meteorologic, topographic, and climatic conditions influence the air quality in the community?

b. Is air quality monitored on an ongoing basis? What pollutants are measured, and what are their levels? Have these levels increased or decreased over the past two years?

c. What are the actual and potential sources of air pollution in the community?

6. *Energy Resources*

a. What is the community's major source of electric power?

b. Are there any health dangers associated with the power sources? What are these dangers?

c. How is energy used in the community? Are there instances when it is wasted?

d. What energy alternatives are available or being developed by the community?

7. *Solid Waste*

a. How much solid waste is produced by the community each year?

b. How are solid wastes collected and disposed of?

c. What are the sources of solid waste?

d. If industrial byproducts contribute to solid waste, are these wastes hazardous? If so, how are they disposed of?

e. What recycling programs are available for solid waste in the community?

8. *Sewage*

a. What type of sewage management program does the community have?

b. What types of sewage treatment methods are used?

c. Where is the sewage treatment effluent discharged?

9. *Radioactive Materials and Waste*

a. What are the sources of low- and high-level radioactive materials and waste products in the community?

b. How are radioactive wastes disposed of?

c. If radioactive materials or wastes are transported through the community, what precautions has the community taken to ensure safety in the event of an accident?

10. In an agricultural community, assess the following:

a. Is there a problem with soil erosion? What methods are being employed to conserve soil?

b. What methods are employed for agricultural pest control?

c. What methods are used to fertilize the land? What are the health hazards associated with these methods?

11. What are the federal, state, and local laws and regulations governing the following and how are they enforced?

a. Water resources.

b. Air quality.

c. Energy resources.

d. Solid waste management.

e. Noise pollution.

f. Radioactive materials and waste.

12. What community agency is responsible for monitoring each of the items in item 11?

13. Does the community have a plan to ensure adequate future consideration of these items? What is the plan?

14. Are there any community groups organized to serve as resources or community advocates if problems occur? What are the groups?

15. What are the major sources of family income in the community? Are these sources tied to environmental pollution? If they are, what is the economic impact of environmental regulation on the community's income sources?

16. Are there endangered species in the community? If so, what is being done to protect them?

17. What conservation or recycling programs are set up in the community for renewable and nonrenewable natural resources?

18. What is the community's philosophy about environmental issues such as pollution, land use, enforcement of standards, and the health aspects of environmental pollution?

19. Do elected and appointed officials support adequate environmental standards, enforcement of standards, and environmental protection? How has their support or nonsupport been demonstrated?

20. Do individuals in the community exhibit actual or potential health problems that can be associated with environmental pollution in either the workplace or the environment? What are these problems and how can they be prevented or alleviated?

21. Are community hospitals and other agencies prepared to cope with disasters resulting from environmental contamination such as a nuclear power plant core meltdown or contamination of homes by hazardous wastes?

Planning

Consider the following when determining if a community is planning with environmental issues in mind:

1. Is environmental protection a priority for the community? How is this demonstrated?

2. What voluntary and public agencies are involved in community planning and development?

3. Are nurses and other health professionals included in planning, particularly when health issues related to pollution are being considered?

4. Does the community currently have a comprehensive plan to solve health problems that are related to environmental pollution? What is the plan?

5. Is there coordination and cooperation between residents of the community and businesses or industries in planning for environmental protection and solving problems associated with pollution?

6. Is there cooperation between national, state, and local levels of government in planning for environmental protection and solving health problems associated with pollution?

7. Are environmental impact statements provided for land use and development projects?

Intervention

Nursing interventions depend upon the specific community environmental contamination, the pollutants involved, and the resources available. The question of nursing interventions has not been adequately addressed in the literature, and interventions are currently being developed on an ad hoc basis. For example, the American Red Cross has recently developed an education module covering nursing response to a radiation disaster such as that which occurred at Three Mile Island. The module will be used to train nurses across the country in how to respond to radiation disasters.

Nurses' Environmental Health Watch, a voluntary membership organization of nurses working to educate nurses and the public about environmental health hazards, publishes a quarterly newsletter, *Health Watch*, that provides information on specific health hazards and includes nursing implications.

When considering the nursing implications of specific environmental health hazards, ask the following questions:

1. What are the signs and symptoms of disease related to the specific pollutant? What is the treatment?

2. How is the general population exposed to the pollutant, and how can exposure be avoided?

3. Should special precautions be taken to prevent pregnant women and children from exposure? What are these precautions?

4. Should precautions be taken to monitor food, water, and air sources for contamination from the toxin? How should this be done?

5. Once a toxin is discovered in the community that threatens public health, what community actions can be taken immediately to prevent continued public exposure? What intermediate and long-term actions need to be taken to continue protection of public health?

6. What nursing actions can be taken to identify and treat the emotional and psychological responses to health threats from pollution?

7. What actions can be taken to rehabilitate a contaminated area?

8. How can nurses work together and with other health professionals in the commu-

nity to educate the public about threats to health from environmental hazards?

9. How can nurses work through their professional association to prevent health hazards associated with environmental pollution?

Evaluation

Evaluation mechanisms must be built into every aspect of the nursing process. Evaluation of the initial environmental assessment and plan is an ongoing process that serves to validate nursing actions and interventions. Current research findings on specific pollutants will provide validation as well as data for revising nursing interventions. It is imperative that nurse researchers investigate environmental health hazards and that findings be reported in nursing literature. Nurses should also assist the public in evaluating public information and make corrections and additions to public knowledge as appropriate.

FUTURE IMPLICATIONS

Within the past few years, there has been an increasing number of incidents related to environmental health hazards. Love Canal, Three Mile Island, and dioxin contamination in Missouri have raised public and official concern over the adequacy of environmental protection and the impact on human resources and health. There are reports in daily newspapers about hazardous waste sites, illegal dumping of toxic materials, and contamination of air and drinking water. Currently, there seems to be an increased flow of information concerning environmental health hazards and protection of natural resources.

As world population increases and more developing countries experience the rewards and problems of technology, there will be an increasing demand placed on the discovery, extraction, and processing of natural resources. The pollution resulting from these processes will add more pollution to the environment.

Solid waste and sewage will increase proportionately with population growth, and better methods must be developed for disposal and recycling of wastes as well as for decreasing the production of solid wastes. Energy needs will also increase proportionately with population growth and consumer demand. With concerted conservation programs, energy waste and production can be significantly reduced. Energy needs are affected by economic factors, consumer demand, and availability of resources. Development of renewable and nonpolluting energy resources such as sun and wind power will occur when it is economically profitable. Individuals may hasten this development by demanding that self-contained, individual energy resources be available for purchase (such as solar energy collectors for home hot water production). As the cost of nuclear power plants continues to increase and the health hazards are identified, strict regulations may force utilities to explore other energy options.

Cutting forests (deforestation) for timber, agriculture, and wood fuel has severely reduced the availability of wood. Deforestation will require that paper be recycled and that forests be replanted to prevent desertification and concurrent climate changes. The impact of acid rain on vegetation, lakes, food supplies, and forests will demand international solutions to this emerging problem. Citizens will continue to insist that stronger laws and regulations be passed to protect air, water, soil, and other natural resources.

Diseases related to environmental factors will continue to emerge, and research will verify that certain diseases are related to artificially produced environmental pollutants. Nurses will be required to develop environmental awareness and expertise so that they can educate the public about disease prevention through environmental protection. By means of nursing models, nursing theory, and nursing research, the interrelationships of pollution, health behaviors, life-style, heredity, and other factors will be determined. Nurses will play an important role in the identification, treatment, and rehabilitation of people afflicted with pollution-related diseases. The nursing profession must take a leadership role in advocating environmental protection, illness prevention, and community awareness of environmental health hazards. The threat of nuclear war will continue to be the most important ultimate environmental concern until nuclear disarmament agreements are reached and enforced.

Inclusion of environmental health issues in undergraduate nursing education and the development of graduate nursing programs that address environmental concerns will hasten the profession's leadership role in this vital area. Nurses should be encouraged to seek graduate education in public health and to focus on environmental health issues so that this expertise can further be developed and implemented in nursing education.

Transcending Space and Time

It is now 2884. Nurse-healers enter the nursing care center dressed in cobalt blue uniforms that entirely cover their bodies. The center's environment is completely sterile and controlled for temperature, humidity, air quality, and visual and auditory stimulation. Messages encouraging self-healing practices and healthful habits interrupt classical electronic music. Soft lighting alternates blue hues with yellows, reds, and violets. The nurses easily distinguish the course of treatment by the color of the light in the client's unit. Blue is used initially for calming treatments and eventually exposures reach violet and ultraviolet (which can now be visualized by those in the healing professions).

No technical equipment is seen in the care center. Clients are suspended on invisible temperature-controlled air cushions. When necessary, clients absorb fluids by adjusting the permeability of their skins. Waste products are eliminated through suction vents in the air cushions. Healing modalities used by the nurses include a variety of highly evolved treatments that resulted from centuries of nursing research. Therapeutic touch is frequently used both for direct healing and for healing at a distance. The nurses working in the center are skilled at using their hands in ways that promote healing and restore wellness.

The humans inhabiting the Earth are called worldlings. They cannot be differentiated culturally, racially, or economically. These differences were eliminated in the year 2059, when atomic weapon explosions destroyed the surfaces of all of the major continents of the Earth. Survivors were forced underground for 35 years. Those who survived were those who had prepared themselves for the anticipated aftermath of the atomic explosions: primarily scientists, economists, government officials, political activists, and health professionals. The political activists had given up the fight against atomic weapons when they realized that an atomic war was inevitable; in 2045 they went underground and prepared themselves for survival. There also remains a camp of descendants of survivors exposed to the radioactive fallout from the blasts. They are evolving with a variety of inherited changes, such as the ability to see and hear higher frequencies. The people in these Atomic Survivors Camps are studied by the scientists; their occupation is that of scientific specimen.

No pollution is now produced on earth. All industrial activities take place on the planet Mars. Energy is produced by nonpolluting solar installations located on space stations and beamed to collection sites on earth. Less energy is needed for heat now, since the earth's atmosphere has warmed up: some areas are so hot that they are uninhabitable by worldlings. As the temperature of the earth increases, several new life forms are evolving, and most of the worldlings are employed by the government as scientists who study these changes.

The majority of the population live in Triton floating cities (Fuller, 1981). Food is farmed underwater, since the agricultural land was destroyed by the atomic blasts and remains radioactive. Some food products are imported from other planets and substitutes for meat and dairy products are now manufactured. Water is produced synthetically and flavored with chemical additives for drinking.

When the worldings leave the indoor environment, which is completely controlled for air quality, temperature, humidity, and the visual, olfactory, and auditory senses, they wear air-conditioned lead-lined suits to protect them from radiation. No other clothing is needed by the worldlings, who are now very vulnerable to the effects of radiation. Exposure is completely restricted. The smallest exposure would require nursing observation for at least three months in a nursing care center.

In 2665 the earth was first visited by beings from other planets. These visitors were able to communicate with worldlings by using computers and mathematical languages. The visitors from outer space told the worldlings that they needed to develop a philosophy of respect for the universe: they stated that pollution from the Earth's industrial parks on Mars was creating hazards on other planets. The extraterrestrial visitors offered to work with worldlings to abolish pollution. The worldlings accepted, and the Universal Council on the Environment was formed.

The Earth has become a center for healing, and other planets send their unwell citizens to Earth for treatment in the nursing care centers. Nurse-healers are known throughout the galaxy for their ability to heal and promote wellness. The nurses are involved in all areas of research as well as in healing, and they work with all other disciplines as experts in healing. The nurses promote wellness not only of individuals but also of the Earth, which is still healing from the atomic blasts of 2059. Several nurses are members of the Universal Council on the Environment and are highly respected by citizens of other planets for their healing abilities.

A great respect for the Earth and the universe is evident now. The worldlings no longer consider themselves to have power over nature; instead, nature is an integral part of their existence. Rituals have developed similar to those practiced by ancient American Indian tribes, and the Earth is once again sacred to the people.

SUMMARY

This chapter has focused on specific environmental hazards, including radiation, water and air pollution, and toxic wastes. The nursing interventions and guidelines presented have demonstrated nursing's unique role in addressing these issues. Based on the future impact of environmental hazards and pollution on health, nurses are urged to take a leadership role in addressing health concerns related to these issues.

DISCUSSION TOPICS

1. What health behaviors can protect people from the damaging effects of environmental health hazards such as radiation, air pollution, water pollution, and pesticides that have bioaccumulated in the food chain?

2. You have decided to participate in a civil defense exercise aimed at preparing people in your city for a nuclear attack. As a nurse, consider the following:

a. What role will you play in the care and treatment of victims?

b. What kinds of injuries and corresponding treatments would be expected after a nuclear invasion?

c. What short- and long-term effects can be expected from radioactive fallout from nuclear weapons?

3. Name one organization in your county or city that addresses environmental health issues and answer the following questions:

a. What is the mission of the organization and what are some major projects currently taking place?

b. How does the organization accomplish its goals?

c. What major issues are addressed by the organization? What is the organization's underlying philosophy in addressing these issues?

d. What publications does the organization provide as educational resources?

4. The staff of a community health nursing agency located in a town that is within five miles of a nuclear power plant has decided to participate in emergency planning in the

event of an accident involving radioactive materials in the plant. You have been selected to chair the committee that will determine the agency's role and to serve as a liaison with the city's emergency planning system. Consider the following when determining your nursing involvement in emergency planning:

a. What actions can be taken to prevent this type of an accident from occurring?

b. If an accident were to occur, what immediate steps should be taken by the nurses in your agency?

c. If orders for evacuation were given, who would be evacuated first and why?

d. Considering the health dangers of radioactive materials that may be released into the environment immediately after such an accident, what public health warnings should be issued immediately?

5. Name one major environmental health hazard in your community and plan a group discussion around the following questions:

a. What is the history of this issue in your community?

b. Is the health of the community threatened? If so, how?

c. What can individuals do on their own to solve the problem?

d. What can individuals do collectively to solve the problem?

e. What are private industry and government agencies doing to alleviate the problem?

f. What will be the long-term health impact if the problem persists?

6. Within the next few years, computer systems will be readily available for information storage, retrieval, analysis, and situation simulation. In what ways will computers be helpful to nurses and other health professionals in determining the effects of environmental pollution on human health?

BIBLIOGRAPHY

Baum, A., & Singer, J., eds.: *Advances in environmental psychology (Vol. 3): Energy: Psychological perspectives.* Hillsdale, N.J.: Lawrence Erlbaum Associates, 1981.

Biddle, W.: Meeting on dioxin soil poisoning reassures Missourians somewhat. *The New York Times,* November 19, 1982.

Biddle, W.: Dioxin's peril to humans: Proof is elusive. *The New York Times,* January 23, 1983, p. 36.

Boffey, P.: Agent Orange: Despite spate of studies, slim hope for answers. *The New York Times,* November 30, 1982, p. 31.

Britain, V.A.: Radiation: Benefit vs. risk. *F.D.A. Consumer,* HHS Publication No. 75-8014, Washington, D.C.; U.S. Government Printing Office, September 1974.

Brittin, W.E., West, R., & Williams, R.: *Air and water pollution.* Boulder, Col.: Colorado Associated University Press, 1972.

Britton, G., Damron, B.L., Edds, G.T., & Davidson, J.M.: *Sludge—Health risks of land application.* Ann Arbor, Mich.: Ann Arbor Science Publishers, 1980.

Brown, M.H.: *Laying waste—The poisoning of America by toxic waste chemicals.* New York: Pantheon, 1980.

Butterfield, R.: Physicians warn of nuclear risks. *The New York Times,* December 10, 1981, p. A20.

Caldicott, H.: *Nuclear madness.* Brookline, Mass.: Autumn Press, 1980.

Carson, R.: *Silent Spring.* Boston: Houghton Mifflin, 1962.

Cionne, E.J., Jr.: Ultrahigh level of poison cited

at Love Canal. *The New York Times*, July 13, 1982.

CIP Bulletin. Carcinogen Information Program, Webster College, St. Louis, Missouri, 1980.

Clark, C.C.: Environmental wellness. *Nurse Practitioner* 6(6), 32–37, 1981.

Cops and dumpers. *The New York Times*, October 7, 1982, p. E5.

Debate over nuclear testing: Where, why, and how? *The New York Times*, September 19, 1982, p. E5.

Ehrlich, P.R., Ehrlich, A.H., & Holdren, J.P.: *Ecoscience: Population, resources, environment.* San Francisco: Freeman, 1977.

E.P.A. agrees to Cleanup of Missouri dioxin sites with U.S. funds. *The New York Times*, November 19, 1982.

Fall Convention Report. *The Reporter* 5 (10), 1981.

Fitzpatrick, M.S.: *Environmental health planning.* Cambridge, Mass.: Ballinger, 1978.

Forstner, U., & Wittmann, G.: *Metal pollution in the aquatic environment.* Heidelberg: Springer-Verlag, 1979.

Franklin, B.: Atom waste disposal issue still unwelcome in Congress. *The New York Times*, August 25, 1982, p. A12.

Fuller, R.B.: *Critical path.* New York: St. Martin's, 1981.

Garmon, L., & Peterson, I.: If it's AVM, this must be France. *Science News*, January 3, 1983, p. 61.

Gofman, J.: *Radiation and human health.* San Francisco: Sierra Club Books, 1981.

Greater New York Council on Energy: *Alternate Currents* 2(3), 2–3, 1980.

Gregerman, S.: *Hazardous waste technologies—Chemical landfills.* Ann Arbor, Mich.: Great Lakes Basin Commission, May 1981.

Gyorgy, A.: *No nukes—Everyone's guide to nuclear power.* Boston: South End Press, 1979.

Hafen, B.: *Man, health, and environment.* Minneapolis, Minn.: Burgess, 1972.

Hesketh, H.E.: *Understanding and controlling air pollution.* Ann Arbor, Mich.: Ann Arbor Science Publishers, 1973.

Kiefer, I.: *Poisoned land—The problem of hazardous waste.* Canada: McClelland & Stewart, 1981.

Kilbourne, E.D., & Smillie, W.G.: *Human ecology and public health.* Toronto: Macmillan, 1969.

Lathrop, J., ed.: *Planning for rare events: Nuclear accident preparedness and management.* Great Britain: Pergamon, 1980.

Lehr, J.H., Gass, T.E., Pettyjohn, W.A., & DeMarre, J.: *Domestic water treatment.* New York: McGraw-Hill, 1980.

Lifton, R.J.: The psychic toll of the nuclear age. *The New York Times Magazine*, September 26, 1982.

Lifton, R.J., & Erikson, K.: Nuclear war's effect on the mind. *The New York Times*, March 15, 1982, p. A17.

Mancino, D.J.: Radiation in the nurse's workplace. *Imprint* 30(1), 35–39, 1983.

McKee, W.D.: *Environmental problems in medicine.* Springfield, Ill.: Charles C. Thomas, 1974.

Metzger, P.H.: Dear sir: Your house is built on radioactive uranium waste. *The New York Times Magazine*, October 31, 1971, p. 14.

Middleton, D.: Study says nuclear war can't be controlled. *The New York Times*, November 18, 1981, p. A11.

Miller, G.T.: *Living in the environment.* Belmont, Calif.: Wadsworth, 1982.

Miller, J.: Senators to check health effects of early U.S. atomic tests. *The New York Times*, September 21, 1982, p. E114.

Nuclear waste primer. League of Women Voters of the United States (Pub. No. 391), Washington, D.C., 1982.

Nuclear weapons: Report of the Secretary General of the United Nations. Brookline, Mass.: Autumn Press, 1980.

Parker, H.W.: *Air pollution.* Englewood Cliffs, N.J.: Prentice-Hall, 1977.

PCB's in the Hudson River—A reclamation program. Pamphlet No. SW-P23, New York State Department of Environmental Conservation, 1980.

PCB's in the land—A remedial program. Pamphlet No. SW-P25, New York State Department of Environmental Conservation, 1980.

People near reactor get pills. *The New York Times*, November 29, 1981, p. 80.

Pierce, J.J., & Vesilind, A.P.: *Hazardous waste*

management. Ann Arbor, Mich.: Ann Arbor Science Publishers, 1981.

Powledge, F.: Water, water, running out. *The Nation*, June 12, 1982, p. 716.

Procedures to minimize diagnostic x-ray exposure of the human embryo and fetus. U.S. Department of Health and Human Services, Public Health Service, Food and Drug Administration, HHS Publication No. FDA 81-8178, 1981.

Purdom, W.P.: *Environmental health* (2nd ed.). New York: Academic Press, 1980.

Radiation protection for medical and allied health personnel. NCRP Report No. 48, National Council of Radiation Protection and Measurements, Bethesda, Md., 1976.

Reinhold, R.: New tests at devastated town to determine if flood spread dioxin. *The New York Times*, December 27, 1982.

Reinhold, R.: Missouri now fears 100 sites could be tainted by dioxin. *The New York Times*, January 18, 1983, p. A27.

Report by the Comptroller General of the United States: Is spent fuel or waste from reprocessed spent fuel simpler to dispose of? EMD-81-78, United States General Accounting Office, Washington, D.C., June 12, 1981.

Rogers, M.E.: *An introduction to the theoretical basis of nursing.* Philadelphia: F.A. Davis, 1971.

Salzman, L.: The five thousand centuries of nuclear garbage. *Business and Society Review* 78 (26), 1978.

Shabecoff, P.: Environmental agency: Deep and persisting woes. *The New York Times*, March 6, 1983, p. 16.

Shapiro, J.: *Radiation protection—A guide for scientists and physicians* (2nd ed.). Boston: Harvard University Press, 1981.

Smoking—A resource to assist hospitals in developing policies on smoking. American Hospital Association, Chicago, September 1982.

Solon, L.R.: Nuclear power—Proliferation and public health. *Health Watch* 3(2), 5–8, 1982.

Sousa, F.: Chemical waste and radioactive materials—Nursing and health implications. *Imprint* 30(1), 30–34, 1983.

Sparks, P.M.: The trash can blues—Environmental health issues related to waste disposal: Its history, management and implications for nursing. *Imprint* 28(5), 46–49, 1981.

State of the environment 1982: A report from the Conservation Foundation. Washington, D.C.: The Foundation, 1982.

Stern, A.C., Wohlers, H.C., Boubel, R. W., & Lowry, W.P.: *Fundamentals of air pollution.* New York: Academic Press, 1973.

Storm over a deadly downpour. *Time*, December 6, 1982, p. A12.

Tickton, S., ed.: *New approaches to energy conservation—New directions for higher education.* San Francisco: Jossey/Bass, 1981.

Trial hinges on safety of atom tests. *The New York Times*, September 27, 1982, p. B5.

Trieff, N.: *Environment and health.* Ann Arbor, Mich.: Ann Arbor Science Publishers, 1980.

Upton, A.C.: Low-dose radiation—risks vs. benefits. *Postgraduate Medicine* 70(6), 34–47, 1981.

Upton, A.C.: The biological effects of low-level ionizing radiation. *Scientific American* 246(2), 41–50, 1982.

U.S. adopts first disposal rule for low-level radioactive waste. *The New York Times*, October 24, 1982, p. 22.

Virginia delays permits for uranium mining. *The New York Times*, April 11, 1982, p. 19.

What do you know about hazardous waste? A citizen's guide to hazardous waste in Maryland. The National Aquarium, Baltimore, Md., 1982.

Williams, S., Jr., Leyman, E., Karp, S.A., & Wilson, P.: *Environmental pollution and mental health.* Washington, D.C.: Information Resources Press, 1973.

Winter, R.: *Cancer-causing agents—A preventive guide.* New York: Crown Publishers, 1979.

APPENDIX A: SOURCES OF
WATER POLLUTION

	Source of Contamination	Disease	Comments
Bacteria			
Salmonella	Fecal contamination water supply.	Typhoid fever; ptomaine poisoning.	
Vibrio cholerae		Cholera	Most serious water-borne disease
Shigella dysenteriae	Contaminated food prepared with infected water.	Shigellosis	Most common water-borne cause of acute diarrhea in the U.S.
Escherichia coli	Fecal contamination of water supply.		Regional variants of *E. coli* cause "travelers' diarrhea."
Bacillus anthracis		Anthrax	Contaminated water causes anthrax in animals, which can be transmitted to humans.
Protozoa			
Giardia lamblia	Fecal contamination of water supply.	Giardiasis	Most common water-borne disease in the U.S. Not destroyed by disinfection, easily removed by fine filtration.
Entamoeba histolytica	Fecal contamination of water supply.	Amebic dysentary	
Parasitic worms[a]			
Nematodes (ascaris)	Ascaris eggs in soil contaminated by sewage in water supply.	Roundworms	Consumption of roundworm eggs or entry through skin. Most common in South.
Trematodes	Fecal contamination of water supply.	Flukes	Enter skin while swimming or wading.
Cestodes	Fecal contamination of water supply.	Tapeworms	Consumption of tapeworm eggs.
Metals			
Mercury	Water contamination from industrial discharge, airborne disposition, landfill	Minamata disease (acute alkyl mercury poisoning).	Symptoms include muscle weakness, vision loss, impairment of cerebral

	Source of Contamination	Disease	Comments
	leaching, pesticides, mercurial fungicides. Bioaccumulates in shellfish and sea fish, fresh water fish, and other aquatic organisms.		function, paralysis, coma, and death. Mercury is regarded as the most toxic metal. Inorganic mercury does not accumulate in human tissues with age and is excreted in urine.
Cadmium	Since cadmium is always associated with the mining of zinc, inefficiently treated zinc mining effluents and flotation sludge can discharge into streams and other water supplies. Industrial discharge from electrical, iron or steel, paper, and plastics industries. Small amount is used in pesticides. Also used in electroplating process, manufacture of rubber and solder in plumbing. Used in manufacture of nickle-cadmium batteries, brazing-soldering alloys, pigments, and as a stabilizer in plastics production. Widest manmade exposure results from contact of water and food with zinc-coated water pipes and galvanized or plated articles. Rainwater collected on galvanized roofs and used for drinking contains cadmium.	Itai-itai disease	Symptoms include painful skeletal deformities.
		Chronic cadmium intoxication	Symptoms develop over a period of 5 to 30 years and include yellow discoloration of teeth, dry mouth, absence of sense of smell, lumbar pain, leg myalgia, kidney damage, and impaired calcium metabolism. Hypertension, glucosuria, alterations in serum enzymes.
		Carcinogen	Linked with cancer of pharynx, esophagus, lung, intestine, larynx, and bladder.
		Mutagen	Chromosomal and DNA damage
Lead	Water contamination from industrial dis-	Acute lead poisoning (rare)	Symptoms include severe vomiting,

	Source of Contamination	Disease	Comments
	charge, landfill leaching, lead piping. Lead is used in a variety of industries, including electrical, foundaries, iron and steel, pulp and paper, nonferrous metals, textile dyeing, pharmaceuticals, waterproofing, varnishes, lead dryers, chrome pigments, gold processes, and insecticides.	Chronic lead poisoning Carcinogen	intestinal cramps, circulatory disorder. Chronic kidney infection, anemia, mental retardation, and convulsions. Higher rates of lung, stomach and large-intestine cancer found in workers in industries that use lead.
Copper	Discharged into surface water from industrial uses, including electrical, foundaries, iron and steel, nonferrous metals, petroleum refining, pulp and paper products. Also enters water through landfill leaching.	Toxic to fish Human toxicity	Has caused serious poisoning of fish in Holland. Small amounts of copper are needed in human diet. Toxicity can cause gastrointestinal irritation and liver damage.
Chromium	Contaminates water supplies by discharges of untreated slimes and factory wastes. Waste materials have been used for construction purposes in Japan. Used as pigment in cosmetics (green).	Toxic to some aquatic invertebrates. Carcinogen	Does not accumulate in the body. Lung cancer from inhalation of dust containing chromium. Also associated with painless perforation of nasal septum and kidney and gastrointestinal damage.
Arsenic	Enters well water supplies through water leaching when sludge is tilled into the land as compost. Surface water supplies can become contaminated from farmland water run-	Chronic ingestion of contaminated drinking water. Carcinogen	Gastrointestinal, skin, liver, and nervous nerve tissue injuries. Arsenic levels can be determined by means of hair analysis. Arsenic plant workers have higher lung

APPENDIX A *(continued)*

Source of Contamination	Disease	Comments
off when sludge is tilled into the soil. Arsenic also occurs naturally in soils, rocks, and minerals. Arsenic is used in the manufacture of pesticides, ceramics, leather, chemicals, and in the preparation of metals.		and lymphatic cancer rates.

[a] The infective forms of all parasitic worms are removed by fine filtration. Disinfectants may not be effective in adequately destroying the eggs.

APPENDIX B: GROUPS CONCERNED WITH ENVIRONMENTAL HAZARDS

American National Red Cross, 17th and D Streets NW, Washington, D.C. 20006. Provides support services to local civil defense programs preparing for radiation disasters and emergency welfare assistance to disaster victims, communities, and local governments during and after a national disaster.

Citizens' Clearinghouse for Hazardous Wastes, Inc., P.O. Box 7097, Arlington, VA 22207. A nonprofit organization established to provide citizen groups, individuals, and small municipalities with information needed to understand and resolve chemical waste problems. Outreach program, speaker's bureau, and registry of technical experts are provided by the Clearinghouse.

Commonwealth of Massachusetts, Department of Public Health, 600 Washington Street, Boston, MA 02111. Provides booklet *Nuclear Weapons—A Public Health Concern* upon request.

The Conservation Foundation, 1717 Massachusetts Avenue, N.W., Washington, D.C. 20036. A nonprofit research and communications organization whose primary purposes are to improve the quality of the environment and to promote wise use of the earth's resources. Request catalog of excellent publications.

Defense Department, Public Information, The Pentagon, Washington, D.C. 20301 (202-697-5753). Answers written and telephone inquiries from the public about Defense Department policies and programs.

Environmental Action, Inc., Suite 731, 1346 Connecticut Ave. N.W., Washington, D.C. 20036. An environmental lobbying and education organization. Environmental Action also has a political action committee (EnAct/PAC) which contributes money to political campaigns. This organization lobbies for a variety of environmental issues, including but not limited to hazardous waste dumps, clean air, clean water, and nuclear wastes.

Environmental Protection Agency, 401 M Street S.W., Washington, D.C. 20460. Administers federal environmental policies, research, and regulations; provides information on many environmental subjects, including water pollution, hazardous and solid waste disposal, air and noise pollution, pesticides, and radiation.

Federal Emergency Management Agency, 500 C Street S.W., Washington, D.C. 20472 (202-287-0300). Provides information on emergency management of natural, manmade, and war disasters, provides technical and financial assistance to state and local governments in response to disasters and emergencies, conducts research, advises the president, and coordinates civil defense community programs.

Friends of the Earth, 1045 Sansome Street, San Francisco, CA 94111. An activist environmental lobbying organization seeking to preserve the natural world not solely for its own sake but to provide an environment hospitable to humans.

Health Network Against Nuclear War, 1855 Folsom Street, San Francisco, CA 94103. Organization of nurses and other health workers that educates the public and health care personnel about the potential health effects of nuclear war.

Natural Resources Defense Council, Inc., 122 East 42 Street, New York, NY 10168. Through legal channels, this organization works to ensure enforcement of environmental laws and regulations. Current pollution campaigns include saving the EPA, the Clean Air Act, and the Clean Water Act, control of toxic substances, clean energy, nuclear nonproliferation, energy conservation, and resource conservation.

Nurses' Alliance for the Prevention of Nuclear War, P.O. Box 319, Chestnut Hill, MA 02167. Organization of nurses who are working to bring awareness of the nursing and environmental effects of war to the general public and to the nursing community on local, state, and national levels.

Nurses' Environmental Health Watch, 1808 Aggie Lane, Austin, TX 78757. This nonprofit association has as its primary purpose educating nurses and the public about the health-related effects of a variety of environmental issues, including but not limited to nuclear war, ionizing radiation, chemical and radioactive waste materials, and air and water pollution.

Public Interest Research Group. National not-for-profit, nonpartisan research and advocacy organization established, directed, and supported by colleges and university students. Environmental issues addressed by the group depend on state and local issues. Check the student activity office on your campus to find out if a PIRG exists in your school or state.

Sierra Club, 330 Pennsylvania Ave. S.E., Washington, D.C. 20003. Citizen's interest group. Promotes preservation of natural resources. Focus is on energy conservation, renewable energy resources, and nuclear energy. Monitors national, state, and local legislation. Headquarters location: 530 Bush Street, San Francisco, CA 94108.

U.S. Arms Control and Disarmament Agency, 320 21st Street N.W., Washington, D.C. 20451 (202-632-9610). Formulates and implements arms control and disarmament policies to promote national security. Negotiates and monitors treaties and agreements, including strategic arms reduction talks (START), intermediate-range nuclear force talks (INF), and nonproliferation of nuclear weapons; monitors agreements on biological and chemical warfare.

Veterans Education Project, P.O. Box 42130, Washington, D.C. 20015. A nonprofit organization dedicated to informing veterans about their rights. Is currently serving as a veterans' advocate for Agent Orange (dioxin) and radiation exposure cases. Publishes *Veterans Rights Newsletter*.

28

Statistical Concepts

Victoria Schoolcraft

There are three kinds of lies: lies, damned lies, and statistics.
DISRAELI

OBJECTIVES

After reading this chapter, you should be able to:

☐ Describe math anxiety and how to overcome it.
☐ Define basic statistical concepts and describe their relationships to each other.
☐ Define and calculate measures of central tendency and measures of variability.
☐ Read and begin to interpret data related to central tendency and variability.
☐ Identify implications for the use of statistical concepts in nursing practice now and in the future.

INTRODUCTION

The quote at the beginning of this chapter shows the suspicion with which many people regard statistics. It is a common claim that people can manipulate statistics to prove their points and to take advantage of the unsuspecting. Statistical information can be presented in ways that are misleading to those who do not understand the underlying concepts. The purpose of this chapter is to help you begin to understand statistical concepts in order to use reports containing such information and also to provide a base upon which to build more sophisticated skills.

Statistics and research have always had a role in public health. Because the focus of public health has been on populations, statistical examination of data has permitted the investigation of many health problems. Therefore, it is quite useful for nurses and other health professionals in the community to understand and be able to use statistical data.

Many people feel threatened by mathematical processes. This fear, which is particularly common among women, has led many women to avoid situations in which mathematics plays a part. This fear has limited women's readiness to include mathematically related activities in the careers they have chosen. Since nursing is predominantly a profession of women, this mathematics avoidance has interfered with the development of nursing in areas such as research and statistical investigations.

Technology is already freeing people from some of the drudgery involved in mathematics as well as from the long involved processes in which small miscalculations can ruin the results of data analysis. Computers are easily programmed to accommodate and analyze data in fairly complex statistical processes. However, in order to know what commands to give the computer, you must first understand what results various statistical methods can produce. Although nurses can rely on consultants for assistance in designing studies and analyzing the results, we will do well to be able to conduct some investigations autonomously. By being comfortable with some simple statistical methods and often with only the assistance of a standard calculator, a nurse can design and conduct small, meaningful studies that can help make good choices about the administration of nursing care.

MATH ANXIETY

The term *math anxiety* is "used to describe the panic, helplessness, paralysis, and mental disorganization that arises among some people when they are required to solve a mathematical problem" (Tobias & Weissbrod, 1980, p. 65). Although it is not the only cause of math avoidance, math anxiety plays a role in the avoidance of mathematical pursuits for both men and women. As the term implies, *math avoidance* refers to the activity necessary to avoid courses, language, or other things associated with the use of mathematics.

Many people practice the avoidance of mathematically related pursuits. Often this can be traced to painful and unfortunate experiences that occurred when they were expected to learn how to understand and use mathematical concepts. Other people have developed a pattern of avoiding mathematics because of a lack of practice with the required skills (Tobias & Weissbrod, 1980). Therefore, math anxiety may be both a cause and an effect of math avoidance.

Although much of the current research about math anxiety has focused on women, some investigators have reported that this problem is also quite common in men (Tobias & Weissbrod, 1980). The difference is that more women practice math avoidance than do men. Such behavior is often reinforced and supported in women, whereas math avoidance is not seen as acceptable for men (Nielson, 1979; Tobias, 1978; Tobias & Weissbrod, 1980).

There are now many programs to help people identify these problems and to cope with them. Some are specifically aimed at increasing skill. Other approaches are aimed at assisting people in becoming more confident in the mathematical skills they must use on a daily basis.

Before you can understand and appreciate the usefulness of mathematics, such as statistics, you must feel fairly comfortable with mathematics in general. Anyone who feels some reservations should acknowledge this bias and take some action to deal with it. This is as good a time as any to come to grips with this perplexing issue. For a beginning examination of the problem and some assistance in tackling it, Sheila Tobias's *Overcoming Math Anxiety* is very useful. Further investigation might take you to the mathematics departments of local schools and universities, where workshops and classes may be offered to help people overcome this problem.

Math anxiety and math avoidance have kept well-qualified women and men from pursuing certain careers or from pursuing advanced education in some fields. This feeling about one's self as being "bad at math" has permeated many people's self-concepts and has affected their feelings of competence and self-confidence.

The purpose of considering math anxiety before beginning the discussion of statistical concepts is to emphasize that although you may be concerned about your ability to tackle these concepts, they are understandable. However, if you have difficulty in understanding them from this chapter, it may be because the text is written at too high or low a level for your experiences and expectations. Do not assume that you are stupid because the ideas and concepts are not immediately obvious.

One thing that may help you tackle any mathematical pursuit is to incorporate both intuitive thinking and logical thinking. In approaching a mathematical problem, it may be helpful first to try to grasp the problem and the potential solution intuitively. For example, considering the concept of "central tendency." The name implies that it has to do with things in the center. It might help, therefore, if you visualize a large field with a central area as you work through the problem. This kind of display helps bolster the verbal or numerical explanations by engaging the intuitive thinking processes.

INTRODUCTION TO STATISTICS

It often comes as a surprise to people to discover how considerable was Florence Nightingale's interest and grasp of the value of statistics in investigating and evaluating nursing and hospital organization. Her extensive and detailed compilations of statistics enabled her to influence those in power on many occasions when she intervened in the interests of soldiers and others whose care interested her. She was able to use the picture that such statistics provided to offer a wide view of health and illness problems and to formulate broadly based interventions. One example of this thoroughness in the use of statistics was the document *Notes on Matters Affecting the Health, Efficiency and Hospital Administration of the British Army*. Among the facts she brought to light was that the death rate of men in the British army was twice that of the death rate for young civilian men (Huxley, 1975). Her efforts to accumulate such information, brilliance at drawing conclusions from them, and perseverance in putting the information in the right hands made her a powerful influence in the design of health and hospital measures to protect soldiers and eventually other British citizens.

As the example indicates, statistics are not merely dry facts: they are useful bits of information that, when compiled, can guide us in assessing and intervening with individuals, groups, and communities. A *statistic* is a single datum which tells us something about a person, a group, or an object. Examples include the number of nurses in the United States, the number of households in a community, the amount of particulate matter in the air, the number of new cases of cancer in a city, and the amount of change in the number of unemployed people from the same month in a previous year. Statistics is also the name of the branch of mathematics in which numerical data are collected, analyzed, interpreted, and presented. Table 28.1 is a glossary of statistical terms.

There are three types of statistical methodology: descriptive, correlational, and inferential. *Descriptive statistics* give information or describe a sample (Downie & Heath, 1974). For example, an investigator might want to describe the level of health knowledge among the adult residents of a given community. The investigator could administer a health knowledge assessment test and calculate the scores. The average score would be computed as well. From these pieces of information, the investigator could describe the average level of health knowledge among members of the community and could compare any given person's performance to the average, high, and low scores. If the test used is one that had been proven valid and reliable with other groups, the investigator could also compare the scores of individuals or the average score to statistics about other groups.

Correlational analysis is the investigation of relationships among two or more variables (Downie & Heath, 1974). A *correlation,* or relationship, that is demonstrated to exist between variables may or may not indicate that one variable is the cause of the other. However, when relationships are discovered between variables, it does permit prediction and encourage further studies. For example, in the use of the health knowledge assessment test mentioned above, the investigator might also gather information about the educational backgrounds, economic statuses, and occupations of those taking the test. Relationships may be found among these various measures that would

---

TABLE 28.1
Glossary of Statistical Terms

Bias: Systematic error introduced by encouraging one outcome over others.

Central tendency: A point in a distribution where scores are concentrated.

Data: Measures or statistics used in calculation.

Inference: A generalization from a sample to a population.

Mean: The point about which the sum of deviations is zero.

Median: The midpoint of a distribution of scores.

Mode: The score that occurs most frequently.

Population: group of persons or a set of scores about which an investigator wishes to draw conclusions.

Random sample: A sample drawn in such a way that every member of the population had an equal opportunity of being included.

Range: The difference between the high score and the low score in a distribution.

Reliability: The degree to which an instrument consistently measures what it is meant to measure.

Sample: A portion of a population.

Standard deviation: The square root of the variance.

Validity: The degree to which an instrument measures what it is supposed to measure.

Variable: A characteristic that takes on different values.

Variability: The extent to which scores in a distribution scatter or cluster.

Variance: The mean of the squares of the deviation scores.

help predict the test scores of other similar groups. Another investigator might study the actual practice of health-oriented behavior and compare that to the level of knowledge about such behavior demonstrated on the test in order to identify knowledge factors that might promote healthy behavior.

In *inferential statistics*, the investigator studies a sample (part) of a population in order to make inferences about the total population (Downie & Heath, 1974). This type of investigation is useful when the total population is too large or too inaccessible to be studied. Samples are selected to be representative of the population. Referring again to the health knowledge assessment test, the investigator might wish to know how knowledgeable the adults in the whole city are about the content of the test. In even a small city, administering such a test to everyone might present numerous difficulties. Therefore, the investigator would draw a sample of people who are representative of everyone in the city and ask them to take the test. After analyzing the results, the investigator could draw some conclusions about the population as a whole.

Data

The basic elements in statistics are data. *Data* are the numbers used in calculation. Data are the actual numbers or facts gathered about the variable one is studying. A *variable* is a quality that may assume different values. In the example of the health knowledge assessment test, the variable is the amount of health knowledge. The data are the scores achieved by those taking the test.

Data may be continuous or discrete. *Continuous data* are that which can be mea-

sured in fractional parts and still make sense. Such data can be converted into measures that are more and more precise, such as converting meters to centimeters or to millimeters. If the data were placed along a line, it would be possible to find a measure at any point along that line. For example, the heights of a group of young women range from 150 to 180 centimeters and are placed on a line. It is conceivable that any measurement along that line could be the height of one of the women in the group.

Discrete data are measurements that can be expressed only as whole units. The number of people in a room, the number of books on a shelf, or the number of automobiles owned by a person are examples of discrete measures. However, in statistical studies, most data are treated as if they were continuous. Therefore, it is possible to end up with such conclusions as, "The average family in this community has 2.6 children." The original measures showed that the families have one, two, three, or more children, but the average may be a fractional number rather than an integer.

Measurement Scales

Data and variables may be placed on four types of scales: nominal, ordinal, interval, and ratio. *Nominal* designation of data means giving a number that identifies the measurement. For example, an investigator might assign numbers to ethnic groups, sexes, occupations, and so forth in order to classify data. Although numbers may be higher or lower than others, the values of the groups classified in this way are not indicated by the numbers. There is no implication, if "nurse" is 10 and "zoologist" is 20 in a list of occupations, that a zoologist is twice as good as a nurse.

An *ordinal* scale is used to place data in rank order. The scale demonstrates the relationship of the measurements to each other in terms of magnitude, but does not indicate the absolute level of merit of the measurements (Minium, 1978). For example, 10 children may be ranked in order of their weights at age 6. The scale shows where each child stands in relation to the other children, but it does not indicate the value of the relative weights. That is, if the child who weighs the least is still overweight for his age, his problem remains even though other children weigh more than he does.

An *interval* scale has the same property as an ordinal scale, in that data are placed in rank order, but it has the additional quality that the distance between individual scores has meaning (Minium, 1978). Calendar years and degrees of temperature are examples of such scales. A person born in 1964 is as much older than someone born in 1974 as he or she is younger than someone born in 1954.

A *ratio* scale has all the properties of the interval scale, but it also has an absolute zero (Minium, 1978). Temperature measured on a Kelvin scale, length, height, and measures of elapsed time are measures that can be put on a ratio scale. A person who is 150 centimeters tall is twice as tall as one who is 75 centimeters in height, for example.

Variables

A *variable* is the object or quality one gathers data about. Variables are either qualitative or quantitative. *Qualitative* variables ''differ from one observation to another in terms of quality or kind'' (Kviz & Knafl, 1980, p. 18). Data about these variables are placed on a nominal scale, because they are differentiated on the basis of their identity and similarity to other data in the same classification. Examples are ethnic group, sex, occupation, or residence.

Quantitative variables ''differ from one observation to another in terms of quantity or amount'' (Kviz & Knafl, 1980, pp. 18–19). These measures are assigned to ordinal, interval, or ratio scales. Examples include any data that are reported in terms of measurable amounts, such as weight, height, test scores, age, and time.

In research activities, independent variables and dependent variables are also distinguished. When an investigator studies a particular problem, the variables are the particular characteristics that are measured. The *independent variable* is the presumed cause of variance, or difference, while the *dependent variable* is the presumed effect. In other words, ''variability in the dependent variable is presumed to *depend* upon variability in the independent variable'' (Polit & Hungler, 1978, p. 38). Change in the independent variable does not necessarily *cause* change in the dependent variable; however, finding a relationship between the two variables enables the investigator to make inferences about the causes of change in the dependent variable. It is usually the dependent variable that the researcher wants to know more about.

Populations and Samples

Population is either ''a group of persons [or objects] about which the investigator wishes to draw conclusions'' or ''the complete set of observations or measurements about which [the investigator] would like to draw conclusions'' (Minium, 1978, p. 15). Thus, a population includes *all* persons or objects in the group. A *sample* is a portion of a population. Taking a sample enables an investigator to study a part of the population in order to draw some conclusions about the entire group. In many of the studies done by nurse-researchers, a researcher would find it difficult to contact or get a response from all the members of a given group. Therefore, a sample is an accessible and economical alternative.

In order to be useful to statistical studies and to provide a basis for valid inferences, a sample must be representative of the characteristics of the group of which it is a part. The way in which this is promoted is by selecting random samples. A *random sample* "must have been selected in such a way that every [individual] in the population had an equal opportunity of being included in the sample" (Minium, 1978, p. 16). For example, an investigator wishes to study an aspect of the elderly population in a given community. There are more than 1,000 people in the community over the age of 70 (the investigator's determination of the lower limit of "elderly"). The investigator determines that a sample of 100 people would be of sufficient size for the study. In order to obtain a random sample, the investigator could do a number of things. The starting point would be to assign every member of the population a number. One method would be to use a computer to generate a list of 100 random numbers up to and including 1,000. Most computers have a program permitting the generation of such a list. The people who had been assigned these numbers would then constitute the sample. Another way would be to write down all the numbers from 1 to 1,000 on individual slips of paper and then to draw 100 slips out of a box. Another method would be to use a random number table (see Rand Corporation, *A Million Random Digits with 100,000 Normal Deviates* and the statistics books listed at the end of this chapter). As the examples demonstrate, there are a variety of ways in which to obtain a random sample. The choice of

method would be determined by the number of members of the population in question and the resources available to the investigator.

It is often helpful to illustrate random sampling with some examples of samples that are not random. Two investigators want to find out how many people in the community realize that a rape crisis center is available. They go through the phone book and call the first and last people listed on each page to get a sample of whether or not the people in the community are informed. There are two factors in particular which make this method invalid. First, anyone in the community who does not have a phone or whose phone number is unlisted has no chance of being included in the sample. Second, anyone whose name appears anywhere on the page but in the first or last position is excluded from the sample. By excluding these people from the survey, the investigators may get an inaccurate picture of the community. There may be factors related to not having a phone or having an unlisted number that are related to the variable under consideration.

Another example of a sample that is not random will further emphasize the importance of this concept. A nurse in a clinic wants to obtain clients' opinions about needs the clinic might meet. She decides to have the first 10 clients each day, for one week, fill out a questionnaire. She feels that this will be a random sample, because people can select the time they want appointments; therefore, it is just "chance" as to who will have appointments at these times. This is not a random selection, however, because as soon as the nurse determines to select the first 10 people each day, she has excluded any clients who must be seen later in the day because of such factors as work schedules, distance from the clinic, or reliance on transportation unavailable earlier.

In addition, she has also excluded any clients who may be seen during other weeks. Thus she will have an unrepresentative sample.

Probability

In inferential statistics, an important concept is probability. "The *probability* of any specified random event is the ratio of the number of ways that event can occur to the total number of possible outcomes" (Kimble, 1978, p. 93). If a person tosses a coin, there are only two possible outcomes: heads or tails. Therefore, the probability of the coin landing heads up is 1 : 2, or one out of two. If the person tosses three coins, there are eight possible outcomes (two possibilities for each coin, or $2 \times 2 \times 2$). One possibility is three heads (HHH), and a second is three tails (TTT). However, there are also three combinations that would produce two tails and one head (TTH, THT, and HTT) and three combinations that would produce two heads and one tail (HHT, HTH, THH).

The face turned up by each coin is a separate event contributing to the final total outcome. That is, no matter what the first coin turns up, the face turned up by the second coin is totally unaffected by the first coin, and the third coin is unaffected by either the first or second coins. Therefore, the probability of getting all three heads is 1 : 8 (one out of eight possibilities), but the probability of getting two heads and one tail is 3 : 8 (three out of eight). If the different ways of getting two heads and one tail or two tails and one head were not considered as different possible outcomes, the erroneous conclusion would be drawn that there are only four possible outcomes: HHH, TTT, HHT, or TTH. In that case, one would expect that each of the four events would have the same probability of occurring, and one would expect to see three heads or three tails coming up just as often as two heads and one tail or two tails and one head. If you flip three coins several times, you will demonstrate that this is not accurate.

The aim of statistics is to test data using certain mathematical processes that allow you to draw conclusions and make inferences within certain limits of probability. Statistical tests have been developed that permit researchers to analyze data and arrive at numerical expressions that make it possible for the researcher to predict that a certain finding is applicable to a population within a given range of probability. This allows us to study and to predict events and outcomes much more significant than how many heads or tails may turn up. For example, a nurse in the community may wonder if there is a relationship between a certain respiratory problem and the proximity of those affected to an industrial site suspected of contaminating the air. A correlational study could be conducted investigating the incidence of this disease in people within a mile of the site and people who live further than a mile away. Such a study might yield results that demonstrated a relationship between the disease and the nearness to the site. Comparing the correlation coefficient with values in an appropriate table would show whether or not this result is likely to have occurred by chance or if it is significant. Statistical tables such as the one referred to greatly simplify analysis of data because they incorporate the ratios of the observed outcomes to the possible outcomes.

MEASURES OF CENTRAL TENDENCY

A measure of *central tendency* is a point in a distribution of measures where scores are concentrated. Central tendency is useful because it allows the comparison of the performance of one group either to a standard of performance or to the performance of another group. The three most commonly used measures of central tendency are mode, median, and mean.

The *mode* is the score that occurs most frequently in a distribution of scores. Table 28.2 lists twenty scores in a hypothetical distribution on a fictitious Health Knowledge Assessment Test (HeKAT). The score that occurs most frequently is 56. Therefore, that score is the mode, sometimes indicated as *Mo*. The *median* is the point in a distribution between the upper half of the scores and the lower half of the scores. In the twenty HeKAT scores in Table 28.2, the median is between 56 and 57, or 56.5. The symbol used for the median is *Mdn*.

The *mean* is the point in a distribution of scores about which the sum of the deviations is zero (Downie & Heath, 1974). The mean is calculated by summing all of the scores and dividing by the number of scores in the distribution. The mean is usually represented with the symbol $\overline{X}$. In mathematical processes, when several scores are summed, the symbol Σ is used to mean "sum of." Table 28.3 shows the distribution

TABLE 28.3
Calculating the Mean and Deviation Scores (Group 1)

X	$X - \overline{X}$[a]
72	15
70	13
68	11
65	8
65	8
63	6
61	4
58	1
58	1
57	0
56	-1
56	-1
56	-1
51	-6
49	-8
49	-8
48	-9
47	-10
47	-10
44	-13
$\Sigma X = 1140$	$\Sigma = 0$

[a] Formula: $\overline{X} = \dfrac{\Sigma X}{N}$

$$\overline{X} = \frac{1140}{20} = 57$$

TABLE 28.2
Scores on Health Knowledge Assessment Test (Group 1)

72	58	49
70	58	49
68	57	48
65	56	47
65	56	47
63	56	44
61	51	

of the HeKAT scores, the formula for calculating the mean, and the substitution in the formula for the scores in the distribution. The figure also shows the deviation scores, which are obtained by subtracting the mean from each score in the distribution. These scores will be used later in other calculations. However, they are shown here to demonstrate that if they are summed, their product is zero, as stated in the definition of the mean.

A common term used to refer to any measure of central tendency is the *average*.

However, in statistical analysis, the precise terms are used: mean, median, and mode. For most statistical work, the measure used is the mean. The use of the term "average" is a good example of ways in which people misinterpret or misrepresent data. For example, Table 28.4 displays another list of scores from a different group that took the HeKAT. What is the average score of the group? The mode is 50, but these scores are concentrated toward the lower end of the distribution, therefore not describing much about the total distribution. The mean is 60.64. However, no score actually appears at that point and only four scores are above it, again not describing much about the total distribution. The median is 53. In this case, the median may give more information about the group's scores, because it shows that as many people scored higher than 53 as scored lower. These differences indicate the importance of knowing the measure being used when the term "average" is used.

The mean enables one to compare the performance of individuals and groups with the performance of other groups or with standards which have been set. For example, if the Health Knowledge Assessment Test was known to be a reliable indicator of knowledge about the material contained in it, the mean obtained for administering it to various groups would result in a standard for comparison. For example, if the national mean was 50, then both groups 1 and 2 are above the national average. Whether or not that really means anything depends upon who is making the interpretations. Further statistical tests could be run to draw further conclusions. For example, the t test is a statistical test that permits us to test means to find out if any difference between them is statistically significant. In this particular instance, a t test was done comparing both groups' means to the national mean of 50. In comparing each group's mean with the other, the results show a significant statistical difference between these groups and the national mean but no statistical difference between groups 1 and 2. The formula for the t test and the calculations involved are shown in Table 28.5. The purpose of including this discussion here is to show that statistical tests can help determine how significant a result is. As you progress through statistics coursework, the details of the t test will become more important. It is mentioned here mainly as an example.

MEASURES OF VARIABILITY

Although means begin to give a picture of the group of scores being studied, an additional dimension is required to increase the usefulness of the data. A *measure of variability* is an expression of the quantitative "extent to which the scores in a set scatter about or cluster together" (Minium, 1978, p. 81). Measures of variability show

| TABLE 28.4 |
| Scores on Health Knowledge |
Assessment Test (Group 2)
79
78
77
75
54
53
52
50
50
50
47
$\Sigma X = 667$

TABLE 28.5
Using the *t* test to Compare Means

Formula for testing a single mean

$$t = \frac{\overline{X} - \mu}{s_{\overline{X}}}$$

Formula for testing two means

$$t = \frac{(\overline{X} - \overline{Y}) - (\mu_X - \mu_Y)}{\sqrt{\frac{\Sigma(X - \overline{X})^2 + \Sigma(Y - \overline{Y})^2}{(n_X - 1) + (n_Y - 1)}\left(\frac{1}{n_X} + \frac{1}{n_Y}\right)}}$$

$\overline{X}$ = Mean of a group
μ = Mean of the criterion group
$s_{\overline{X}}$ = Standard error of mean = $\dfrac{s}{\sqrt{n}}$
$\overline{Y}$ = Mean of second group
n = Number of scores in group
df = Degrees of freedom; calculated by $n - 1$
p = Level of statistical significance

Comparing group means to "national average" for HeKAT
Group 1 (19 df; $p = .05$; critical $t = \pm 1.729$)

$$t = \frac{57 - 50}{2.29} = 3.06$$

Group 2 (10 df; $p = .05$; critical $t = \pm 1.812$

$$t = \frac{60.64 - 50}{3.16} = 3.37$$

Comparing two group means
Groups 1 and 2 (29 df; $p = .05$; critical $t = \pm 1.699$)

$$t = \frac{(57 - 60.64) - (50 - 50)}{\sqrt{\frac{1314 + 1629.06}{19 + 10}\left(\frac{1}{20} + \frac{1}{11}\right)}} = -.97$$

something about how much alike or how different the scores in a distribution are.

The *range* is the simplest measure of variability. It is the difference between the high score in a distribution and the low score. What are the ranges for the distributions in Tables 28.2 and 28.4? To arrive at these figures, subtract 44 from 72 for the Group 1 to obtain the range of 28. For Group 2, the range is 30. In this instance, the two groups are being compared on the same scale for the same test; therefore, it is legitimate to draw conclusions about the relative performance of these groups. However, if the two ranges pertained to two different tests, such comparisons would be meaningless. For example, Group 1 had a range of 28 on the HeKAT. The same group took another test, Knowledge of Home Safety, and the scores ranged from 87 to 115. This resulted in a range of 28. Since the tests have different scales of scoring, even though the same group got the same range of scores, the scores are not comparable.

The range is a useful statistic because it indicates how much difference there is between the highest and lowest scores. However, it does not reveal how much the scores within the distribution were alike or different. Look at the following distributions, all with ranges of 20:

14, 15, 15, 17, 20, 21, 25, 34

116, 128, 132, 135, 136, 136, 136

2, 3, 4, 5, 6, 7, 7, 8, 10, 11, 13, 14, 16, 17, 18, 18, 20, 22

The scores in the first row are concentrated somewhat toward the lower end, and there is a gap between the highest and second highest scores ($\bar{X}$ = 20.13). The scores in the second row are concentrated toward the upper end ($\bar{X}$ = 131.29). The scores in the last row are fairly evenly distributed along the range ($\bar{X}$ = 11.33). When you determine both the range and the mean of a given set of scores, this gives more depth to understanding the distribution.

Another measure of variability is the *deviation score*. This measure "expresses the location of a score by indicating how many score points it lies above or below the mean of the distribution" (Minium, 1978, p. 84). Table 28.3 shows the deviation scores for Group 1 on the HeKAT. These scores tell more about each individual score than does the raw score by itself and contribute to the calculation of more useful measures. Deviation scores are indicated either by the expression $X - \bar{X}$ or by χ.

The most useful measures of variability in statistical studies are variance and standard deviation. *Variance* is "the mean of the squares of the deviation scores" (Minium, 1978, p. 85). It is symbolized either with σ^2 (the lower-case Greek letter *sigma*) to represent the variance of a population or with S^2 for the variance of a sample. The formulas for calculating these statistics are shown in Table 28.6. Variance is most useful in inferential statistics. The value of this measure is limited in descriptive statistics because it is expressed in terms of a squared unit of measurement (Minium, 1978).

TABLE 28.6
Variance

Variance of a population	σ^2	$\dfrac{\Sigma \chi^2}{N}$
Variance of a sample	S^2	$\dfrac{\Sigma \chi^2}{n}$

The problem of the variance expression is remedied by taking the square root of that number, which yields the statistic known as the *standard deviation*. This is the most important and widely used measure of variability. It is symbolized by σ or S, for the population and for a sample, respectively. The formulas for calculating these values are shown in Table 28.7. Once the standard deviation is calculated for a group of scores, that and the mean of the scores give a good idea of the performance of the group on the particular instrument of measurement. Tables 28.8 and 28.9 show the calculation of the variance and standard deviation for groups 1 and 2 on the HeKAT.

Measures of variability offer the same opportunities for comparisons as do measures of central tendency. They permit you to compare a group with a standard as well as to compare groups with each other. Vari-

TABLE 28.7
Standard Deviation

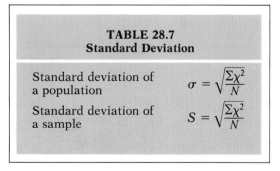

Standard deviation of a population	$\sigma = \sqrt{\dfrac{\Sigma \chi^2}{N}}$
Standard deviation of a sample	$S = \sqrt{\dfrac{\Sigma \chi^2}{N}}$

TABLE 28.8 Variance and Standard Deviation for Group 1 on the HeKAT[a]		
X	χ	χ^2
72	15	225
70	13	169
68	11	121
65	8	64
65	8	64
63	6	36
61	4	16
58	1	1
57	0	0
56	−1	1
56	−1	1
56	−1	1
51	−6	36
49	−8	64
49	−8	64
48	−9	81
47	−10	100
47	−10	100
44	−13	169
$\Sigma X = 1140$		$\Sigma \chi^2 = 1314$

$$^a S^2 = \frac{1314}{20} = 65.70$$
$$S = \sqrt{65.70} = 8.11$$

TABLE 28.9 Variance and Standard Deviation for Group 2 on the HeKAT[a]		
X	χ	χ^2
79	18.36	337.09
78	17.36	301.37
77	16.36	267.65
75	14.36	206.21
54	−6.64	44.09
53	−7.64	58.37
52	−8.64	74.65
50	−10.64	113.21
50	−10.64	113.21
50	−10.64	113.21
49	−11.64	135.49
$\Sigma X = 667$		$\Sigma \chi^2 = 1629.06$

$$^a S^2 = \frac{1629.06}{11} = 148.10$$
$$S = \sqrt{148.10} = 12.17$$

tion allows you to determine where a certain percentage of scores falls in relation to the mean, regardless of the number of scores. The usefulness of this will become clearer in the next section.

ability measures give another dimension to describing a set of scores in addition to the mean. For example, in comparing groups 1 and 2 to the standard for the HeKAT, you would use both the mean and the standard deviation to examine the distributions. If the standard deviation for the national group was 10, Group 1 varied less than the national group and Group 2 varied more than the national group.

As the comparison of the standard deviations indicates, this statistic is useful descriptively for comparing groups of different sizes. Furthermore, the standard devia-

NORMAL DISTRIBUTIONS

When scientists and mathematicians began to notice that many measures of human differences tended to conform to the same kind of distribution, they were amazed and delighted. This tendency has continued to be extremely important in statistics. Many variables in every field of science fall into *normal distributions*. The pervasiveness of this phenomenon is what makes it such a useful concept in statistics. The realization that various measurements fit into normal distributions is the basis for much of inferential statistics and for the theory used for sampling populations.

The Normal Curve

Scarcely anyone has gotten far in the formal education system without becoming aware of the normal curve. The *normal curve* is an abstraction that mathematically describes the normal distribution. All normal curves have some of the same properties, even though they may not be identical in shape. For example, Figure 28.1 shows two different curves, both of which are of normal distributions. The actual shape of a curve is affected by the units of measurement on the x and y axes. On the curve marked A, the scores are not grouped as

closely and the increments in frequency are smaller than on the curve marked B. This shows why it is important to be a careful reader of statistical reports. It would be possible to intentionally or unintentionally emphasize or deemphasize some aspect of the data shown in Figure 28.1.

The standard deviation of a distribution also affects the shape of the curve. Figure 28.2 shows the curves for two groups that took the same test. The groups have equal means but unequal standard deviations. Group A has a smaller standard deviation than does Group B.

Characteristics of the Normal Curve

Regardless of the shape or the scale, all normal curves have certain characteristics that help to define them. The normal curve is:

1. *Symmetrical:* The left and right halves are mirror images of one another.
2. *Unimodal:* The distribution has only one mode at the center. Mode, mean, and median are all the same value.
3. *Asymptotic:* The curve never touches the horizontal axis.
4. *Continuous:* There are no gaps in measurements; they run continuously from one value to another.

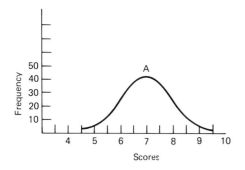

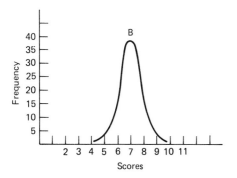

Figure 28.1 Two graphs of one normal distribution.

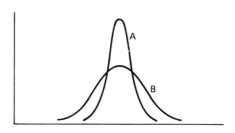

Figure 28.2 Distributions of two groups on the same test.

5. *Proportional:* The proportion of area under the curve is the same regardless of the actual values. That is, approximately 68 percent of the area is within one standard deviation on either side of the mean, 95 percent falls within two standard deviations on either side of the mean, and 99.7 percent falls within three standard deviations on either side of the mean (Minium, 1974, pp. 94, 107).

Figure 28.3 shows a normal curve.

Using Normal Distributions

Knowing that certain things are normally distributed helps you make predictions about the likelihood of certain events. It also helps you make plans and decisions. The following example indicates some of the ways a nurse can use knowledge of normal distributions:

Shelba Morris, RN, knows that according to a standardized assessment test, 20 months is the mean age at which children begin to construct sentences of two or more words. If there is a standard deviation of ±2 months, she knows that nearly any child will be able to accomplish this verbal skill by 26 months (three standard deviations above the mean). With this information, she could expect that she will see fewer than one child in 100 who does not achieve this skill level by 26 months. Shelba uses this information to teach and counsel parents so that they

know there is a range of almost a year within which children develop this skill. (Three standard deviations below the mean would mean that 14 months is the earliest age at which this skill develops. Fewer than .015 percent of children develop this ability earlier than 14 months.)

The example shows how useful standardized data is in teaching and counseling. What would it mean if Ms. Morris started noting that she was seeing a higher percentage than .015 percent of children with a delay of this ability? It could mean that she or whoever is reporting on the children's language ability is unreliable in noting the skill. Perhaps people who suspect a problem are more likely to be seen by Ms. Morris, whose specialty is child development. There may be sociocultural factors within the community that affect language development. There are many possible explanations, all of which would warrant further investigation before Ms. Morris can identify the actual problem. Similar concerns would be investigated if Ms. Morris saw one or more children who began using sentences earlier than 14 months.

Validity and Reliability

There are some important cautions to be observed when applying standardized data. For one thing, the person using a standardized test must investigate the background of the test to determine that the norms have been appropriately set. This includes obtaining information from a variety of sources, not just the designers of the test, to demonstrate that the same distribution fits samples from various geographical areas, from the correct age group, and from the same sociocultural mix. One of the greatest errors in past application of standardized tests was using norms set by one kind of group for a different group. For example, many intelligence tests have been found to be biased against certain racial, ethnic, or

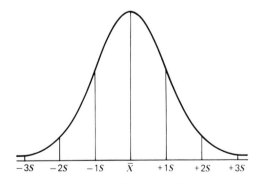

Figure 28.3 The normal curve.

even geographical groups. Such tests include language or concepts characteristic of the white middle class and do not include experiences or idioms familiar to other groups. This example relates to the validity of the instrument. *Validity* is the degree to which a test or other instrument measures the quality it is supposed to measure. In the above example, what may actually have been measured by the intelligence tests was knowledge, not intelligence.

The other aspect of assessing an instrument is reliability. *Reliability* is the degree of consistency with which an instrument measures what it is supposed to measure. For example, a reliable assessment test given to the same children on different days would produce essentially the same results on each administration.

An instrument that is not reliable is also not valid. If an investigator cannot always depend on obtaining the same results when a test is administered to the same group, the measurements on the test must be affected by things other than what it is supposed to measure.

Tom Shipman, RN, wants to investigate nurses' reactions to prolonged isolation such as might occur during space flight. In trying to develop an instrument, Tom gives a group of nurses a proposed questionnaire that includes questions about their feelings about being alone and being in closed spaces. The results fall into a normal distribution; however, when he gives the same group a standardized test pertaining to isolation, the group's scores do not conform to the standard distribution.

The example shows one of the most common ways to establish reliability and validity: to administer the prospective instrument in conjunction with an instrument with known reliability and validity and see if the distributions are consistent. In the example, although the questions on Mr. Shipman's proposed questionnaire seemed relevant to isolation (valid), the results were unreliable.

Interestingly enough, an instrument can be reliable without being valid. The discussion earlier of the intelligence tests represents a good example of this kind of problem. Some tests consistently yield the same kinds of results but do not actually measure intelligence, in many people's opinion. A further example is the question of the validity of some instruments that assess growth and development. The nurse must be certain that the groups used to establish the normal distribution are appropriate. Consistent results that fall outside the published norms may be attributable to gradual change in ability within the age group being assessed. For example, United States norms for height and weight at various ages need periodic revision as children and adults improve their health status.

FUTURE IMPLICATIONS

The dawn of the space age, marked by the 1957 launch of Sputnik, had a great impact on mathematics and science teaching. Over the years, higher-level science and math have been introduced in earlier grades. Sensitivity and creativity in motivating and teaching students in these content areas have not advanced rapidly enough; therefore, students are being labeled and are labeling themselves in ways that interfere with their ability to learn mathematics and science. The future will bring more versatile approaches to learning in all areas.

Already, young people are becoming familiar with computer technology at very early ages. Instead of asking "Read me a story," little children are requesting, "Load me in a program." Such early interaction with computers is enabling young people to become knowledgeable and creative with the technology. Computers offer two particular benefits in teaching science and mathematics. One is that they make self-paced, self-directed learning possible. Once people overcome their initial shyness about interacting with computers, they can set a self-directed pace and proceed unhampered by other learners or the patience of a teacher.

Another asset of computer-assisted learning is computer graphics. A computer program not only can describe the normal distribution but also can display data graphically. The examples used in this chapter can be demonstrated pictorially and sequentially by computers, making the explanations easier to follow. Computer technology is advancing so rapidly that predictions made now may easily become outdated. However, it seems likely that the technology will continue to become more versatile and sophisticated. Units will become more accessible, not only in homes but also in areas designed for inexpensive use by the public, such as libraries.

A principal concern of some people is the potential inequity in computer access between girls and boys (Kiesler, 1983). For example, in some schools, boys tend to take over computer terminals and keep girls from using them or to make fun of girls in order to discourage their use of computers. This kind of situation must be remedied and efforts extended to foster girls' comfort with technology. Programs and games that appeal to girls will become increasingly common. Companies that manufacture computer software may respond to an untapped market and produce materials that will interest and involve girls in computer use.

In order to strengthen the quality of life for each individual, everyone must have some concern for the ability of all people. Fostering the abilities of our young people in mathematics and science will help society as a whole. If educators and parents continue to treat problems with mathematics as personal problems of the students, the older generation will contribute to intellectual and emotional waste. The future must include a real commitment to understanding math learning problems and to creating innovative solutions.

As statistical studies help people to describe populations better, this will contribute to prediction and planning. At present, forecasting the future by means of statistics has variable success. However, as more things are discovered which do or do not conform to normal distributions, it will be possible to be more effective in forecasting. New studies will give new sets of data to replace the old.

As resources change, notions about the significance of certain statistics will also change. For example, one prediction is that by the year 2000, the U.S. population will be about 250 million people. If resources are limited for developing a cure for a disease that afflicts one percent of the population, that group of 2.5 million people will have no recourse. On the other hand, the cure for a disease such as the so-called common cold which afflicts nearly 100 percent of the population recurrently may continue to be high on the list of funded research projects.

Access to computers will increase the opportunities nurses have to conduct research. As nurses increase their confidence with the mathematical aspects of research, they will be able to devote their time to the design and implementation of studies on populations. Their computers will enable them to handle large amounts of data, draw random samples, and study significant variables. As they become more comfortable with technology, they will begin to design their own programs to meet their needs as well as to serve the needs of populations.

Computer networks already exist that enable people vastly separated by space to communicate quickly and efficiently. The growth of these systems will enable statistics to be rapidly available. Skarnulis (1982) cites an example in which a writer filed an article with his publisher via The Source, a subscription network. It took about four and half minutes and cost 50 cents to transmit a 2,500-word article. This kind of activity will revolutionize the system of compiling and disseminating data. Coresearchers from different parts of the United States could collaborate much more easily and inexpensively. Consultants could have a complete visual representation of the statistical information in a matter of minutes and could give assistance in a much more timely fashion than via telephone or conventional mail services.

Mathematics is as much a part of our lives as the air we breathe, and taken as much for granted, until something goes wrong. Early experiences can create both positive and negative attitudes about mathematics. For those who have developed negative attitudes and have avoided math new experiences designed to be positive and curative can reverse these attitudes.

We should all make every effort to build and support an educational system that fosters security and interest in mathematics. Every nurse will benefit from his or her own math skills as well as from the skills of others. Understanding basic statistical concepts will provide a strong foundation for finding meaning in the mountains of data a nurse encounters.

SUMMARY

This chapter has described the problem of math anxiety and some of the implications for nursing of this difficulty. Basic statistical concepts have been introduced to enable the student to understand their application

in nursing practice. Some projections for the future have been discussed to permit consideration of nursing's continued need for mathematical skills.

DISCUSSION TOPICS

1. Describe your early experiences with math. If you have a history of math avoidance, how has it affected you? If you have experienced math anxiety, how have you dealt with it? How has it affected you?

2. If you have math anxiety or math avoidance, what are you going to do about it?

3. How do you feel about the questions below that ask you to do calculations? Will you attempt to solve the problems? What will you do if you have difficulty in applying the material in this chapter to solve the problems?

4. For a study of the students in your nursing program, how would you arrive at a random sample that included 20 percent of the students? Discuss your suggestion with others and decide whether or not the criterion for a random sample has been met.

5. What is the total possible outcomes of tossing four coins? What is the probability of tossing two heads and two tails?

6. How are the mean, median, and mode alike? How are they different?

7. What are the mean, median, and mode of the following sequence of scores? (Answers follow the Bibliography.)

60, 72, 75, 75, 76, 77, 79, 80, 82

8. Describe variance and standard deviation, and tell how they are related to each other.

9. What are the range, variance, and standard deviation for the scores in question 7?

10. What is the normal distribution? How

is it related to the normal curve? Describe the normal curve.

11. When have you used normally distributed data in your nursing activities?

12. What is the significance of the concepts of validity and reliability in statistics?

13. How much have you used computers in your educational experience? In your personal experience?

14. Do you own a personal computer? If you do not own one, how could you get access to a computer on a regular basis?

15. What could you do if you had more time with a computer than at present?

16. How might you be using statistics in the future?

BIBLIOGRAPHY

Coates, V.T.: The potential impact of robotics. *The Futurist* 17(1), 28–32, 1983.

Downie, N.M., & Heath, RW.: *Basic statistical methods* (4th ed.). New York: Harper & Row, 1974.

Huxley, E.: *Florence Nightingale*. New York: Putnam, 1975.

Kiesler, S.: Second-class citizens? *Psychology Today*, March 1983, pp. 40–43, 46–48.

Kimble, G.A.: *How to use (and misuse) statistics*. Englewood Cliffs, N.J.: Prentice-Hall, 1978.

Kviz, F.J., & Knafl, K.A.: *Statistics for nurses*. Boston: Little, Brown, 1980.

Minium, E.W.: *Statistical reasoning in psychology and education*. New York: John Wiley & Sons, 1978.

Nielsen, L.: Feminism and factoral analyses: Alleviating students' statistical anxieties. *College Student Journal* 13(1), 51–56, 1979.

Polit, D.F., & Hungler, B.P.: *Nursing research:*

Principles and methods. Philadelphia: Lippincott, 1978.

Rand Corporation: *A million random digits with 100,000 normal deviates*. Glencoe, Ill.: The Free Press, 1955.

Schrier, J.: Travels in the network nation. *Technology Illustrated* 3(2), 56–61, 1983.

Six population surprises and the future. *The Futurist* 16(6), 72, 74, 1982.

Skarnulis, L.: Is there an electronic byline in your future? *The Futurist* 16(6), 40–46, December 1982.

Sweetnam, G.: Computer kids: The 21st-century elite. *Science Digest* 90(11), 84–88, 1982.

Tobias, S.: *Overcoming math anxiety*. New York: Norton, 1978.

Tobias, S., & Weissbrod, C.: Anxiety and mathematics: An update. *Harvard Educational Review* 50(1), 63–70, 1980.

Vallee, J.: The computer grapevine. *Science Digest* 91(2), 36, 1983.

ANSWERS TO DISCUSSION TOPICS

If you have trouble, reread the relevant part of the text, look at another book that explains what you do not understand, ask a teacher or friend to help you—but *keep trying.*

5. Total outcomes = 16
   Probability of 2 head, 2 tails = 6 : 16

7. Mean = 75.11
   Median = 76
   Mode = 75

9. Range = 12
   Variance = 36.56
   Standard deviation = 6.05

29

Epidemiology and Communicable Disease

Evelyn E. Ramming

All interest in disease and death is only another expression of interest in life.

THOMAS MANN

OBJECTIVES

After reading this chapter, you should be able to:

☐ Define the science of epidemiology.
☐ Describe the epidemiological trends in the study of infectious and noninfectious diseases.
☐ Define the theories of disease causation.
☐ Define the methods of epidemiological study.
☐ Describe three ways the nurse participates in the epidemiological process.
☐ Identify future concerns in epidemiology.

INTRODUCTION

Epidemiology is the basic science of community health. It is both an academic discipline and a method of scientific inquiry. In contrast with clinical medicine and nursing, which study the effect of disease or injury on individual clients and families, the science of epidemiology focuses on the patterns and distribution of health and disease in a given population or community. It attempts to consider all causal factors and relationships surrounding health and disease so that effective programs can be developed to control or prevent the effects of illness or injury and promote optimum conditions for health. This chapter will discuss the basic methods and tools utilized in epidemiological study, some of the progress that has been made in controlling and pre-

527

venting health problems, and the use of the epidemiological method to study present and future health care needs. A glossary of terms relating to epidemiology is presented in Table 29.1.

TABLE 29.1
Glossary of Epidemiological Terms

Agent: Factor whose presence or absence may cause disease; may be biological, chemical, or physical.

Communicable: Able to be transmitted from one host to another.

Endemic: habitual or usual (as the presence of a disease or infectious agent) within a geographical area.

Environment: The external conditions that may enhance or inhibit the interaction between host and agent; they may be physical, biological, social, cultural, and economic.

Epidemic: The occurrence in a community or region of an illness or a group of illnesses of similar nature clearly in excess of normal expectation.

Etiology: Cause of a disease or condition.

Host: A vertebrate or invertebrate species (humans, animals, etc.) capable of being infected or affected by an agent.

Immunity: Insusceptibility to disease or condition; may be natural or acquired.

Incidence: A measurement of the number of new cases of a disease or other event occurring in a population during a given period.

Infection: A result of successful invasion of an infectious organism and its multiplication and growth on or in living tissue; *not* synonymous with disease.

Morbidity: Illness or some other condition, *not* including death.

Mortality: Death.

Pandemic: An epidemic over a wide geographical area, or even worldwide.

Prevalence: Measurement of all cases (old and new) of disease or other condition present in a population at a given time.

Vital statistics: Data about births, deaths, marriages, divorces, illness.

TRENDS IN EPIDEMIOLOGY

To the uninitiated, the term *epidemiology* often evokes a mental picture of the study of communicable disease epidemics such as the black plague and typhoid fever. In some respects, this is accurate, since the science of epidemiology flourished as a result of the need to study and control communicable and infectious diseases. Until a few decades ago, this was the primary focus of the epidemiologist. The leading causes of death in the late nineteenth and early twentieth centuries were communicable diseases, such as tuberculosis and pneumonia. As late as the middle of the twentieth century, large municipal hospitals and sanitariums functioned primarily for the treatment of persons afflicted with severe and often fatal diseases, such as diphtheria, pertussis, poliomyelitis, smallpox, and tuberculosis. Other diseases, such as measles (once considered a benign childhood disease), while not necessarily requiring hospital treatment, frequently had devastating consequences for populations. Complications of measles, such as pneumonia and encephalitis often caused death and disability among children. Communicable disease control was therefore the major concern of clinical medicine as well as of community health or population medicine.

As a result of research and development in the improvement of diagnosis and treatment methods, the advent of immunization against some diseases, improved nutritional status, and better living conditions and sanitation control, there has been considerable reduction in morbidity and mortality from communicable disease. Probably the most significant event in the control of communicable diseases, such as typhoid fever, was not the discovery of antibiotics and medications used to treat the illness but the primary method of water and sewage treatment to help prevent the disease from occurring at all. Outbreaks of communicable disease still challenge the health care practitioner in community health as well as in other areas of practice. We have witnessed the passing of smallpox, and diseases such as poliomyelitis and rubeola (measles) are being eradicated in this country as a result of intensive immunization efforts. However, the threat of epidemics of communicable diseases still is present in areas of the world where unsanitary conditions are the norm or where people are apathetic about immunization programs. For example, in spite of a vigorous and well-planned immunization program in one state, during the spring and summer of 1982 an outbreak of rubeola caused alarm among health care professionals and lay persons alike. This was a result of unimmunized young children being exposed to a school-aged boy who also had never been immunized and who contracted the disease. Rubeola is a severe illness and can cause serious problems for persons who contract it. It is also highly preventable through immunizations.

Other communicable diseases, such as hepatitis, salmonella, and meningitis remain perplexing problems to community health workers. Sexually transmitted diseases, including syphilis, gonorrhea, and herpes II, among others, continue to occur in epidemic proportions in some communities. Although antibiotic therapies are available for syphilis and gonorrhea, newer strains of both diseases have developed that are resistant to standard treatment. These diseases remain major health problems, although public education and treatment efforts have intensified. Herpes II, or genital herpes, emerged in the 1980s as a critical problem. To date, no effective treatment or cure has been discovered. These and other infectious and communicable diseases continue to be the subject of epidemiological study and research.

While some communicable diseases continue as serious threats to public health, they have, for the most part, taken a back seat to chronic diseases as the leading causes of death and disability in the world. Emergence of these diseases closely followed the control and eradication of the severe effects of infectious diseases. Cardiovascular diseases, cancer, and accidents rank as the current leading causes of morbidity and mortality in the United States (Hancock, 1982).

The prevalence of chronic illnesses has increased significantly over the past few decades as a result of continued improvement in the treatment and management of diabetes, heart disease, stroke, and many other life-threatening diseases. Many people who might have died from these conditions now survive. Problems related to lifestyle and stress are achieving prominence in our concern for the public health. In the broadest sense of the term, these problems may be considered to exist in epidemic proportions. Although historically epidemics have involved communicable diseases, now and in the future health care workers need to be concerned about these new epidemics, which affect all aspects of the human condition—physical, mental, emotional, and social.

The focus of epidemiological study should be on those conditions that affect the health of a given population at any given time. If the word "epidemiology" is broken into its component parts, we see this quite clearly: *epi-* meaning down or on; *-demos,* relating to people; *-ology,* study or knowledge. *Epidemiology* then can encompass the study of anything that befalls or comes upon people. Accordingly, there has been a shift in the focus of epidemiological study toward the causal factors and relationships involved in noninfectious health problems. Problems such as automobile accidents, mental illness, suicide, drug addiction, and rape have joined the ranks of communicable diseases and chronic diseases as the targets of epidemiological study. In the future, it is reasonable to expect epidemiologists to focus their attention on those health problems related to increased leisure time, hazards of space travel, and computer technology.

THE EPIDEMIOLOGICAL PROCESS

Causation of Disease

The goals of epidemiological studies are to gain knowledge about the etiology of a disease or health problem and then to utilize that knowledge in the development of preventive measures and public health practices. A number of serious diseases—both infectious and noninfectious—will continue to occupy the interest and time of epidemiologists for years to come. Many of the fundamental epidemiological concepts have evolved from studies of infectious or communicable diseases, but they are equally

applicable to noninfectious diseases and conditions (Lilienfield & Lilienfield, 1980).

The Epidemiological Triangle

A traditional approach to the study of the natural history of a disease or health problem has been to analyze the interaction between a pathogenic or causative agent, a susceptible host, and the environment. This ecological model evolved through the study of infectious diseases and is depicted frequently as a triad (Figure 29.1) in which the agent, host, and environment are in dynamic equilibrium (Dever, 1980). In this model, the *agent* is considered to be the primary factor (bacteria, fungi, virus) without which a specific disease cannot occur. The *host* refers to humans or animate beings that come in contact with the agent. Host factors that influence the interaction with the agent and the environment include biological factors, such as age, sex, race, immunity, and genetic makeup, and behavioral factors relating to habits and customs. The *environment* includes all that is external to the host and agent but that may influence interaction between them. When there is a change in any one of these components, the balance or equilibrium is disrupted and the possibility of disease occurrence is increased or decreased. For

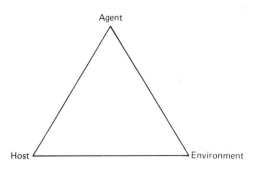

Figure 29.1 The epidemiological triangle.

example, an environmental change, such as heavy flooding of a town, can increase the likelihood that the area water supply will be contaminated with waste products. This increases the possibility that the population of the town (hosts) could be infected by disease-causing organisms (agents). Other examples of disruption that could increase the possibility of disease occurrence include the mutation of a virus, which might increase its virulence and subsequent ability to infect the human host, and conditions in the host, such as severe malnutrition or immunosuppressive disease, that increase his or her susceptibility to disease.

This model of disease causation has been particularly useful in efforts to control infectious diseases. Development of vaccines that increase the immunity of the host and improvement of sanitation and waste disposal (environmental measures) help to control or prevent the transmission of several infectious diseases. However, control of many serious diseases or conditions (both infectious and noninfectious) is difficult, since the causation of these problems is not a single entity. Epidemiological studies of other kinds of disease, such as mental illness, cardiac disease, and cancer, reveal no specific agent or cause. Even with diseases that have an identifiable agent (bacteria, virus), there are often many other factors related to the host and environment that inhibit or facilitate development of an active form of the disease. This necessitates the use of another model of disease causation.

Multiple Causation

The *multiple-causation* approach to the study of disease is based on the idea that effects of disease are not the result of single agents but rather develop as a result of several important and significant factors acting together. This occurs with infectious as well as noninfectious diseases.

Tuberculosis is frequently cited as an example of this model. The primary agent in tuberculosis is the tubercle bacillus, which does exist outside of a host. Not everyone who comes in contact with the agent develops an active form of the disease. Factors related to development of tuberculosis include such things as the virulence of the agent, the characteristics of the environment, and the characteristics of the host, such as genetic makeup, nutritional status, and immunity to the disease. In this instance, the agent (the tubercle bacillus) is a necessary but not sufficient cause of tuberculosis, since other conditions of the host and environment must be present for the active clinical disease to occur.

Having to take into consideration a variety of factors makes control of the disease or condition more difficult. However, it is not necessary to be knowledgeable about all the etiological mechanisms involved in the disease process to take preventive measures. Knowledge of one or two components involved may allow for significant strides in prevention. This is especially true in the control of chronic noninfectious diseases, such as coronary disease and myocardial infarction, for which no single causative agent has been identified. Research has shown a definite relationship between heart disease and certain life-style activities, such as smoking, ingestion of food containing high levels of cholesterol, and increased mental and emotional stress. Control of diet, regular exercise, and use of effective stress management techniques have been shown to reduce a person's risk of experiencing a myocardial infarction. There has also been a positive association established between cigarette smoking and the development of lung cancer and chronic pulmonary disorders. It is thus possible to achieve significant reduction in morbidity and mortality from these problems by not smoking. Even so, there are many instances of people who violate all of these sensible rules and still escape the consequences of serious life-threatening diseases or, in contrast, of people who follow good health habits but die at early ages of heart attacks.

METHODS AND TOOLS OF EPIDEMIOLOGICAL STUDY

Epidemiological study can be summarized generally under the following headings: descriptive, analytic, and experimental.

Descriptive Epidemiology

Descriptive epidemiology is the study of the amount and distribution of disease within a population by person, place, and time (Dever, 1980). Its purpose is to provide a statistical overview of public health problems and to give clues about the etiological factors involved. This method yields a description of who is affected by a particular health problem, where the cases occur, and when they occur. Data are obtained from such sources as vital records and statistics, census information, surveys, and disease reports. The data collected are then presented as percentages or in the form of rates. *Rates* are fractions in which the numerator (top term) contains the number of people affected by a disease or condition and the denominator (bottom term) is comprised of the population at risk for that specific disease or condition. Some rates commonly used in public health reports are shown in Table 29.2.

Use of rates is helpful in comparing and contrasting disease frequency in population groups and in measuring the health of a community. While there is always the danger of misuse of statistical data, there are also valid uses for them in the work of community health. For example, proportionate mortality rates give information about the damage a disease can do. They are the basis for the data on leading causes of death, and they can be used by the epidemiologist in selecting areas for further study and by the health administrator in

TABLE 29.2
Determination of Rates

Rate	Fraction	Multiplied by
Age-specific death rate:	Number of deaths of a specified age group / Estimated midyear population of that age group	× 1000
Case fatality rate:	Number of deaths from specified disease / Number of persons with the disease (old and new)	× 100
Cause-specific rate:	Number of deaths from specific cause / Estimated midyear population	× 100,000

TABLE 29.2 (*continued*)

Rate	Fraction	Multiplied by
Crude birth rate:	$\dfrac{\text{Total number of live births}}{\text{Estimated midyear population}}$	× 1000
Crude death rate:	$\dfrac{\text{Total number of deaths during a given year}}{\text{Estimated midyear population}}$	× 1000
Fertility rate:	$\dfrac{\text{Number of live births}}{\text{Estimated number of females aged 15–44 at midyear}}$	× 1000
Fetal death rate II (*stillbirth rate*):	$\dfrac{\text{Number of fetal deaths at 20 weeks or more gestation}}{\text{Number of live births plus fetal deaths of 20 weeks or more gestation}}$	× 1000
Incidence (*crude rate*):	$\dfrac{\text{All new cases occurring during a period of time}}{\text{Estimated midyear population}}$	× 100,000
Infant mortality rate:	$\dfrac{\text{Number of deaths under one year of age (in defined populations)}}{\text{Number of live births}}$	× 1000
Maternal mortality rate:	$\dfrac{\text{Number of deaths from puerperal causes (pregnancy, postpartum)}}{\text{Number of live births during that year}}$	× 10,000
Neonatal mortality rate:	$\dfrac{\text{Number of deaths under 28 days of age}}{\text{Number of live births}}$	× 1000
Postneonatal mortality rate:	$\dfrac{\text{Number of deaths at ages 28 days to 1 year}}{\text{Number of live births minus neonatal deaths}}$	× 1000
Prevalence (*crude rate*):	$\dfrac{\text{All cases (old and new) existing at a given time}}{\text{Estimated population at that time}}$	× 100,000
Proportionate mortality rate:	$\dfrac{\text{Number of deaths from specific cause}}{\text{Total number of deaths from all causes}}$	× 100
Sex-specific death rate:	$\dfrac{\text{Number of deaths of males or females}}{\text{Estimated male or female population at midyear}}$	× 1000

determining priorities for planning purposes (Lilienfield & Lilienfield, 1980). Similarly, maternal mortality rates and neonatal and infant mortality rates can provide valuable information about the need for programs designed to promote optimum perinatal care.

Analytic Epidemiology

Analytic epidemiology goes beyond the descriptive phase to test a hypothesis about the nature of a health problem. Data derived from descriptive studies often provide clues or findings about a problem that lead an investigator to make a guess or formulate hypotheses for further study. Two methods of analytic study are the retrospective method and the prospective method.

Retrospective Method

In the *retrospective method*, often referred to as *case–control*, a group of people who have been definitely diagnosed as having a particular health problem (cases) are compared with a group of people who are free of that particular problem (controls). The proportion of the specific characteristics being studied is compared between the two groups.

The retrospective approach looks backward to analyze data to see if a disease or other health problem is preceded by or related to some condition more frequently than would be expected to occur by chance. Retrospective studies are relatively inexpensive to carry out, are easily repeatable, and have the advantage of allowing the investigator to study the association of a specific disease or condition with as many characteristics as possible. In a retrospective study, however, one has to depend for information either upon the individual's

memory or on the availability of some record (Lilienfield & Lilienfield, 1980). Also, the retrospective method allows the researcher to make associations between certain characteristics or health practices and the development of disease, but it cannot give a direct estimate of an individual's risk of developing a disease. The following is an example of use of the retrospective method:

As a result of a descriptive epidemiological study, the high incidence of an unusual problem among school-age children in a certain community was discovered. The epidemiologist wanted to discover what factors might have influenced the development of that problem. Through a retrospective approach, he identified and selected a number of children (cases) with the disease in question and compared those cases with a group of children with similar characteristics but without the disease (controls) by questioning the children and their families, reviewing records, and other methods of inquiry. The investigator attempted to make an association between the problem (disease) and certain factors, such as diet, living conditions, or habits.

A retrospective study that has had long-standing importance in the field of maternal and child nursing is the discovery by an Australian ophthalmologist of the relationship between congenital cataracts in children and the contracting of rubella by their mothers early in their pregnancies. Another retrospective study of great importance was the association of heavy cigarette smoking with lung cancer.

Prospective Method

The *prospective method* of study begins with a disease or condition and watches it over a period of time to see what develops. This approach is useful in confirming any association observed from a retrospective study. A prospective study is sometimes called a *cohort study*. A *cohort* is a specific group of people at a certain time. For example, a class of nursing students could be considered a cohort. In a cohort study, an epidemiologist selects a group of people for study and gathers information about those who do and those who do not have the characteristics in question. For example, in a study about smoking and lung cancer, those who smoke would be considered the experimental group and those who do not would be the control group. This population group, or cohort, would be followed over a period of time, probably several years, to see how many of the smokers developed lung cancer. Smokers would be compared with nonsmokers as to incidence of disease.

The prospective approach is time consuming and fairly expensive to carry out. The method does provide a direct estimate of the risk of developing a particular condition in the presence of a certain characteristic. It also enables an investigator to study the relationship of the characteristic to other diseases or problems.

Experimental Epidemiology

In the *experimental method,* the conditions are under the careful control of the investigator. The experiment follows a study protocol and allows for control of variables, random allocation of subjects, and elimination of bias on the part of the experimenter. There are two forms of epidemiological experiments (Lilienfield & Lilienfield, 1980, p. 256):

1. *Clinical trials,* in which the efficacy of a preventive or therapeutic agent or procedure is tested on individual subjects.
2. *Community trials,* in which a group of individuals as a whole is used to determine the efficacy of a drug or procedure.

An example of a clinical trial would be the administration of BCG vaccine as a prophy-laxis for tuberculosis. A community trial could involve the evaluation of fluorides in preventing dental caries.

EPIDEMIOLOGY AND THE NURSING PROCESS

The epidemiological process is based on the problem-solving approach. It compares in several ways to the nursing process. When one uses the epidemiological process, one identifies a health problem or concern, gathers data relevant to the situation, formulates and tests hypotheses regarding causal factors, and then seeks ways of intervening in the situation to prevent the problem or reduce the risk of its occurrence. The nurse can participate in epidemiological studies in many ways. In his or her own practice, a nurse may be the person who identifies a situation that requires further investigation. The problem may be one that the nurse can study independently or with minimal help or one for which a large-scale investigation by the health department is required. The following is an example of an alert nurse's reporting and the ensuing investigation:

A nurse in the health service of a midwestern university was alarmed one morning to see the health service waiting room full of students with similar complaints of nausea, vomiting, and diarrhea. All the students lived in the same dormitory, and all reported becoming ill within a few hours after eating the evening meal in the dormitory cafeteria the preceding evening. Further questioning of the students revealed that there were many more students at the dormitory who had similar symptoms but who were not seeking aid from the health service. The nurse called the local health department medical officer, who initiated an investigation of the complaint. A community health nurse and an epidemiologist interviewed both affected and nonaffected students, cafeteria personnel, and some other campus and dormitory personnel. Food samples were taken, as well as cultures of some of the kitchen equipment. The outbreak of gastroenteritis was linked directly to ingestion of improperly cooked roast beef. Fortunately, none of those affected were seriously ill or had to be hospitalized, but the incident was of grave concern. Cafeteria personnel were instructed in proper preparation, safe handling, and proper storage of all foods served.

In the above case, the nurse in the health service and the community health nurse each contributed to the epidemiological process by participating in the collection of data in collaboration with other health department personnel. By being knowledgeable about the disease process and the importance of the data to the investigation, the nurses were instrumental in assuring that the information was collected accurately and thoroughly.

The nurse must also know which diseases are designated by law as reportable to the local or state health department. These generally include communicable diseases such as measles, mumps, chickenpox, smallpox, rabies, hepatitis, and venereal disease. Prompt reporting of any case of such diseases is imperative. The nurse should take notice of any unusual occurrence of certain illnesses and should gather data on who is affected, when the illness began, and the nature of the problem. The nurse can further promote control of communicable disease by encouraging parents to immunize their children and by educating the community about treatment and preventive measures for disease control.

During the data-collection phase of epidemiological investigations, the nurse can also inform and educate the target population about the need for cooperation with the investigation so that they and others can benefit from the results. Many research or epidemiological studies have been hampered by the study subjects' failure to continue to participate. The nurse's support and guidance of participants could be the determining factor in a study's being carried to completion and considered valid.

The nurse can contribute to the epidemiological process by using data obtained from his or her own practice in the community. For example, epidemiological studies have demonstrated repeatedly the relationship between certain host factors, such as excessive weight, smoking, lack of exercise, and type-A personality traits to the incidence and prevalence of coronary artery disease. Some community health nurses have initiated programs designed to help clients with weight reduction and proper diet intake, cessation of smoking, development of a proper exercise regime, and reduction of stress. By using epidemiological data meaningfully, nurses can help reduce the morbidity and mortality rates of such chronic diseases and improve the quality of life in the community.

Knowledge of the basic concepts involved in the epidemiological process is essential for any nurse, not just one who practices in a community health setting. Nurses play a key role in prevention of disease as well as in restoring and maintaining optimum health wherever they practice.

The tools and techniques that are employed in the epidemiological process, such as rates and other statistics, will be unfamiliar to the novice practitioner. With an increased knowledge base and continued practice, the nurse can achieve a better understanding of their use in appraising and evaluating health problems of the community.

The role of the nurse in epidemiological investigations is important and should not be taken lightly. From initiation of the study to implementation of health programs based on the results of the investigation, the nurse has a great deal to contribute to the control and prevention of many health care problems and to promotion of health in the community.

PLANNING FOR HEALTH: MANDALA OF PUBLIC HEALTH

An innovative approach to studying health and illness in a community has been proposed by Trevor Hancock and his colleagues in Toronto (Hancock, 1982). Hancock's model speaks to the need to consider multiple causation and the relationship of internal and external factors that influence health. This mandala of health (a mandala is a circular symbol of the universe) portrays the human ecosystem in all its complexity as it affects the health of the individual (Figure 29.2). The model shows that people exist within and as a part of nature and of the natural and social ecosystems, influenced by them and capable of influencing them (Hancock, 1982). For example, Hancock's model shows how family influences an individual through four factors:

1. *Human biology,* including genetic predispositions and traits and the degree of the immune system's competence.

2. *Personal behavior developed in child-*

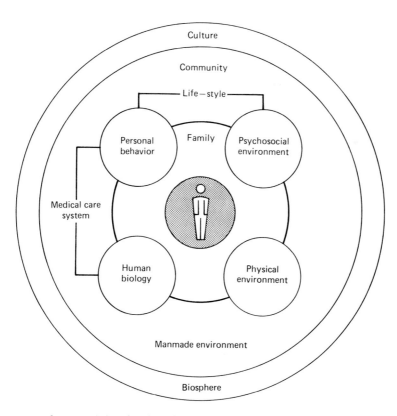

Figure 29.2 The mandala of public health (From Hancock, T.: Beyond health care. *The Futurist* 16(4), 6, 1982. Reproduced by permission.)

hood, including such things as risk taking, eating habits, self-care, and response to stress.

3. *Psychosocial environment of the individual and family,* including school, work, workplace, and the impact of media.

4. *Physical environment,* not only in the home but also in the workplace and the neighborhood.

Hancock defines life-style as personal behavior modified and influenced by a lifelong process of socialization. He cites as an example that the decision to smoke is influenced by a complex set of factors including influence of peers, behavior of parents, and the social image of smoking portrayed in the media.

Thus any attempt at changing people's habits apart from the context of their psychosocial environment may be futile. The mandala shows the limited role that the medical care system plays in determining an individual's health (Hancock, 1982): the community environment is far more influential. Furthermore, individuals are affected by the planetary biosphere (including air, water, soil, and all living things) and by their cultural system, which is based on Judeo-Christian tradition, a scientific approach, democratic political thought, and a technological emphasis and which imposes its own philosophy, world view, and values on our perceptions (Hancock, 1982). The mandala illustrates the human ecosystem of health. It is being utilized by the City of Toronto Department of Public Health as a model for the complexity and the interrelationship of factors that affect health and illness and thus as a way of determining what interventions are needed to improve the public's health. This model is discussed further in Chapters 23 and 30.

FUTURE IMPLICATIONS

Epidemiology has made great strides toward discovering the etiology of diseases and the identification of preventive measures. The greatest successes have been in the area of communicable diseases. There is also better understanding of causal mechanisms of noninfectious and chronic diseases. In the future, epidemiologists will still be concerned about the prevention and control of communicable diseases. There will be continued health department surveillance of diseases that are currently kept under control by means of immunization and sanitation measures. The emergence of new strains of known pathogens that are resistant to standard therapy will require intense study to discover a method of control. Diseases such as acquired immune deficiency syndrome, which is believed to be caused by an as yet unknown virus, will continue to be the focus of long-term epidemiological study. There is also the possibility of human contact with new microorganisms as a result of space exploration. Communicable disease control will undoubtedly be a major focus of epidemiology for years to come.

Study of chronic noninfectious diseases will be affected by several societal changes. One of these is the increasing proportion of elderly people in the population. By the year 2030, the percentage of the world's population over 65 years of age is expected to be from 18 to 20 percent (Bezold, 1982). The proportion of people with health problems generally increases with age. As a group, the elderly are more likely than the young to suffer from the effects of multiple, chronic, and often disabling conditions. The *Surgeon General's Report on Health Promotion and Disease Prevention* (1979) states that 80 percent of our older people have one or more chronic conditions; their medical treatment accounts for about 30 percent of the nation's health care expenditures. Certainly epidemiological studies will continue to explore health problems related to aging and the elderly and to use the information gained through such studies to improve the health and quality of life for older adults.

Study will continue of the effect of environmental pollution on human health. Toxic factors in the environment currently present great challenges to public health personnel. Large numbers of people are exposed to chemicals designed for industrial and agricultural use. Air pollution remains as a major health hazard. Radiation is a serious health concern for many people. Exposure to these toxic compounds and to ionizing radiation can have serious effects on human populations that may not be realized for 20 years or more. Current clinical and epidemiological research has helped to identify harmful substances by finding unusually high rates of disease occurrence in certain population groups with histories of exposure to toxic environmental agents. Epidemiological teams of the twenty-first century will continue to uncover more data about the effects of exposure to hazardous elements on the physical and mental health of human populations.

The effect of the communications revolution on the health of individuals has already aroused some concern. For example, increasing use of computers and related equipment in houses and offices has led some experts to ask whether sitting in front of an electronic screen for long stretches of time will become a major health hazard by the end of the century (Bezold, 1982).

The growing American interest in nutrition, exercise, and health promotion could have an effect in the future on reduction of morbidity and mortality from some chronic diseases. The probability of extra-terrestrial travel and life on a space station will provide additional areas of study for the epidemiologist in relation to physical and mental health of the travelers.

SUMMARY

Epidemiology is the basic science of community health. An understanding of its concepts and principles is vital for nurses in the community or hospital setting. This chapter has described the broad scope of epidemiology in the study of infectious and noninfectious diseases as well as other significant health-related events. Theories of disease causation and some methods and tools of epidemiological study were discussed. The epidemiological process was compared with the nursing process, and the importance of the role of the nurse was emphasized. Future applications of the epidemiological process were discussed.

DISCUSSION TOPICS

1. Select a noninfectious health problem in your community, such as motor vehicle accidents or alcoholism. Analyze the problem according to the theory of multiple causation. Identify possible areas of intervention to alleviate the problem.

2. Meet with an epidemiologist from your local health department. Discuss with him or her the process of investigation of an actual outbreak of a communicable disease in your community. Identify factors related to host, agent, and environment that influenced the course of the disease and the method of control.

3. Obtain statistics from your local health department about death rates and morbidity. What are the leading causes of death and disability in your community? What

health programs are available through the health department or other agencies to reduce morbidity and mortality from these problems?

4. Consider the trends in health care delivery today and the possible impact on the health of people at the turn of the twenty-first century. Discuss some potential areas for epidemiological study at that time.

5. What are some possible health problems that may emerge with the opening up of extraterrestrial travel and space colonies?

BIBLIOGRAPHY

Bezold, C.: Health care in the U.S. *The Futurist* 16(4), 14–18, 1982.

Dever, G.E.A.: *Community health analysis.* Germantown, Md.: Aspen Systems, 1980.

Ferguson, M.: *The aquarian conspiracy.* Los Angeles: J.P. Tarcher, 1980.

Hancock, T.: Beyond health care. *The Futurist* 16(4), 14–18, 1982.

Healthy people: The Surgeon General's report on health promotion and disease prevention. U.S. Department of Health, Education and Welfare, DHEW Publication No. 79-55071, Washington, D.C., U.S. Government Printing Office, 1979.

Lilienfield, A., & Lilienfield, D.: *Foundations of epidemiology* (2nd ed.). New York: Oxford University Press, 1980.

MacMahon, B.: Epidemiologic methods. In D. Clark & B. MacMahon, eds., *Preventive and community medicine.* Boston: Little, Brown, 1981.

Wigley, R., & Cook, J.R.: *Community health—Concepts and issues.* New York: D. Van Nostrand, 1975.

30

Health Planning

Victoria Schoolcraft

> The health of nations is more important than the wealth of nations.
>
> WILL DURANT

OBJECTIVES

After reading this chapter, you should be able to:

- [ ] Discuss the importance of a health model.
- [ ] Discuss the implications of the components of the mandala of public health.
- [ ] Describe the characteristics of the soft health path.
- [ ] Describe the contrasts between public health policy and healthy public policy.
- [ ] Identify policy areas that affect community health.
- [ ] Give examples of healthy public policy in various policy areas.
- [ ] Identify ways of becoming involved in health planning.
- [ ] Identify appropriate preparation and participation in health planning groups.
- [ ] Identify behaviors that incorporate awareness of the political nature of health planning.
- [ ] Describe the steps in health planning strategy.

INTRODUCTION

The concept of health planning grew out of the report of the National Commission on Community Health Services in 1966. The commission emphasized the role of the professional who served as a volunteer outside of his or her usual area of employment in order to participate in health planning for the community (Simmons, 1974). The Partnership for Health Act, passed in 1966, promoted the involvement of citizens in plan-

541

ning for health care delivery and in making recommendations about health resources (Foley, 1981).

The National League for Nursing (NLN) established a Council on Community Planning in 1967 but abolished it in 1971. At that time, the Council's responsibilities were to be assumed by the constituent leagues. Simmons (1974) noted this apparent lack of conviction within the NLN about the role of nursing in community health planning. He also drew attention to two important publications about nursing. The report of the National Commission for the Study of Nursing and Nursing Education (1970) did not recommend that nurses become involved in community planning. Brown's well-received study of nursing in the hospital and in the community (1970 & 1971) encouraged nurses to function independently of other health care providers and consumers.

The National Health Planning Resources and Development Act (Public Law 93-641) was passed in 1974. Congress intended this mechanism to bring order to the fragmented health care system, promote better allocation of services, foster continuity of services, establish standards for evaluation of care, and help control health care costs. This act established local health systems agencies (HSAs), which are responsible for planning and developing services, manpower, and facilities to improve the health of communities. The system provided that at least 51 percent of the governing board members be consumer representatives. In addition, nurses were designated, among other caregivers, to serve on HSA boards.

Henry A. Foley, former administrator of the Health Resources Administration, identified some of the benefits of the Health Planning Program (1981): more than 200 health systems agency plans have been developed, over 50,000 citizens have become involved in the health planning process, state and local officials are much more conscious of cost containment and access to health care, business and labor have become involved, and some unnecessary acute care hospital beds have been eliminated.

Recent problems within the system have included uncertainty about federal support because of change in administrations and new priorities, domination by providers of health care, failure to come to grips with the real issues of cost containment, and difficulty in addressing the issue of access effectively. The greatest problem is the continual intertwining of the health system with the illness system.

As long as power in the health care system is wielded by people whose primary affiliation is with illness care, our society will continue to have an expensive burden to bear. There will always be a need for appropriate resources for acute, episodic care. However, now and in the future, most people spend the greatest part of their lives outside acute care settings. The quality of that part of their lives must be ensured by comprehensive and effective planning.

A HEALTH MODEL

The scientific approach to the study of medicine and disease has been a mixed blessing. The identification of causes of disease and the vigorous pursuit of cures have been an obvious boon to the developed nations. The unfortunate aspect has been the disregard for any but the biological factors in disease. Research and investigation have been oriented around disease—either prevention or cure—resulting in a negative definition of health as the absence of disease. This seems comparable to thinking of light as the absence of darkness. Does it not seem logical to define disease as the absence of health, just as darkness is the absence of light?

Does our perspective on disease and health make a difference? Identifying health as a state to be promoted, attained, maintained, and valued demonstrates a positive approach. In the disease-centered medical model, health is a transient state that is regained or restored and human beings are seen as passive and as having little or no power over the onset of disease. This fosters a reactive, dependent client role in which people seek out a medical practitioner to treat them, cure them, and make them well.

Several of the preceding chapters have discussed the importance of acknowledging the influence of numerous factors in the development or deterioration of individuals, groups, and environments. However, the so-called health care system has persisted in emphasizing single factors or the exclusive role of each individual in his or her health. Nursing must recognize the importance of a model of health to provide a rational framework for health planning.

Trevor Hancock, associate medical officer of health for the city of Toronto, has designed a "mandala of health" (1982; see Figure 29.2 in Chapter 29). The most important aspect of the model is the relatively minor place it gives to the medical care system. Of much greater significance are the family, the community, and culture. Within these constructs are the other environmental determinants that interact to influence an individual's health status (see the network model Figure 24.1 in Chapter 24).

Both Figures 24.1 and 29.1 are holistic models with synergistic implications. There is no way to predict the behavior of the whole system or to appreciate the impact of the interrelationships within these models by examining only one part of the system. Both models present holistic views. *Holism* is the perception of human beings as whole persons "made up of physiological, emotional, intellectual, and spiritual dimensions that dynamically interact" (Carlson, 1981, p. 231). Further, the environment must also be regarded holistically, as both models indicate.

There is a desperate need for nurses to move nursing's focus away from illness care toward the factors that affect health. For example, many people are becoming involved in health-promotion activities. At present, these pursuits, even though frequently done in groups, are individualistic. Since such activities as personal exercise programs, sensible nutrition, and stress reduction are helping many individuals, there is an immense need for research on them. Nurses need to develop a body of knowledge to provide a basis for encouraging and supporting particular styles of self-health promotion.

As societal values evolve so that self-care and holistic health become the norm for individuals and families, nurses will become more involved in program development and resource networks. They will develop teaching modules in a variety of formats and media to permit self-directed individuals to remain independent and healthy.

To make any real differences in the future of health, nurses must participate in planning for societal change. For example, nurses must support environmental movements, promote research to discover why healthy people are healthy, and use their assertive and political skills to promote health for all people. Nurses must both promote individual autonomy and initiative and ensure the integrity of the environment.

AN AGENDA FOR HEALTH

Soft Health Path

Hancock (1980) coined the phrase *soft health path* to describe a "flexible, resilient, sustainable and benign" approach to health. Some of the characteristics of the approach are (Hancock, 1982):

· The health model
· Focus on prevention
· Locally based health centers
· Support for effective alternate healing methods
· Concern with quality of life rather than quantity
· Use of community development approaches
· Community approach
· Protection for victims
· Emphasis on the social environment
· Active involvement of the client
· Promotion of self-care
· Sensitivity to the environment
· Concern for global issues

Other writers have characterized approaches as "holistic health" or a "new health paradigm." A variety of these concepts are integrated in Table 30.1.

   The soft health path, the holistic health movement and the new health paradigm are similar ways of approaching health care. The approaches synthesize environmental health, public health, primary care, and self-care. Advocates come from varying backgrounds. Many are health professionals, but vast numbers are people who are simply concerned with their own wellness and with the health of their communities and their planet. The soft health path provides a foundation for planning healthful

TABLE 30.1
Soft Health Path/New Health Paradigm

Qualities
   Health-centered
   Promotion and prevention oriented
   Cost-contained
   Uses minimal amounts of technology
Approaches
   Holistic/integrated
   Acceptance of alternate methods
   Uses new modalities
   Community-based
   Community-oriented
   Planetary perspectives
   Proactive and planned
   Future-oriented
Human Orientation
   Autonomy and self-care
   Body, mind, and spirit in dynamic equilibrium
   Interpersonal relationships emphasized
   Life-style emphasized
   Interaction with environment
   Multiple determinants of health
Attitude Toward Disease
   Seen as a process
   Multiple causation
   Need to strengthen host
Characteristics of Providers
   Facilitators
   Teachers
   High-touch and caring

SOURCE: Ardell, D.B.: Holistic health planning. In *The holistic health handbook.* Berkeley, Calif.: And/Or Press, 1978; Ferguson, M.: *The aquarian conspiracy.* Los Angeles: J.P. Tarcher, 1980; Hancock, T.: Beyond health care. *The Futurist* 16(14), 4–13, 1982; Snyder, R.D.: Health hazard appraisal. *The Futurist* 16(14), 25–29, 1982.

living conditions and for reducing the risks and stresses that lead or push people to live unhealthy lives.

Healthy Policies

In order to plan on the broad scale necessary to improve the health of the nation, it is necessary to start with health-oriented public policy. Hancock (1982, p. 7) offers a contrast between the present "public health policy" and a "healthy public policy." This dichotomy is shown in Table 30.2.

The policy areas in need of attention are energy, transportation, nutrition and agriculture, employment, economics, education, family and social planning, and the medical care system. The overriding belief is that ensuring the health of all will benefit the individual. This contrasts with the traditional approach of caring for individuals and hoping that the result will be general. Suggestions of how to improve all of the areas of concern follow. These paragraphs integrate the ideas of many futurists, particularly Donald Ardell (1978), Marilyn Ferguson (1980), Trevor Hancock (1982), Jennie Popay, Jenny Griffiths, Peter Draper, and John Dennis (1980), and E.F. Schumacher (1973).

Energy

Energy use affects health both directly and indirectly. Direct effects include the pollution of the environment and overreliance on technology. Its incidental and long-term potential for diminishing health include extensive processing of food, the fast pace of life, and the eventual exhaustion of nonrenewable resources. Needed policies and strategies include development and use of nonpolluting energy resources; promotion of simpler life-styles based on limited consumption of energy and material goods; and stricter regulation and monitoring of pollution and waste disposal.

Transportation

Most Americans use private vehicles as their main or only form of transportation. This choice has environmental, energy, and personal implications. Frequent use of private vehicles that burn hydrocarbon fuel combine to degrade the environment. Furthermore, accidents are the major cause of death of Americans from 1 to 44 years of age. Of these, nearly half are motor vehicle accidents, many of which involve alcohol

---

TABLE 30.2
Public Health Policy versus Healthy Public Policy

Public Health Policy	Healthy Public Policy
Chiefly concerned with the health-care system	Chiefly concerned with creating a healthy society
Dominated by the hard health path (care, cure, medical model, high-tech, individual-oriented, dependent clients)	Dominated by the soft health path (prevention, health model, low-tech, community-oriented, autonomous clients)
Sectoral/analytical	Holistic
Present-oriented	Future-oriented
Accepts the givens	Questions the givens

SOURCE: Hancock, T.: Beyond health care. *The Futurist* 16(4), 4–13, 1982.

consumption. Useful policies related to transportation would support safe, nonpolluting public transit; slower, smaller, less-polluting private vehicles; vehicle pools; local distribution of goods; and better pedestrian and cycling routes.

Nutrition and Agriculture

Our American diet features a high reliance on animal sources of protein. This requires us to use large areas of land to produce grain to nourish these animals. Other agricultural land is used to grow nonfood items such as tobacco or crops used in the production of alcohol. Much of the food Americans consume is highly processed and includes a greater amount of salt, sugar, fat, and calories than most people need. Too few people have knowledge and incentive to alter their nutritional patterns. Health-oriented policies would encourage restrictions on production of crops used to produce animals for slaughter or used in tobacco and alcohol production; incentives for local or home-grown sources of food; and consumer education in nutrition and agriculture.

Employment

Chronic unemployment as well as unhealthy work environments are both implicated in reducing the quality of life. Healthy employment policies focus on encouragisng full employment; developing new jobs; and developing systems that place value on the services performed by people not usually considered to be part of the work force, such as homemakers, retired people, and community volunteers. Healthy work environments are promoted by providing work that is meaningful, relevant and satisfying; giving workers determination over some aspects of their work environments; and maintaining physically and psychologically safe working environments.

Economics

The American economy is consumption oriented. People are encouraged to make money and to spend it. The emphasis on production of material goods encourages unwise expenditure of energy resources, the development of nondurable products, and a sense of value predicated on the acquisition of possessions.

Policies promoting healthy economics would include small-scale production for local consumption; self-reliance and interdependence within the community; emphasis on quality and durability of products; limits to growth that threatens the quality of life in an area; and equalizing the resources available to all members of the community.

Education

Our educational system rarely contributes to the development of health values and community identification, often because it overemphasizes traditional curricular concerns, avoids current issues, and rejects the concept of life-long learning. Healthy education policies would promote inclusion of relevant, interesting health teaching and activities aimed toward nutrition, physical fitness, stress management, and environmental awareness in the formal educational system; and provision of alternate learning experiences for people of all ages to enable them to discover healthy components of life-style (e.g., wellness fairs, conferences, and workshops).

Family and Social Issues

Stable families and coherent social policies help to build and maintain healthy people and communities. People need groups to identify with in order to have healthy emotional, spiritual, and physical lives. Promotion of support and cohesion in the areas of family and social policy include encouragement of community self-reliance and development of community projects; facilitation of networks to link families for economic and emotional support; promotion of interaction and understanding among generations; and fostering of self-esteem and feelings of competence and community responsibility.

Medical and Health Care Systems

The current medical care system, with its emphasis on care and cure rather than change and prevention, is far from cost effective. Medical care will always be needed when health care is unsuccessful or untried; but there must be a fundamental realization that the medical care system is not the same as the health care system.

Public policy must differentiate medical and health care. When monetary resources are available for what is presently called health care, those who allocate funds may, for example, be comparing a research project to develop artificial livers with a research project to promote reduction in alcohol consumption. All too often such decisions are decided in favor of tertiary medical treatment rather than primary health endeavors. It is not sensible to keep looking at ways to treat the few at the expense of the many.

Healthy medical policy would include providing links and incentives to minimize the uses of medical treatment in favor of health promotion; defining the limitations of medicine realistically; deemphasizing the role of the medical care establishment within society; making hospitals and other institutions healthier places; and promoting the client's role as a partner in care rather than merely a recipient.

Policy relating to the health care system would include providing incentives for staying healthy; teaching self-health skills; promoting the use of ambulatory and home care; developing decentralized local community health centers; and promoting research into healthy life-styles and alternative health practices.

GETTING INVOLVED

Nurses in local communities can begin their involvement in health planning by determining what community group has the most comprehensive view of health planning and becoming involved in it. This may be a local health systems agency or a community-wide or state-wide planning group. McLemore (1980) identifies several ways in which one can become involved. The first way is to attend the meetings. This will enable you to learn about the workings of the group and will make the group aware of your interest. Some HSA and similar governing boards are elected by community members, whereas others are appointed by professional organizations with designated seats on the board. A nurse who is interested in an elected seat can run in an election or ask his or her professional organization for the appointment if seats are filled in this way.

Other boards, which are self-perpetuating, fill openings by appointing people whom the board members or staff members know. Nurses can get involved in agency committees and activities or furnish resumes to acquaint these people with nurses' interests and backgrounds.

While awaiting an appointment and after getting appointed, the nurse should prepare for participation by doing the following (McLemore, 1982):

- Know relevant law
- Study parliamentary procedure
- Read health care literature from a variety of sources and disciplines
- Learn specifics of health planning
- Know the organization's mission, bylaws, and goals
- Read the organization's recent annual reports
- Become familiar with the organization's activities
- Participate in orientation and training programs for board members
- Maintain current knowledge of relevant political and legislative activity
- Maintain alliances with consumer groups
- Maintain alliances with the nursing community, particularly among nurses involved in health planning

Health planning is a political process, and those involved in it should recognize this. Whenever there are numerous people competing for limited resources and limited power, political activity results. Whenever people differ in their values and goals, political activity will come into play. Some guidelines for functioning in a political situation are:

- Observe the group to determine who has power and influence and how they use it.
- Review past decisions that might affect current issues.
- Be familiar with issues to be discussed; clarify your own position.
- Discuss complex issues with other members before meetings.
- Determine what is and what is not negotiable.
- Inform and educate other members in advance.

- Form coalitions.
- Encourage brainstorming, negotiation, and collaboration.
- Learn to identify and deal with people who force overly rapid decisions or encourage inordinate delays.
- Balance talking with listening.
- Learn how much openness and candor is acceptable in the group.
- Be reliable about preparing for and attending meetings.
- If you are expected to speak for a constituency, make periodic assessments of its members' priorities and needs.
- Involve other people on the board who are interested in health initiatives.

Nurses can also join other groups that include health planning among their concerns. For example, many cities and states have citizens' groups that are formally constituted to advise mayors, governors, or government officials on such needs as the status of women, the welfare of children, the aging, mental health services, physical fitness, nutrition, or environmental protection. Although these groups tend to promote fragmentation and duplication of services and competition for resources, they do provide another route for promotion of health.

Until health planning becomes vested in comprehensive, locally centralized groups, there will continue to be difficulties in promoting coherent community-wide approaches. One way to bring about harmony within the present system is for nurses to form alliances among themselves and with other health-oriented groups to discuss and identify the health priorities of specific communities. Alliance members can then work to influence adoption of the same priorities within their respective groups.

HEALTH PLANNING STRATEGY

Health planning strategy follows the same steps as the nursing process. It is continuous and cyclic. As presented here, the steps seem to be distinct and to succeed one another smoothly. In reality, there may be many stops and starts. Furthermore, there may be frequent setbacks if health planning is done by the group that oversees the illness care system.

Organizing

Organizing is the preliminary phase that takes place before assessment. At this time, the group members begin to settle into their roles as planners, the overall strategy is defined, and all participants receive background information on health and health planning. Those who are comfortable with the health orientation are identified. Those who are not are encouraged and educated so that they will be able to assume this responsibility. If necessary, additional consumers and health professionals may be included.

In order to ensure that health planning will take place it is valuable to establish a rule within the group that certain blocks of time will be set aside in advance for this process. If a planning period must be preempted, an alternate time should be set up.

Assessment

The health of the community is next assessed, particularly in terms of the factors listed earlier in this chapter and in Chapter 23 on health promotion with individuals and families. The group identifies resources in the community that promote health or that can be integrated into health-promo-

tion activities. The group develops policies on health and goals related to each policy.

The group also sets priorities and establishes time parameters for dealing with the priorities. Ardell (1978) suggests three criteria for identifying key health priorities:

1. The significance of the problem for the health status of area residents.
2. The prospects for success and the significance of anticipated results.
3. The relative cost of implementing the recommendation in relation to the benefits.

Planning

During planning, the group identifies ways of meeting its goals. These may include public education, advisement, consultation, development of incentives, mobilization of interest groups, or identification of research funding. The group's greatest task will undoubtedly be to motivate individuals and groups in the community to subscribe to and implement programs related to the health priorities that have been determined.

One strategy might be to select one key priority with special significance in the community, plan a visible campaign that has a high likelihood of success, and publicize the results widely. Ideas for such key interventions can be garnered from the community health literature and modified to suit the priorities within another community. One example of this is the health fair. Until fairly recently, health fairs were organized by nurses or consortiums of service groups, and many still are. However, a recent trend has been the organization of health fairs by television stations. The resultant link with broadcast media makes the health fair highly visible and raises the community's level of health awareness for a period of time. This example is not meant as a model program. On the contrary, health fairs tend to emphasize screening—a secondary-prevention activity—rather than health promotion. The merit of the health fair is that it is highly visible.

Planning must be done deliberately and must include attention to detail. In order to promote success and good will for future programs, one must provide high-quality, well-designed services that meet the set goals of promoting health.

Implementation

With a realistic plan based on genuine needs within the community, the implementation phase can proceed. The planning group is seldom the same group that implements the plan. Therefore, it is essential that the plan be meaningful to those who must make it work. It is likely that implementation will take place in stages, since goals may be long-term. The planners and the implementers may meet at the inception of the plan and periodically thereafter in order to clarify the plan, as well as to discuss progress and identify problems. This kind of interaction will increase the overall success.

Evaluation

The evaluation plan is set in conjunction with the goals, policies, and priorities. In addition, the particular implementation strategies used are evaluated. The evaluation data are used to continue the planning activities. Research may be conducted on health planning, and this will help in short- and long-term evaluation of the effects of planning.

Evaluation must be realistic. Since many of the factors related to health are linked to societal institutions and to life-style,

changes take time. Popay et al. (1980) point out that traditional approaches to prevention, such as exhortations against smoking, overeating, or alcohol abuse, have had little success in changing those patterns, which are essentially symptoms of underlying problems. Instead, attention must be directed at "removing or reducing the conditions that pressure people to lead unhealthy lives" (p. 367).

OTHER INFLUENCES ON PLANNING

Because the factors that influence health are related to public policies, societal values, and governmental funding, there are other ways to have an effect on planning besides direct involvement. The chapters in this book on political action and governmental influences include recommendations of ways to influence legislation. These can include strategies ranging from monitoring proposed and enacted laws to drafting health-promotion legislation.

It is important to be familiar with health planning activities on the community, state, and national levels. Nurses can volunteer their information and may even be solicited as consultants on health issues. Nurses can sensitize friends and colleagues to health promotion by stimulating discussions about health issues. Another avenue to pursue is writing articles for professional journals as well as nonprofessional periodicals.

The most important thing to remember in contacting an official, a planning group, friends, colleagues, or a reading audience is to be accurate and clear. The facts about most threats to health are dramatic. Generate concern and interest, raise questions, issue challenges, but do not criticize or exaggerate.

FUTURE IMPLICATIONS

Alvin Toffler (1981, p. 442) advocates an *anticipatory democracy,* or a future-oriented participative approach in political, economic, and social systems. Some existing groups encourage this to some extent, but far too often, democratic processes are turned into so-called majority rule, and all too frequently, the "majority" simply has more wealth, more formal education, and more official power than the sometimes more numerous "minorities." Perhaps the United States will always have a class system, but with effort, it can be restructured in ways that do not dehumanize and debase the lower classes. Healthy public policies can promote quality in life-style regardless of material possessions.

Some communities already use techniques that involve as many community members as possible in making healthy public policies and in determining their own futures. For example:

The state of Alaska conducted a "Town Meeting in the Air." Using television, telephone, and the consensor (a computer link), citizens were enabled to register their opinions on various topics. Voters expressed preferences for government support of the development either of carpooling through the use of incentives or of mass transit. Over 80 percent of Alaska's citizens participated in responding to 122 questions. (Linderman, 1980)

Saint John, in New Brunswick, Canada, adopted a Comprehensive Community Plan to guide the city's physical growth. The approach used was the Delphi technique. As the planners applied this technique, they sought expert opinions from individuals and groups in the community. This phase resulted in the tentative identification of issues. In the next phase, community residents responded to and verified or expanded on these issues. Finally, goals were set that related to the identified issues, and a long-term implementation design was developed. Citizen participation was comprehensive and extended over a period

of several months. (D'Amore & Rittenberg, 1980)

The Colorado Front Range project involved over 3,000 citizens from the 13 counties on the eastern slope of the Rocky Mountains. A task force developed five scenarios for the future development of the area. Participants in forums held in each county were guided through "visioning" exercises in which they considered the implications of each scenario. In quality-of-life workshops, participants brainstormed about the "desired future" for each county. The input from the forums was used by the task force to develop a desired-future statement. This was presented to a representative group and approved with minor changes. This has served as a guide for policies (many of which have health implications), to promote the realization of the future the people want.

(Ellison, 1981)

These successful efforts at participative planning can serve as guides for health planners. It is possible to interest and involve people in their communities and in community health. There are other similar examples in the literature.

Future-oriented literature is becoming quite well-accepted. Books such as Ferguson's *Aquarian Conspiracy* and Naisbitt's *Megatrends* have become best sellers. Futures courses are cropping up in universities around the country. These trends indicate the readiness of many people to look at and study the future. These people will be able to serve as guides for others.

In order to have a healthy future, everyone is going to move toward a new kind of life-style. Schumacher (1973) characterized it as "small is beautiful." Gregg (in Elgin, 1982) referred to it as "voluntary simplicity." This life-style incorporates personal values consistent with the healthy public policy described earlier. We are quickly discovering that the only way to have everything we could ever want is to be satisfied with wanting only what we need.

SUMMARY

It is possible for nurses to have a significant role in health planning. This chapter has outlined some of the policies that affect the health of the public. Suggestions have been offered for directions in which these policies might change. Guidelines for involvement and participation in health planning were presented, as were some successful community planning activities and their implicit promises for the future in the hope that the reader will use these tools and others in this book to make even better tools to build healthy tomorrows.

DISCUSSION TOPICS

1. Discuss the two models described in this chapter (public health mandala and interacting environmental determinants of health). Construct a model that incorporates both.
2. What characterizes the soft health path? What are the characteristics of the hard health path?
3. Give two examples of activities, practitioners, or services in your community that exemplify the soft health path.
4. Identify a public health policy in your community that could be changed into healthy public policy.
5. Identify two examples of healthy public policy in your community.
6. What health planning bodies exist in your community? Are nurses involved in these groups?
7. Identify interpersonal skills and strategies you could use as a member of a health planning group.
8. Give examples of activities that take place during each phase of the health planning process.

9. Give an example of legislation that has recently been passed or is being considered in your state legislature that affects health planning. Discuss the effects this legislation can have on planning.

10. In order to get an idea of how community members might feel about areas of lifestyle affected by health planning, consider the following statements yourself. Respond to each of the items with "yes," "no," or "not applicable." Discuss your responses with your classmates.

  a. I participate in a car pool.
  b. I think there are more disadvantages to carpooling than advantages.
  c. I use tobacco products.
  d. I think rules restricting tobacco use are unfair.
  e. I consume alcohol at least once a week.
  f. I think it is appropriate that laws limit alcohol consumption to certain groups and certain situations.
  g. Industry is responsible for cleaning up its own pollution.
  h. People are a lot more concerned about the quality of the environment than they need to be.
  i. External controls don't have much affect on life-style.
  j. Nurses do not have to be involved in political action.
  k. My personal health is affected by the health of the planet.
  l. Satisfaction with work affects my health.
  m. I would be willing to do the following if it would contribute to the health of my community.

   (1) Give up the use of tobacco.
   (2) Consume less alcohol.

(3) Limit my use of private transportation.

(4) Use mass transit.

(5) Participate in a physical fitness program.

(6) Change my dietary patterns.

(7) Notify legislators of my concerns about health.

(8) Boycott products of companies that pollute the environment.

11. What do the responses to the parts of topic 10 indicate about your own health-related attitudes? Discuss your responses and the responses of others.

12. What reactions might you get to the above survey if you asked community residents to respond? What are some ways you can change attitudes and actions of community residents to promote a healthy environment?

BIBLIOGRAPHY

Ardell, D.B.: Holistic health planning. In Berkeley Holistic Health Center, *The holistic health handbook*. Berkeley, Calif.: And/Or Press, 1978.

Bezold, C.: Health care in the U.S. *The Futurist* 16(4), 14–18, 1982.

Binstock, R.H.: Effective planning through political influence. *American Journal of Public Health* 59(5), 808–813, 1969.

Brown, E.L.: *Nursing reconsidered: A study of change*. Part 1. Philadelphia: Lippincott, 1970.

Brown, E.L.: *Nursing reconsidered: A study of change*. Part 2. Philadelphia: Lippincott, 1971.

Cain, H.P., II: Health planning in the United States: The 1980's—A protagonist's view. *Journal of Health Politics, Policy and Law* 6(1), 159–171, 1981.

Carlson, R.: Health care. In A. Villoldo & K. Dychtwald, eds., *Millenium: Glimpses into the 21st century*. Los Angeles: J.P. Tarcher, 1981.

Checkoway, B.: The empire strikes back: More lessons for health care consumers. *Journal of Health Politics, Policy and Law* 7(1), 111–124, 1982.

Cohen, P.D.: Community health planning from an interorganizational perspective. *American Journal of Public Health* 72(7), 717–721, 1982.

D'Amore, L.J., & Rittenberg, S.: Shaping urban futures through public participation. In F. Feather, ed., *Through the 80's: Thinking globally, acting locally*. Washington, D.C.: World Future Society, 1980.

Elgin, D.: *Voluntary simplicity*. Toronto: Bantam, 1982.

Ellison, J.: Anticipatory democracy in action. *The Futurist* 15(6), 10–14, 1981.

Falkson, J.L., & Leavitt, H.A.: The real lessons of national health planning. *Journal of Health Politics, Policy and Law* 7(1), 125–127, 1982.

Feingold, E.: The changing political character of health planning. *American Journal of Public Health* 59(5), 803–808, 1969.

Ferguson, M.: *The aquarian conspiracy*. Los Angeles: J.P. Tarcher, 1980.

Foley, H.A.: Health planning—Demise or reformation. *New England Journal of Medicine* April 16, 1981, pp. 969–972.

Fuller, R.B.: *Critical path*. New York: St. Martin's, 1981.

Gordon, L.J.: Popullution (The 1981 APHA Presidential Address). *American Journal of Public Health* 72(4), 341–346, 1982.

Green, L.W., Wilson, R.W., & Bauer, K.G.: Data requirements to measure progress on the objectives for the nation in health promotion and disease prevention. *American Journal of Public Health* 73(1), 18–24, 1983.

Hancock, T.: The soft health path: An alternative future for health in the 80's. In F. Feather, ed., *Through the 80's: Thinking globally, acting locally*. Washington, D.C.: World Future Society, 1980.

Hancock, T.: Beyond health care: Creating a healthy future. *The Futurist* 16(4), 4–13, 1982.

Healthy people: The Surgeon General's report on health promotion and disease prevention. Washington, D.C.: U.S. Government Printing Office, 1979.

Jaffe, R.M.: Health in the 80's: Toward optimum human existence. In F. Feather, ed., *Through the 80's: Thinking globally, acting locally.* Washington, D.C.: World Future Society, 1980.

Kaufman, H.: The politics of health planning. *American Journal of Public Health* 59(5), 795–797, 1969.

Kinlein, M.L.: Point of view/on the front: Nursing and family and community health. *Family and Community Health* 1(1), 59–68, 1978.

Laessig, R.E., & Urkowitz, A.G.: The environmental health matrix: Information for use in planning. *American Journal of Public Health* 72(4), 373–375, 1982.

Linderman, M.S.: Community decision-making in the future. In F. Feather, ed., *Through the 80's: Thinking globally, acting locally.* Washington, D.C.: World Future Society, 1980.

McLemore, M.M.: Nurses as health planners. *Nurse Educator* 5(5), 20–23, 1980.

Mott, B.J.F.: The myth of planning without politics. *American Journal of Public Health* 59(5), 797–803, 1969.

Naisbitt, J.: *Megatrends.* New York: Warner, 1982.

National Commission for the Study of Nursing and Nursing Education: *An abstract for action.* New York: McGraw-Hill, 1970.

Newman, O.: *Community of interest.* Garden City, N.Y.: Doubleday/Anchor, 1981.

Palmiere, D.: Types of planning in the health care system. *American Journal of Public Health* 62(8), 1112–1115, 1972.

Popay, J., Griffiths, J., Draper, P., & Dennis, J.: The impact of industrialization on world health. In F. Feather, ed., *Through the 80's: Thinking globally, acting locally.* Washington, D.C.: World Future Society, 1980.

Ruybal, S.E.: Community health planning. *Family and Community Health* 1(1), 9–18, 1978.

Schumacher, E.F.: *Small is beautiful.* New York: Harper & Row, 1973.

Simmons, H.J., III: Community health planning—With or without nursing? *Nursing Outlook* 22(4), 260–264, 1974.

Snoke, A.W.: What good is legislation—or planning—if we can't make it work? *American Journal of Public Health* 72(9), 1028–1033, 1982.

Snyder, R.D.: Health hazard appraisal. *The Futurist* 16(4), 25–29, 1982.

Toffler, A.: *The third wave.* New York: Bantam, 1981.

Vladeck, B.C.: Interest-group representation and the HSA's: Health planning and political theory. *American Journal of Public Health* 67(1), 23–29, 1977.

GLOSSARY

accountability Being responsible for and answerable to the consequences of one's behavior.

adaptation The dynamic process of change in response to life events.

ageism Bias against people for no other reason than their age.

agent A factor whose presence or absence causes disease; may be biological, chemical, or physical.

aggression A type of interpersonal behavior in which an individual acts in such a way as to infringe on the rights of others; may include manipulation, domination, or humiliation of the other person.

anger–dismay syndrome Being perplexed, shocked, and at a loss about how to cope with the angry expressions of another; feeling powerless and overwhelmed and unable to change these responses.

anxiety A feeling of tension or apprehension that seems out of proportion to the situation at hand; brought on by an unspecific, vague threat.

Aquarian conspiracy A leaderless network working to bring about change in society; sees humankind embedded in nature and made up of autonomous individuals who are self-determining.

assertiveness A type of interpersonal behavior

that enables individuals to act in their own best interests without anxiety and to exercise their own rights without denying the rights of others.

automation The technique of making an apparatus, process, or system function automatically, without human intervention.

autonomy Freedom to govern oneself and to make choices according to one's own moral or professional principles.

bill A proposal for the enactment of a new law.

change Any planned or unplanned alteration in the status in an organism, situation, or process.

changing The second phase in the change process, during which implementation of an idea or plan takes place.

client A person who engages the professional services of another person or agency; a person capable of directing or collaborating in matters determining his or her own life.

community A social system whose members have significant relationships with each other.

conflict An expressed struggle between at least two interdependent parties who perceive incompatible goals, scarce rewards, and interference from one another.

consultation A collaborative effort on the part

of the consultant and consultee using problem solving to bring about change.

contract A mutual agreement between two or more parties concerning their expectations of each other in regard to a specified objective or goal.

creative thinking Thinking that is innovative and imaginative.

creativity Behavior that is novel and to some extent adaptive to reality; it must solve a problem, fit a situation, or accomplish a goal, and the idea must be sustained and elaborated to its fullest.

crisis An individual's response to an obstacle that results when his or her usual problem-solving strategies are ineffective in meeting interpersonal needs.

cultural imposition Subtle and less-than-subtle ways in which an outsider imposes his or her own values, beliefs, and practices upon others.

culture The patterns of human behavior (thought, speech, action, and technology) that are learned and transmitted from one generation to another; customs, social forms, beliefs, and traits characteristic of a racial, religious, or social group.

cybernation The employment of computers in bringing about automation.

depression A clinical syndrome characterized by an alteration of affect; expressed as feelings of sadness and loss of interest in daily activities.

disease A specific physical or emotional malady linked to selected causal factors.

ecosystem The interaction of organisms within the environment; a self-sustaining and self-regulating system.

endemic Habitual or usual presence of a disease or infectious agent within a geographical area.

environment All that is external to the human body.

epidemic Occurrence in a community or region of an illness or a group of similar illnesses clearly in excess of normal expectation.

epidemiology The study of the causal factors and relationships that affect the health of people.

ethics The branch of philosophy concerned with what is good and bad; the study of principles of conduct.

ethnicity Social characteristics of a more or less cohesive subgroup with similar biological origins that is in a diverse cultural setting.

4th dimension thinking Thinking that is "cosmic," holistic, and intuitive.

future shock The stress and disorientation experienced by individuals when they undergo too much change in too short a time.

futurism A philosophical orientation toward studying the future.

generalist A practitioner who has basic preparation in professional nursing and is able to apply the content included in the basic curriculum to a certain area of practice.

gerontology The study of human aging.

group Two or more people interacting and influencing each other toward some common purpose or goal.

health A relative state that represents the degree to which an individual can operate effectively within the circumstances of heredity and the physical and cultural environment; the expression of the extent to which the individual maintains in readiness the resources required to meet the exigencies of the future.

high-level wellness An integrated method of functioning that is oriented toward maximizing the potential of which the individual is capable within the given environment.

holism Consideration of a human life as consisting of a dynamic, continuous interaction among biological, emotional, intellectual, and spiritual dimensions.

hospice care A sheltering institution or visiting team of helpers designed to control and relieve the emotional and physical suffering of the terminally ill and their families.

host A vertebrate or invertebrate species capable of being infected or affected by an agent.

human determinants Factors that determine human needs.

human needs Factors that must be satisfied to permit an individual to function in a given milieu in order to guarantee survival with pride and pleasure.

incidence Measurement of the number of new cases of a disease or other event occurring in a population during a given period.

individualism A doctrine that individual interests are or ought to be ethically paramount.

individuality The total character peculiar to and distinguishing one person from others.

inference A generalization from a sample to a population.

lateral thinking Thinking that is unexpected and not sequential.

law A standard of human conduct established and enforced by the authority of society through its government.

leadership The attributes or personal characteristics that contribute to influencing others; may include influencing the activities of others in attaining goals.

learning A change in insights, behavior, perceptions, or motivation, or a combination of these; gaining knowledge, understanding, or skill through study, instruction, or investigation.

life-style The aggregation of decisions by individuals that affect their health and over which they more or less have control.

morals Activities and institutions that societies use to preserve and enhance social order and welfare.

morbidity Refers to illness or some other condition; does not include death.

mortality Death.

motivation The desire to learn or to accomplish something.

network Structured relationships between individuals or collectives; linkages among the elements of an individual's environment.

networking The process of developing and using a network for support or assistance.

norms Standards or rules that develop within a group; expectations for the members' behavior.

pandemic Epidemic over a wide geographical area.

paradigm A typical example or archetype; a model of behavior.

passiveness An interpersonal behavior in which an individual denies his or her own rights.

patient A person under medical care who lacks full self-awareness and self-control.

pollution Artificially produced contaminates that threaten the health and well-being of humans.

power The ability of an individual or group to influence the behavior of others.

prevalence Measurement of all cases (old and new) of a disease or other condition present in a population at a given time.

primary health care Prevention of illness and promotion of maximum health.

queen bee syndrome A set of behaviors through which a woman leader strongly identifies with men in a situation and refuses to be helpful to other women.

readiness A learner's ability to achieve outcomes deemed appropriate; includes physical, psychological, intellectual, cultural, social, and value factors.

refreezing The third and last phase of change; takes place when the organization settles in and functions at the new desired level.

religion A personal or institutionalized system of spiritual attitudes, beliefs, and practices.

rights Guidelines for moral activity that designate relationships among people; includes both duties and responsibilities.

role The dynamic or behavioral aspect of a status position.

role conflict Incompatibility between two or more roles that an individual is expected to perform in a given situation.

screening Administration of tests for early identification of health problems.

social control The influencing of human behavior to maintain social order.

socialization The learning of social roles that prepares one for adult and other specific kinds of role performance.

specialist A practitioner who has undertaken advanced education in order to gain breadth and depth of knowledge in a specific area of practice.

spirit The animating but intangible principle that gives life to the physical organism.

spiritual Those motivations and loyalties which are intangibly directive in the lives of those persons who exercise religious faith in their reach for supreme values.

standard A means of determining what a thing should be and what is necessary for a high quality of practice.

statistic A measured fact expressed as a number.

statistics The scientific discipline used for examining, interpreting, and reporting research results.

status a collection of rights and duties that go with a given position in a group.

stress The nonspecific physiological response of an organism to any demand made upon it.

synergy Behavior of whole systems unpredictable by the behavior of their parts taken separately; the principle that the product of the whole is greater than the sum of its parts.

teaching A process that enables others to learn.

thinking Forming or having something in mind.

unfreezing The first phase of change, during which recognition of the need for change in a situation occurs.

values Traditional institutions and ideals of a society that are highly esteemed.

variable A characteristic that takes on different values.

vertical thinking Thinking that is expected, logical, and progressive.

Index